Introduction to Research in the Health Sciences

To the memory of Dr George Varnai and Dr George Polgar
To Elizabeth Kearney and June M. Thomas

Introduction to Research in the Health Sciences

Stephen Polgar BSc (Hons) MSc
Lecturer, School of Behavioural Health Sciences,
Faculty of Health Sciences
La Trobe University, Melbourne, Australia

Shane A. Thomas BA (Hons) Dip Pub Pol PhD
Reader, School of Behavioural Health Sciences,
Faculty of Health Sciences
La Trobe University, Melbourne, Australia

THIRD EDITION

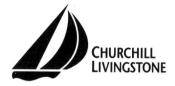
CHURCHILL
LIVINGSTONE

MELBOURNE EDINBURGH LONDON MADRID NEW YORK TOKYO 1995

CHURCHILL LIVINGSTONE
An imprint of Harcourt Brace and Company Limited

© Pearson Professional Ltd 1998
© Harcourt Brace and Company Limited 1998

First edition 1988
Second edition 1991
    Reprinted 1991
    Reprinted 1992
Third edition 1995
    Reprinted 1996
    Reprinted 1998
    Reprinted 1999
A catalogue record for this book is available from the British Library.

National Library of Australia Cataloguing in Publication Data
Polgar, Stephen.
    Introduction to research in the health sciences.

    3rd ed.
    Bibliography.
    Includes index.
    ISBN 0 443 05039 2.

    1. Medicine – Research – Methodology. 2. Medical sciences –
    Research – Methodology. I. Thomas, Shane A. II. Title.

610.72

A Library of Congress Cataloguing in Publication record is available for this title

For Churchill Livingstone in Melbourne
Publisher: Judy Waters
Editorial: Pam Lewis
Copy Editing: Marta Veroni
Desktop Preparation: Sandra Tolra
Typesetting: Friedo Ligthart, Designpoint
Indexing: Max McMaster
Production Control: Bob Stagg
Design: Jan Schmoeger, Designpoint
Produced by Churchill Livingstone in Australia
Printed in China
NPCC/05

Preface to the third edition

Over the past decade and since we wrote the first edition of Polgar and Thomas major changes have taken place in health care delivery and the education of health professionals. For the most part, these changes have been driven by technological advances and increasing demands to evaluate the cost, effectiveness and quality of health services. Therefore, the education of *all* health professionals (not only potential researchers and administrators) ought include a sequence of research methods subjects so as to ensure that they are in a position to understand and utilize advances in their areas.

Our aim has been to write a text in this area which could be used by all health sciences students. This third edition of *Introduction to research in the health sciences* was made possible by the continuing support for this text in various countries including Australia, Canada and the United Kingdom. Also, the second edition was translated for Spanish speaking readers, under the title *Introduccion a la investigacion en las ciencias de la salud*. The book is used by students and practitioners across a broad range of health professions, including behavioural sciences, medical records, administration, medicine, nursing, occupational therapy, orthoptics, pharmacy, physiotherapy, podiatry, prosthetics and orthotics, and speech pathology.

We are grateful for our readers' suggestions concerning improvements to the book. In response, we have included introductions to each of the seven sections in order to facilitate the reader forming an overview of the research process. A major improvement is the addition of 'discussion questions' at the end of each section. The discussion questions invite readers to examine more complex issues such as theory formation and models, the ethics of evaluating novel treatments, or the development of assessment instruments.

In order to maintain the simplicity of the text, we decided against substantial increases in the scope of contents of the book, such as including additional statistical tests or expanding the current treatment of qualitative methods. It must be remembered that this is an introductory text, designed to provide the student with the foundations for further work in the area.

S.P.
S.A.T.

Melbourne, 1994

Preface to the second edition

We have been most gratified by the positive responses of our readers to the first edition of Polgar and Thomas. In response to our readers' suggestions, we have included several new features in the second edition. These include an extensive glossary of research terms and additional sections on observation, interviews and qualitative methods. Improvements have also been made in other chapters.

In the production of the second edition, we would like to thank Carol Greene for her diligent and excellent word processing and our students and colleagues for their many helpful suggestions. We would especially like to thank Dr Felicity Allen, Dr Ken Greenwood and Ian Story for assisting with the development of the glossary.

Melbourne, 1991

S.P.
S.A.T.

Preface to the first edition

The aim of this text is to introduce students in the health sciences to research methods. The form and content of the book reflect the authors' experience in teaching research methods to health sciences students, including those studying nursing, physiotherapy, podiatry, medical records administration, medicine, pharmacy, prosthetics and orthotics, psychology, occupational therapy and orthoptics. In addition, the book draws on the authors' experience in research supervision, research consultancy and collaborative research with a variety of health professionals.

In preparing the text, we have taken into account both the educational needs of the students and the current trends in professional practice and research. While far too numerous to discuss or even to list, the issues which were considered included: the varied maths/science backgrounds of health science students, time pressures on students arising from clinical practice, pervasive problems in numeracy, changes in current professional education in the health sciences, interdisciplinary practices in health care, problems in published health sciences research, the need to introduce ethics, and conceptual shifts from biomedical to more holistic models of health care.

In order to present a simplified and integrated overview of the material, we found that key issues had to be left out or condensed. These include measurement theory, qualitative methods and multivariate statistics.

We are very grateful to our students whose critical feedback and performance was fundamental in shaping this book. We are also particularly grateful to Dr Christina Lee for the contributions she has made to the writing of this book.

Some of the material in Chapter 21 was based on work by Dr. Jon Russell, and we are grateful for his permission to use this material. We are very grateful to Dr Tom Matyas for his guidance and encouragement. We are also grateful to Dr Felicity Allen, Ms Colette Browning, Mr Peter Foreman, Dr Kay Patterson, and Dr Marcelle Schwartz for providing encouragement and criticism which were extremely useful for preparing this book.

S.P.
S.A.T.

Melbourne, 1988

Contents

The scientific method

In this section we will examine some of the basic characteristics of the scientific method. A 'method', in the present context, refers to a systematic method for acquiring knowledge and establishing its truth. Health providers justify their theories and practices on the grounds that they are 'scientific', that is, based on scientific methodology. While not everything we do as health providers is, nor for that matter should be, 'scientific', the scientific method is essential for conducting research and evaluation aiming to improve the effectiveness and cost-effectiveness of health services.

A common view of the scientific method is that it enables us to describe, predict, explain and perhaps to control events in the world. As an example, consider how researchers and practitioners in the health care system responded to the outbreak of the AIDS (acquired immuno-deficiency syndrome) epidemic. One of the first signs of this epidemic was the clinical observation that young men presented with a deadly cancer (Kaposi's sarcoma) which was previously found only in the elderly. It was *hypothesized* that the premature failure of the immune system was responsible for the disorder. A hypothesis is a testable prediction about the relationship between observed events. Subsequent clinical evidence supported this hypothesis, leading to a clear definition of the disease as 'AIDS'. As more cases of AIDS were identified it became evident that certain groups in the population were most at risk: persons who were involved in multiple homosexual relationships or persons who were intravenous drug users, or those who required blood products, for instance for haemophilia. An important development was the confirmation of the hypothesis that the disease was caused by a specific virus labelled 'HIV' (human immuno-deficiency virus). On the basis of the above clinical, epidemiological and virological evidence it was hypothesized that the HIV was transmitted through body fluids such as blood or semen. In this way it became possible to predict which practices in the population involved a high level of risk for transmitting the virus.

The above findings and hypotheses contributed to constructing **theories** of AIDS, providing systematic and integrated conceptual frameworks for explaining the transmission and integrating the clinical features of the disorder. These theories also inform current practices aimed at controlling the epidemic, such as testing blood products for HIV, or promoting 'safe sex' behaviours in the population. The effectiveness of these practices (at least in some countries) for containing the epidemic is evidence confirming the accuracy of our understanding of the problem. At the same time, we remain sceptical about certain aspects of our theories, recognizing that there are no vaccines or pharmacological cures for AIDS as yet available.

You might have recognized that the above brief account of attempting to contain AIDS is deficient in an essential way: in excluding the personal experiences and actions of persons at risk or having HIV. The above account represents a quantitative approach to the scientific method aiming to provide a mechanistic or reductionistic explanation of health and illness. This method is not adequate for researching and theorizing how persons, their families and the community respond to health related issues and problems. It has been argued that our methods should also include qualitative or interpretive approaches to discover the personal meanings involved in being at risk of or suffering from diseases or disabilities. Qualitative methods are also appropriate for researching the cultural context and social construction of a disorder, for instance, discovering the 'images' of AIDS sufferers communicated by the media in a given community.

The position taken in the present book is that the scientific method as applied to health care must include both quantitative and qualitative methods. This more inclusive view of the scientific method may not be supported by all researchers, but in our view the 'biopsychosocial' approach to health care requires both methods for research and theory formation. Regardless of controversies regarding the nature of science and its methodology, there is a broad consensus concerning the conventions and rules for conducting and reporting health sciences research, as outlined in the present book. Our goal is to convey these to our readers.

1

The scientific method

INTRODUCTION

The primary aim of this chapter is to outline the scientific method and to compare it with other methods for conducting enquiry. Special emphasis is placed on the method as a means for conducting research and justifying practices in the health sciences.

The general aims of this chapter are to:

1. Define what is meant by 'method', and outline some common methods of enquiry
2. Outline the scientific method
3. Draw attention to some controversies concerning the nature of the scientific method
4. Discuss how the scientific method is applied to the conduct of health sciences research.

METHODS AND KNOWLEDGE

Patient care involves the acquisition of a set of specific skills, the practice of which is justified in terms of a systematic and shared body of professional knowledge. Any system of knowledge is based on the use of appropriate methods. The term 'method' refers to a systematic procedure for carrying out an activity, and in the present context implies a set of rules which specify:

1. How knowledge should be acquired
2. The form in which knowledge should be stated
3. How the truth or falsity of the knowledge should be evaluated.

Before we begin discussion of the scientific method it is useful, as a means of contrast, to look at some of the other methods of knowing used in the health sciences.

Authority. According to this method, knowledge is considered true because of tradition, or because an experienced and distinguished clinician says that it is true. As a student, you are asked to accept statements as true because your teachers and clinical supervisors say they are true. To maintain their authority, the 'sources' of knowledge acquire and cultivate various signs of expertise, such as the appellation of 'Professor', or encourage the performance of status rituals. For instnace, consider the 'Consultant' who sweeps into a hospital ward followed by a retinue of students, registrars and nurses. Who would dare to question the truth of any of the consultant's sacred utterances? There are problems with this method of authority. What happens when the statements arising from one authority are contradicted by those made by an equally prestigious authority? Say, Authority X claims that in their experience psychoanalysis is effective, while Authority Y states that the technique is useless. How can we resolve such conflicting claims? In practice, unless objective and acceptable criteria for resolution can be found, we will have unending disputation, *ad hominem* (personal) attacks, or, in instances of some religious or political disagreements, violence. That is, the controversy is resolved by denigrating or silencing the dissenting authority. In contrast, the scientific method emphasizes the examination of the empirical evidence for establishing the truth of statements.

Rationalism. Reasoning is commonly used to arrive at true knowledge. It is assumed that if the rules of logic are applied correctly, then the conclusions are guaranteed to be valid. As an example, let us look at the following syllogism:

(a) All persons suffering from heart disease are males
(b) Person X has heart disease
(c) Therefore, person X is a male.

Logic guarantees that the conclusion (c) is true, provided the syllogism is in a valid form and the premises (a) and (b) are true. Clearly, the limitation of formal (that is, 'content independent') reasoning is that it works in practice only if we have means for establishing the factual truth of the premises. In the above example, conclusion (c) might be empirically false, given that the premise (a) is factually false.

Of course, logic and mathematics are very much a part of science. But we require evidence to be collected to support logic and mathematical operations.

Intuition. Knowledge is sometimes acquired by sudden insights which arise without conscious reasoning. Truth is judged by the clarity of the experience and its emotional content (the 'Eureka!' experience). For instance, after working with a patient without success, you might have a sudden insight about how to change your treatment program. Unfortunately, even the strongest intuitions are sometimes proven false when put to an empirical test. You might find that your brilliant clinical insights often fail.

Sometimes new scientific discoveries are resisted because they seem counterintuitive. For instance Ignaz Semmelweiss, a perceptive and humane 19th century physician, noticed appalling levels of puerperal fever and maternal death at his hospital. He reasoned that the infection was spread by medical students and staff who went to delivery rooms from the morgue, without adequately washing their hands. In 1848 Semmelweiss introduced antiseptic procedures in his wards, and demonstrated a substantial reduction in mortality from puerperal fever. However, his colleagues were offended by the notion that physicians were carriers of disease. Semmelweiss was dismissed from his post, ostracized by the medical establishment and died in pitiful circumstances. Clearly, in the light of current evidence we can say that Semmelweiss' contention was correct, while his colleagues' intuition was mistaken. Authority, logic and intuition all have their places in health care. In a general way, the scientific method can be contrasted with other methods in that it emphasizes the need for empirical evidence.

THE SCIENTIFIC METHOD AND THE POSITIVIST VIEW

The scientific method crystallized over a period of several centuries, concomitantly with the growth of scientific research. The beginnings of modern Western science are generally traced to the 16th century, a time in which Europe experienced profound social changes and a resurgence of great artists, thinkers and philosophers. Gradually, scholars' interests shifted from theology and armchair speculation to systematically describing, explaining and attempting to control natural phenomena. These changed circumstances allowed philosophers like Descartes and Francis Bacon to challenge tenets of mediaeval thinking, and scientists like Galileo, Newton and Harvey to propose new models of natural phenomena.

The approaches of such great thinkers had three basic elements, which are the basis of scientific method:

1. *Scepticism.* The notion that any proposition or statement, even when made by great authorities, is open to doubt and analysis.
2. *Determinism.* The notion that events in the world occur according to regular laws and causes, not as a result of the caprices of demons or witches.
3. *Empiricism.* The notion that enquiry ought to be conducted through observation and verified through experience.

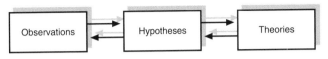

Fig. 1.1 The scientific method

The scientific method is represented in a simplified form in Figure 1.1. This view is consistent with a view of natural science methodology called 'positivism' by the 19th century philosopher Comte, as well as 'reductionism', a concept introduced in Chapter 8. Both these terms have acquired multiple meanings in the area of philosophy of science. Our meaning is explained below.

1. Observation, description and measurement

The description of phenomena involving the precise, unbiased recording of observations of aspects of persons, objects and events forms the empirical basis of all branches of science. Observations can be expressed as either verbal descriptions or sets of measurements. The personal perceptions of the investigator must be transformed into descriptive statements and measurements which can be understood and replicated by other investigators. Some research is based on observation made with instruments (such as recording electrodes, microscopes and standardized clinical tests) while other research calls for observation unaided by instruments. Even though advances in instrumentation have contributed enormously to scientific knowledge, the use of complex instrumentation is not a necessary feature of scientific observation. Rather, the key attributes of scientific observation are accuracy and replicability by other scientists. When observations are appropriately summarized and are confirmed by others, they form the factual bases of scientific knowledge.

2. Generalization and induction

Statements and measurements representing observations are integrated into explanatory systems called hypotheses and theories. The logic underlying scientific generalizations is called induction. Induction involves asserting general propositions about a class of phenomena on the basis of a limited number of observations of select elements. For example, having observed that penicillin is useful for curing pneumonia in a limited set of patients, we make the generalization 'The administration of penicillin cures pneumonia (in all patients)'.

3. Hypotheses

The statement 'The administration of penicillin cures pneumonia' is called a hypothesis. Scientific hypotheses are statements which specify the nature of the relationship between two or more sets of observations. In this instance, the first set of observations relates to the administration of penicillin, the second set is related to changes in clinical observations or measurements concerning pneumonia. As we shall see in subsequent sections, an important feature of scientific hypotheses is that the terms used must have clear-cut, observable referents. When these hypotheses acquire strong empirical support, they may be called 'laws'.

4. Theories

Scientific theories are essentially conjectures representing our current state of knowledge about the world. Hypotheses are integrated into more general explanatory systems called theories. A theory will clarify the relationships between diverse classes of observations and hypotheses. For instance, a theory to explain why drugs called antibiotics are effective in curing some infectious diseases will integrate evidence from diverse sources, such as microbiology, pharmacology, cell physiology and clinical medicine. Other examples of theories are the heliocentric theory of the solar system, the DNA theory of genetic inheritance, and the neuronal theory of central nervous system functioning. It is an essential feature of scientific theories that they are statements based on the correct use of language and logic. Some theories entail a model, which is a mathematical or physical representation of how the theory works. In this way, theories specify the causes of events, and provide conceptual means for predicting and influencing these events. In health care, theories are important for explaining the causes of health and illness and predicting the probable effectiveness of treatment outcomes.

5. Deduction

A scientific theory should lead to a set of empirically verifiable statements or hypotheses. Hypotheses are deduced logically from the statements and/or mathematical models which specify the causal relationships postulated by a theory. For instance, if we hold the theory that a set of neurones in the occipital lobe mediates visual sensation in humans, then the hypothesis follows that the activation of these neurones (say, by electrical stimulation) will lead to the report of visual sensations. Such hypotheses have been the bases for subsequent spectacular clinical advances such as artificial vision through cortically implanted electrodes.

6. Controlled observation

It is desirable that hypotheses are tested under controlled conditions. The aim of control is to discount other competing hypotheses for explaining the predicted phenomenon. For example, if we intend to show that occipital lobe stimulation causes the visual sensations, we must show that we are 'controlling for' any type of brain stimulation causing such changes. Conversely, we would need to show that occipital lobe stimulation doesn't lead to a host of other types of sensations. Only by discounting alternative explanations through control can we have confidence in the relevance of our observations for our research hypothesis.

7. Verification and falsification

After the evidence has been collected, the investigator decides whether or not the findings are consistent with the predictions of the hypothesis. If the hypothesis is supported by the evidence, then the theory from which the hypothesis was deduced is strengthened, or verified. However, when the data do not support the hypothesis, the related theory is falsified. If a theory can no longer predict or explain evidence in its empirical domain, it becomes less useful, and is usually later discarded in favour of new, more powerful theories. Therefore, scientific theories are not held to be absolute truths, but rather as provisional explanations of available evidence.

The application of the above process has contributed to the spectacular growth of scientific knowledge. Observation and measurement, facilitated by new instrumentation, have resulted in an increased number of accurate and reproducible facts. These new facts both challenge existing theories and call for the creation of novel, more powerful theories. The new theories serve as impetus for more research, resulting in new instrumentation and observations. Advances in scientific knowledge have been applied to creating new technologies, which in turn contribute to advances in scientific knowledge. For instance, the invention of computers was possible because of advances in electronics, chemistry and mathematics. In turn, the use of computers is now contributing to making and summarizing scientific observations or formulating explanatory models. In addition, the use of computers as information processing systems has generated useful metaphors for theoretical advances, such as explaining the human brain and mental functioning. In this way, the scientific method contributes to furthering our aims by helping us to describe, explain, predict and sometimes control the world in which we live.

CONTROVERSIES CONCERNING THE NATURE OF THE SCIENTIFIC METHOD

It would be false to claim that the above description is the only interpretation of the scientific method. Rather, there are good reasons why there are controversies concerning the nature of the scientific method as described above.

Firstly, the scientific method is a set of rules devised and applied by individual scientists. They are not eternal truths, but conventions believed to be useful for conducting scientific enquiry. In this way, not only the content but also the methodology of science is open to criticism, debate and change.

Secondly, the interpretation of what constitutes the scientific method is an activity pursued by philosophers of science and epistemologists. In adopting different conceptual frameworks (Realism, Instrumentalism, Anarchism, Idealism, etc.) concerning the nature of reality and knowledge, these philosophers generate unending controversies concerning the nature of the scientific method.

As scientists or health professionals, we can't sit around forever waiting for philosophers to decide on the appropriate way of gathering knowledge. However, as the following points exemplify, it would be churlish not to take into account some of the important ideas arising from the history and philosophy of science.

The theory-dependence of observation

Critics such as Chalmers (1976) argued that it is simplistic to believe that observations are made independently of theoretical notions held by the observer. The observer is selective with regard to what is recorded as evidence. Our observations and facts are 'theory-dosed', that is, theories specify what observations are of importance and what aspects of these observations should be recorded or ignored. Schatzman and Strauss (1973) put this point elegantly when they stated that the researcher 'harbours, wittingly or not, many expectations, conjectures and hypotheses which provide him with thought and directives on what to look for and what to ask about'. For instance, in observing the EEG (electroencephalogram) of an epileptic patient, our perception is guided by theories of the electrical activity of the brain and the nature of brain pathology. We will also hold ideas how the EEG machine works (for example, electrode sensitivity, amplification) and identify 'artifacts' in the evidence. What is observed as evidence of epilepsy by an expert could be perceived as meaningless squiggles by a naive observer. We shall take account of this point in Chapter 12, when we discuss the reliability and validity of measurement.

The validity of induction

Philosophers of science have questioned the logical validity of making general claims on the basis of a limited set of observations. To quote Chalmers (1976): 'any observational evidence will consist of a finite number of observation statements, whereas a universal statement makes claims about an infinite number of possible situations'.

For instance, we might have observed that the administration of penicillin cured pneumonia in 100 000 patients. This doesn't necessarily guarantee the *logical* truth of the universal statement 'penicillin cures pneumonia', or that patient 100 001 will be cured. We will look at the theories related issue of generalization from samples in Chapter 3. Scientific theories are seen as probabilistic, in the sense that new, inconsistent evidence might emerge in the future, challenging the generality of the theory. Also, it has been argued by some philosophers of science, that hypotheses *need not* be based on induction, but may arise from any source, provided that they have falsifiable empirical consequences.

What constitutes falsification?

It was stated earlier that when novel empirical evidence is inconsistent with the predictions of a theory, the theory is 'falsified' and is eventually modified or discarded. Commentators such as Lakatos (1970) argued that theories are not, in fact, so readily modified or discarded by scientists. Rather, they are structures which have an inner hard core of assumptions protected by an outer belt of auxiliary, modifiable hypotheses. Consider, for instance, the 'germ' theory of infectious disease, on the basis of which one would predict that penicillin (which kills germs) will cure bacterial infections. Suppose that we administer penicillin to a number of patients with an infectious disease and find no clinically useful changes, contrary to what was predicted. On the basis of this falsification, will we discard the germ theory of disease? No. Rather, we will utilize an auxiliary hypothesis to explain our findings, such as 'the development of penicillin resistant bacteria'. The methodological issue which remains controversial is the logical basis for discarding one theory and accepting its rival (see Feyerabend 1975). As we shall see in Chapter 22, we judge the outcome of a research program in the context of an overall pattern of related findings and theories.

SCIENCE AND THE CULTURAL CONTEXT

Science as a human activity

Scientific enquiry is conducted in particular social settings, by individuals with personal aims and values. Some more recent formulations of methodology take into account the social and interpersonal conditions which influence scientists' professional activities (Kuhn 1970, Feyerabend 1975). In this text, we will pay attention to social values, in the context of ethical considerations for designing and conducting research (Ch. 2). Also, we recognize that the formulation of hypotheses and theories are creative acts, rather than the outcomes of the automatic application of induction. In this way, the questions asked by health researchers and the ways in which they explain their findings are influenced in subtle ways by the cultures in which they participate.

The social context of health care research

To understand the nature of scientific research in general, and health care research in particular, it is useful to examine how they fit into an overall social context. That is, the way in which persons living in a society view health and illness and the ways in which health workers carry out their professional roles influence the range and scope of health care research (e.g. Taylor 1979).

Until recently, the 'medical model' was by far the most dominant approach to understanding illness in western society. Briefly, in terms of the medical model, illness is represented by a particular 'lesion' or dysfunctioning within the human body. The role of the health professional is to identify the location and nature of the lesion or the clinical imbalance and to implement appropriate measures to correct the problem. The patient is assigned a rather passive role in this process; as being the 'locus' of the lesion or imbalance and as a person complying with the health professionals' recommendations. In the context of the medical model, the most appropriate research is seen as that which improves the technical effectiveness and, therefore, the social power of the health professional.

In Western society the medical model has been, and will continue to be, an influential model for guiding clinical practice and health research. Nevertheless, there have been gradual changes in health care that require the questioning of the generality of the medical mode for the following reasons:

1. There have been important changes in the roles and status of health professionals such as nurses, occupational therapists, physiotherapists, speech pathologists and podiatrists. Rather than taking an ancillary, paramedical position, these individuals are becoming directly and independently responsible for a broad range of health care functions, including prevention, assessment, therapy and rehabilitation. However, the perspectives and practices of these health professionals is at times quite different from that involved in the medical model and may require quite different approaches to research and theory. The gradual establishment of university based education for these professionals has provided

an increased opportunity for relevant research, which is not necessarily guided by the medical model.

2. From the 1970s onwards it had become evident that there had been a significant increase in the cost of health care; in part due to the adoption of very expensive diagnostic procedures and the increasing trend for specialisation among medical practitioners (Taylor 1979). Attempts to contain health care costs have resulted in several lines of approach including:

(a) increased focus on preventive health care; as evidenced by anti-smoking campaigns, or drink driving legislation to contain the incidence of road trauma;
(b) increased efforts to enhance the cost effectiveness of current treatment strategies; for instance by improving communications between clinicians and patients or managing patients' fears concerning treatments by the application of psychological techniques;
(c) increased support for self help groups and community managed health centres with a more active involvement of individuals in understanding and managing their own health.

3. Preventative and educational approaches require somewhat different views of the client and the professional to that implicit in the medical model. In turn, research is required which can clarify the relationships between community lifestyles, individual behaviours, health and illness and general economic and social circumstances (e.g. Gardner 1989).

The more holistic approach, which also informs health care research is called the **psychosocial** or **biopsychosocial** model (see Engel 1977), and currently has considerable influence in how we conceptualise health care and how we plan and carry out research. At the same time, the medical model remains influential in research aimed at understanding the workings of the human body and improving the technical aspects of health care, such as clinical assessments and interventions.

QUANTITATIVE AND QUALITATIVE METHODS

The introduction of a biopsychosocial approach has raised questions about the combination of methodologies relevant to health sciences research. We perceive patients or clients in two different but interrelated frameworks: firstly as broken down or malfunctioning biological systems; secondly, as persons, like ourselves, living in a society and who are attempting to make sense of, and cope with, their particular health care problems.

As argued earlier, the first view informs a reductionist or **quantitative** approach to research and knowledge. That is, we view our patients objectively, as natural objects, and attempt to identify and measure important variables which represent the causes and expressions of a clinical condition. We develop models and theoretical frameworks which systematically explain how these variables are interrelated and undertake therapeutic actions which serve to diminish the variables representing illness or disability. Our therapeutic actions are the *technical* applications for our scientific theories; their outcomes and effectiveness should be tested under controlled conditions.

The second view informs a **qualitative** or interpretive approach to research and knowledge. We view our patients as persons and attempt to gain insights into their subjective experiences and the reasons for their actions in particular situations. We develop theories for interpreting the nature and development of their personal points of view, and to inform our therapeutic actions so that they seem meaningful and appropriate to our patients. (These concepts are further discussed in Ch. 8).

Take, as an illustration of the above approaches, a patient with cancer. In a quantitative analysis we attempt to quantify the problem by using appropriate instrumentation which measure variables such as the size and location of the tumour and the extent of its spread within the organism. Consistent with current theories of the nature of cancer, various techniques such as surgery, radiology or chemotherapy might be brought into play, the effectiveness of which will be judged in terms of controlling specific variables associated with the condition, such as levels of pain, the weight or time of survival of the patient.

With a qualitative perspective, we would address the meaning of the condition from the patient's personal point of view, within the context of his or her family setting and social circumstances. That is, the patient's value systems must be clarified and understood before actions such as assessments and therapeutic actions are undertaken. Enquiry might uncover conflicting values, for instance, concerning the implementation of a program of chemotherapy. From the clinician's point of view, a radical program of chemotherapy might seem appropriate, as probably quantitatively extending the patient's life by several years. However, from the patient's point of view, the quality of life under chemotherapy might seem inadequate, and also they might not wish to be a burden on their families. Clearly, both in clinical practice and in related research, evidence from both quantitative and qualitative enquiries should be integrated for insuring effective health care. This text covers both quantitative and qualitative orientations with an emphasis upon the quantitative orientation. The authors use both approaches in their own research, often in the same project.

THE RESEARCH PROCESS

Although there are differences in how health scientists approach problems, Figure 1.2 shows the sequence of procedures commonly involved in quantitative research. The term 'data' refers to the complete set of observations or measurements recorded in the course of a research process. You will find that the organization of this book follows the steps and stages of the research process, as outlined below.

1. Planning. As we shall show in Section 2, research planning involves selecting appropriate strategies and measurements to answer questions or to test

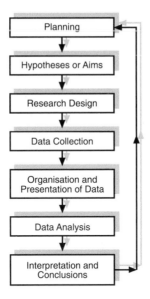

Fig. 1.2 The research process

hypotheses. It will be argued in Chapter 2 that planning must take into consideration previous research evidence as well as ethical and economic factors before the appropriate research strategy and measurement is selected, and the precise research hypothesis or aim is stated.

2. Research design. The usefulness of research depends on plans specifying appropriate sampling methods for ensuring the generalizability of the results. Appropriate designs are selected for ensuring controlled observation in order to demonstrate causal relationships. Chapters 3–4 in Section 2 and Chapters 5–8 in Section 3 examine how the uses of appropriate designs and sampling methods ensure the generality and validity of investigations across a variety of research strategies. Chapters 8–11 also outline some basic issues in the collection and interpretation of evidence in the context of qualitative research.

3. Data collection. The next step in the research process is collection of data (Section 4). Chapters, 9, 10 and 11 examine data collection methods commonly employed in health research. Chapter 12 is concerned with appropriate ways for carrying out measurements, and different types of measurement scales available for research and clinical assessment.

4. Organisation and presentation. Section 5 introduces descriptive statistics representing the conventions for summarizing and describing the data. Chapters 13–16 examine basic concepts in this area, outlining how graphs and various descriptive statistics are used to condense and communicate research and clinical findings.

5. Data analysis. Data analysis involves applying the principles of probability for calculating confidence intervals and testing hypotheses. The area of inferential statistics, involving decisions concerning whether the data support experimental hypotheses, is outlined in Chapters 17–19 in Section 6.

6. Interpretation. The final step in any research project involves interpreting ones findings. The findings may support existing theories or practices; suggest that new techniques may be more effective, or new theoretical notions which are more able to explain phenomena. It is rare that the findings from any single research project are completely definitive, and often the results may suggest the need for further investigation in related subject areas or contexts. This issue will be examined in Sections 6 and 7.

7. Publication. For research to be scientifically meaningful, investigators must present their results in the form of publications in professional journals. Research findings become part of scientific knowledge only if they stand up to methodological critique and replication. In Chapter 21 we will discuss conventions for preparing publications. In Chapter 22 we will outline steps for critically evaluating published research.

The above steps and stages of research represent a logical sequence which is followed in most research projects. An exception, as we mentioned earlier, is in the case of 'qualitative' research (Chapter 8) where a more flexible sequence might be employed. Also, in qualitative research the empirical evidence is not normally summarized and analysed through statistical methods, but through the use of language and the analysis of narratives.

RESEARCH AND CLINICAL PRACTICES

Research methods cover a wide variety of skills and techniques aimed at the methodologically valid investigation of questions of interest to the researcher. These methods of enquiry are not restricted to research laboratories, nor need they involve expensive equipment or large research teams. Rather, these methods imply an approach to stating and answering questions in any setting.

Applied research in the health sciences focuses on issues such as the prevalence and causes of illness, the usefulness and accuracy of assessment techniques, or the effectiveness of treatments. Applied research which is published, aims at producing findings which are of a general interest to groups of professionals working in the health area.

Research methods interact with health practices in multiple, and mutually productive ways. An important general aim of this textbook is to discuss the relationships between theories, practices and the ways in which research methods contribute to these in the area of health care.

Instrumentation and measurement

Individuals working in a modern health care setting are often called upon to use and interpret the results of complex measuring instruments. These instruments include 'high-technology' diagnostic products as well as a variety of standardized clinical tests and measures.

Effective diagnosis involves acquiring skills for using such instruments, understanding the criteria for selecting specific instruments, and being able to interpret the clinical significance of the measurements produced by them.

Therefore, the first aim of this text is to introduce to the student the concepts of validity and reliability, and the procedures involved in interpreting the results of various tests and measures.

Data presentation and analysis

Much of our knowledge of patients, disease processes, or the functioning of health care institutions, is expressed numerically; through the use of descriptive and inferential statistics. The student needs to understand statistical concepts for two reasons:

1. To produce and communicate sets of measurements about patients and treatment outcomes for both clinical and administrative purposes
2. To be able to interpret research and evaluate data presented in a statistical form.

There is an increasing emphasis on interprofessional interaction in health care. Therefore, it is unfortunate when practising clinicians are unable to present or understand clinically relevant evidence which has been presented in a quantitative form. Much important information is missed this way, often to the detriment of patients.

The second aim of this text is to introduce the student to fundamental procedures in presenting and interpreting quantitative (and to a minimal extent, qualitative) evidence in the health sciences.

Evaluation of treatment procedures

Research and evaluation techniques are typically used by the health professional at two levels:

1. To evaluate the effectiveness of particular treatment techniques in order to improve the quality of therapy available to the client
2. To evaluate the relative effectiveness of health care programs in order to determine the allocation of resources in health settings.

Governments and health care consumers now routinely want to see evidence that their money is well spent. To survive as a therapist in the coming years, it will be necessary to provide hard empirical evidence to justify professional effectiveness. The third aim of the present text is to introduce the student to research strategies appropriate for treatment evaluation.

Conceptual basis for clinical practice

Research methods are based on the application of the scientific method to the conduct of enquiry. As the terms 'health sciences' or 'clinical sciences' imply, there is a close relationship between clinical practice and the scientific approach. Much (although not all) of the systematic knowledge underlying modern health care is based on science. Therefore, an adequate understanding of the basis for current professional knowledge and practices presupposes some insight into scientific methodology.

The fourth aim of this text is to introduce students to scientific methodology by examining how health related research is planned, conducted and interpreted.

Research contribution

Traditionally, the majority of systematic research contributions to the health sciences emerged from the faculties of Science and Medicine. However, this situation has changed with the emergence of college or university based education for health care workers.

In recent years, in areas such as nursing, occupational therapy, physiotherapy and speech pathology, there has been a substantial increase in the quantity and quality of published research. It should be recognized that, to a considerable extent, the growth, effectiveness and prestige of the allied health professions depend on the production of research of a high standard. We recognize that only some health professionals have the motivation, interest and opportunity to become involved in research. Nevertheless, the emergence of motivated individuals capable of contributing to professional knowledge requires an introduction to research methods during their education.

The fifth major aim of the present book is to introduce students to basic features of the research process, in preparation for further studies in this area of health care. Although not all health practitioners are actively involved in research, it is a necessary condition for professional development that one is able to critique published research.

SUMMARY

There are several common methods used for acquiring, stating and establishing knowledge. The scientific method is one of these methods, useful in justifying the validity of diagnoses and clinical interventions in the Western health care system. Scientific method is concerned with applying a set of rules or conventions that will allow us to produce scientifically valid knowledge. These rules specify how observations should be made, and theories and hypotheses stated and evaluated.

Theories and hypotheses obtained and verified through scientific enquiry are not held to be absolutely true. An inherent part of the scientific approach is scepticism, regarding both the contents of knowledge and the underlying methodology. We have pointed out that there are controversies concerning what constitutes scientific methodology.

It was argued that the scientific method is directly applicable to conducting research in the health sciences. In general, the stages for research include planning, stating aims or hypotheses, and formulating designs; collecting, summarizing and analysing the data; and drawing conclusions. This process can be applied to ensuring advances in health care and to problem-solving in specific clinical settings. There is a close relationship between professional practices and health sciences research. The rest of the book is organized to follow the stages involved in performing research.

SELF ASSESSMENT

Explain the meaning of the following terms:

authority	intuition
deduction	observation
data	qualitative
determinism	quantitative
empiricism	rationalism
falsification	scepticism
hypothesis	theory

True or false

1. A 'method' specifies how knowledge should be acquired, stated and tested.
2. Very strong intuitions always turn out to be true.
3. The method of authority depends on the status and credibility of the source.
4. When a syllogism is in a valid form, the conclusions should be factually true provided the premises are true.
5. Rationalism calls for correct reasoning for acquiring truth.
6. The case of Ignaz Semmelweiss illustrates that medical decisions are based on the scientific method.
7. Scepticism refers to the notion that all knowledge is false.
8. Empiricism refers to the notion that events in the world occur according to regular laws and causes.
9. Scientific observations are different from ordinary observations because they depend on the use of instruments.
10. Scientific observations must be recorded as numbers.
11. Hypotheses are unproven theories.
12. Hypotheses are statements which specify the nature of the relationship between two or more sets of observations.
13. The logic underlying scientific generalization is called induction.
14. Scientific theories represent notions of natural events and their causes.
15. A good scientific theory is one that can not be, in principle, falsified.
16. Controlled observation aims to identify the causes of events.
17. Scientific theories should enable the deduction of empirically verifiable hypotheses.

18. When the empirical evidence is found to be consistent with the implications of a hypothesis, we can say that the theory from which ~~the hypothesis was deduced is absolutely true.~~

19. When we say that a theory was falsified, we mean that hypotheses deduced from it were not supported by empirical evidence.

20. We can question the content but not the methodology of science.

Multiple choice

1. A scientific theory is a set of statements:
   - *a* conforming to the rules of logic
   - *b* explaining the relationships which pertain among apparently diverse phenomena
   - *c* which lead to empirically testable hypotheses
   - *d* all of the above.

2. The statement 'Persons who are highly anxious do not perform well on learning tasks' is:
   - *a* a theory
   - *b* hypothesis
   - *c* false
   - *d* in principle empirically untestable.

3. A scientific hypothesis:
   - *a* should be verified through the use of logic and disputation
   - *b* should be open to empirical verification
   - *c* can not arise through intuition
   - *d* *a* and *c*.

4. The results of scientific research:
   - *a* should be made available for critique and replication
   - *b* should not be used to support existing theories
   - *c* must be obtained in controlled laboratory situations
   - *d* must conform to public expectations about the outcome.

5. Descriptive statistics:
   - *a* are based on the principles of probability
   - *b* represent conventions for planning research
   - *c* represent conventions for summarizing and organizing data
   - *d* specify the selection of appropriate measurement scales.

6. The scientific method is a set of rules specifying how:
   - *a* scientific knowledge should be acquired, stated and tested
   - *b* scientists should conduct their life
   - *c* how society should conduct its affairs
   - *d* all of the above *a*, *b*, and *c*.

7. Authority, as a method, is:
   a   no longer relevant to the conduct of health care
   b   the fundamental source of the scientific method
   c   neither *a* nor *b*
   d   both *a* and *b*.

8. A therapist without formal medical qualifications treated cancer patients using an 'alternative' regimen of herbs, massage and medication. Say that there is no scientific evidence available that such a treatment is effective. It follows that:
   a   the treatment was ineffective because it lacks scientific evidence
   b   the treatment was ineffective because the practitioner was unqualified
   c   both *a* and *b*
   d   neither *a* nor *b*.

9. As evidence for the effectiveness of the treatment, the therapist provides a hundred signed statements from current or former patients claiming that they were satisfied with the treatment. One reason such evidence lacks scientific validity is that:
   a   the opinions of patients can not, in principle, constitute scientific evidence
   b   it was not acquired in a manner consistent with the principles of scientific observations
   c   we can not, in principle, generalize from only a hundred observations
   d   it pertains to an 'alternative', non-scientific treatment regimen.

10. In the context of the scientific method, evidence which would be most indicative of the effectiveness of the treatment would be:
   a   the support of medically qualified people
   b   the argument that each patient has the right to select their own form of treatment
   c   that the survival times of the patients were better than those of equivalent patients being treated with conventional therapies
   d   that the patients were willing to pay money to receive the treatment.

11. The statement 'If my theory of schizophrenia is true, then the sun will rise tomorrow morning' is:
   a   probably based on the invalid use of deduction
   b   untestable
   c   based on the method of authority
   d   *a* and *b*.

12. According to an astrologer, people who were born under a particular star sign are 'basically kind and very intelligent, although because of their modesty not sufficiently appreciated by others'. To test the truth of this statement, the astrologer asks a group of individuals if this description fits their personality. 95% of the sample agrees that the description is accurate. One of the problems with this enquiry is that:
    a astrology is inherently false, therefore the evidence must be wrong
    b 'personality' is inherently a misunderstood concept
    c in this case a 100% agreement is required for acceptable evidence
    d it is contrary to the principles of controlled observation.

13. The notion that facts are 'theory-dependent' implies that:
    a what is recorded as evidence is independent of the event being studied
    b theories and hypothesis have no relationship to empirical observations
    c what is recorded as evidence can be influenced by the theoretical notions of the observer
    d only our minds exist, rather than a material world.

14. Lakatos argued that:
    a theories are discarded only when their 'hard core' of assumptions are falsified
    b a 'belt' of auxiliary hypotheses protect the fundamental 'hard core' assumption of a theory
    c theories can not be refuted or falsified on the basis of empirical evidence
    d both a and b.

15. Which is the least controversial statement concerning the scientific knowledge?
    a There is only one acceptable form of the scientific method independent of the phenomenon being investigated.
    b Scientific theories are derived from the use of induction, rather than creative insights.
    c The principles of the scientific method can be usefully applied to conducting systematic research.
    d Scientific enquiry is conducted independently of the personal values and social environment of scientists.

16. Which of the following problems might be best approached through the scientific method?
    a The clinical effectiveness of a new instrument needs to be evaluated.
    b The hospital budget is cut by 10%.
    c Personnel refuse to staff an abortion clinic on moral grounds.
    d The nursing staff go on strike.

DISCUSSION, QUESTIONS AND ANSWERS

These questions ask you to examine issues concerning the applications of the scientific method to various aspects of health sciences research. Unlike the multiple-choice or true or false questions, these discussion questions do not necessarily have a single correct answer. Rather, they are aimed at promoting a critical, integrative view of conducting research.

Our first discussion question involves theories and examines the relationships between theories, models, hypotheses and empirical observations. Theories are conceptual frameworks as we discussed in Chapter 1 integrating a range of related observations and explanatory hypotheses. We may deduce empirically testable hypotheses from our theories.

On the basis of observations, in particular when the observations are carried out under controlled conditions, we establish the probable truth of our hypotheses, and thereby support or falsify the theories which were originally the sources for the hypotheses.

Some theories include models which represent specific aspects of a theory. Models are used for explaining real situations and predicting novel empirical outcomes. Models can be as follows:

1. Physical models. These models are constructed from materials, for example a 'pump' model of the heart for showing how the circulatory system works, or a construction of the DNA molecule to show how different nucleotides are organized in order to replicate genetic information.

2. Mathematical models. These models contain a series of equations that represent our theoretical interpretations of real life situations. For example, epidemiologists may employ mathematical models to predict how a given epidemic might spread in a population, or a physiologist may employ a mathematical model of neuronal membranes to predict the behaviour of action potentials in a neurone. When our theories and related models are sufficiently detailed and well formed, we may use these in simulation research. Nowadays we use computers, which are capable of carrying out the complex calculations necessary for the simulation of a real life situation and predicting numerical outcomes.

3. 'Paper and pencil' models. Often our theories are not sufficiently detailed for making precise numerical predictions. Here the models are 'sketches' of a particular system; defining the key elements of the model and showing how these elements interact to produce various outcomes. Such models enable us to make testable predictions concerning the effects of variables as shown by the following model (Fig. D.1) of the 'Gate Control Theory' of pain (Melzack & Wall 1965).

(Note that for teaching purposes this model is an incomplete and modified representation of the original. If you are interested in understanding pain problems, you should consult Melzack and Wall's original work).

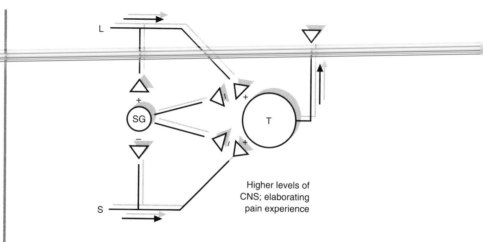

Fig. D.1 Model of spinal gating of nociceptive input
(adapted from Melzack & Wall, 1965)

Elements of the systems

(a) L: 'Large' diameter axons of receptors, which convey information concerning mechanical stimuli, such as pressure and vibration.

(b) S: 'Small' diameter axons of receptors, which convey information concerning noxious (tissue damaging) stimuli.

(c) SG: Neurones within the 'substantial gelatinosa' (SG) of the spinal cord. These receive converging information from L and S axons. The SG neurones control, or 'gate' through pre-synaptic inhibition, the information flowing through to the 'T' neurones.

(d) T: 'Transmission' neurones in the spinal cord, which receive information from both L and S axons. The pattern of activity of T neurones is projected to higher levels of the CNS (Central Nervous System), where this information is elaborated into the experience of pain.

(e) ◁: Synapses, which may be either excitatory (+) or inhibitory (–). Excitatory synapses increase, while inhibitory synapses decrease the activity of the post-synaptic neurones.

(f) →: Arrows showing the direction of the information flow; in this case from the periphery towards the spinal cord and, subsequently, to higher levels of the CNS.

The above model is an attempt to produce a representation of the events which take place in the mammalian nervous system when receiving and processing nociceptive input at a spinal cord level. The model integrates a broad range of research in the neurosciences and has been applied to explain aspects of pain control in clinical settings.

Questions

After this rather prolonged introduction to the model, we are ready to ask questions how it may be applied to explaining and predicting observations about pain.

1. Use the above model to describe what happens in the nervous system during noxious (tissue-damaging) stimulation.
2. How would we use controlled observations to demonstrate that small (S), rather than large (L) neurones convey nociceptive information. (Assume that we have instrumentation for measuring the activity of single neurones in response to different kinds of stimuli.)
3. Explain how we would use evidence obtained by recording the activity of single neurones to demonstrate that T neurones are in fact involved in nociception.
4. Describe the effects of large (L) and small (S) axons on the activity of SG neurones.
5. Explain the mechanism by which SG neurones function as a 'pain gating' system.
6. Propose a hypothesis for predicting the effects of selectively damaging T neurones on subsequent pain experience.
7. Propose a hypothesis for predicting the effects of damaging large axons (L) on subsequent pain experience.
8. A virus is identified which damages SG neurones. As a hypothetical case, imagine that people who have this virus report greatly reduced pain sensitivity. What would be the implication of this observation for the validity of the Gate Control theory of pain?
9. Would you discard the Gate Control theory on the bases of the hypothetical observations described in question 8? Explain.
10. A clinical technique called TENS for relieving pain involves the gentle peripheral electrical stimulation of painful areas. Explain in terms of the model how TENS might work to reduce pain. (Hint: TENS does not directly reduce the activity of S axons).

Answers

1. Small diameter 'S' axons convey nociceptive information towards spinal cord neurones, including the SG and the T neurones. The SG neurones are inhibited through nociceptive inputs while the T neurones are excited by the stimulation. Information concerning tissue damage is then conveyed by the axons of the T neurones to higher levels of the CNS. There it is elaborated into the experience of pain.
2. By showing that the activity of T neurones was correlated to the levels of peripheral noxious stimulation.
3. Mechanical stimuli—show S axons not responsive while L axons change rate of activity.

Noxious stimuli—show S axons change rate of activity while L remain unresponsive

4. Large axons excite (increase the rate of activity of SG neurones) while small axons inhibit the rate of activity of the SG neurones.

5. The SG neurones inhibit the effect of the S axons on the T cells. As L axons excite the SG neurones, the action of L fibres is to 'close' the pain gate. The S fibres 'open' the pain gate by inhibiting the SG neurones. In effect the model is telling us that mechanical stimulation, such as gently scrubbing an injured area will reduce nociceptive input. On the other hand, noxious stimulation seems to maintain the effects of subsequent nociceptive inputs.

6. The T cells are crucial for transmitting nociceptive information to higher levels of the CNS. Hypothesis: Selectively damaging T neurones will reduce or eliminate pain experience following nociceptive stimulation.

7. Damage to L axons will result in reduced excitatory stimulation of the SG neurones, opening the spinal gate to noxious stimulation. Hypothesis: Damaging L axons would increase the pain experienced following nociceptive stimulation.

8. As the model proposes that SG neurones are involved in the gating of noxious stimuli, we would predict that damage to the SG neurones would increase pain sensitivity. Reduced pain sensitivity is evidence which would falsify the Gate Control theory.

9. Probably not; as we discussed in the context of Lakatos' ideas. Theories have a 'protective belt' of assumptions; which means that a single empirical falsification need not result in the rejection of the theory. In this case, we may look for additional effects of the virus; say in destroying CNS tissue involved in elaborating pain experience. However, in the long run, such disconfirmations will lead to discarding the theory.

10. In terms of the model TENS works by stimulating the L axons, and thereby 'closing' the pain gate, as outlined in 4 and 5.

Research planning

The first stage of research involves the detailed planning of the project. The plan for what is to occur in the project is written up in a document called the research protocol. Before the research project may proceed, the protocol is examined by ethics committees and funding bodies to ensure that it conforms with general methodological and ethical principles. The three chapters of Section Two aim to outline the basic considerations for the successful preparation of a research protocol.

The primary reason for carrying out a research project is to obtain empirical evidence that will advance theory and practice in the health sciences. Before all else, we must be sure that we are asking the right questions, that is, raising issues and problems which are central to progress in contemporary health care. We must convince the critical reader that our aims or the hypotheses which we are attempting to resolve are in fact of central importance. Asking the right research questions depends on being creative; for instance identifying previously ignored patterns in the data; or the construction of novel theories that predict new, as yet unobserved phenomena. Of course, we are not suggesting that researchers are geniuses, or that only brilliant, ground-breaking research is funded. Much important research is carried out by perfectly ordinary men and women, who are interested in their patients and their problems, who have a good knowledge of their professional practices and who understand research methods.

To justify the research proposal it is necessary to write a 'literature review'. The literature review is a summary and critical evaluation of previous research and theory relevant to the problem which we are intending to investigate. In this way the literature review both provides a conceptual background for our proposal and justifies the need for further empirical evidence by identifying 'gaps' in our knowledge.

The proposed research may be descriptive, for example collecting information concerning health needs of a community and/or the impact of illness or injury on a group of patients. In Chapter 3, non-experimental research strategies are described. Non-experimental research which includes both quantitative and qualitative surveys (Section 3) aims to provide a clear picture or description of the health of individuals, groups or whole communities. Experimental research strategies are appropriate when we are testing hypotheses about the causes of illness, and when we attempt to gain control over extraneous variables which may influence treatment outcomes. The notions of causality and control are central for health research; and are explored in Chapter 4. Of course, when we write a research protocol, we must be sure that we select the appropriate research strategy.

No research can proceed unless it is judged to be ethical by an appropriate committee. A research proposal is judged ethical if it conforms with our rules and values concerning caregiving. These rules and values are made explicit in documents representing the standards of professional groups and of institutions (e.g. hospitals, universities and research councils). The research protocol must be described in sufficient detail so that a decision can be made as to whether any harm might occur to participants in the research project.

Economic considerations, or the availability of resources also has a strong influence on research planning. For example, you may have designed a qualitative research project which involves one hundred 'in depth' interviews with persons suffering from a disorder. Say you have only one year and a very limited amount of money to complete your project. You would be advised either to reduce your sample size, or, if this is not possible, change your topic. Obviously, ethics or funding committees only approve projects which are feasible to be completed with the available resources.

The way in which samples are selected is discussed in Chapter 3. Selection of an appropriate sample is crucial for the generalizability (or external validity) of your findings. Our aim is to select a representative sample of the population but this may not be always possible in health sciences research. We need a sample size which is sufficiently large to identify the phenomena in which we are interested, but not too large or we are simply wasting resources.

Thus, research planning is a process, by which we transform our ideas into well planned, ethical and economically feasible projects, as is described in a research protocol.

2

Research planning

INTRODUCTION

Before the actual data collection begins, researchers invest considerable time and effort in the planning of their investigations. The first step is to select and to justify the selection of the research problem. The second step for quantitative research is to transform the problem into a clear researchable aim or hypothesis. Research planning includes the selection of an appropriate research strategy for providing required empirical evidence. The selection of the appropriate research strategy depends not only on the questions being asked, but also on identifying ethical issues and resource constraints which define the scope and form of the investigation.

The specific aims of this chapter are to:

1. Discuss how research questions are selected and justified
2. Specify how questions are transformed into empirically testable hypotheses or aims
3. Broadly outline research strategies available for specific types of investigations
4. Discuss the ethical and economic constraints on the planning and execution of research.

SOURCES OF RESEARCH QUESTIONS

Advances in health sciences research depend on the identification of questions and problems which promote the development of more powerful theories of health, illness and disability, and then devising more effective ways of assessing, treating and preventing health problems. This advancement depends very much on researchers asking the 'right' questions and identifying solvable problems.

The formulation of research questions depends on the expertise of women and men who have a combination of theoretical knowledge and practical experience for identifying problems and asking the right questions. The professional backgrounds of researchers is an important consideration, to the extent that one's educational background and practices will in part determine what are seen as theoretically and professionally interesting problems.

Whatever the researcher's professional background, it is understood that they are strongly (even passionately) interested in a particular area of the health sciences. The formulation of even apparently simple research questions is often the culmination of intensive preliminary observations, spending long hours in the library reading through and critically analysing related research, and thinking through the various issues. It is assumed that the researcher already has, or intends to develop, a specialized area of expertise, which is normally a precondition for advancement in health theory or practice.

The health care setting in which the researcher works often has a strong influence on the formulation of research questions. For example, it is an important consideration if the researcher works in a laboratory, a hospital, a community clinic or in private practice. These settings will influence how the patients' problems are perceived, and how researchers define professionally relevant solutions to these problems.

In many areas of health care, such as rehabilitation, community health and neurosciences, researchers sharing similar interests may join together in multidisciplinary research teams. Because of the broad range of expertise and perspectives such teams may be in a position to formulate interesting research questions.

Unfortunately, because of professional rivalries and interpersonal conflicts, such multidisciplinary research groups are sometimes not as productive as they should be. Good research often requires interpersonal and communication skills.

THE FORMULATION OF RESEARCH QUESTIONS

There is a variety of valid sources for formulating research questions. These include:

1. Hypotheses logically deduced from existing theories, as discussed in Chapter 1
2. Hypotheses suggested by clinical observations and insights such as that of Semmelweiss, discussed in Chapter 1
3. Questions raised by previously conducted research which was inconclusive, invalid or not complete. These questions arise from the critical evaluation of published literature, as outlined in Chapter 22
4. Questions raised concerning the effectiveness of currently used or new treatment or assessment techniques. These questions arise in the context of evaluating or attempting to improve the outcome of health care
5. Solutions required to pressing problems faced in professional settings including problems reported by patients. In effect much of applied health sciences research may be seen as a process for identifying, clarifying and solving problems.

Whatever the source or sources of the questions or problems, it is understood that they can be answered or resolved by collecting and analysing relevant empirical evidence.

THE JUSTIFICATION OF RESEARCH QUESTIONS

When researchers call on public funds to conduct their investigations, they must explain in what way their intended investigation will contribute to scientific knowledge or clinical practice. In 'pure' scientific research, a proposed investigation is justified in terms of its potential contribution to existing knowledge. In the context of 'applied' health research, the investigator may be required to demonstrate that the empirical evidence will in some way contribute to the improved practice of health care, and benefit patients.

Before embarking on the design and conduct of a research project, the investigator must review previous publications relevant to the aims of the intended project (see p. 25). This process is essential, both for providing the appropriate background and context for the investigation, and for justifying the investigation in contributing to existing knowledge.

Literature searching is carried out at appropriate research centres or libraries where scientific and professional journals are stored. There are nowadays various computerized literature search methods which can simplify the search. Professional library staff can help to locate the relevant literature. However, the critical evaluation of the literature depends on the application of research methods (see Ch. 22) for the identification of controversies or 'gaps' in the available evidence.

FORMULATION OF RESEARCH AIMS OR HYPOTHESES

Hypotheses

A frequent goal in quantitative research is to test a hypothesis. Hypotheses are propositions about relationships between variables or differences between groups that are to be tested. Hypotheses may be concerned with relationships between observations or variables (for example, 'Is there an association between level of exercise and annual health care expenditure for Australians?') or differences between groups (for example, 'Do patients treated under therapy x exhibit greater improvement than those treated under therapy y'?) A **variable** is simply a property that may vary from case to case, for example, the room temperature, the ages of the patients, or their improvement on a measurement scale.

Some research projects do not have a hypothesis to be tested in any formal sense. For example, if you are measuring the health needs of a local community, there need not be any expectation or hypothesis to be tested. This does not mean the research is deficient, it just means it has a different objective from other types of research projects. In fact, for qualitative research, holding clear cut hypotheses may prejudice the investigation (see Ch. 8). In these cases, we talk about the research having aims or objectives, rather than hypotheses. An obvious and necessary condition for formulating research aims or hypotheses is that the research questions should have empirical referents. In planning research, the investigator is required to give observable referents to vague and ambiguous concepts. That is, investigators must decide on precisely how the variables are going to be measured. This is called the operational definition of a variable, and will be discussed in Chapter 12 in the context of measurement. Clearly, when formulating research aims or hypotheses we must specify the variables being studied, and how these variables are to be observed or measured.

Let us look at an example for illustrating how concepts should be specified in terms of empirical (observable) referents. Consider the concept 'coronary disease'. What are its observable referents (or symptoms)? They include:

- Severe periodic pain in the chest and upper left arm
- Occlusion (blockings) of coronary arteries, reducing blood flow
- Sudden death

Now suppose a new drug, x, is introduced to help people with coronary disease. The researchers hypothesize that 'The new drug x is effective for helping patients with coronary disease'. Using the observable symptoms as referents, the research hypothesis is then restated:

Patients diagnosed with coronary disease taking drug x will report fewer incidents of pain in the chest and upper left arm than patients taking traditionally used drug y

or

Patients diagnosed with coronary disease taking drug x will have greater volume of blood flow through their coronary arteries than patients taking traditionally used drug y

or

Fewer patients diagnosed with coronary disease taking drug x will die during a five year period than those taking traditionally used drug y.

A published example of formulating hypotheses

Let us look at a published example for illustrating how concepts can be defined in operational terms. This paper is titled: *Effects of preoperative teaching on postoperative pain: a replication and extension,* by Morgan, Wells and Robertson (1985).

Firstly, the proposed intervention 'preoperative teaching' is a rather vague concept. What do the authors mean by this? In effect, this involved 'brief relaxation training', which is more precise. However, there are a variety of possible brief relaxation techniques. Therefore, quite appropriately, the authors explained that: 'The present study was designed to replicate, at least conceptually, and extend a method...described by Flaherty and Fitzpatrick (1978)' (Morgan et al 1985).

Now by reading through the reference, and noting the modifications of the authors described in the paper, we are in a position to understand the precise nature of the intervention.

Secondly, we may ask how the outcome (postoperative pain) was defined and measured? After all, as the authors pointed out, pain is a subjective experience and its quality and meaning may be different for patients. Having reviewed the relevant literature, Morgan, Wells and Robertson (1985) decide to operationally define pain in terms of:

(i) The amount of analgesic required by individual patients following surgery: in general, the less pain the smaller the quantity of analgesic required

(ii) The self-reports of patients on a 10 point pain rating scale, reporting the 'sensory' and 'distressing' aspects of pain.

Although we may argue about the validity of these means for measuring pain, the authors provided operational definitions for the variables studied in their clinical experiment. The following hypotheses guided their research:

1. Patients taught a relaxation technique will have lower vital signs (blood pressure, pulse and respiration) than those not taught a relaxation technique.

2. Patients taught a relaxation technique will experience less pain than those not taught a relaxation technique as indicated by:
   a. consuming fewer analgesics
   b. less self-reported pain sensation
   c. less distress from these sensations

3. Patients taught a relaxation technique will be discharged from the hospital earlier than those not taught a relaxation technique (Morgan et al 1985:269-270).

The formulation of an adequately formed research hypothesis or aim is a process during which the researcher gradually refines a broadly based issue into specific operationally defined statements. This process must take into account the logical requirements of designs for the data collection and ethical standards for conducting health sciences research. In addition, the aims or hypotheses must inform a realistic data collection procedure which can be supported by the resources available for researchers. We will examine these issues in the rest of this chapter.

RESEARCH STRATEGIES

Research planning also involves the selection or formulation of research strategies. Research strategies are established procedures for designing and executing research. Research strategies outlined in this book include experimental and quasi-experimental strategies, single case research, surveys, and qualitative field research. Before detailed discussion of the differences between these strategies is undertaken in following sections, it is instructive to compare the basic structures of non-experimental (surveys) and experimental research. As we shall see in subsequent sections, these are fundamentally different ways of conducting research.

Non-experimental strategies

The three essential steps involved in non-experimental strategies are shown in Figure 2.1.

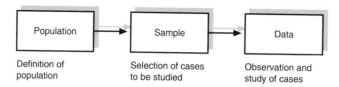

Fig. 2.1 Structure of a non-experimental study

You will note in Figure 2.1 that the researcher defines the population of interest, selects the cases to be studied (this process is described in some detail in Chapter 3) and then observes or studies them, generating the data. There is no active intervention in the situation by the researcher. Indeed, intervention that would change the phenomenon being studied is discouraged and avoided. In this type of research strategy there is a constant tension between the requirements for close and detailed observation and the possibility that the behaviour of the cases may change because they are being studied. There are techniques for dealing with this problem, such as the use of unobtrusive measures and participant observation, which will be discussed in subsequent chapters. An important class of non-experimental research strategies are called 'qualitative' or 'interpretive' (Ch. 8).

Experimental strategies

Experimental research strategies involve more steps, as illustrated in Figure 2.2. As with the non-experimental strategy, cases are selected for study from a defined population. However, these cases are then assigned (generally by chance or random method) to a treatment or non-treatment group, and then treated. (The term 'treatment' is used here in the sense that the subject or event is being systematically influenced or manipulated by the investigator; that is, in a broader sense than as medical or physical treatment). The two groups are then observed and compared. If everything went according to plan, any differences in the data of the treatment and non-treatment groups should be a result of the effects of the treatment. Unfortunately, there are often other factors (sources of error) that are responsible for the differences. Good experimental technique attempts to eliminate these errors through control (Ch. 4).

Thus, there is quite a difference in the structure of experimental and non-experimental research strategies. Cook and Campbell (1979) have proposed a third class of *'quasi-experimental'* strategies (which are really just tightly structured non-experimental strategies) that we will also cover later (see Ch. 6).

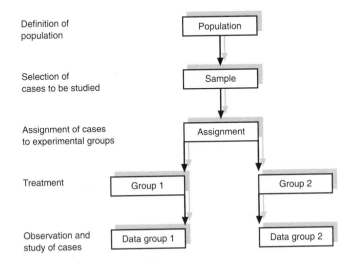

Definition of population — Population

Selection of cases to be studied — Sample

Assignment of cases to experimental groups — Assignment

Treatment — Group 1 — Group 2

Observation and study of cases — Data group 1 — Data group 2

Fig. 2.2 Experimental research strategies

The decision of the investigator to adopt experimental or non-experimental strategies depends on the phenomenon being studied and the specific question type of research (causal or descriptive) being investigated.

RESEARCH PLANNING: ETHICAL CONSIDERATIONS

In health research, where the health and lives of people participating in the study may be at stake, ethical considerations play a decisive role in research planning and execution. For instance, consider the question of the effects of cigarette smoking on health. A convincing way of investigating this question would be through experimental strategies, which (as we will see) are best suited for establishing causal relationships. However, it would be ethically unacceptable to have a number of people randomly assigned to a group involved in long term, heavy cigarette smoking. Clearly, evidence must come from quasi- or non-experimental strategies, where investigators observe the effects of smoking in persons who have themselves chosen to smoke.

A research process is judged to be *ethical* by the extent to which it conforms to or complies with the set of standards or conventions in the context in which the research is to be carried out. Most health settings and higher education institutions now have ethics committees to oversee health research involving humans and/or animals. Ethics committees along with the researcher are responsible for interpreting and enforcing ethical standards. It should be noted, however, that even when a given research proposal is judged to be ethical, it may not be seen as *moral* by specific individuals or groups in a community. A good example is animal experimentation when the research involves painful or stressful procedures such as surgery. According to the value systems of some persons and groups, such work is considered to be intrinsically immoral. From this viewpoint, there may be no justification for inflicting suffering on animals, even when the results may be beneficial for humans. Others argue that such procedures are morally justified, given that they are necessary for the advancement of the biological and medical sciences and provided that reasonable steps are taken to limit the suffering of the animals. There are no absolute solutions for such controversies, but often discussing these issues in public helps to establish a degree of consensus in the community and guidance for the ethical decisions of researchers.

It is beyond the scope of this sub-section to examine in full the ethics of health research, but the following issues are central to making decisions in these areas:

1. Benefits. Who is to benefit from the research? One likes to think that 'humanity', 'the subjects', or 'health science' are going to be the beneficiaries. A slightly more cynical analysis points to the investigators as having the most to gain, at least in the short term. After all, given a successful outcome for the research project, they stand to satisfy their curiosity, improve their career prospects, or to raise their esteem before colleagues. In practice, benefits accruing to the investigator, the participants and health science have to be carefully weighed in relation to the conduct of any project. The protection of the rights and welfare of the participants is the primary consideration of scientific ethics.

2. Informed consent. Informed consent by human participants is a necessary condition for ethically acceptable research. This means that all the risks involved in the investigation must be explained, as well as the possible benefits. Honest explanation of the procedures to the participant takes considerable skill, if disclosing the design of the study (say with placebo treatments) influences the expectations and performances of the participants. Also, special care needs to be taken when the participants are in some way limited in understanding the risks; for example, people who are intellectually disabled, or confused under the influence of drugs. Informed consent implies a freedom of choice: the participant must feel confident that refusal to participate will not prejudice their subsequent clinical treatment.

3. Protection of participants. It is the investigator's responsibility to minimise the chances of long-term deleterious effects to subjects. Dangers can arise from administering new interventions or treatments with unknown side-effects, denying treatments of known effectiveness, or using invasive assessment techniques. The welfare of laboratory animals must not be ignored. There are nowadays enforceable constraints on the conditions for using non-human subjects in research.

4. Minimizing discomfort. The investigator must also minimize even short term pain, anxiety, discomfort or embarrassment involved in an investigation, especially if it is not part of routine therapeutic practice. This is an important issue, as some therapists and researchers take a mistakenly 'proprietary' view of their patients, imagining that they should put up with some discomfort for the good of medical science. In the past, patients in public wards of hospitals and long-term prisoners have been most vulnerable to questionable ethical practices.

5. Privacy. Health care research may involve collecting information which can lead to the embarrassment or stigmatisation of the participants. The identity of participants must be protected; for instance by 'coding' their real names.

6. Community values. Some research, such as that involving the assessment of sexual functioning or the investigation of human fetuses, calls for very sensitive planning. Anatomical research involving the use of human cadaver material must be planned to ensure respectful handling and disposal. Even if the investigator does not agree, the values and taboos of groups in the community must be taken into consideration when planning the investigation.

7. Conservation of resources. A fundamental value is that the time and effort of researchers and subjects and the resources of the community should not be wasted on a badly planned investigation. Of course, there is never a guarantee that an investigation will produce clinically useful results. However, some poorly designed projects are doomed to failure even before the data collection begins, and lead to confusion and controversy in the professional literature. Therefore, the correct use of research methods is not only useful for solving problems, but constitutes an ethical necessity. Many ethics committees also vet projects for scientific merit before the project is approved.

A responsible investigator is required to take into consideration ethical principles and to plan research projects accordingly, so that no harm is caused. Therefore, the health researcher must use considerable ingenuity in designing valid investigations, while maintaining ethical values. One of the roles of ethics committees is to guide investigators on complex issues, and to ensure that research is conducted in accordance with accepted community principles.

SELECTION OR RESEARCH STRATEGIES: ECONOMIC CONSIDERATIONS

Selection of appropriate research strategies is also influenced by the resources of investigators. Some projects involving the evaluation of the safety and effectiveness of new drugs, or the identification of risk factors in cardiac disease, have taken tens of millions of dollars to finance. Research planning takes into account economic issues, such as:

Availability of participants. Here the investigator has to consider if enough people can participate in the project under the required conditions. Attention has to be paid to issues such as the frequency of the disorder in the community, problems in identifying participants, and their level of voluntary participation. As it will be shown in Chapter 3, selection of participants is crucial for the validity of a study.

Availability of equipment. Some equipment is costly to acquire or to operate (for example, CT scanners, biochemical assays, experimental drugs). Research planning should take these expenses into account.

Availability of expertise. Specialized assessment techniques and the administration of clinical treatments require professional expertise. If these are beyond the investigator's competence or if the experimental design requires an unbiased, 'blind' therapist or assessor (see Ch.5), there must be means for securing them.

Availability of time. Research projects have a tendency to take considerably longer than an inexperienced researcher might expect, due to the erratic and at times disastrous workings of Murphy's Law: 'If anything can go wrong, it will'. Equipment breaks down and needs to be repaired, subjects 'disappear', collaborators might not deliver services promised. Research planning should take into account possible problems and how these might affect the time scale of investigations. This is a particularly important issue for post-graduate students.

The availability of resources strongly influences the scope of the research program and also the research strategy selected by the investigator. A research project must be shown to be economically feasible before it is initiated. It is only after the ethical constraints and economic resources have been evaluated that the researchers' questions can be transformed into clearly defined hypotheses or aims.

STEPS IN RESEARCH PLANNING

The following steps should be considered in quantitative research before actual data collection begins. The term 'data' refers to the set of observations recorded during an investigation.

1. Identification of the research problem
2. Retrieval and critical evaluation of relevant literature for justifying and giving the context of the research problem
3. Formulation of precise research aims or hypotheses in the light of:
    a. the relevant variables selected for study
    b. the appropriate research strategies
    c. the ethical restraints necessary to protect subjects
    d. the projected cost of the project.
4. In addition, as to be discussed in this book, research planning takes into account:
    a. how the sample is to be selected (Ch. 3)
    b. the design of the investigation (Chs 4–8)
    c. how the data is to be collected (Chs 9–12)
    d. how the data is to be analysed (Chs 13–20)

The above points are written up in the form of a **research protocol**. This is submitted to supervisors, colleagues or ethical committees, for scrutiny of methodological and ethical problems. It is only when the protocol is acceptable that the actual data collection begins. It is often desirable to carry out a small scale preliminary study, called a 'pilot' This is an economical way of identifying and eliminating potential problems in the large scale investigation.

SUMMARY

The planning of a research project requires the transformation of a vague question or problem into clearly stated aims or hypotheses. To achieve this, the researcher should review the relevant literature and evaluate ethical considerations and economic constraints in conducting the investigation. Next, an appropriate research strategy needs to be selected. On the basis of the above, the researcher is in a position to state precisely the aims or hypotheses being investigated.

Before data collection begins, a protocol for the complete investigation is scrutinized by colleagues to correct methodological problems, or to prevent unethical research.

SELF ASSESSMENT

Explain the meaning of the following terms:

ethics
informed consent
literature review
Murphy's law
non-experimental study
pilot study
research strategy
variable

True or false

1. Scientific research always involves the testing of hypotheses.
2. A sample is a sub-set of the data.
3. The population being studied is defined after the sample has been selected.
4. A research protocol is a summary of the data obtained in an investigation.
5. A pilot is a small-scale research program to demonstrate the feasibility of an investigation.
6. Human cadavers are not sentient beings, therefore their treatment falls outside the scope of medical ethics.
7. Planning quantitative research includes specifying the variables to be studied and how these are to be measured.
8. Abstract constructs, like 'intelligence' or 'motivation' cannot have empirical referents.
9. A literature review is necessary for providing the appropriate background and rationale for an investigation.

10. Well-established data collection techniques are called research findings.
11. A non-experimental design involves the assignment of subjects to treatment groups.
12. Both experimental and non-experimental designs involve the drawing of an appropriate sample from the population being studied.
13. An anthropologist studying how ethnic groups relate to illness would tend to adopt a quantitative research strategy.
14. The clear explanation of the risks involved in a research project is a necessary condition for obtaining informed consent from a subject.
15. The use of correct research methods does not constitute an ethical necessity.
16. A hypothesis is a proposition about the relationship existing between variables or prediction of differences between groups.
17. Some scientific research projects do not involve the testing of hypotheses.
18. Existing theories are the only appropriate sources for experimental hypotheses.
19. In a non-experimental study there is no need to pay attention to sampling.
20. Experimental designs involve the assignment of the sampled subjects into treatment groups.
21. Experimental designs are more appropriate than non-experimental designs for demonstrating causal relationships.
22. The subjects participating in medical research are generally the most likely beneficiaries of the project.
23. Informed consent of human subjects is necessary even when the investigation is not apparently embarrassing or dangerous.
24. It is unethical to study human sexual behaviour because people find it embarrassing to serve as subjects.
25. Medical researchers should expect that patients who receive free hospital treatment should participate in medical experiments.
26. The correct use of research methods in conducting an investigation is useful, but not an ethical necessity.
27. A well designed, relevant research project will be always financed, regardless of the expense.
28. A variable is a property or attribute which varies from subject to subject.

Multiple choice

1. The aim of research planning is to:
   a   generate appropriate aims or clear-cut research hypotheses
   b   select an appropriate research strategy
   c   identify possible ethical or economic limitations in conducting the investigation
   d   a and b
   e   all of the above.

2. A 'literature review':
   a is a list of research publications relevant to an investigation
   b should discredit research findings which are inconsistent with the hypothesis
   c should include only findings which directly support the hypothesis being investigated
   d should be a critical review of findings relevant to an investigation.

3. Which of the following is common to both experimental and non-experimental research strategies?
   a assignment
   b selection of cases to be studied
   c experimental hypothesis
   d participant observation
   e field research.

4. Which of the following is unique to the experimental research strategy?
   a assignment
   b selection of cases to be studied
   c definition of population
   d participant observation
   e field research.

5. The availability of resources to conduct an investigation:
   a is not the concern of a scientific researcher
   b has an influence on the scope and design of the investigation
   c is determined by Murphy's Law
   d none of the above.

6. 32 degrees Centigrade is an example of:
   a a variable
   b the value of a variable
   c a ratio
   d a null hypothesis.

7. A variable is:
   a a property which can take different values across different individuals
   b a property which can take different values within an individual
   c both a and b
   d neither *a* nor *b*.

8. Which of the following represents the most explicitly formulated research aim?
   a The aim of the present project was to investigate if health care workers were satisfied with their current rates of pay
   b The aim of the present project was to identify the number of persons living in the Newcastle metropolitan area
   c The aim of the present project is to examine pay rates.

9. Which of the following represents the most explicitly formulated research aim?
   a   The aim of the present project was to investigate if health care workers in Gotham City were satisfied with their pay and career prospects
   b   The aim of the present project was to investigate if emotionally disturbed persons living in Gotham city received adequate medical care
   c   The aim of the present project was to identify the reasons why health professionals in Gotham city leave their professions, and turn to other types of employment
   d   The aim of the present project was to identify the proportion of teenagers in Gotham city smoking more than 10 cigarettes a day.

10. A research protocol should make explicit:
   a   the justification for undertaking the research project
   b   the way in which the data is to be collected
   c   the empirical evidence provided by the investigation
   d   a and b.

11. Which of the following represents a non-researchable problem (in the context of the scientific method)?
   a   Is aspirin preferable to steroids in reducing the symptoms of arthritis?
   b   Does the use of alcohol result in greater levels of brain damage than the use of marijuana?
   c. Are painful experiments involving animals justified if they lead to benefits to patients?
   d   Do people coming from a low socioeconomic class receive poorer health care than people from a higher class?

3

Sampling methods and external validity

INTRODUCTION

Research in the health sciences usually involves the collection of data on a sample of cases, rather than on the entire population of cases in which the investigator is interested. A sample is studied because it is usually impossible or extremely costly to study complete populations. For instance, when individuals suffering from conditions such as diabetes, cerebral palsy or emphysema are being investigated, it is not possible to study everyone because of the large size of such populations, and because many people do not seek treatment or may be wrongly diagnosed. Therefore, in both experimental and non-experimental investigations, the researcher routinely studies a subset or sample of the population, and then attempts to generalize the findings to the population from which the participants were drawn.

The aim of this chapter is to examine ways samples should be drawn so as to ensure that they permit the investigator to make valid generalizations from the sample to the population.

We will also consider the question of generalizing the findings of an investigation to other samples and situations. This is referred to as 'external validity', a concept related to induction, as discussed in Chapter 1.

The specific aims of this chapter are to:

1. Define what is meant by sampling and representative samples
2. Outline the relative advantages and disadvantages of commonly used sampling methods
3. Discuss the relationship between sampling error and sample size
4. Examine the concept of external validity for generalizing research findings to other settings.

WHAT IS SAMPLED IN A STUDY

This chapter will focus on the selection of the research participants or subjects in a study. However, in most studies, many other things are also selected or sampled. These include:

1. the information to be collected
2. the procedures for the collection of the information
3. where the research is conducted
4. the clinicians and researchers who are involved.

Many researchers focus on the selection of the research participants and do not pay enough attention to the other factors they are sampling. It is not at all unusual to see studies that employ large and sophisticated participant samples with only one or two clinicians involved in the research in one health setting. Although it does not have to be the case, many quantitative studies are very weak in their consideration (and sampling) of research context but strong in participant sampling. Many qualitative studies, again unnecessarily, have strong consideration of context but are weak in their sampling of research participants.

BASIC ISSUES IN SAMPLING

Often, because of the number of cases involved, it is not within the resources of the researcher to study the whole population. In any event, in most situations it would be wasteful to study all the population. If a sample is representative, one can generalize validly from the sample's results to the population.

The population is the group of individuals in which the researcher is interested. For example, all English women under 25; all children with diagnosed spina bifida in the state of Alberta; all the students at a particular Australian college. The researcher defines the population to which he/she wishes to generalize. Note that a population need not consist of human or animal subjects. Objects or events can he also sampled, as shown in Table 3.1.

As shown in Table 3.1, a **population** is an entire set of persons, objects or events which the researcher intends to study. A **sample** is a subset of the population. **Sampling** involves the selection of the sample from the population.

Table 3.1 Examples of populations and samples

Population	Possible sample selection
All working podiatrists in a state	50 podiatrists selected for a study of job satisfaction
All working pathologists in a state	25 pathologists selected for detailed tax evaluation by an inspector
The temperature of a patient during a 24 hour period	Hourly measurements of patient's temperature recorded by staff
Stuttering in a child's speech	Number of stutters made during 5 minutes of reading a standard piece of material
All patients in a state with frontal lobe damage	30 patients with frontal lobe damage selected for evaluating a rehabilitation program
All surgical gauzes held by a given hospital	10 gauzes selected by a bacteriologist to test for sterility

REPRESENTATIVE SAMPLES

There is a variety of different ways by which one can select the sample from the population. These are called sampling methods.

The aim of all sampling methods is to draw a representative sample from the population. The advantage of a representative sample is clear: one can confidently generalize from a representative sample to the rest of the population without having to take the trouble of measuring the rest of the population. If the sample is biased (not representative) one can generalize less validly from the sample to the population. In addition, this might lead to quite incorrect conclusions or inferences about the population. This would mean that the results obtained in the study would not necessarily generalize to other experiments or studies using the same population. Figure 3.1 illustrates the concept of a representative sample.

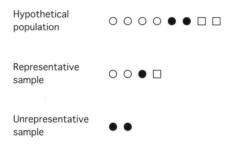

Fig. 3.1 A simple representative sample

Figure 3.1 illustrates a hypothetical population composed of three different types of elements. A representative sample is a precise miniaturized representation of the proportion of elements of the population. An unrepresentative or biased sample does not represent the elements in correct proportions, leading to mistaken conclusions about the state of the population.

The selection of the appropriate sampling method depends upon the aims and resources of the researchers. For instance, if someone is designing a very expensive social welfare program on the basis of a survey of clients' needs, it is imperative that the researcher uses a good sampling method and obtains a representative sample, so that appropriate inferences may be made about the population. Good sampling methods are more expensive and more difficult to implement than poor methods. The main sampling methods used in scientific and clinical research are incidental and random sampling.

INCIDENTAL SAMPLES

1. Incidental sampling is the cheapest and easiest sampling method to use. It involves the selection of the most easily accessible members of the target population. For example, a political scientist who stands in the middle of a city street and quizzes people about their voting intentions is practising incidental sampling. However, it is likely that this sample would not be representative of the general voting population. There would probably be an over-representation of businessmen and white-collar workers, and an under-representation of factory workers and housewives. Thus the political scientist's predictions of any election results might not represent the actual results because of these sampling anomalies. The sample is likely to be unrepresentative and biased.

A further example of incidental sampling might involve a researcher surveying the needs of a group of spina bifida children at a local community health centre. Their measured needs may be representative of those of other spina bifida children but then again they may not.

Thus, incidental sampling is cheap and easy to implement but may give a biased sample that is not representative of the population.

2. Quota sampling. Sometimes it is known in advance that there are important subgroups within the population that need to be included in the sample because they may affect the study's results. Two important groups within the human population are males and females. Further, it is known that they occur in the ratio of approximately 49: 51 in the general population. Our intrepid researcher might decide that it is very important that the sexes are proportionally represented in the sample. Thus, the researcher would set two quotas (of 49 male and 51 female respondents in a sample of 100 and sample accordingly in a city street. This is still a form of incidental sampling but has some advantages over simple incidental sampling. Even more complicated examples involving more than 2 groups can be accommodated as shown in Table 3.2.

Table 3.2 Distribution of percentages of gender and occupational variables in the general population

	Blue collar	**White collar**	**Not employed 'no collar'**	**Total**
Male	19	21	9	49
Female	15	15	21	51
Total	34	36	30	100

We can see from Table 3.2 that if we were to be representative regarding both sex and occupational status, in a sample of 100 people we would need 19 blue collar males, 15 blue collar females, and so on.

Quota sampling still has a number of shortcomings: before it can be used, one has to know which population groups are likely to be important to a particular question and the exact proportions of the various groups in the population. Also, the members of the sample are still incidentally chosen. The blue collar males, for example, selected in a city centre on a weekday may still be quite different from those working elsewhere.

RANDOM AND SYSTEMATIC SAMPLES

1. Random sampling. This is one of the best but most difficult sampling methods to implement. A random sample is one in which all members of the population have an equal chance of selection. Thus a random sample is more likely to be representative of the relevant population than an incidental sample.

The procedure for drawing a random sample involves:

(a) The construction of a list of all members of the population
(b) Using a method such as dice, coins or random number tables to select randomly from the list the number of members required for the sample.

A simple example of a random sample is provided by a common raffle, where names on equal size papers are put in a hat, shaken and selected 'blind'. Many lotteries use numbered balls that are drawn randomly from a barrel. Another way to draw a random sample is to construct a list of all the members of the population and assign a number to each element. Then a table of random numbers, generated by a computer, could be used to select a random sample. Nowadays, computers can do this efficiently, even when large populations are involved.

The cases selected from the list constitute a random sample. Sometimes, because of refusal to participate in the study, mortality, etc. it is necessary to select replacements for some cases. This can introduce bias into the sample, as the refusers may differ consistently from those who accept. An example of this would be seen in a survey of sexual behaviours: persons who would refuse to participate might have different sexual behaviours from those who consent to participate.

However, random sampling methods have a number of important advantages over incidental or non-random methods:

• Because the exact sizes of the sample and population are known, it is possible to estimate exactly how representative the sample is, that is, the size of the sampling error. This cannot usually be done with non-random sampling methods.
• Because random samples are usually more representative than non-random samples, the sample size needed for good representation of the population is smaller.

The major disadvantages of random sampling methods are:

• The researcher needs to be able to list every member of the population. Often this is impossible because the full extent of the population is not known. For example, it would be very difficult to sample randomly from the population of Australians with coronary disease, because no such list exists.
• Cost. It is much easier to use conveniently available groups. Random sampling usually involves considerable planning and expense, especially with large populations.

2. Stratified random sampling. This is the same as quota sampling, expect that each quota is filled by randomly sampling from each subgroup, rather than sampling incidentally. For example, if one was drawing a sample stratified with respect to sex, one would have to prepare a list of all females and all males in ~~the population and then sample randomly from those lists with the numbers of~~ each group in the sample corresponding to the population proportions.

The advantages of stratified random sampling are:

- All the important groups are proportionally represented. This is particularly important when key sub-groups in the population occur in low proportions.
- The exact representativeness of the sample is known. This has important statistical ramifications.

The disadvantages are:
- A list of all members of the population, their characteristics and the proportions of the important groups within the population need to be known.
- Cost.
- The gain in accuracy is usually very small in comparison to simple random sampling.

3. Area sampling. In area sampling, one samples on the basis of location of cases. For example, on the basis of census data, the investigator may select several areas in a city or county with known characteristics, such as high or low unemployment rates. The areas could then be further divided into specific streets and the occupants of, say, every third house contacted for participation in the study. In other words, the locations are randomly selected and then one interviews the occupants of those locations. This can be a very effective, cheap method of sampling in social surveys. It does not require a list of the individual members of the population, merely the location where they live.

4. Systematic sampling. This involves working through a list of the population and choosing, say, every tenth or twentieth case for inclusion in the sample. It is not a truly random technique but will usually give a representative sample. It is based on the (usually justified) supposition that cases are not added to the list in a systematic way which coincides with the sampling system. Provided a list of cases is available, systematic sampling is an easy and convenient sampling method. In clinical practice we are using systematic sampling when, for instance, we measure temperature and blood pressure every hour.

SAMPLE SIZE

One of the most poorly understood aspects of sampling is the optimal number of cases that should be included in a sample.

It is obvious that in one sense the more cases selected the merrier, but the costs associated with the data collection must be weighed up against the greater accuracy of making inferences with larger samples. Also, some health related studies involve discomfort, pain, or even danger to patients or laboratory animals. Therefore it is ethically necessary (see Ch. 2) to ensure that no more than the bare minimum of subjects is used. The fact is that clinical researchers 'walk a tightrope' in deciding the optimum sample sizes for these kinds of studies. However, there are some principles available to guide the researcher.

First of all, let us say quite definitely that there is no magic number that we can point to as an optimum sample size. We cannot say what percentage of the population should be sampled. Rather, the optimum number in the sample depends on the characteristics of an investigation, in the context of which the sample is drawn. In general, the optimum sample size is one which is adequate for making correct inferences from a sample to a population. Let us try to illuminate this in relation to the concept of sampling error.

Sampling error

Sampling error is reflected in the discrepancy between the true population parameter and the sample statistic. For example, if I happen to know from census data that the average age of males in a district is 35 years and the average age of a sample of males I have surveyed from the district is 30 years, then I have a sampling error of 5 years. However, if we do not know the actual population parameters, we can only estimate the probable sampling error.

Sampling error is related to sample size by the following relationship:

$$\text{Sampling error} \quad \propto \quad \frac{1}{\sqrt{n}}$$

What the above equation claims is that the greater the sample size (n), the smaller the probability sampling error. In fact, the sampling error is inversely proportional to the square root of the sample size. For the calculation of probable sampling error see Chapter 17.

From this relationship it can be seen that doubling the sample size would only result in a reduction of the error by a factor of the square root of 2 (1.414). Similarly, a ninefold increase in sample size would result in only a threefold reduction in the sampling error. Figure 3.2 illustrates this point by showing the graphical relationship between probable sampling error and sample size.

It can be seen from this graph that not much is gained from a sample size of over, say, n_1. Yet the cost of the sampling and data collection can be very high with large numbers, (such as n_2) for relatively little gain in reducing sampling error. In some research situations, even large probable sampling errors have relatively little potential influence on our decisions. In such situations, we can live with a relatively small sample size. In other situations, we need large samples to justify our confidence in the truth of our decisions.

As an illustration, suppose that we are attempting to predict the outcome of an election fought between two political parties: A and B. A representative sample of 100 respondents is polled before the election. Say the outcome is as follows:

Intends to vote for A	Intends to vote for B	Estimate sampling error
25%	75%	10%

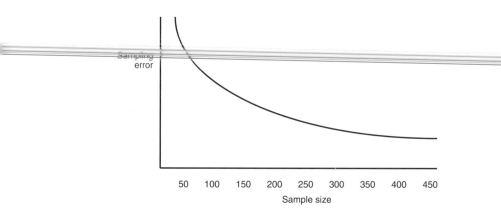

Fig. 3.2 The relationship between sample size and sampling error. The scaling but not the form of the curve will alter with the variability of the data

In this instance, the estimated sampling error is very small in relation to the size of the *effect* (that is, the difference between the % of intended votes for the two parties). We can predict confidently, assuming that the respondents were truthful and don't change their minds before the elections, that political party B will romp into government. Increasing sample size, say to 10 000 would enormously increase the cost of the survey. The corresponding reduction in sampling error would not justify this cost, as we would still come to the same conclusion. However, say the following sample statistics were obtained in the pre-election poll of n = 100 respondents:

Intends to vote for A	Intends to vote for B	Estimate sampling error
48%	52%	10%

Now, the same level of estimated sampling error is too large, in relation to the apparent size of the effect, to make a decision concerning which party is likely to win the election. The poll would have to be repeated using a substantially increased sample size to reduce the sampling error.

The example illustrates the notion that the adequacy of the sample size is affected by the specific investigation in which we are making inferences. A sample size which is adequate in one situation might be inadequate in another. One benefit of a pilot study is that it allows the investigator to estimate the size of the effect, and thereby make an educated guess of the sample size required to demonstrate it. In addition, a pilot study indicates the adequacy of the sampling model being employed by the investigator.

EXTERNAL VALIDITY AND SAMPLING

The term **external validity** refers to the extent to which the results of an investigation can be generalized to other samples or situations. External validity can be classified into two types: **population** and **ecological** (Huck et al, 1974).

Population validity refers to generalizing the findings from the sample to the population from which it was drawn. We have already examined the importance of having a representative sample in the generalizing of results from a sample to a population. However, an investigator in the health sciences might face another problem: that the accessible population from which the sample was taken might not be the same as the target population, that is, the one of general interest. Let us illustrate this point with an example:

A physiotherapist working in a large private maternity hospital intends to examine the effectiveness of a new antenatal exercise procedure for pregnant women for controlling levels of pain during delivery. A random sample of 50 pregnant women is chosen for the investigation from the population attending the hospital. The sample is then randomly assigned into two groups: one receiving the new antenatal exercise procedure, the other receiving the traditional program. The researcher finds a statistically and clinically significant difference between the two procedures, such that the new program is shown to be effective.

Strictly speaking, these findings can be generalized only to the population of women who attend the hospital. However, if the target population is *all* women having babies, then the generalization lacks external validity, because women attending different hospitals or having children at home had no chance of being included in the sample. They might have different characteristics in relation to the variable measured and these different characteristics may interact with the treatment in different ways to that of the sample. For instance, women who chose to deliver at home might respond better to the traditional intervention.

Ecological validity. There is also another limitation to external validity: the situation in which an investigation is carried out might not be generalizable to other situations. This is called ecological validity. Consider the following examples:

1. It has been shown that for clinical pain (due to disease or injury), morphine is an excellent analgesic. However, in laboratory studies of pain induced by electric shocks, morphine had little effect on subjects' reports of pain threshold. Clearly, generalizing from laboratory to clinical settings, or vice versa has to be done with extreme caution (Beecher 1959).
2. Coronary arteriography involves the insertion of a small-gauge catheter into the coronary arteries, and injecting a dye for X-ray visualization. It was initially reported that the mortality rates for this rather dangerous-sounding practice were only 0.1% (1 per 1000) in a first-class medical institution. However, later reports from various other institutions showed mortality rates as high as 8% (80 per 1000) (Taylor 1979). Clearly, the effectiveness of treatments or the usefulness of clinical evaluations can well depend on in whose hands they are carried out.

The above examples illustrate the caution necessary in generalizing findings.

SUMMARY

Appropriate sampling strategies ensure the external validity of both experimental and non-experimental investigations. The aim of sampling strategies is to ensure the selection of a sample which is *representative* of the population of objects, persons or events the investigator aims to study. Incidental and quota samples are chosen for convenience, but these sampling strategies do not guarantee a representative sample. Random and stratified random sampling methods ensure that all elements of the population have a chance to be selected. Random sampling strategies are the most desirable to obtain a representative sample, although unfortunately random sampling is not always possible in health sciences research. Area sampling and systematic sampling are also strategies which can be used to obtain representative samples.

An adequate sample size reduces the probability of random sampling error. More precisely, the probable sampling error is inversely proportional to the square root of the sample size. It was argued that optimum sample size is not the maximum number of obtainable subjects or a constant number or proportion. Rather, it has to be estimated for a specific investigation on the basis of the parameters of the phenomenon being studied. Two types of external validity were discussed: population and ecological. External validity is related to inference, which involves using evidence from a limited set of elements to formulate general propositions.

SELF ASSESSMENT

Explain the meanings of the following terms:

area sample	population validity
biased sample	random sample
ecological validity	random sampling
external validity	representative sample
incidental sample	sample
population	sampling error (probable)

True or false

1. The basic idea underlying sampling is to select a representative sample from which the investigator can make inferences to the population.
2. A sample is said to be random when it is not representative of the population.
3. If a population contains 50% males and 50% females, and our sample has 10% males and 90% females, then our sample is said to be biased.
4. When you take a patient's blood pressure daily, you are in fact sampling from a population of potential blood pressure readings.
5. If the patient's blood pressure fluctuates considerably during the day, then a single reading will be an inadequate sample.
6. Stratified random sampling involves the selection of the most accessible elements of the population.
7. Say that important sub-groups of the population are known and subjects are sampled incidentally in proportion to these sub-groups. This sampling method is known as area sampling.
8. A random sample is one in which 50% of the elements of a population have equal chances of being sampled.

9. Random sampling in health sciences is the least expensive and time consuming strategy for selecting a sample.
10. When you take blood pressures hourly, you are in fact using a random sampling method.
11. The larger the sample size, the larger the sampling error.
12. The problem of internal validity might emerge when we generalize results obtained in one research setting to another.
13. An incidental sample can not be, in principle, representative of the population .
14. If a sample is representative, it yields valid data for making generalizations about the population from which it was drawn.
15. The main difference between random and quota sampling is that in quota sampling particular sub-groups of the population are represented proportionately .
16. Incidental sampling generates less bias than systematic sampling.
17. Area sampling involves selecting an area at random and assessing the inhabitants of that area.
18. A sample that is unbiased is a representative sample of the population from which it is drawn.
19. Sample error decreases as the sample size increases.
20. If the sample size is halved, the sampling error will be doubled.
21. If a sample is large (say $n > 500$) then the sample must be representative.
22. Generalizing findings from laboratory to clinical settings raises questions of ecological validity.
23. The problem of population validity refers to a population which contains invalid elements.

Multiple choice

1. As sample size increases
   a the sampling error decreases
   b the ecological validity of the investigation increases
   c the population becomes more accessible
   d the sample becomes more biased.

2. A representative sample
   a consists of at least 500 cases
   b must be a random sample
   c is defined as the inverse of the square root of the sample size
   d reflects precisely the crucial dimensions of a population.

3. An incidental sample is
   a not necessarily biased
   b generally obtained through costly and difficult sampling procedures
   c used only in non-experimental investigations
   d none of the above.

An investigator wishes to study individuals suffering from agoraphobia (fear of open spaces). The investigator places an advertisement in the paper asking for subjects. 100 replies are received, of which the investigator randomly selects 30. However, only 15 subjects actually turn up for their appointment. Questions 4-6 refer to the above information.

4. Which of the following statements is true?
   a The final 15 subjects are likely to be a representative sample of the subjects selected by the investigator
   b The final 15 subjects are likely to be a representative sample of the population of agoraphobics
   c The randomly selected 30 subjects are likely to be a representative sample of those agoraphobics who replied to the newspaper advertisement
   d None of the above is true.

5. The problem with drawing a representative sample of subjects with clinical conditions such as agoraphobia is that
   a The subjects who consent to participate may be unrepresentative of the target population
   b no sampling strategies are appropriate
   c no complete lists of sufferers' names are usually available
   d a and c.

6. The basic problem confronted by the investigator is that
   a the accessible population might be different from the target population
   b the sample has been chosen using an unethical method
   c the sample size was too small
   d agoraphobics are impossible to study in a scientific way.

7. Say that it is known that coronary disease occurs twice as frequently among males as females and three times more commonly among over 50-year-olds than those under 50. Given a sample of 120 obtained by quota sampling, how many subjects would you expect to be female and under 50?
   a 60
   b 40
   c 30
   d 10

8. Referring to the population in Question 7, and given a sample obtained by stratified random sampling, how many females over 50 would you expect in the sample?
   a 40
   b 30
   c 10
   d 5

9. If a study is externally valid then
   a its results can be generalized to other equivalent settings
   b it must have been an experiment
   c quota sampling must have been used
   d all the subjects in the sample must have been equivalent.

10. A random sample is one in which
   a all the elements had an equal chance of selection
   b a chance method was used to select the elements included in the sample
   c both *a* and *b*
   d neither *a* nor *b*.

11. When we say that a study lacks ecological validity we are implying that
   a the study was carried out in a laboratory
   b the results cannot be generalized to other settings
   c the target population is different to the accessible population
   d all of the above.

12. Pilot studies are useful for establishing
   a the approximate sample size necessary for the investigation
   b the appropriateness of the sampling model being employed
   c both *a* and *b*
   d neither *a* nor *b*.

13. If a pilot study indicates that the effect is likely to be small in relation to the sampling error then the investigator should
   a abandon the research project
   b use a relatively small sample
   c use a relatively large sample
   d use an incidental method of sampling.

4

Causal research
and internal validity

INTRODUCTION

Some types of research are purely descriptive: the aim of the investigator is to
gather descriptions and measurements about phenomena. For example, we may
gather statistics on the incidence of schizophrenia or neonate deaths. However,
in the health sciences much research is aimed at identifying the causes of illness
and disabilities. It is by understanding these causes that we can formulate and
justify our assessments and treatments. Furthermore, we can justify the treatments
we use in that we can point to empirical evidence that demonstrates that the
treatments are causing the beneficial changes in patients' symptoms. In scientific
research, the concept of internal validity is related to the design of research
projects.

The specific aims of this chapter are to:

1. Examine the concept of causality
2. Examine how threats to internal validity generate plausible alternative
   explanations
3. Discuss how control arising from correct designs increases internal
   validity
4. Discuss some limitations of control in clinical research.

CAUSALITY

In scientific research, we look for the following important criteria for the
demonstration of causality:

1. Antecedent occurrence of cause to effect (C occurs before E)
2. Covariation of cause and effect (if C occurs then so does E)
3. Elimination of rival causal explanations of the effect (If C does not occur,
   then E does not occur).

The first criterion is quite obvious. For instance, if we say that injury to the
person's arm is the cause of their reported pain, we assume that the injury was

sustained prior to the onset of the pain. Clearly, if the pain had been already present, the injury would not be seen as the cause of the pain. Secondly, we assume that there will be concomitant variation between the injury and the pain. The worse the injury, the more severe the pain. As the injury clears up, a decrease in the level of pain can be expected. In general, we are establishing a lawful functional relationship between the cause and the effect.

However, observing a relationship between two events is not enough to demonstrate causality. Night follows day in a predictable, lawful fashion. But we don't say that day causes the night. In scientific research, we look for *control* over phenomena, so that we can reproduce or change them at will. Of course, such control is not always possible; for instance, in the fields of astronomy, geology and cultural anthropology. One cannot invoke an earthquake or a supernova at will, or return to times past. All we can do is to describe, point out patterns or covariations, and then formulate hypotheses and theories which offer a causal explanation for the findings. In particular, we must attempt to eliminate plausible alternative explanations or hypotheses which offer rival causal explanations for the findings. What constitutes plausible alternative explanations changes from situation to situation. However, we will examine some in the next sub-section, in the context of threats to internal validity.

THREATS TO INTERNAL VALIDITY

Cook and Campbell (1979) defined a number of threats to the internal validity of experiments and quasi-experiments. These threats to internal validity compromise the ability of the researcher to conclude that the different treatments administered to groups of subjects are in fact responsible for the differences or lack of differences observed. Threats to internal validity are in fact sources of alternative explanations for the outcome of an investigation.

These threats to internal validity include:

1. History. This refers to events that intervene between the pre-test and post-test (see Ch. 5) that do not form part of the treatment being investigated by the researcher. For example, in a study of the effects of an exercise program on hypertension, some of the patients might take up additional exercise, such as playing tennis.

2. Maturation. In a study over time, the patients may naturally mature. This is a particular problem with paediatric and geriatric populations and studies that are conducted over an extended time period (so called longitudinal studies). In a more general sense, maturation refers to any time-dependent internal changes in patients; for instance, an infection clearing up by 'itself', naturally.

3. Testing. The patient may, as a result of familiarity with the testing procedures, appear to improve spontaneously. These are sometimes called practice effects. For instance, the re-administration of an IQ test might lead to better performance without an actual improvement in the subjects' intellects. Alternatively, a test may so boring that upon second administration, the patients apparent performance may decline due to boredom and fatigue.

4. Instrumentation. During the time between measurements, the measuring instrument might change, for example, start reading heavier or lighter, leading to apparent improvement or deterioration when no such change has occurred.

5. Regression to the mean. This is a special effect that originates from the unreliability of test measures. Often, clinical research involves the selection for study of patients who have achieved particularly low or high scores on one or more measures, for example the most depressed patients or those with the highest measured cholesterol levels. It is often found that such patient groups when retested will show apparent spontaneous improvement or regression towards the mean. This happens because, on the second measurement, the measurement error tends to be less than on the first measurement. If patients are chosen on the basis of very good or very poor performance on an initial assessment, they are likely to include a number of cases in which measurement error is quite high, and proportionately few with small measurement error. In such cases the regression to the mean phenomenon is a possibility, as on the second measurement there is likely to be less extreme measurement error, on average.

6. Selection or assignment errors. The groups being compared may, due to inadequate assignment or selection procedures, be different at the outset, rather than as a result of any treatment effects. This might well happen if the subjects were not randomly assigned into treatment groups. If the groups differ before treatment, it is very difficult to attribute differences after treatment to the treatments alone.

7. Mortality. You don't have to have anyone die in a study to have mortality. Mortality in a study refers to when a participant withdraws from the study before its completion. There may be more dropouts in one group than in others, leaving the groups to be different. For instance, subjects in a placebo group might reject an ineffectual treatment and refuse to participate to the conclusion of the study. As the subjects who drop out might be different to those who stay, the experimental and the control group no longer remain equivalent. Once again, if the groups are different, it is difficult to ascribe these differences to their different treatments.

The following investigation illustrates the effects of some of the above threats to validity:

A recent study attempted to demonstrate the effects of an exercise program in patients with occlusions (blockage) of some of the major arteries in the leg. The **dependent variables** measured included the distance walked by the patient to 'limit of pain tolerance'. The **independent variable** was the exercise program, which included daily walking, with encouragement to increase the distance daily. Patients were also strongly advised to stop smoking and were given a diet low in animal fats and carbohydrates.

More than half the patients were smokers and reported that their smoking declined markedly by the end of the program. The method of the experiment involved pre-tests on the dependent variables (including walking), the administration of the treatment, and then a re-test six weeks after the program commenced. The results were not evaluated statistically, but the results (Fig. 4.1) appeared to indicate an increase in the walking distance. The study was done under the guidance of a vascular surgeon, who also selected the patients.

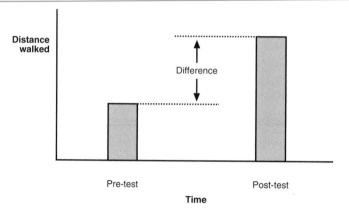

Fig. 4.1 Walking tolerance: before and after exercise program

Figure 4.1 shows that there was an increase in the patients' average walking distance. The question here is: 'Was this change in the dependent variable caused by the independent variable or by other uncontrolled extraneous variables?' To answer this question, let us examine some of the possible threats to the internal validity of the study.

1. History. The threat here is due to simultaneous changes in walking, smoking pattern, and diet; any of which might have been responsible for some or all of the changes in the dependent variable reported in the study.

2. Maturation. The degree of this threat depends on the natural history of the illness. Natural improvement in the condition might account for at least some of the difference in walking.

3. Testing. Both the pre-test and the exercise program included walking. It might be that the difference between pre-test and post-test is simply due to practice effects; the patients becoming more confident in walking to real tolerance limits.

4. Instrumentation. This threat is not relevant in this instance, in that no sophisticated or potentially inaccurate measuring devices were used to measure the dependent variable.

5. Regression to the mean. Possibly, the vascular surgeon selected extreme cases for the study: those most in need of treatment. Their performances might have drifted back towards the mean on the post-test.

6-7. Selection errors and mortality. These threats are not relevant, as no control group was included in the study.

We have not shown that the extraneous variables described above necessarily caused the reported difference. Rather, the point is that, because of the lack of control, the investigator cannot claim that the differences found in the dependent variable *necessarily* reflect changes due to the independent variable; that the change observed in the outcome measure was *caused* by the treatment.

THE NEED FOR CONTROL

We have seen how uncontrolled extraneous variables can result in plausible alternative explanations for the outcomes of an investigation. In causal research, the adoption of an appropriate design enables us to remove the confounding influences of extraneous variables. If we can do this—correctly attribute any effects we observe and eliminate the effects of other factors—we can say that the experiment is internally valid or has *internal validity*.

In the context of laboratory research, an investigator can use several types of strategies to achieve control over extraneous variables. For instance, a physicist studying electrical phenomena will make sure that the apparatus is insulated against extraneous electrical disturbances. Also, a researcher studying bio-feedback would make sure that the subjects were in a noise insulated, temperature controlled room. In 'field' research, in applied clinical settings, such tight control is not feasible. Other methods, such as the inclusion of control groups in the design are utilized to ensure internal validity.

A **control group** consists of subjects who undergo exactly the same conditions as the group receiving the treatment, the causal effect of which is being investigated. For instance, in drug trials control groups will often receive an injection of saline solution if the experimental treatment is administered via injection, in order to control for the effects of actual injection. If the medication were administered orally, similar-looking inert tablets would be used for control subjects. It has been found that if people receive any form of 'therapy', improvement may occur even when the 'treatment' is physiologically and biochemically inert. The effect is called a **placebo effect.** The control group allows the experimenter to measure the size of this and other effects, and to control for these effects.

If we are to include a control group in our experiments, it is essential that at the outset the experimental and control groups are as similar as possible. We have to take the group of subjects participating in the study and split them up into the experimental and control groups as equally as possible.

The methods we use to decide to which groups the subjects are to be assigned are termed **assignment procedures**. As we have seen in Chapter 2, the assignment of subjects to their groups by the investigator is an essential feature of an experiment. The two main assignment methods used will be discussed in more detail in Chapter 5.

In later chapters, we will see that control is possible for non-experimental designs as well as experimental designs. Control is a matter of degree, rather than an absolute. Even some tightly designed investigations allow for plausible alternative explanations arising from unexpected extraneous variables. Furthermore, a trade-off exists between internal and external validity. In order to maximize internal validity of an experiment, the researcher ought to eliminate as many external influences as possible. In a hypothetical study of resident psychiatric patients, this could include suspension of visits, removal of furniture, cessation of all other medication, elimination of contact with other patients and so on. How representative would this be of everyday life? Could these results be usefully generalized to any other context? Therefore, to ensure the ecological validity of the investigation, we may sacrifice control and, to some extent, internal validity. The inclusion and appropriate use of control groups improves the internal validity of an investigation.

THE USE OF CONTROL GROUPS IN CLINICAL RESEARCH

Let us re-examine the investigation outlined on page 57 and see how it stands up to threats of internal validity, with the use of a control group included in the study.

1. Select the sample of subjects with arterial occlusions to participate in the study. To ensure external validity we would need a better sampling strategy than some surgeon's say-so. However, for ethical reasons the subjects might need to be checked out, to minimize possible adverse side effects of the treatment.
2. Assess the walking distances of the patients in a pre-treatment test.
3. Assign subjects into experimental or control groups by matching on basis of pre-test performance, and random assignment within pairs. We will examine such research designs in Chapter 5.
4. Administer: (a) experimental treatment (total package of exercise plan, walking, diet and smoking reduction) and (b) control treatment (an alternative activity, walking, diet and smoking reduction). The *only* difference between the two groups is that one group receives the exercise program, and the other some alternative activity.
5. Test both groups on walking distance, following the treatment.

The results of this fictional study are presented in Figure 4.2.

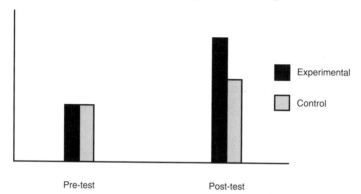

Fig. 4.2 Hypothetical results of a pre-test post-test study

Let us examine how this new design stands up to threats of internal validity in contrast to the original investigation outlined on page 57.

1. History. Both groups had walking, smoking decrement and diet; it is unlikely that the difference between post-test results shown in Figure 4.2 is due to these variables.

2. Maturation. Both control and experimental groups had the same time to recover or deteriorate; it is unlikely that this factor explains the difference .

3. Testing. Both groups had the pre-test and the walking; unlikely that this factor explains difference.

4. Instrumentation. Not relevant, as discussed on page 58.

5. Regression to mean. Both groups were similar on pre-test performance, given that they were matched.

6. Selection error. Random or matched assignment would have controlled for this, so initial differences between the two groups is minimized.

7. Mortality. This depends on the actual data; internal validity is preserved if drop-out rates are equivalent in the two groups.

We can see that using a design with a control group resulted in an improvement of the internal validity of the investigation. Note that the use of a control group has not removed the effects of history and other extraneous variables in this study. It is still possible, but much less likely, that the differences in the outcomes for the two groups were *not* a result of the different treatments they received. Now the investigator has a much sounder basis for deciding whether or not the exercise program was effective.

It should be noted that there are ways, other than control groups, to minimize the effects of uncontrolled extraneous variables. For instance, if 'noise' is a possible extraneous variable in administering a test, we may 'insulate' from it by using a quiet setting. However, if noisy settings are the norm in real life, then the search for higher internal validity may be at the cost of external validity.

SUMMARY

The demonstration of causality involves the discounting of plausible alternative explanations for the outcome of an investigation. When uncontrolled extraneous variables generate alternative explanations to the research hypothesis then the investigation lacks internal validity. The aim of designing an investigation is to reduce the threats to internal validity. It was shown that when the design includes an appropriate control group, the causal effects of the treatment on the outcome becomes more convincing.

However, in field research involving human subjects, complete control over the phenomena is not possible. To some extent, control might have to be sacrificed in order to ensure the external validity of the results. In the next chapter, we examine a variety of research strategies and the designs used within these strategies aimed at maximizing internal and external validity.

SELF ASSESSMENT

Explain the meaning of the following terms:

assignment errors	instrumentation
causality	internal validity
causal explanations	maturation
control	mortality
history	regression to the mean
	testing

True or false

1. It is possible to have an effect occur prior to its cause.
2. If a group of children were found to have improved their reading skills in a long term treatment program, it would be easy to eliminate maturation as a rival explanation to treatment for their improvement.
3. If two groups in a study start off on an unequal basis, this would probably be an example of assignment errors.
4. In a test of skill that is easily learnt, testing effects are unlikely to be a problem.
5. Control groups will eliminate assignment errors.
6. If the researcher can attribute the outcomes in a study to the treatment programs employed and not other factors, then the study is internally valid.
7. If a study is internally valid then it must be externally valid.
8. Mortality refers to the difficulty of patients dying while undergoing the treatment program.
9. Regression to the mean occurs mainly in studies where groups have been selected to participate on the basis of some form of extreme score in a pre-test.
10. Control refers to the need to eliminate alternative conflicting explanations for the outcomes observed in a study.

Multiple choice

1. If a group of participants in a study are selected on the basis of a particularly poor pre-assessment, it is likely that they will appear to 'improve' when re-assessed soon after, without any treatment. This phenomenon is known as:
   a regression to the mean
   b maturation
   c history
   d assignment error.

2. If, after a twelve month program, a group of children with reading problems had improved their reading ages by an average of nine months, a viable alternative explanation for the results, other than the effectiveness of the program, would be:
   a regression to the mean
   b maturation
   c history
   d assignment error.

3. If, after the evaluation of the effectiveness of two different rehabilitation programs, it was found that the participants in the 'best' program had all attended a disability workshop together, a viable alternative explanation for the results other than the program would be:
   a regression to the mean
   b maturation
   c history
   d assignment error.

4. If, after the evaluation of the effectiveness of two different rehabilitation programs, it was found that the participants in the 'best' program were selected from a less impaired group, then a viable alternative explanation for the results other than the program would be:
   a regression to the mean
   b maturation
   c history
   d assignment error.

5. The advantage of including a control or comparison group in a study of treatment effectiveness is that:
   a effects such as maturation can be eliminated
   b effects such as maturation can be reduced
   c effects such as maturation can be measured
   d effects such as maturation can be ignored.

6. If a well designed study demonstrates a convincing advantage of one therapeutic technique over another, but is based on a sample of five people in the two groups, then the study is likely to have:
   a high internal and low external validity
   b high external and low internal validity
   c low internal and external validity
   d high external and internal validity.

7. Those patients who receive inert treatment in a control comparison group yet respond as if they had received real treatment are demonstrating:
   a the placebo effect
   b external validity
   c internal validity
   d regression to the mean.

8. In a long term treatment study with a single group with no comparison or control group, it is possible to attribute any improvements observed to:

  a the treatment
  b history effects
  c maturation
  d all of the above.

DISCUSSION, QUESTIONS AND ANSWERS

Our next discussion question takes us back over fifty years in time, to the setting of the closed psychiatric institutions where persons with serious mental illnesses were often confined under dismal and overcrowded conditions. Psychiatric researchers were desperately seeking new and effective treatments which could enable the residents to return to the community and thus to relieve the pressure on the institutions. A team of Italian researchers, lead by the psychiatrist Cerletti, were working on a new technique which they hoped would provide a quick and effective treatment for schizophrenia.

Unfortunately, their research program was guided by what was later shown to be a false hypothesis; that persons who suffered from epilepsy did not develop schizophrenia. On the basis of this false hypothesis it was predicted that inducing epileptic convulsions would help to reduce the signs and symptoms of schizophrenia. Thus, in the late 1930s thousands of mentally ill persons were administered convulsants, such as the drugs cardiazol and metrazol. The drugs induced convulsions that were difficult to control and proved to be very dangerous. Cerletti argued that the use of electrical shocks to induce epileptic convulsions would be a safer approach than the drugs.

In an article which outlines the historical development of electroshock, Krzyzowski (1989) reported what happened when Cerletti and his assistant Bini first presented these ideas to their colleagues.

> Bini, at a conference in Munich in 1936, and Cerletti in the same year in Milan, mention the possible application of electric current to cause therapeutically desired epileptic attacks. The idea was almost unanimously rejected on the grounds of its barbarity and associated hazard. It should be noted that the electric chair had just been introduced in America.
>
> *(Krzyzowski 1989, p. 51).*

Regardless of this hostile reaction, Cerletti and his team continued research into electric shock, experimenting with animals in Rome's slaughterhouses. According to Krzyzwoski (1989, pp. 51-52) the team was ready for their first human subject by the year 1938.

> On April 15 1938, a patient manifesting distinct symptoms of mental illness was admitted into the clinic in Rome after having been arrested by the police for travelling on a train without a ticket. The condition of the patient was then as follows: fully normal orientation, expressed distinct introversion, and persecution delusions often using neologisms. He considered himself to be under telepathic influence directing his behaviour. At the same time he exhibited hallucinations thematically related to the delusions. He was depressed and altered neurological conditions were found. Schizophrenia was diagnosed.

65

Having selected their first subject, the team administer the first ECT (electroconvulsive therapy) procedure.

Two electrodes were attached symmetrically in the vicinity of the crown and forehead and then a relatively low 80 V current was passed for 1.5 seconds. On switching the current on, the patient sat upright on the bed, his muscles contracted and he fell back onto the bed, not losing consciousness, however. He cried out for a while and then became quiet.

It appeared that the voltage applied was too low to induce the convulsion required for the therapeutic effectiveness of the ECT procedure. What happened next is discussed by Krzyzowski:

Continuation of the treatment was postponed until the next day. The patient, on hearing of such suggestions, roused himself and shouted normally: 'No more. It could kill me'. The words were spoken aloud normally, while previously he used only a specific and hardly understandable jargon, self-devised and full of neologisms. This normal utterance confirmed and assured Cerletti of the effectiveness of the method and, in spite of the strong reservations of his assistants, he decided to repeat the ECT without delay. This time a 110 V current with a pulse duration of 1.5 s was used. Once again a short lived, general contraction of all muscles was observed followed by a full classic epileptic type attack of convulsions. All those present uneasily watched the pallidness and cyanosis accompanying the attack, relaxing as the patient gradually recovered.

The story, you will be pleased to hear, had a happy ending.

After prolonged treatment consisting of 11 full and 3 incomplete shocks, the patient was discharged from the clinic in good health. At follow-up a year later, the mental state of the patient was seen to be good and stable. Subsequent years evidenced a widening application of ECT.

(Krzyzwoski 1989, p. 52)

As a matter of interest, ECT is still used by contemporary psychiatrists, but in a greatly modified fashion:

- It is used with anesthesized patients, with electrodes placed only on one side of the head.
- It is not used with persons with schizophrenia (for whom it was found to be ineffective) but rather with persons who are profoundly depressed.
- It is used as a 'last resort' when current pharmaceutical treatments are ineffective.

Questions

The following questions concerning research planning are related to the above narrative:

1. On the basis of the information given propose aims and/or hypotheses which might have guided the above study.
2. Given the state of psychiatric knowledge and practice of the late 1930s; do you think the above study was justified?
3. Give 3 or 4 reasons why a contemporary ethics committee might reject such a research project.
4. By present ethical standards, what should have been done after the patient shouted 'No more, it could kill me'?
5. Cerletti proceeded with a more severe shock on the grounds that the previous shock 'improved' the patient's condition. Comment on this logic, in the context of scientific methodology?
6. Do you think such dangerous experiments are ever justified in the context of health care? If yes, under what conditions?
7. Discuss 2 or 3 problems with the 'internal validity' (Ch. 4) of this study. Suggest simple changes in 'control' which may help to improve internal validity.
8. Comment on the 'external validity' of this study in the light of the fact that subsequent ECT was shown to be ineffectual as a treatment for schizophrenia.
9. Do you think Cerletti and his colleagues were guided by a rather simplistic 'paradigm' of schizophrenia? Explain, by comparing the biomedical and 'biopsychosocial' approaches in Section One.

Answers

1. The research seems to have been guided by several interrelated aims and/ or hypotheses.
   (i) The first aim was to find the electrical shock intensity which was sufficient to induce an epileptic seizure in a human.
   (ii) The second aim was to demonstrate that the seizure did not result in death or disability; that is, that the treatment was 'safe'.
   (iii) The hypothesis implicit in the research might be stated as: 'A course of ECT is effective for reducing the signs and symptoms of schizo-phrenia'.
   You may be able to suggest other aims and hypotheses. None of the outcomes was stated precisely in the paper quoted.
2. As you may have judged from this brief excerpt, the state of knowledge concerning the biological causes of mental illness was confused and had a weak empirical basis. Biological treatments, such as drug induced epileptic seizures were poorly theorized, dangerous and generally ineffective. In this context, in the late 1930s, it could be argued that experimenting with new and safer treatments was justified.
3. We outlined some relevant ethical guidelines in Chapter 2 in terms of which the present study would be judged as problematic, e.g. questionable benefits for patients, lack of informed consent, dangerous and painful

intervention, lack of consultation with the relatives/guardians of a mentally ill person.

4. Obviously, discontinue the research. Even though the person was confused when admitted to the hospital, his request was rational and reasonable. There was no doubt whatsoever concerning the patient's desires, and by present ethical standards researchers must comply with such requests.

5. The first electrical shock did not induce the epileptic convulsion which was postulated as the factor 'causing' the therapeutic change. As the first shock simply hurt the man, there was no theoretical or empirical justification for his apparent improvement being due to this shock.

6. One could argue that risking people's health and lives in the context of 'heroic' medicine is never justified. Rather we should look to prevention or gentler, more natural treatments.

   The other point of view is that aggressive medical treatment is justified if there are incapacitating and chronic problems, such as schizophrenia. According to this approach, painful and potentially harmful experimental treatments are justified provided the study is well designed and the participants are well informed and have consented.

7. The issue is whether or not the apparent improvement in the patient's condition was due to the ECT or to other 'extraneous' factors or variables. There are several possibilities which provide plausible alternative explanations, such as:

   (i)   *History*. The patient may have been frightened by the treatment and 'pretended' to be better to escape the situation

   (ii) *Maturation*. The patient may have recovered anyway, his condition may be cyclical

   (iii) *Testing or instrumentation*: There may have been inaccuracies and bias in the way in which the patient's condition was assessed.

   Control may be introduced by using groups of persons who have (i) no treatment and/or (ii) another treatment for schizophrenia.

   The appropriate designs for showing causal effects are outlined in Section Three. But because of the poorly designed research in the area, it was almost two decades of useless treatments before it became evident that ECT was not an effective treatment for schizophrenia.

8. Clearly, there was no evidence that the improvement claimed in this study was caused by ECT. In addition, it is tricky to make inferences from unrepresentative samples to populations. In this study, the patient may have shown symptoms of depression, which perhaps responded to the treatment. But this may not be generalizable to persons who show other patterns of schizophrenia. External validity is ensured by appropriate sampling procedures (Ch. 3) and clear operational definition and assessment of the condition, as outlined in Chapter 12. Without appropriate sampling and assessment procedures, we may use inappropriate treatments, unsuitable for the specific needs of our patients.

9. The researchers were working in the context of a 'biomedical' model, assuming that schizophrenia was simply a biological disorder which could be suddenly cured by a heroic treatment such as ECT. A 'biopsychosocial' approach takes a more complex view of chronic disorders, and research programs include identifying and treating both psychological disabilities and social handicaps entailed in schizophrenia. Biopsychosocial research may involve both quantitative and qualitative methods.

Research designs

In the previous section, we identified broad categories of descriptive (non-experimental) and causal (experimental) strategies for conducting research. The aim of Section 3 is to discuss these issues in more detail, by examining various research designs and outlining their applications for conducting health sciences research.

The conceptual basis for experiments is the need for control, as outlined in Chapter 4. In experimental research (see Ch. 5) we manipulate one or more variables (independent variables), while controlling the extraneous variables, by using appropriate controls such as control groups. If the experiment is well designed and properly conducted, we are in a position to demonstrate the causal effects of the independent variables on the outcome or dependent variables. The random assignment of subjects to experimental groups is a common way to achieve control. However, health and illness outcomes often have multiple and interacting causes requiring multivariate experimental designs.

Another issue we need to address is reactivity of human beings to social situations, such as being involved in research. Well designed experiments attempt to control for the biases of both the subjects and the experimenters involved in a research project.

There are situations where for practical or ethical reasons we cannot randomly assign subjects to control or treatment groups. Here we use quasi-experimental methods which involve comparing pre-existing groups undergoing different treatments (see Ch. 5). There are other research designs discussed in Chapter 6, including naturalistic comparisons, correlational designs and surveys. Naturalistic comparisons and correlational designs enable us to describe and predict relationships among variables, but should be used only with extreme caution in attempting to understand causal effects. Surveys include the use of questionnaires and interviews to study a person's knowledge, attitudes and beliefs concerning aspects of health and illness; are essentially a tool for descriptive research. The accuracy of non-experimental designs depends on appropriate sampling strategies being used in selecting the subjects.

An interesting and commonly used design in clinical settings is the n = 1 or 'single case' design. The advantage is that using n = 1 designs we may be able to demonstrate causal effects using only one or two subjects, without the need for separate control groups. The major limitation of n = 1 (and other types of clinical case studies) is that the findings may not be generalizable to other cases or situations.

Chapter 8 describes some of the elementary characteristics of qualitative 'field research' designs. This chapter aims to compare and contrast quantitative and qualitative research, and describes the importance of qualitative research for understanding the personal experiences of our clients and/or patients. Specific qualitative designs (such as in-depth interviewing and participant observation) and strategies for interpretive data analysis are outlined in Section Four.

5

Experimental designs

INTRODUCTION

Experimental research involves the active manipulation of variables under the control of the researcher. These are termed **independent variables**. The experimental approach attempts to study how subjects or phenomena will react to the manipulated conditions through monitoring one or more outcome measures. The outcome variables are termed **dependent variables**. If an experiment is well designed, the experimenter may, in principle, detect causal relationships between the independent and the dependent variables. However, there are many threats to the satisfactory detection of such relationships.

The experimental approach has been used extensively in the 'hard' sciences and therefore is worthy of close study.

The specific aims of this chapter are to:

1. Examine the basic structure of experimental research designs
2. Consider threats to the validity of the results obtained from experiments
3. Discuss how researchers and participant may react to experimental situations.

EXPERIMENTAL RESEARCH

Experimental studies involve the following steps:

1. Definition of the population. Researchers define the population to which they wish to generalize. For example, this might be males over 55 years with coronary heart disease or the local community or a certain type of health care organization.

2. Selection of the sample. Using an appropriate sampling method, the sample is selected from the population. It is important that the sample is representative of the population. (It is important to note that steps 1 and 2 are common to most research designs and have been previously discussed in detail.)

3. Assignment procedures. Using an assignment procedure, the participants are allocated to groups. For example, in an experimental study of the effectiveness of different types of weight-loss procedures, one group might receive an instructional manual, another might receive supervised dietary training, and others may receive no treatment. The purpose of the assignment procedure is to ensure that the groups are as similar as possible or equivalent to begin with. If they are substantially different, it will be very difficult to attribute any differences in final outcome to the 'treatments' administered. That is, internal validity will be under threat.

4. Administration of intervention (treatment). The researcher then administers the intervention(s) to the various groups participating in the experiment. This is called the independent variable(s). It is important that the intervention is administered in an unbiased way, in order that a fair test of any differences in outcomes may be provided. As will be discussed later, awareness of the expected outcomes on the part of participants often leads to a spurious promotion of the phenomena under study. Therefore, the true aims and expectations of the researcher are sometimes concealed from the participants.

5. Measurement of outcomes. The researcher assesses the outcome of the experiment through measurement of the dependent variable. Sometimes, the dependent variable is measured both before and after the experimental intervention (pre-test, post-test) and other times only afterwards (post-test only).

Thus, in an experimental study the researcher actively manipulates the independent variable(s) and monitors outcomes through measurement of the dependent variable(s).

Assignment of subjects into groups

The most straight forward approach is to assign the subjects randomly to *independent* groups. Say, for instance, we were interested in the effects of a specific drug (we'll call this Drug A) in helping to relieve the symptoms of depression. Also, we decide to have a placebo control group, which involves giving patients an capsule identical to A, but without the active ingredient.

Given a sample size of say 20, we would assign each subject randomly to either the experimental (Drug A) or the control group (placebo control). In this case, we would end up with the following two treatment groups:

	Levels of the independent variables	
	Control group (Placebo)	**Experimental group** (Drug A)
Number of subjects	$n_C = 10$	$n_E = 10$

Here n_C and n_E of course refer to the number in each of the groups, given that the total sample size (n) was 20.

Matched groups

Random assignment *does not guarantee* that the two groups will be equivalent, rather the argument is that there is no reason that the groups should be different. While this is true in the long run, with rather small sample sizes even chance differences among the groups may have an impact on the results of an experiment. Matched assignment of the subjects into groups minimizes group differences due to chance variation.

For instance, following the hypothetical example discussed previously, say that the experimenter required that the two groups should be equivalent for the measure of depression being used in the experiment. Here the subjects would be assessed for level of depression before the treatment and paired for scores from highest to lowest. Subsequently the two subjects in each pair would be randomly assigned to either the experimental groups or the placebo. In this way, the two groups would be the same for the average pre-test scores on depression.

DIFFERENT EXPERIMENTAL DESIGNS

Three types of experimental design will be discussed. These are the pretest/post-test, post-test only and factorial designs.

Pre-test/post-test design

In this design, measurements of the outcome or dependent variables are taken both before and after intervention. This allows the measurement of actual changes for individual cases. However, the measurement process itself may produce change, thereby introducing difficulties in the clear attribution of change to the intervention on its own. For example, in an experimental study of weight loss, simply administering a questionnaire concerning dietary habits may lead to changes in those habits by encouraging people to scrutinize their own behaviour and hence modify it. Alternatively, in measures of skill, there may be a practice effect such that without any intervention, the performance on a second test will improve. In order to overcome these difficulties, many researchers turn to the post-test only design.

Post-test only design

At first glance it may appear that this would make measurement of change impossible. At an individual level this is certainly true. However, if we assume that the control and experimental groups were initially identical and that no change had occurred in the controls, direct comparison of the post-test scores will indicate the extent of the change.

This type of design is fraught with danger in clinical research and should only be used in special circumstances, such as when pre-test measures are impossible or unethical to carry out. The assumptions of initial equivalence and of no change in the control group may often not be supported and, in such cases, interpretation of group differences is difficult and ambiguous.

Factorial designs

A researcher will often not be content with the manipulation of one variable in isolation. For example, a clinical psychologist may wish to manipulate both the type of psychological therapy and the use of drug therapy for a group of patients. Let us assume he/she was interested in the effects of therapy versus no psychological treatment, and of drug A versus no treatment. These two variables lead to four possible combinations of treatment (see Table 5.1).

This design enables us to investigate the separate and combined effects of both independent variables upon the dependent measure(s). If all possible combinations of the values or levels of the independent variables are included in the study, the design is said to be **fully crossed.** If one or more is left out, it is said to be **incomplete.** With an incomplete factorial design, there are some difficulties in determining the complete joint and seperate effects of the independent variables.

In order that the terminology in experimental designs is clear, it is instructive to consider the way in which research methodologists would describe the example design in Table 5.1 This is a study with two independent variables (sometimes called factors), namely, type of psychological therapy and drug treatment. Each independent variable or factor has two levels or values. In the case of psychological therapy, the two levels are Rogerian therapy and no psychological therapy. This would commonly be described as a 2 by 2 design (each factor having two levels). There are 4 groups (2 × 2) in the design.

Table 5.1 Example of a factorial design

	Drug A	**No drug**
Rogerian therapy	1	2
No psych. treatment	3	4

If a third level, drug B, was added to the drug factor, then it would become a 2 by 3 design with six groups required. Two groups, drug B with Rogerian therapy and drug B with no psychological therapy, would be added. It is possible to overdo the number of factors and levels in experimental studies. A 4 × 4 × 4 design would require 64 groups! That is a lot of subjects to find for a study.

Repeated measures and independent groups

In order to economize with the number of subjects required in an experimental design, the researchers will sometimes re-use subjects in the design. Thus, at different times the subjects may receive, say, drug A or drug B. If it were the case that every subject encountered more than one level of the drug variable or factor, then 'drug' would be termed a repeated measures factor. An important consideration is using a 'counterbalanced' design to avoid series effects. For instance, half the subjects should receive drug A first, and half drug B. If *all* the subjects received drug A first and then drug B, the study would *not* be counterbalanced and we would not be able to determine whether the order of administration of the drugs was important. Time is a common repeated measures factor in many studies. A pre-test post-test design involves the measurement of the same subjects twice. If 'time' is included in the analysis of the study, then this is a repeated measures factor. In statistical analysis, repeated measures factors are treated differently from factors where each level is represented by a separate, independent group (see Ch. 19). This is true *both* for matched groups discussed earlier as well as for repeated measures discussed above.

Multiple dependent variables

Just as it is possible to have multiple independent variables in an experimental study, it is also permissible to have multiple outcome or dependent measures. For example, in order to assess the effectiveness of an intervention such as icing of an injury, factors such as extent of edema and area of bruising might both be important outcome measures. In this instance, there would be two dependent measures.

It is nevertheless true that the statistical treatment of studies with two or more outcome measures (multivariate designs) can be somewhat problematic, and hence researchers are often more disposed towards multiple independent variables than multiple dependent variables.

EXTERNAL VALIDITY OF EXPERIMENTS

We have already discussed external validity in Chapter 3. There are further criteria for ensuring the generalizability of an investigation, depending on the procedures used, and the interaction between the patients and the therapist.

The Rosenthal effect

A series of classic experiments by Rosenthal (1976) and other researchers have shown the importance of expectancy effects, where the expectations of the experimenter are conveyed to the experimental subject. This type of expectancy effect has been termed the **Rosenthal effect** and is best explained by consideration of some of the original literature in this area.

Rosenthal and his colleagues performed an experiment involving the training of two groups of rats in a maze learning task. A bright strain and a dull strain of rats, specially bred for the purpose, were trained by undergraduate student experimenters to negotiate the maze. After a suitable training interval, the relative performances of the two groups were compared. Not surprisingly, the bright strain significantly out-performed the dull strain.

However, what is surprising is that, in fact, the two strains were not different! The two groups of rats were genetically identical. The researchers had deceived the student experimenters for the purposes of the study. The students' expectations of the rats had resulted in different methods of treatment which had affected the rats' learning ability. These results have been confirmed time and time again in a variety of experimental settings, and with a variety of subjects.

If the Rosenthal effect is so pervasive how can we control for its effects? One method of control is to ensure that the subjects do not know the true purpose of the study, that is, the experimental hypothesis. This can be done by withholding information—just not telling people what you are about—or by deception.

Deception is riskier and less ethical. Most organisations engaged in research activity have ethics committees which take a dim view of this sort of approach. Whatever the mechanism, if the subjects are unaware of the hypothesis being tested we say that they were **blind** to the hypothesis.

Often, however, blinding of the subjects is not enough. In many studies it is critical that the person taking the measurements, administering the treatments, etc. is blinded also. Thus if both the experimenter (not the researcher) and the subjects do not know the researcher's hypothesis, we say that **double blinding** has been employed. Both subject expectations and experimenter expectations are Rosenthal effects.

Hawthorne effect

Quite apart from the issue of the expectations of participants in experimental studies, there is the issue of whether the attention paid to subjects in the experimental setting alters behaviour.

In the late 1920s, a group of researchers at the Western Electric Hawthorne Works in Chicago were investigating the effects of lighting, heating and other physical conditions upon the productivity of production workers. Much to the surprise of the researchers, the productivity of the workers kept improving independently of the actual physical conditions! Even with dim lighting, productivity reached new highs. It was obvious that the improvements observed were not due to the manipulations of the independent variables themselves, but some other aspect of the experimental situation. The researchers concluded that there was a facilitation effect caused by the presence of the researchers. Perhaps the workers were afraid they would lose their jobs! This type of effect has been labelled the Hawthorne effect and is prevalent in many settings.

Of particular interest to us is the manifestation of the Hawthorne effect in clinical research settings. It must be taken into account that even 'inert' treatments might result in significant improvements in the patient's condition. The existence of the placebo effect reinforces the importance of having adequate controls in applied clinical research. Although we cannot eliminate it, at least we can measure the size of it through observation of the control group, and evaluate the experimental results accordingly.

WHEN SHOULD EXPERIMENTAL STUDIES BE USED?

Some philosophers and methodologists would say 'never'. This position is adopted by those who argue that by intervening in the situation under study, the experimenter irrevocably changes it. This is an extreme position and not a terribly popular one in the health sciences, as intervention in natural situations in an attempt to ameliorate conditions may be considered to be the primary activity of health scientists.

There are many situations in which the experimental approach is the best available. The study of the effectiveness of interventions is an area of particular suitability, often allowing definitive conclusions about the relative effectiveness of different treatment approaches to be reached. The control of extraneous factors provided in a well designed and executed experiment strengthens the conclusions reached.

There are many situations in which other approaches are better suited. For example, if it is wished to estimate the health needs and wants of a community, experimental methods would be less suitable than, say, survey or observational approaches.

It is a matter of matching the research aims with an appropriate investigation method. If these aims include the study of the effects of interventions, especially in clinical populations, then experimental methods are a prime candidate. However, in many studies, experimental designs are implemented with an emphasis upon the maximization of internal rather than external validity. That is, the results are methodologically pure but of doubtful validity in the field. This is not an inherent feature of the experimental approach, but a common failing.

SUMMARY

The experimental approach involves the active manipulation of the independent variable(s) and the measurement of outcome through the dependent variable(s). Good experimental design requires careful sampling, assignment and measurement procedures to maximize both internal and external validity.

The Hawthorne and Rosenthal effects are important factors affecting the validity of experimental studies, and we attempt to control for these by 'blinding', when ethically possible.

Common experimental designs include the pre-test/post-test, post-test only and factorial approaches. These designs ensure that investigations can show causal effects.

SELF ASSESSMENT

Explain the meaning of the following terms:

control group	maturation
factorial design	mortality
Hawthorne effect	physical model
history	pre-test/post-test design
independent variable	post-test only design
internal validity	random assignment
instrumentation	Rosenthal effect
matching	selection error
mathematical model	

True or false

1. ~~The dependent variable is the variable measured by the investigator.~~
2. Selection or assignment error arise when, after the assignment of the subjects, the groups are not equivalent.
3. If in a clinical investigation more people die in the control group than the experimental group, the investigation lacks internal validity.
4. Ideally, the control group and the experimental group should receive exactly the same treatments.
5. Given that a placebo is an inert substance, its administration has no effects on the subjects' behaviours.
6. The random assignment of subjects is always preferable to assignment by matching.
7. Persons can serve as their own controls.
8. We reduce the effects of subject and experimenter expectancies by blindfolding.

Multiple choice

1. The aim of controlled observation is to:
   a remove the effects of confounding influences
   b identify the effects of the independent variable on the dependent variable
   c establish causal relationships
   d all of the above.

2. To say that an investigation lacks internal validity means that:
   a the independent variable had no effect
   b the dependent variable wasn't measured
   c uncontrolled variables may have affected the outcome
   d there were several dependent variables.

3. Which of the following is most representative of a placebo effect?
   a Headache is reduced when an anti-depressant is administered
   b Headache is reduced one second after swallowing an analgesic, well before it is absorbed by the body
   c Headache is increased after a fierce argument with a 'significant other'
   d Headache is decreased after the use of biofeedback.

A researcher is studying the effect of a new drug on healing of ulcers. Patients are assigned randomly, by the physician who treats them, to receive either the standard treatment or the new drug. Patients are informed that they are being studied, but they do not know which treatment they are getting. The measure of rate of healing is the number of days until the ulcer is completely healed.

4. The independent variable in the above study was:
   a   ulcers
   b   the new drug
   c   type of treatment
   d   rate of healing.

5. The dependent variable in the above study was:
   a   ulcers
   b   the new drug
   c   type of treatment
   d   rate of healing.

6. This study is:
   a   double blind because the patients do not know what treatment
       they are getting or which is expected to be more effective
   b   double blind because neither the researcher nor the patients know
       what treatment each person is getting
   c   single blind because the patients don't know what treatment they
       are getting but the physician who treats them does
   d   not blind at all as the patients know they are being studied.

7. Which of the following threats to internal validity is not controlled for
   in this study?
   a   maturation
   b   regression to the mean
   c   repeated testing
   d   history
   e   none of the above.

8. This investigation is an example of:
   a   an experiment, because patients are assigned randomly
   b   a study, because the treating doctor did the assigning
   c   an experiment, because two treatments are compared
   d   a study, because there is no control group.

9. If an experiment is internally valid, this means that:
   a   the study's results cannot be generalized to other equivalent settings
   b   the sampling method is appropriate
   c   the study is not really an experiment
   d   the independent variable is responsible for any trends observed
   e   the dependent variable has face validity.

A researcher wishes to study the effectiveness of a new drug for treating
arthritis. Subjects are selected randomly from patients attending a clinic and
are assigned randomly to treatment with the new drug (A) or with the current
standard treatment (B). A pre-test/post-test design is used. A number of
arthritic symptoms is assessed using a checklist of seven items.

10. The dependent variable in this study is:

    a the number of arthritic symptoms

    b the new drug

    c the method of assignment

    d the type of treatment.

11. The independent variable in this study is:

    a the number of arthritic symptoms

    b the new drug

    c the method of assessment

    d the type of treatment.

12. The actual outcome of the study is illustrated by the following graph. Even though the subjects were assigned randomly, the graph indicates possible threat(s) to internal validity due to:

    a maturation

    b regression to the mean

    c assignment

    d *b* and *c*

    e all of the above.

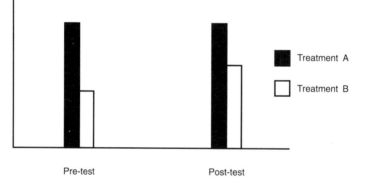

13. A factorial design involves:

    a more than one independent variable

    b more than one dependent variable

    c only one independent variable, but with more than one level

    d no control group

    e none of the above.

14. Simulation research means:

    a using computers to analyse data

    b studying differences between different artificial limbs

    c studying a model of a situation to reach conclusions about a situation

    d pretending to research one behaviour while actually studying another.

15. An appropriate design for an investigation will be one which:
    a minimizes all possible sources of error
    b is experimental
    c gives you the answer you expect
    d none of the above.

16. If a study is externally valid, then:
    a it must have been an experiment
    b the dependent variable has face validity
    c it cannot be internally valid
    d its results can be generalized to other equivalent settings.

17. The placebo effect:
    a happens only in drug studies
    b occurs in experimental as well as control groups
    c is another name for relaxing subjects
    d occurs only if you don't have double blinding.

18. Random selection of subjects in a study is typically employed to:
    a maximize generality of the results
    b minimize random measurement error
    c control assignment errors
    d minimize Rosenthal effect
    e minimize Hawthorne effect.

19. Random assignment of subjects in an experiment is typically employed to:
    a minimize random measurement error
    b minimize Rosenthal effect
    c minimize Hawthorne effect
    d ensure that the experimental and control groups are similar at the outset
    e maximize generality of the results.

20. The principal advantage of a factorial design is that:
    a all important factors are taken into account
    b only one factor is considered
    c the dependent variable is more reliable
    d the joint effects of two or more independent variables may be assessed
    e the independent variable has more levels.

6

Surveys and quasi-experimental designs

INTRODUCTION

In the previous chapter, the basic features of the experiment were presented. Experiments, when properly designed and implemented, allow the study of causal relationships between variables. However, the detection of causal relationships may not be the goal of the researcher and, even if it is, experimental procedures may not be feasible. Most health sciences research does not use the experimental design. Bloch (1987) reported that of the 757 articles on back pain published in 1985, only eight employed a randomized control (experimental) design. In this chapter we will examine a variety of 'naturalistic' approaches used for investigation of phenomena which do not lend themselves to true experimental designs.

The specific aims of this chapter are to:

1. Examine the uses of naturalistic designs
2. Discuss the use of surveys in health sciences research
3. Outline the characteristics of designs involving naturalistic comparisons, correlations and quasi-experiments
4. Identify some of the limitations of naturalistic designs.

NATURALISTIC DESIGNS

If experimental designs provide the tightest possible control, why should we resort to alternative methods? There are a number of reasons why non-experimental research designs may be employed instead of experimental designs.

1. Many variables are not amenable to experimental manipulation. For example, if the research question is concerned with sex differences in responses to heart surgery, then sex cannot be manipulated by the researcher. Similarly, if the researcher is interested in age differences, the ages of the participants cannot be altered by her or him. Many such

variables cannot be manipulated and hence cannot be incorporated in this way in an experimental study.

2. Often it is ethically inappropriate to investigate research questions using an experimental design. For example, if a researcher wished to perform a study on the effects of smoking upon health, to do this in an experimental design would require the experimenter to randomly allocate participants to the smoking or non-smoking group i.e. force people to smoke and others to not smoke. In experimental designs using a non-treatment control group, valuable and effective treatment might be withheld from participants. Would you agree to be harmed for the sake of science?

3. Experiments are best used to study simple causal relationships between variables. Yet, many human diseases and illnesses are not determined by a single cause but rather by a number of causes interacting in a complex fashion. For instance, heart disease may be caused by factors such as smoking, excessive stress, inappropriate diet or genetic factors. To identify such possible causal (or risk) factors, we need to study systems as they function in nature. That is, we should investigate patients in their natural setting, even with the difficulties this entails.

Therefore, we use naturalistic designs when experimental methods are inappropriate, as a result of the nature of the characteristics of the variables or individuals being investigated.

SURVEYS

Surveys are investigations aimed at describing accurately the characteristics of populations for specific variables (see Fig. 2.1). Surveys are commonly used in health care research for the following purposes:

1. To establish the attitudes, opinions or beliefs of persons concerning health related issues. The data collection techniques often include questionnaires or interviews (see Chs 9 & 10).
2. To study characteristics of populations on health related variables, such as utilization of health care, blood pressure, emotional problems or drug use patterns.
3. To collect information about the demographic characteristics (age, sex, income, etc.) of populations. A government census can be an important source of knowledge concerning population characteristics.

The statistics obtained from the above types of surveys present us with an overview of the state of health, illness and treatment patterns in a given community. In this way, we can gain insights into issues such as the prevalent causes of death or the health related requirements of the population. The above statistics might present us with patterns in the data, that is, significant differences or interrelationships. Such patterns can be the bases for hypotheses and theories concerning the causes of illness in a community. The area of health science concerned with such matters is called **epidemiology.**

NATURALISTIC COMPARISONS
AND CORRELATIONAL STUDIES

We can use surveys to study differences or interrelationships between health related variables in select populations.

Naturalistic comparison

Essentially, this type of survey or study involves the comparison of two or more naturally occurring groups or populations, in relation to one or more measures.

For example, a researcher may be interested in the relative performances of males and females on a test of spatial abilities. The researcher might take a sample of each sex studying at a university, and then compare the relative performances of the males and females on the test.

Or, a researcher might be interested in whether people growing up in different cultures have different pain reactions. Here, the researcher would select a sample of volunteers from the cultural groups of interest and compare their pain responses to standard noxious stimuli.

There are extraneous variables which can be controlled in this type of investigation. In both studies, the researcher could (and should) control variables such as the ages or educational backgrounds of the subjects. Note, however, that the researchers have not manipulated the variables being studied. All that has been done is to measure differences between naturally occurring groups, whereas in a true experiment, the independent variable is actively manipulated by the researcher. One could not seriously claim that the researcher had manipulated the sexes or the cultures of the participants! It is important to maintain this distinction between experimental and natural comparison studies. Although there is a similarity in that groups are compared, in the experiment the researcher actively controls who receives what treatment. In a natural comparison study, there is no such control and groups may differ in many uncontrolled variables other than the one, chosen by the researcher.

To relate this back to our first example, if our researcher determines that there is indeed a statistically significant difference in the performance of males and females on the measure(s) chosen, well and good. If our researcher then claims that biological factors are solely responsible for the differences, this is another matter altogether. This inference is only one of a number of alternative explanations that could be advanced to account for the differences observed. It could be, for instance, that males and female in a sample have been exposed to different types of toys and games during their development, so that males might perform better or worse on some tasks. In the second example, any significant results in the pain responses might not be due to 'culture', but rather perhaps to systematic biological differences among the groups or a complicated interaction between these factors.

The simple fact of the matter is that it is impossible to unequivocally determine causation in natural comparison studies. However, with logically interrelated studies, investigators may gain crucial information about the differences between groups on clinically relevant measures. Natural comparison studies are vital components of the researcher's methodological tools.

Correlational studies

The aim of correlational studies in the health sciences is to identify **interrelationships** among clinically significant variables. The term 'correlation' will be examined in detail in Chapter 16. At this point, let us just say that correlation expresses numerically the strength of association that might exist between two or more variables.

Let us look at a simple illustration of correlational studies. Say that clinical observations indicate that people who suffer from coronary heart disease tend to be overweight. Such observations might generate the hypothesis:

> There is a significant positive correlation between being overweight and the probability of coronary heart disease.

Here, the investigator will need to draw a representative sample of the population of interest (500 men and 500 women randomly selected from a population of healthy men and women aged 40 living in a specified district). The next step would be to determine the values of the first variable, that is, the subjects' weights and heights. These measures might be monitored over a period of time to check for drastic changes in weight. The second variable would be measured by the criterion of whether or not the subject suffered from heart disease during a specified period (say 10 years) representing the length of the study. The incidence of coronary disease can then be converted into a probability for a particular category of weight (see Table 6.1.)

You can see from Table 6.1 that the higher an individual scores on one variable (percentage overweight) the higher the scores on the other variable (probability of coronary heart disease). In this way, the fictional data presented in Table 6.1 are consistent with the predictions of the hypothesis stated above.

Table 6.1 Fictional data representing the relationship between variables 'percentage overweight' and 'probability of coronary heart disease' (for a 10 year period)

Percentage overweight	Number of subjects	Number suffering coronary heart disease	Probability of coronary heart disease
Underweight or normal	600	30	30/600 = 0.05
10–19% overweight	200	20	20/200 = 0.10
20–29% overweight	100	15	15/100 = 0.15
30–39% overweight	75	20	20/75 = 0.27
40% or more overweight	25	10	10/25 = 0.40

Two points should be considered at this stage. First, no evidence has been presented that one variable is *causally* related to another.

This sort of investigation does not, by itself, allow us to conclude that, for instance, 'Being overweight causes coronary heart disease'. There are several alternative hypotheses, such as 'Stress causes both being overweight and heart disease', which can also account for the findings. Secondly, it is clear that, at least for the period of the investigation, the variable 'Percentage overweight' doesn't account for all of the other variable 'Probability of coronary heart disease'. That is, according to the data presented in Table 6.1, there are normal or underweight individuals who suffer from coronary heart disease, and very overweight people who do not. Clearly, there must be other variables which are also related to the incidence of coronary heart disease. In fact, we find that there is a host of other variables, such as smoking, blood cholesterol level, personality type, stress, and family history of heart disease, which also correlate with the probability of coronary heart disease.

Some human diseases, for example, lung cancer and chronic back pain have complex, interacting causes. Natural comparisons and correlational designs can help us to identify risk factors, that is, variables which *might* be causally related to the onset or progress of these illnesses.

QUASI-EXPERIMENTAL DESIGNS

If clinical interventions are to be undertaken to reduce the risk factors associated with a disease, then clinicians require reasonable evidence that these factors are, in fact, causally related to the disease. Quasi-experimental designs are often used for this purpose.

Quasi-experimental designs can resemble experiments, with the important difference that there is no random assignment into treatment groups. However, the investigator can control the time at which a treatment is introduced or withdrawn. One such method is time-series design.

Time-series designs

Time-series designs involve repeated observations before and after a given treatment. In this way, changes in the sequence of observations following the introduction of a treatment may represent the effects of the treatment on the observed variable. Let us look at an example illustrating the use of time series designs in health sciences research.

Returning to the risk factor of 'being overweight' we discussed previously, the following investigation using a time-series design could provide evidence for a causal relationship between this variable and cardiac disease.

1. Select an appropriate population to study.
2. Specify the dependent variable, that is, some clear-cut measure of 'coronary heart disease'. A commonly used measure may be the incidence

of the disease. By 'incidence' we mean the number of new cases of the disease reported in relation to the population within a specified period of time (for example, 50 per 100 000, 1 year).

3. Introduce an appropriate treatment which reduces the magnitude of the risk factor. In our example, a health promotion package could be introduced, emphasizing exercise and good eating habits. Let us assume that this intervention is adequately financed and a significant proportion of the population adheres to the program. Then it could be hypothesized that:

   Introduction of the health promotion package will result in a decrease in the incidence of coronary heart disease in the community.

4. Monitor the dependent variable, over a period of time. It is essential to have readings of the variable both before and after the introduction of treatment. In this instance, the incidence of coronary illness would be determined from the medical records of hospitals, clinics and physicians. Also, public health authorities often gather and make available such statistics.

Figures 6.1A and B represent two of the many possible empirical outcomes using time-series designs. We will assume that the incidence of the illness was monitored for six years before and after the introduction of the treatment.

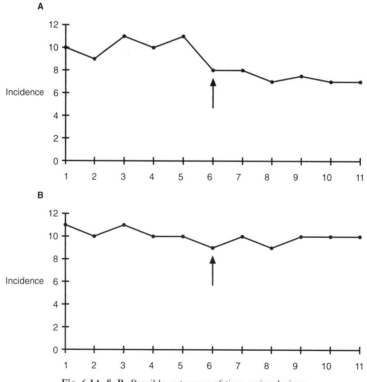

Fig. 6.1A & B Possible outcomes of time-series designs

There are, of course, other possible outcomes. However, in this case, Figure 6.1A would be consistent with the predictions of our hypothesis, while the outcome shown on Figure 6.1B would be inconsistent with our hypothesis. Discussion of the way in which data generated by time-series designs are analysed is beyond the scope of the present text. However, briefly, it involves the analysis of trends (increase or decrease) found in the dependent variable.

Time-series designs suffer from various problems of internal validity. What assurance have we, after all, that the decrease in the incidence of coronary heart disease, shown in Figure 6.1A, was caused by the introduction of the health promotion program? Maybe there was another cause, such as the introduction of drugs to control high blood pressure.

Multiple-group time-series designs

The introduction of multiple-group time-series designs involves the comparison of two or more naturally occurring groups. Let us examine a simple illustration of such designs by a fictional further investigation of the coronary heart disease problem.

Using a multiple-group time-series design, the investigator would select a community which is as similar as possible on demographic variables: socio-economic classes, age, size of the community etc. to the community being studied. In this way we would have:

Community A. Control. Do not introduce health promotion program.
Community B. Introduce health promotion program.

Figure 6.2 shows two of the several possible outcomes for such an investigation.

Where the two communities show different trends, the outcome shown on Figure 6.2A, is consistent with our previously stated hypothesis. However, in Figure 6.2B there is a trend for decrease in both A and B, therefore the evidence is not consistent with the prediction of the hypothesis.

Even with multiple-group time-series designs, some threats to internal validity remain. There are no guarantees that the communities A and B were equivalent on all relevant factors, or that there were no important changes during the study in the communities which might have influenced the incidence of coronary heart disease. The best that researchers can do is to identify and try to estimate the effect of such extraneous factors on the dependent variable. There are problems such as insulating the two groups: when people in Community B learn about the program being carried out in Community A they, by themselves, might initiate aspects of the program.

THE INTERNAL AND EXTERNAL VALIDITY
OF NATURALISTIC DESIGNS

We have noted several types of problems concerning the internal validity of investigations using natural comparison, correlational and time-series designs.

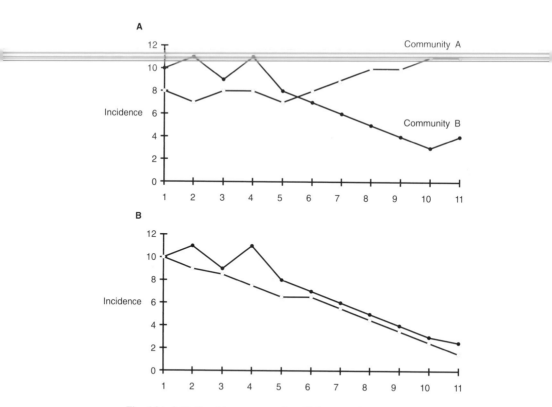

Fig. 6.2A & B Possible outcomes of multiple-group time-series designs

These are similar to the problems of internal validity found in experimental investigations. However, because researchers have generally less control over the phenomena being investigated, the use of natural comparison designs makes it more difficult to evaluate causal hypotheses. That is, given uncontrolled extraneous variables, a variety of plausible alternative hypotheses might be offered to account for the findings (Ch. 4). Therefore, in areas such as epidemiology, researchers use evidence arising from a variety of investigations using different types of designs to evaluate their theories and models of the causes of human diseases.

When evaluating evidence from natural comparison designs, the external validity of the findings must be considered. In Chapters 3 and 5, we stated that external validity refers to the generalizability of the results of an investigation. Strictly speaking, the results of an investigation should be generalized only to the population from which the sample was selected. For instance, consider the example discussed previously, where a sample of male and female students were compared on a test of spatial ability. Any differences between these two groups can be generalized validly *only* to the population of students from which the samples were drawn. Sometimes investigators forget this obvious point, and try to make inferences about males and females in general. Such sweeping generalizations are quite invalid. For instance, other cultures with alternative child rearing practices might well have males and females with completely different relative spatial abilities. Just because a variable is found to be a risk factor in one community, does not guarantee that it will have the same influence on diseases in another community. Clearly, the finding that cigarette smoking is a serious risk factor for coronary heart disease in Western societies doesn't *necessarily* mean that cigarette smoking is a risk factor for coronary heart disease among Zulus. Given the complex, interacting causes of coronary heart disease, it might be that there are different risk factors in communities which follow different lifestyles or have different physical constitutions.

It is not surprising, therefore, that advances in knowledge concerning systematic differences between culturally, racially, or sexually different groups have been slow and controversial.

SUMMARY

Descriptive surveys were shown to be important for establishing the attitudes, behaviours and health problems of a community. These statistics might be used to propose theories or hypotheses of the nature and causes of illness. We examined several types of non-experimental research designs, including naturalistic comparisons, correlational designs and time-series designs. It was argued that these designs are appropriate when experimental designs can not be used, having the advantage that we can study systems as they are in nature.

Just as with true experimental designs, investigations using natural comparison designs must confront problems of internal and external validity. Unlike experimental designs, quasi-experiments do not involve subject assignment into treatment groups. However, we can control the nature of the treatments and the times at which they are introduced. Because control over subject selection and the administration of treatments is more difficult, evaluation of causal hypotheses using naturalistic designs tends to be more controversial than with experimental designs. This does not mean, however, that their use is invalid. Rather, researchers and clinicians working in areas such as epidemiology need to integrate evidence arising from investigations using a range of research designs.

SELF ASSESSMENT

Explain the meanings of the following terms:

correlational studies
epidemiology
multiple-group time-series
naturalistic comparisons
risk factors
surveys
time-series
quasi-experimental designs

True or false

1. If it is impracticable to manipulate an independent variable, the investigator might adopt a non-experimental design.
2. The finding that the incidence of birth abnormality has increased in a community since the fluoridation of the water supply is sufficient evidence that fluoridation caused the birth defects.
3. If there is a high correlation between levels of stress and heart disease, we can say that stress is a risk factor in heart disease.
4. Time-series designs involve the repeated observation of subjects before and after treatment.
5. An important difference between experimental and quasi-experimental designs is that in a quasi-experimental study the subjects are not assigned into treatment groups by the investigator.
6. A quasi-experimental design affords greater control over extraneous variables than an experiment.
7. It might be invalid to infer that there are general differences between males and females on the basis of findings involving a sample.
8. An investigator compares the IQs of two ethnic groups, but does not control for systematic differences in socioeconomic status. Therefore, the study lacks internal validity.
9. When we speak of the 'insulation' of one group from another, we mean attempting to prevent subjects in a control group learning about and adopting the treatment given to an experimental group.
10. If a risk factor is, in fact, a cause for a disorder, we can predict that reducing the risk factor should lead to a reduction in the incidence of the disorder.
11. Surveys are utilized in the social, but not in the medical sciences.
12. 'Naturalistic' designs are useful when it is physically or ethically impossible to manipulate the independent variable.
13. The advantage of naturalistic designs over experimental designs is that they enable the investigator to exercise more control over the independent variable.
14. Naturalistic designs should not be employed to investigate conditions which have complex, interacting causes.
15. Naturalistic comparisons yield data which unequivocally establish the causal effects of the independent variable.
16. A risk factor is a possible cause of a disease.
17. Quasi-experimental designs can involve the production of 'time-series'.
18. Time-series designs involve the calculation of correlation between time and space.
19. A multiple-group time-series design involves the comparison of two or more naturally occurring groups over a period of time.
20. A multiple-group time-series design can be employed only if the subjects can be randomly assigned into treatment groups.

21. For a factor to be recognised as a 'risk factor' it must be shown that it correlates with aspects of a disorder across cultures.
22. Epidemiologists are interested in the frequency and causes of diseases.

Multiple choice

1. Naturalistic designs are appropriate when:
   - *a* it is ethically inappropriate to manipulate the independent variable
   - *b* when only a small sample of subjects is available
   - *c* when the independent variable is extremely difficult or impossible to manipulate
   - *d* *a* and *c*
   - *e* all of above.

2. Naturalistic comparisons differ from experimental designs in that:
   - *a* random selection of subjects is not possible with naturalistic comparisons
   - *b* random assignment of subjects is not necessary with naturalistic comparisons
   - *c* naturalistic comparisons lack external validity
   - *d* all of the above.

3. A risk factor is:
   - *a* a sufficient cause for a complex disorder
   - *b* a necessary cause for a complex disorder
   - *c* both *a* and *b*
   - *d* neither *a* nor *b*.

We compare a representative sample of Kamchatkans and Patagonians currently resident in Australia on a test of visual acuity. Questions 4 and 5 refer to the above.

4. The design employed in the above investigation is:
   - *a* a naturalistic comparison
   - *b* a true experiment
   - *c* a factorial design
   - *d* a time-series design.

5. Given that the sample of Kamchatkans are found to have higher visual acuity than the sample of Patagonians, we can conclude that:
   - *a* Patagonians have poor eyesight
   - *b* Kamchatkans have higher visual acuity than Patagonians
   - *c* living in Kamchatka improves one's visual acuity
   - *d* Kamchatkans living in Australia probably have higher visual acuity than Patagonians living in Australia
   - *e* both *a* and *d*.

6. We employ correlational designs in order to:
   a establish the magnitude and direction of association between variables
   b to establish unequivocally causal effects
   c to identify the possible causes of disease entities
   d both a and c.

7. We intend to investigate if the use of ice is more effective than an exercise program in treating a particular type of physical injury. The design most appropriate for investigating this problem is:
   a an experimental design
   b a correlational design
   c a model
   d a time-series design.

8. An investigator intends to establish if there is a relationship between levels of atmospheric lead and learning deficits in children. The design most appropriate for investigating this problem is:
   a an experimental design
   b a correlational design
   c a model
   d a time-series design.

   The following graph summarizes changes in infant mortality rates over a period of years in two communities, A and B. In community A, a program of intensive fetal monitoring was introduced at the time indicated by the arrow. No such program was introduced in community B.
   Questions 9-10 refer to the above information.

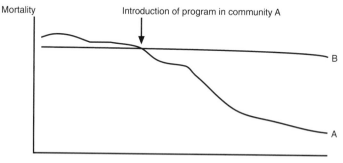

9. The investigation should be described as:
   a a correlational study
   b an experiment
   c a time-series design
   d a multiple-group time-series design.

10. The findings summarized in the above graph appear to be consistent with the conclusion that:
    a the introduction of fetal monitoring had no effect on infant mortality rate
    b the introduction of fetal monitoring decreased mortality rate
    c the introduction of fetal monitoring increased infant mortality rate
    d none of the above conclusions is consistent with the data.

11. Risk factors of diseases:
    a can be identified by correlational designs
    b are not necessarily the sole causes of diseases
    c are not necessarily the same across cultures
    d all of the above.

A multiple-group time-series design is introduced to study the effects of an insecticide on the number of spontaneous abortions. The insecticide was introduced (not by the investigator) in Community A, but not in a similar Community B. The following graph represents the hypothetical data.

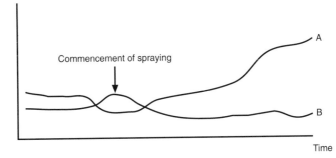

12. On the basis of the above graph, one can conclude that:
    a there is evidence that the introduction of the insecticide increased spontaneous abortions in Community A
    b there is no evidence that the introduction of the insecticide increased spontaneous abortions in Community A
    c there appears to be a contamination of Community B by the insecticide
    d a and c.

13. An investigator distributes a questionnaire to a sample of ex-nurses in an attempt to discover their reasons for leaving the profession. This is best described as:
    a a quasi-experiment
    b an experiment
    c a survey
    d a social model.

14. In an attempt to demonstrate the causal relationship between intake of animal fat and heart disease, an investigator studies the eating habits and heart disease rates of demographically defined groups. Which of the following (hypothetical) findings, is most inconsistent with the hypothesis that 'The intake of high levels of animal fats causes heart disease'.

    a   Vegetarians have a lower rate of heart disease than meat eaters
    b   Canadian males have a lower rate of heart disease than Canadian females
    c   The increase of protein and fat intake in China has correlated with an increased incidence of heart disease
    d   Eskimos, whose diet consists mainly of animal fats, have lower incidence of heart disease than Egyptians who eat mainly grains.

7

Single subject (n = 1) designs

INTRODUCTION

We have previously discussed designs involving the comparison of groups of subjects. These designs can provide evidence concerning the general causes of diseases, or the overall effectiveness of treatment. However, as clinicians we most commonly work with individual patients. We need to understand the specific causes of their problems and the effectiveness of treatments as applied to them as individuals.

The aim of the present section is to examine single subject (n = 1) designs, as applied by a variety of health professionals in natural settings. You will recognise close similarities between these designs, and the quasi-experimental designs discussed in Chapter 6.

The specific aims of the present chapter are to:

1. Examine the use and comparative advantages of AB, ABAB, and multiple-baseline designs
2. Comment on the validity of n = 1 designs.

AB DESIGNS

Let us look at a simple example to illustrate the basic procedures involved in using n = 1 designs. Say that a patient is admitted to your ward suffering from a condition which involves having a high temperature. Before an appropriate treatment is devised, the patient's temperature is recorded every 15 minutes, for 2 hours. Following this time interval, the patient is given medication to reduce their temperature. The question here is: 'How do we show that the medication was effective for reducing the patient's temperature?' Obviously, we need to show that the patient's temperature had fallen following the administration of the medication. Figure 7.1 illustrates a possible outcome.

Let us assume that the drug is known to act quickly, say in 20 minutes. The evidence shown in Figure 7.1 would be clearly consistent with the hypothesis that the medication caused a decrease in the patient's temperature. Let us

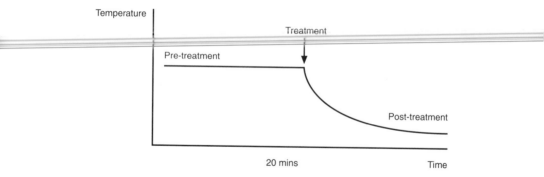

Fig. 7.1 Possible outcome of an AB design

generalize this example to n = 1 designs used in various settings. Figure 7.2 illustrates the general conventions used in n = 1 designs.

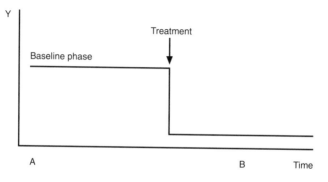

Fig. 7.2 General structure of *n* = 1 designs

1. We can see that the Y axis represents a dependent variable; observations made of specific physical characteristics of behaviours.
2. The X axis represents the time over which the observations were carried out.
3. The period A represents the sessions during which no treatment was administered. The observations recorded during A form the **baseline**.
4. Period B represents the sessions during which the independent variable (treatment) was administered.
5. The observations taken during A are compared with those taken during B. Systematic changes between A and B (increases or decreases) are assumed to reflect the influence of the treatment.

Therefore, an AB design involves the taking of observations during A, introducing an appropriate treatment, and then taking observations during B.

It might have occurred to you that several of the threats to validity (outlined in Chapter 4) can be identified in AB designs. An obvious one is maturation, that is, changes occurring in the patient which might influence the dependent variable. Another possible threat is history, that is, influences on the patient other than the actual treatment. In the example we just looked at, one could also argue that perhaps the patient's temperature would have gone down, even without the drug, because of the condition improving by itself, or the environment of the ward (maturation). Next, we shall look at ABAB designs, which provide stronger control for extraneous variables than AB designs.

ABAB DESIGNS

The basic feature of ABAB designs is the introduction of a reversal condition. That is, the researcher attempts to re-introduce the conditions pertaining under A. In this way, the design allows the examination of the observations as they occur when the treatment variable is withdrawn again and, therefore, control for threats to validity discussed above.

Developing the above example, an ABAB design would involve the withdrawal of the drug and its subsequent reintroduction. Figure 7.3 illustrates this procedure.

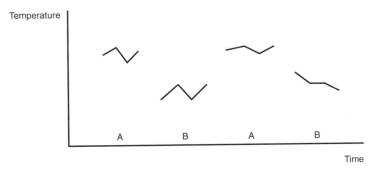

Fig. 7.3 Graph of patient's temperature under different treatment conditions

Figure 7.3 illustrates the outcome that when the drug is withdrawn (second A) the patient's temperature returns to previous levels. When the drug is reintroduced (second B), the patient's temperature declines. Clearly, such an outcome is consistent with a causal relationship between the independent variable (treatment) and the dependent variable (observations of temperature). Figure 7.4 demonstrates the graph expected using ABAB designs.

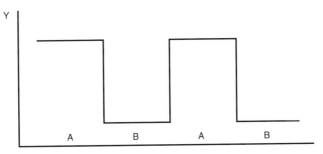

Fig. 7.4 General structure of ABAB designs

Although the above design is useful for demonstrating causal effects in a single individual, there are situations where it is inappropriate. ABAB designs are less useful when there is a good reason to expect that the variable underlying the observations is irreversible following the treatment. For example, if the medication used in the previous example involved antibiotics, then the discontinuation of such drugs after a period might not result in the re-emergence of the symptoms. After all, the antibiotics might well cure the underlying problem. Even when reversal is possible, it might not be ethical. Clearly, if we have succeeded in establishing desirable effects in our client during the first B period, we might well be reluctant to reverse this for the sake of establishing causal relationships.

MULTIPLE BASELINE DESIGNS

Multiple baseline designs involve the use of concurrent observations to generate two or more baselines. Given two or more baselines, the investigator has the opportunity to introduce treatment affecting only one set of observations, while using the other(s) as a control. We will examine a hypothetical clinical problem to illustrate these designs.

Say that we have a brain-damaged client showing aggressive behaviours which disrupt therapy. Therapy is offered in two situations, say occupational therapy (Situation 1) and speech therapy (Situation 2). A behavioural program is devised, aimed at reducing the frequency of the aggressive outbursts. A multiple baseline design involves the observation of the frequency of the target behaviour in both Situations 1 and 2. After establishing a baseline, the treatment is introduced firstly in one of the situations and then in the other. Evidence demonstrating the effectiveness of the behavioural treatment is shown in Figure 7.5.

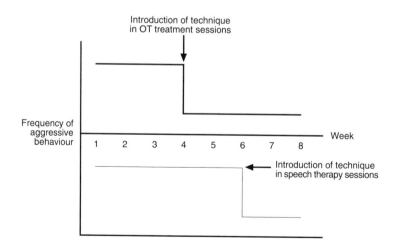

Fig. 7.5 Aggressive behaviour of a brain-damaged patient in two situations

The fictional data presented in Figure 7.5 indicates that the frequency of the target behaviour (aggression) declined in Situation 1 when the treatment was introduced, while it remained stable in Situation 2. The subsequent introduction of the treatment in Situation 2 resulted in a decrease of the behaviour.

Multiple baseline designs can be introduced also by generating baselines for two or more behaviours, or for two or more individuals. Just as in the example involving the different situations, the treatments would be introduced first for one of the behaviours or individuals and, subsequently, for the others. Figure 7.6 illustrates a general example for multiple baseline designs.

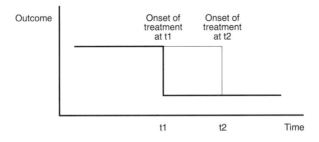

Fig. 7.6 General structure of multiple baseline designs

Clearly, by introducing the treatment at different times, we are controlling for the effects of extraneous variables which might influence our dependent variable. Both ABAB and multiple baseline designs are appropriate for demonstrating the benefits of therapeutic procedures in individual patients.

THE VALIDITY OF n = 1 DESIGNS

We examined three (AB, ABAB, multiple baseline) designs in the previous sub-sections. As a matter of fact, there are more complicated, 'mixed' designs available for n = 1 investigations. The mixed designs include elements of both reversal and multiple baseline strategies. We are not going to discuss these in detail in this text; interested readers are referred to Hersen and Barlow (1976).

A basic requirement for the valid interpretation of all n = 1 designs is the production of a stable baseline. Unless this requirement is met, the interpretation of the results is extremely difficult. In some clinical situations, the production of a stable baseline might be unethical as it would involve witholding treatment. Also, the treatment phase must be long enough for the effectiveness of the treatment to emerge. Some treatments, such as those involving physical rehabilitation or psychotherapy, might need to be administered for months before their effectiveness, or lack of it, becomes apparent.

It is essential that the observations should be valid and reliable. Some observations are straight-forward, such as those based on taking temperatures. However, given a more complex variable such as 'aggression' we need to establish with clarity that different observers agree on the type of behaviours we are going to observe. After all, behaviours which might seem 'aggressive' to one observer might not be classified as such by another. This issue is discussed further in Chapters 9 and 12.

We have already discussed how n = 1 designs attempt to control for the influence of extraneous variables. Although the n = 1 designs can be conceptually adequate to demonstrate causality, the patients, being in their natural setting, can be influenced by all sorts of uncontrolled events. After all, it is not possible (or really desirable) to insulate individuals from their environment. Therefore, sources of invalidity must be evaluated with respect to each n = 1 investigation. It must also be remembered that no matter how sophisticated the n = 1 design, the observed outcomes for any given case may not generalize to other cases. Using techniques known as meta-analysis it is possible to combine the data from a number of such single case studies to investigate overall trends. Thus n = 1 designs do not sidestep sampling nor generalizability issues.

SUMMARY

In this chapter, we examined three (AB, ABAB and multiple baseline) of the designs available for studying single individuals in their natural settings. It was argued that ABAB and multiple baseline studies provide a valid means for evaluating the causal effects of variables on therapeutic outcomes. These n = 1 designs are particularly useful for establishing the usefulness of treatment procedures for individual patients. Although some limitations and ethical constraints might emerge in conducting n = 1 studies, they provide a useful tool for the practising clinician interested in evaluating the effectiveness of treatments.

Although the statistical analysis of n = 1 studies is beyond the scope of this introductory text, it should be noted that graphing our observations, as discussed in this chapter, provides evidence for possible causal relationships. A precondition for interpreting the results of n = 1 studies is, of course, having a sufficient number of stable observations across the various conditions.

The n = 1 designs are quite similar to quasi-experimental designs, in that the investigator has control over the type and timing of the treatments.

SELF ASSESSMENT

Explain the meaning of the following terms:

AB design
ABAB design
baseline
multiple baseline
designs reversal

True or false

1. n = 1 designs are most appropriate for conducting epidemiological investigations.

2. The graphing of n = 1 findings involves graphing the magnitude of the dependent variable along the Y axis and time or sessions along the X axis.

3. With an AB design, the time period A represents the time period during which the treatment is introduced.

4. A 'baseline' is a series of observations recorded during a period when the treatment is administered.

5. With an AB design, a treatment is introduced, withdrawn and then reintroduced .

6. A limitation in using ABAB designs in clinical investigations is that it might be possible, but quite unethical, to withdraw a treatment.

7. Using multiple baselines across two situations involves establishing baselines, then administering treatments simultaneously in both situations.

8. An advantage of using multiple baseline designs over AB designs is the increased control over threats to internal validity.

9. AB designs involve a period of initial treatment followed by the withdrawal of the treatment.

10. For n = 1 designs, the 'B' period is when the treatment is administered.

11. n = 1 designs can not, in principle, indicate causal effects.

12. The major advantage of n = 1 designs is that no ethical issues need to be taken into account in planning such research.

13. An ABAB design involves introducing the treatment twice.

14. An ABAB design provides a more powerful control over possible extraneous variables than an AB design.

15. ABAB designs are particularly useful when changes in the symptoms following treatment are irreversible.

16. The production of a stable baseline might be unethical in some clinical situations.

Multiple choice

1. Quasi-experimental and n = 1 designs are similar in that:
   a they can both involve time dependent sets of observations
   b both can involve control over the time at which a treatment is introduced
   c both a and b
   d neither a nor b.

2. An ABAB design:
   a involves the use of two individuals, A and B
   b has two baseline periods
   c depends on manipulating A and measuring B
   d involves correlating AA with BBC.

Consider the following outcome for an n = 1 type investigation.

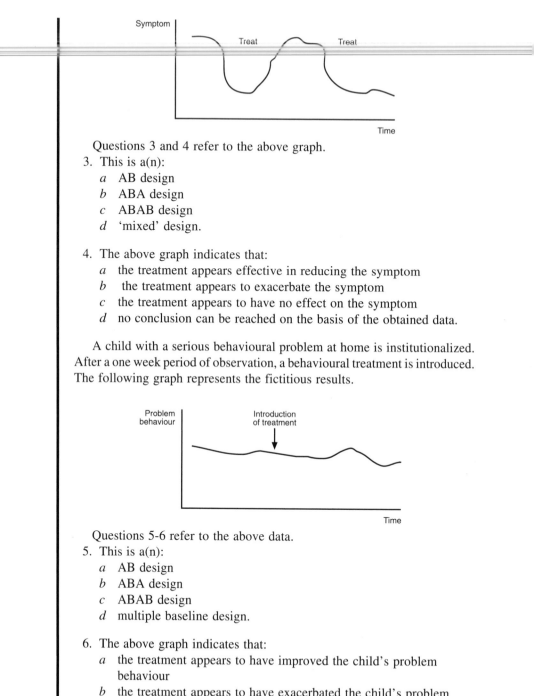

Questions 3 and 4 refer to the above graph.
3. This is a(n):
   a   AB design
   b   ABA design
   c   ABAB design
   d   'mixed' design.

4. The above graph indicates that:
   a   the treatment appears effective in reducing the symptom
   b   the treatment appears to exacerbate the symptom
   c   the treatment appears to have no effect on the symptom
   d   no conclusion can be reached on the basis of the obtained data.

A child with a serious behavioural problem at home is institutionalized. After a one week period of observation, a behavioural treatment is introduced. The following graph represents the fictitious results.

Questions 5-6 refer to the above data.
5. This is a(n):
   a   AB design
   b   ABA design
   c   ABAB design
   d   multiple baseline design.

6. The above graph indicates that:
   a   the treatment appears to have improved the child's problem
       behaviour
   b   the treatment appears to have exacerbated the child's problem
       behaviour
   c   the treatment appears to have had no effect on the child's behaviour
   d   a factorial design should have been used.

7. Treatment is undertaken to attempt to reduce anxiety in an individual. An ABAB design is used to evaluate treatment effectiveness. Because of different shifts at a hospital, six different observers are used to record the anxiety related behaviours. Problem(s) with this investigation is (are) that:
   a the observers might not record exactly the same behaviours as reflecting 'anxiety'
   b the presence of the different observers might influence the behaviours in different ways
   c both a and b
   d neither a nor b.

A new technique to improve running speed in athletes is evaluated. The following graph represents fictional results for two athletes.

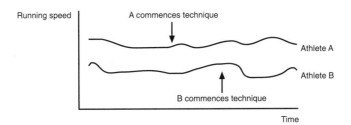

Questions 8 and 9 refer to the above data.

8. This design is a(n):
   a AB
   b ABAB
   c multiple baseline
   d factorial.

9. The above graph indicates that:
   a the new technique appears to improve running speed
   b the new technique appears to reduce running speed
   c the new technique appears to have no effect on running speed
   d further investigations on the effects of the technique are necessary.

10. The use of an ABAB design is most useful for reducing threats due to:
    a placebo effects
    b experimenter expectancy
    c maturation
    d assignment.

8

Qualitative field research

INTRODUCTION

The research strategies discussed in previous chapters can be called 'quantitative' in that the data obtained consists of measurements which can be statistically treated. It has been argued by some researchers that such quantitative statistical portrayals miss the essence of what constitutes health and illness in human beings. Qualitative or interpretive field research involves the investigation of specific individuals in their social settings. The investigator seeks to understand the thoughts, feelings and experiences of individuals, focusing on direct, face-to-face knowledge of patients or clients as human beings coping with their conditions and treatments in a given social setting. The use of evidence from qualitative studies has traditionally been a fundamental source of knowledge in the clinical and social sciences.

The specific aims of this chapter are to:

1. Outline different conceptual approaches to qualitative research
2. Compare and contrast specific dimensions of qualitative and quantitative approaches to research
3. Examine the scope and limitations of qualitative research in health sciences.

WHAT IS QUALITATIVE FIELD RESEARCH?

Qualitative field research is disciplined enquiry examining the personal meanings of individuals' experiences and actions in the context of their social environments.

'Qualitative' refers to the nature of the data or evidence collected. Qualitative data consists of detailed descriptions, based on language or pictures recorded by the investigator. 'Field' research indicates that the investigation is preferably carried out in the natural environment in which the phenomenon occurs, rather than in controlled laboratory settings. By 'disciplined' we mean that the enquiry is guided by explicit methodological principles for defining problems, collecting and analysing the evidence, and formulating and evaluating theories.

'Personal meaning' refers to the way in which individuals subjectively perceive and explain their experiences, actions and social environments. Qualitative field research provides systematic evidence for gaining insights into other person's views of the world, 'putting ourselves into someone else's shoes', as it were.

There are a variety of approaches to qualitative field research, which take somewhat different positions concerning how data should be collected and analysed. Also, there are several diverse schools of thought which have contributed to the historical development of qualitative field research. The most noteworthy contributions were made in the following areas (for brief reviews, see Taylor and Bogdan 1984, Cohen and Manion 1985):

1. *Phenomenology.* Phenomenology, which is both a system of philosophy and an approach to psychology, emphasizes the direct study of personal experience and the understanding of the nature of human consciousness. Research in this area involves 'bracketing' or putting aside the usual preconceptions and prejudices that influence everyday perception so that we can uncover the pure constituents of conscious experience. Conscious experience, is in turn, seen as the basis for personal meaning, as we reflect on our experiences in the context of our goals and purposes. An important concept adopted from phenomenology is the notion of 'multiple realities', that is, different people may consciously experience the world in quite diverse ways. In order to understand the meanings of a person's actions, we must become adept, through empathy, at seeing things from their point of view.

2. *Symbolic Interactionism.* Symbolic interactionists emphasize that a social situation has meaning only in the way people define and interpret what is happening. That is, people don't react to 'objective' aspects of their environments, but rather their actions are guided by their personal interpretations of the situation. It follows that different people, on the basis of their past experiences and their particular social positions may come to interpret a specific situation in quite divergent ways, and act in conflicting fashions. For instance, a male obstetrician might view childbirth in quite a different way to a female midwife, and in turn their views might be quite discordant with that of a woman giving birth. In social and health care settings, it is useful to explore different perceptions of events, as it is clear from the work of symbolic interactionists that 'shared perspectives' among people cannot be taken for granted.

3. *Ethnomethodology.* Ethnomethodologists study the processes associated with the way in which people perceive, describe and explain the world. Ethnomethodologist argue that the meanings of specific actions and events are not necessarily obvious to a person, but are in fact rather ambiguous and problematic. People select and apply specific rules and principles in order to define and give meaning to situations in which they find themselves and in order to justify their actions in a given situation. Research carried out by ethnomethodologists demonstrates that in our everyday communications and social interactions, we take an enormous amount of cultural context, such as norms and rules, for granted and we tend to 'bracket' this as obvious or common sense. It

must be remembered, however, that when the cultural backgrounds of individuals diverge, the understanding of personal meaning becomes less obvious or commonsense.

Although taking somewhat different views of personal meanings, the above three approaches have common themes and all have contributed to the development of qualitative field research. Table 8.1 shows key aspects of qualitative field research, in contrast to quantitative approaches.

DATA COLLECTION AND INTERPRETATION IN QUALITATIVE FIELD RESEARCH

The fundamental aim of planning and designing qualitative field research is to position the investigator close to the participants, so as to gain access to and describe personal experiences, and to interpret their meanings in specific social settings. The following subsection develops in more detail the corresponding points presented in Table 8.1. Illustrative examples will be discussed later, when we review data collection strategies in Chapters 9, 10 and 11.

Table 8.1 Contrast between quantitative and qualitative methods

	Quantitative	**Qualitative**
Perception of the subject matter	reductionistic; identification and operational definition of specific variables	holistic; persons in the context of their social environments
Positioning of researcher	objective; detached observation and precise measurement of variables	subjective; close personal interaction with subjects
Data base	quantitative; inter-relationships among specific variables	qualitative; descriptions of actions and related personal meanings in context.
Theories	normative; general propositions explaining causal relationships among variables	interpretive; providing insights into the nature and social contexts of personal meanings.
Theory testing	controlled; empirically supporting or falsifying hypotheses deduced from theories	consensual; matching researcher's interpretations with those of subjects and other observers
Applications	prediction and control of health related factors in applied settings	interacting with persons in a consensual, value consonant fashion in health care settings.

Adapted from McGartland & Polgar (1994)

Perception of subject matter

1. Qualitative field research is carried out in a natural setting, and there is no attempt made by the investigator to control for extraneous influences. Furthermore, there are no operational definitions provided for the dependent or independent variables, but rather the phenomenon being studied is perceived and described as a whole.

2. Strong preconceptions or fixed hypotheses are not advantageous for qualitative field research. This is a different situation to that in quantitative research, where there are precisely defined hypotheses or aims guiding the research. Of course, qualitative researchers do have general aims and theoretical notions pertaining to the phenomena being studied; but these are tentative and are open to modification as the data collection proceeds.

3. Qualitative field research focuses on the in-depth understanding of specific individuals, rather than studying the general characteristics of a large population of individuals across specific variables. It should be kept in mind, however, that some quantitative designs may address single cases, as we have seen in Chapter 7 in relation to n = 1 designs. The difference is that n = 1 designs address specific variables representing aspects of the individual's behaviour or clinical symptoms, rather than attempting to describe and understand the individual holistically in the context of their natural social settings. Such an approach is called 'idiographic' (describing a specific individual) as opposed to the 'nomothetic' (describing general phenomena) view of research in quantitative research.

Positioning of the researcher

1. As discussed in Chapter 12, accurate and replicable measurements are valued in quantitative research. The fundamental positioning of the researcher is 'objective', that is aiming to perceive and record events without any personal bias or distortion. The situation in qualitative field research is far more complex, as the researcher is more a part of the phenomenon being investigated than the detached observer in quantitative research (see in Ch. 11). It is argued here that to understand personal meanings and subjective experiences one has to become involved with the lives of the subjects being studied. That is, some degree of empathy must develop between the researcher and the subject. By empathy, we mean the ability to 'put ourselves in the other person's shoes', to see things from their perspective(s).

2. A particular reason for the advancement of quantitative research has been the development of instrumentation that has enabled the collection and recording of data to be more precise. It has also given access to phenomena not naturally accessible to unaided human senses, as for instance the development of light and electronic microscopy. However, when standardized tests and measures are used to study a person, they become 'enframed' within the limitations of the instrument, and their possible unique self-expression remains outside the scope of the enquiry. The qualitative researcher may find a measurement instrument intrusive, one which might restrict and confine the possibilities of understanding of a person.

There are advantages to a human 'measuring instrument' which are exploited in qualitative research. After all, we are more adaptable and multi-purpose than even very sophisticated machinery, and can observe subtle behavioural changes and verbal and nonverbal cues in our subjects. In addition, as the investigation progresses, the human 'instrument' becomes more aware of what is happening and thus the data collection becomes more accurate.

Data base

1. The data obtained in quantitative research consists of sets of measurements of objective descriptions of physical and behavioural events. These are summarized and analysed in accordance with statistical principles outlined at an introductory level in Sections 4 and 5 of this book. The data in qualitative research is descriptive, a 'thick' or thorough description of what people said, their actions and activities, non-verbal behaviours and interactions with other people. 'The reality of the place should be conveyed through representation of its mundane aspects in a straight forward manner' (Lofland, 1971, p.4). An important aspect of field research is keeping thorough, up to date field notes. These should be recorded as closely as possible to the time of occurrence of the phenomena under study. The field notes should contain direct quotations from the participants and the settings in which the statements and actions were recorded. Where possible (if this is not inappropriate or intrusive), the researcher may use audio and video recordings, as outlined in Chapter 10. This helps to record events, and improves accuracy in conveying what was said and done in a given setting, as it is possible to review the obtained information.

2. Even though 'objectivity' does not mean remaining detached from the situation, it is essential in qualitative research that the reports of events should be truthful. The investigators should not allow ideological biases to distort or censor their observations, or deliberately lie to place their subjects in a good or bad light. This is a particularly important point, as given the close personal interaction with the subjects, one may be predisposed to report favourably. An extreme of this in anthrophological research is called "going native", when one completely adopts the views of the subjects being studied.

3. By 'data base', we mean the overall empirical evidence that forms the basis for theory formation and specific applications for health care. In quantitative research, the data base will consist of the statistically treated data which will enable us to see how specific variables are interrelated. In terms of qualitative field research, the data base is essentially a narrative (or a story if you like) that reports what has happened to people, what they did or said in specific situations. This narrative should be adequately detailed so as to illuminate for the reader the personal meanings that the reported events had for the subjects.

Theories

Theories are representations of our current state of knowledge about the state of the world. Theories are abstract logical coherent explanatory systems which integrate a broad range of research findings (i.e. the facts). Theories may be constituted of premises stated in everyday language, with particular attention paid to the appropriate use of concepts and the logical development of the premises.

Theories based on quantitative evidence integrate patterns of findings concerning the interrelationships among variables. Such theories often contain 'models', which may be mathematical and or systems representations of the patterns of findings. For instance, models of anatomical and physiological processes, such as that of the circulatory or nervous systems are good examples of successful quantitative models.

On the other hand, theories integrating evidence from qualitative field research do not address facts about how objects are constituted and interact, but rather are interpretations of personal meanings emerging in specific social settings. In qualitative field research there are several different approaches to theory formation. We will discuss some of these further in Chapter 10, in the context of interpreting data arising from unstructured, in-depth interviews.

1. Some commentators (Guba & Lincoln 1983) argue that data collection and theory formation should be intrinsically integrated rather than being different stages of the research process. In addition, it is suggested that personal meanings should be seen as unique and idiosyncratic, and thus no attempt should be made to systematically integrate such diverse personal positions. Theory, from an idiographic position, is seen essentially as the accurate presentation of the situation from a particular person's perspective.

2. Other qualitative researchers approach theory formation by attempting to identify common 'themes' or categories of meanings emerging from the data. The important point here is that the theoretical categories are developed from evidence expressing personal meanings, rather than 'facts' derived from the statistical treatment of objective measurements concerning variables (Ch. 11). In this way, theory is said to be 'grounded' in the narratives of particular individuals.

3. Some researchers stress the broad, culture interpreting aspects of qualitative field research. The formation of **critical theory** explains how personal meanings and actions emerge and are influenced by the person's social and cultural milieu. Critical theories identify the extent to which individual's self-perception and freedom for action may become distorted and limited by the operation of power and coercion within society (e.g. Grundy 1987, pp. 15–19, 106–114).

Theory testing

Theories based on quantitative evidence lead to clear cut, empirically testable predictions or hypotheses logically deduced from the theories (see Ch. 1). Theories are supported or falsified by empirical evidence collected under controlled conditions. Testing qualitative theories is somewhat different, as no causal mechanisms may be included in the theoretical framework. The simplest verification of qualitative interpretations is to go to the subjects themselves, in order to establish if the researcher's interpretations make sense to them. The extent to which a consensus develops between researchers and their subjects is one of the important indications of the truth of qualitative theories.

Applications for health care delivery

The applications of quantitative evidence and theories are essentially *technical;* providing mechanisms in terms which we can predict and control specific health related variables. That is, we apply quantitative approaches for discovering the causes and progress of diseases and disabilities, for developing and validating assessment procedures and for evaluating the effectiveness of interventions (see also Ch. 1).

In contrast, qualitative field research provides evidence and theories which enable us to better understand our clients as human beings. This research discloses how illnesses, disability and health care delivery affects people's lives as interpreted from their points of view. In the following subsection, we will examine some of the applications of qualitative field research for improving health care delivery.

QUALITATIVE FIELD RESEARCH IN HEALTH CARE

When there are significant differences in the cultural backgrounds and experiences of persons, the understanding of personal meanings becomes problematic. For instance, an anthropologist might need to spend decades immersed in, and systematically studying, a different culture before they are in a position to accurately interpret the actions and traditions of the participants.

There are numerous areas of health care where research involving the interpretation of personal meanings is essential for ensuring effective practices. The following three examples illustrate areas where qualitative field research is making strong contributions for clarifying personal meanings, in situations where 'shared perspectives' of health care issues can not be taken for granted.

1. *Understanding cultural differences between health workers and clients.* In countries such as Australia, Canada or the United Kingdom we live in multicultural societies. There is persuasive evidence that the way people experience their bodies, or events such as childbirth, pain or illness depend to a large extent on their cultural backgrounds. When health practitioners misconceive their clients' view concerning their illness or injury, the outcome may be erroneous diagnoses, useless interventions, and an inappropriate treatment of clients. A particularly important area of qualitative field research is to clarify personal meanings of clients and therapist with regard to health care problems, in an attempt to improve communications and enhance treatment outcomes.

2. *Evaluating the effects of health care environments.* Health care institutions, such as general and mental hospitals, can be seen as 'subcultures' having strong influences on the lives of both staff and clients. Persons with chronic illnesses and disabilities requiring long term care might come to view themselves and their life situations from an 'institutionalized' perspective. The development of critical theories in these areas is particularly relevant for understanding the influences of health care environments. Research findings in this area have been applied to devise strategies for empowering people such as those with intellectual disabilities to live and participate in the community.

3. *Relating to people with neurological or psychiatric problems.* People diagnosed as suffering from problems such as schizophrenia, intellectual disability or brain disorders may, to some extent, experience themselves and the world in ways different from 'normal' people. How such persons experience aspects of their world is by no means obvious, as these clients may demonstrate severe information processing impairments, such as delusions, hallucinations or memory problems, which may make it extremely difficult to establish empathic relationships. However, in order to ensure that persons with such severe impairments or disabilities are treated appropriately and with understanding as persons, health professionals must learn to see things from their perspectives. Qualitative field research has provided evidence which has helped to clarify the personal perspectives of people with severe disabilities.

The above are some obvious examples where qualitative research is appropriate for clarifying personal meanings, and enhancing understanding and communication in health care settings. Of course, personal meanings are relevant to *all* health care situations, not only in the obviously difficult area discussed above. The following exemplify questions which are appropriately approached through field research strategies:

- What is it like to have a speech disorder; in what ways does it disrupt the person's life, from their points of view?
- How do caregivers interact with terminally ill patients? How do health professionals experience the death of a patient?
- How do health professionals break the news of unfavourable diagnoses, such as heart disease, to their patients? How are such situations seen from the perspectives of the health professional or the patients?

Qualitative field research is particularly relevant in professional areas such as occupational therapy, nursing or family medicine where a personal closeness and understanding between the health professional and the client is an essential part of the therapeutic process. In other areas, such as surgery, radiography or pathology, the technical aspects of the practice are seen as more important and this is reflected in the predominance of quantitative approaches.

We are arguing that quantitative and qualitative field research should be seen as complementary; the former contributing to the technical development of practices and the latter defining the personal and social frameworks in which health care is delivered.

THE INTEGRATION OF QUANTITATIVE AND QUALITATIVE METHODOLOGIES

When used jointly, quantitative research tools can be particularly powerful. One of the authors has recently conducted a study of how people evaluate primary health services (Thomas et al 1993a). The first step in this process was to conduct focus group interviews (see Ch. 10) with 20 groups of eight participants specifically selected from a wide range of ethnic backgrounds, ages and sexes. The groups were conducted by a facilitator who presented nine questions concerned with knowledge and opinions of, and satisfaction with, health services. The discussions were recorded and transcribed.

One set of analyses of the transcripts involved consideration of everything that had been said about the health services with regard to satisfaction or dissatisfaction. This resulted in 39 separate categories or themes. These themes, therefore, were directly derived from the participants' own words and interpretations of their experiences.

The themes were then framed in the form of questions that sought information from people about their satisfaction and dissatisfaction with health services. The questions were then incorporated into a questionnaire (see Ch. 9). When the questionnaire was piloted with a sample of 500 people who attended several doctors' surgeries over a period of three weeks, it was found that none of the participants nominated new factors that affected their satisfaction and dissatisfaction. Thus, the procedure used in developing the questionnaire had very effectively captured how people decided whether they were satisfied or dissatisfied with their health services. This study is an example of where qualitative and quantitative research methodologies can combine powerfully.

THE VALIDITY OF QUALITATIVE FIELD RESEARCH

It should be noted that the unstructured and descriptive nature of the data collection process in field research often sits uneasily with those favouring 'quantitative' research strategies. The major problem with the unstructured data collection techniques is that observer bias may cloud or distort the data being collected. As previously discussed, there are well known observer effects such as the Rosenthal effect and the Hawthorne effect. Structured data collection methods are most likely to control for these effects, although there are not guarantees that they will be eliminated.

Furthermore, the sampling processes involved in qualitative field research are complex. Most social phenomena are profoundly affected by their participants. 'Real' situations may not reflect these biases. An important issue in understanding qualitative research is the specific culture dependence of the findings; what is true in one social setting may not be true in another.

Therefore, as in other types of research, qualitative field studies also have to confront problems of external and internal validity. Guba and Lincoln (1983) recommended a variety of strategies to ensure the validity and reliability of field studies. These strategies included:

- Asking subjects if the observations about them are credible (believable)
- Prolonged engagement by the observers to minimize distortions caused by their presence
- Triangulations, which involved pitting against each other different data and theoretical interpretations, so as to provide cross checks of observations and interpretations.

Therefore, in spite of controversies in the area, qualitative field researchers pay considerable attention to methodological issues to ensure the adequacy (that is, validity and reliability) of their investigations. The situation is essentially no different to quantitative research, although qualitative researchers take somewhat ~~different steps to ensure the accuracy and generalizability of their empirical~~ findings.

SUMMARY

Qualitative field research strategies include data collection which is aimed at understanding persons in their social environments. Rather than generating numerical data supporting or refuting clear cut hypotheses, field research aims to produce accurate descriptions based on face-to-face knowledge of individuals and social groups in their natural settings. The role of the observer in this context is crucial, and usually involves physical and social closeness between the subject and the observer. Data collection involves objective and accurate reporting of the activities and appearances of persons in their natural environments. As with other strategies of research, investigators must pay considerable attention to the external and internal validity of field research. We briefly looked at some ways in which field researchers can cross check their descriptions in an attempt to ensure the validity of their reports and interpretations.

Different research designs may be used to generate evidence of the same processes, although from different perspectives. For instance, any complex clinical phenomenon, such as schizophrenia, may be studied using any of the research strategies outlined in Chapters 4–8. In fact, to understand the scope of the problems and the effectiveness of the appropriate treatments, it is desirable to use a variety of research strategies. Conversely, a comprehensive theory of a clinical problem should generate any number of hypotheses within the realm of the research strategies discussed in this book.

SELF ASSESSMENT

Explain the meaning of the terms:

personal meaning
qualitative field research
quantitative research
ethnomethodology
critical theory
phenomenology
empathy

True or false

1. Qualitative field researchers focus on individuals behaving in their natural environments.

2. According to Lofland (1971), the field researcher should maintain a 'distance' from subjects in a physical and social sense.
3. A problem with unstructured data collection techniques is the possible distortion of the evidence through observer bias.
4. The basic aim of qualitative field research is to test clearly defined hypotheses.
5. It is essential in qualitative field research to place disadvantaged or oppressed people in a 'good light', to further their needs or causes.
6. Qualitative field researchers need not concern themselves with issues of validity.
7. Qualitative field research generally involves the use of precision instruments to measure specific subject variables.
8. Qualitative field research generally produces intimate, face-to-face knowledge of other individuals.
9. Phenomenologists are concerned with the understanding of the nature of human conscious experience.
10. Quantitative research produces data well suited to the formulation of causal models.
11. Quantitative research is most appropriate for interpreting personal meanings in social settings.
12. Quantitative research is best suited to discovering how biological systems work.

Multiple choice

1. Qualitative field research involves:
    a the testing of clear cut hypotheses by employing sophisticated measuring instruments.
    b empathy with subjects of view
    c structured data collection
    d carrying out of research in the open air.

2. Which of the following is not an example of qualitative field research?
    a A researcher studying nursing conditions in major hospitals spends a week working as a nurse aide at Prince Henry's Hospital.
    b An anthropologist goes to live with a New Guinea tribe to find out about their religious practices.
    c A psychologist studying therapeutic processes attends group therapy as a client.
    d A speech pathologist compares two rival methods of treatment for stuttering.
    e A physiotherapy student spends a day in a wheelchair and uses this experience to write a report on some of the problems of the physically handicapped.

3. Which of the following disciplines would most likely employ qualitative designs?
   a nuclear physics
   b anatomy
   c genetics
   d sociology.

4. The medical model, as discussed in Chapter 1, is best supported by:
   a qualitative field research
   b quantitative research
   c philosophical speculation
   d all of the above.

5. Which of the following is *not* a characteristic of quantitative research?
   a A holistic approach to persons
   b Precise definition of variables being studied
   c Prediction and control of phenomena
   d Theories including causal models.

6. An important basis of qualitative field research is:
   a phenomenology
   b numerology
   c measurement theory
   d the medical model.

7. A psychiatrist is interested in research to identify the relationship between brain dopamine levels and the occurance of specific well defined abnormal behaviours. This research would be:
   a based on phenomenological principles
   b a project in an ethnomethodological framework
   c a quantitative project
   d best described as qualitative field research.

DISCUSSION, QUESTIONS AND ANSWERS

The health sciences clinical researcher has a rich variety of research designs from which he or she may choose; including the experimental, survey, single case and qualitative field approaches. Each approach has its unique strengths.

The experimental and single case designs are particularly suited to studies of the effects of health interventions. These are studies that are concerned with the clinical impact of administering different types of interventions (or non-intervention) upon people. In the classical two group experimental study, similar groups of people are administered with either an intervention or a non-intervention condition and their outcomes are compared. The use of non-intervention with people who are ill has moral and ethical implications. So, often the experimental method is used to study the relative effects of two or more different types of intervention. There has been an affinity between the professions where health interventions are the norm and a form of enquiry which also involves intervention (i.e. the experimental and single case types of research design). However, much high quality health sciences research involves other types of research design.

Sample surveys are frequently employed to study the opinions of large groups of people concerning health services and their experiences of health and illness. Epidemiological research, which is aimed at studying the distribution of health and illness and associated risk factors in populations, generally involves large scale sample surveys. These surveys often draw upon hospital and other health agency records.

Qualitative field research involves the disciplined examination of the personal meanings of individuals' experiences and actions in the context of their social environment. The emphasis in such research is upon depth of interpretation rather than extent of sampling. Therefore such studies typically employ much smaller samples of participants than, for example, sample surveys.

It is useful to consider examples of the application of the various techniques to the same type of research questions.

Let us consider the situation of people with back injuries associated with manual labour. The major problem associated with back injuries is disability arising from pain. In countries such as the United States and Australia older workers who come from non-English speaking backgrounds are over-represented amongst people with these injuries. This is probably because such people are over represented in jobs that have a greater risk of back injury and the effects are cumulative over a long period of time.

Experimental example

Let us consider an example of where a clinical researcher is interested in comparing the effectiveness of two alternate interventions for treatment of the back injury. There are two common approaches: a conservative approach

121

such as physiotherapy, and surgery. So if we took 20 workers with back injuries and, after random allocation, 10 of them were treated with a conservative intervention such as physiotherapy and 10 were treated with surgery, we could compare their outcomes.

To achieve a true experimental design, the people need to be randomly allocated to surgery or physiotherapy. Incidentally, to implement this procedure in real life would require a lot of talking to the relevant ethics committees. All the participants would have to volunteer.

As far as the measurement of outcome is concerned, most experimental studies would employ a quantitative measure of outcome. For example, the workers could fill in a pain questionnaire, perhaps on several occasions after the intervention, in order to compare the outcomes for the two groups. The use of a written questionnaire, especially if it is provided in English only to people from a non-English speaking background, makes assumptions about the literacy of the participants which may or may not be valid.

Natural comparison example

If the clinical staff had chosen the interventions for the patients on a non-random basis, the study as described above would be a natural comparison study. Simply comparing groups does not mean we have an experimental design. Otherwise, the study could be structured in an identical fashion to the experimental example described above.

Single case example

A single case design involves the administration and withdrawal of interventions in a systematic fashion in order to observe their impact upon the phenomenon under study. The person in the single case trial is usually challenged with varied interventions to compare the effects of each. This type of design closely approximates the natural clinical history of interventions with many patients, particularly those with chronic illness. However, the interventions in a single case study are structured much more rigorously.

In the present context, while it would be possible to administer and withdraw physiotherapy and to have baseline phases of no treatment, the surgical intervention cannot be withdrawn. Once the surgery is done, it permanently and drastically changes the person's body. Therefore a single case example could involve the alternation of baseline (no treatment) and physiotherapy and then, as the last link in the chain of events, the surgery. This is not a methodologically strong design, as there could be carry-over effects from the previous interventions that interact with the surgery, and the order of the administration of the surgery could not be readily altered.

Survey example

An alternative way of conducting the study of workers with back injuries would be to select a large group of such people and survey them concerning the different types of interventions they have had for their injury. The outcomes for different groups could then be compared, because, as in a natural comparison study, we can compare groups in a survey design. For example, we could compare men and women respondents. We could even give them the same pain questionnaire as in the types of study previously discussed.

Surveys, of course, do not necessarily involve the use of questionnaires. One could bypass the patients and survey their medical records (with the necessary approvals) and use a coding schedule. Alternatively, the information could be collected in the form of a structured survey interview.

Qualitative field research example

An additional way of studying this issue would be to conduct in-depth interviews with a small number of injured workers to study their interpretations of their situation. Workers who had surgery, as well as those who had physiotherapy, could be interviewed. The interviews would normally be recorded verbatim, transcribed and then exhaustively analysed for the theoretical constructs needed to describe the experiences of the participants. The use of checklists, survey inventories and the like is normally avoided, although it is usual to have a list of issues to be introduced by the interviewer. The respondent typically describe their experiences and perceptions in their own natural discourse.

In studies which use questionnaires, there is limited interaction between the researcher and the respondent. As is suggested by their name, the respondents respond to the questions framed solely by the researcher. Such an approach can be useful in eliciting factual information in an economical manner. However, it places the respondent in a relatively passive role. If the researcher and the respondent do not share the same constructs, ideas, feelings and motives, the 'wrong' questions may be asked. Schatzman and Strauss (1973, p. 57) note that the researcher 'harbors, wittingly or not, many expectations, conjectures and hypotheses which provide him with thought and directives on what to look for and what to ask about'. The respondent in most questionnaire studies has very little opportunity to contribute to the research agenda. Generally, a token 'any other comments' section is the extent of the invitation for the respondent to contribute to this agenda.

Questions

1. What would be the 'best' design to study the impact of physiotherapy and surgery upon the pain of workers with back injuries?
2. If the participant has been measured frequently over an extended time period, what type of data analysis is required?
3. What type of research design does an epidemiologist typically employ?
4. What special arrangements should be made for participants in research studies with low literacy in English?

5. Is it possible to use an experimental design with in-depth interviewing techniques?

Answers

1. No doubt this question will generate much lively debate. The authors' view is that there is no single 'best' method to conduct such investigations. Each of the methods listed has legitimate insights to offer, which provide a perspective different from that of the others, provided the study is conducted well. Vive la difference!
2. This type of design requires an analysis method that can handle repeated measures data, i.e. this is a repeated measures design.
3. Although they may use a variety of different designs, the epidemiologist is likely to use large scale surveys, often of clinical records. The goal of epidemiologists is to determine the patterns of distribution of illnesses and their relationship with risk factors. Although the modelling may be complex, the research design is simple. Do a big survey.
4. Clinical researchers, who are often fluent in English, frequently do not make appropriate arrangements for participants with levels of literacy in English lower than their own. Such arrangements could include the provision of interpreters, translated instructions and questionnaires, and interviewers to read the questions to the participants.
5. Yes it is possible to do so, however, it is very unusual. Experimenters typically employ quantitative outcome measures and researchers who use in-depth interviews tend to be disinclined to use experimental research designs. Perhaps both could learn from the other?

Data collection

There are numerous methods available for data collection. The appropriate methods are chosen depending on the aims, design and resources of the research project.

Questionnaires are commonly used with survey designs. In Chapter 9 we examine a number of ways in which we can draw up and validate questionnaires. There are different types of questionnaires ranging from highly structured, standardized scales to unstructured open-ended formats.

An interview (see Ch. 10) is, in a sense, a conversation between the interviewer and the person being interviewed. As they require the presence of an interviewer, this increases the cost and effort needed to obtain data. Also, the presence of an interviewer may, in various situations, influence the respondent's answers. Qualitative research studies often employ in-depth interviewing techniques which are preferably carried out in the 'natural' settings (homes, hospital, etc.) in which the respondents are living or receiving treatment.

Observational methods are also commonly used strategies for data collection. They may range from highly structured observational protocols, indicating precisely which behaviours or clinical signs should be recorded, to unstructured records of the experiences of participant observers, as used in qualitative research.

Depending on how the data is recorded and analysed, interviews and observations may be used for both quantitative and qualitative research. However, the use of instrumentation to produce numerical data is most appropriate for quantitative research. There is today a variety of standardised measurement instruments available for measuring biological and psychological functions (see Ch. 10).

Whatever data collection strategy is being used, we must ensure that it is reliable (replicable) and valid (accurate). Otherwise, as discussed in Chapter 12; the measurement error due to unreliable and invalid data collection strategies may prevent the researchers from achieving their goals.

9

Questionnaire design

INTRODUCTION

In research investigations, information can be collected through the application of a variety of techniques such as interviews, questionnaires, observation, direct physical measurement and the use of standardized tests. This chapter focuses on questionnaires and questionnaire design, since they are frequently used to collect data in health sciences research.

The specific aims of this chapter are to:

1. Introduce basic concepts in questionnaire design
2. Discuss the construction and administration of questionnaires.

QUESTIONNAIRE CONSTRUCTION

A questionnaire is a document designed with the purpose of seeking specific information from the respondents. Questionnaires are best used with literate people. The design of the questionnaire is crucial to its success. The process of design and implementation is usually termed questionnaire construction.

Questionnaire construction usually involves the following steps:

1. The researcher defines the information that is being sought. This may involve a lot of thinking and discussion. Inspiration for selection of the required information comes from the investigator's research objectives, discussions with others, reading and other sources. At this stage, the document is typically a list of information yet to be translated into specific question form.

2. Drafting of the questionnaire. The researcher next takes the list of information they wish to obtain from the respondent and attempts to devise draft questions. As is discussed later in this chapter, the phrasing and design of the questions and the overall design of the questionnaire are important for the validity of the obtained information. If the questionnaire is badly designed, then the responses may not accurately reflect the real situation for the respondents.

3. Questionnaire pilot. It is wise to pilot or trial a new questionnaire with a small group of the intended respondents and with clinical or research colleagues, in order to improve its clarity and remove any problems, before the main survey. The pilot respondents may be asked whether the questions were clear.

4. *Redrafting of the questionnaire*. If the pilot phase uncovers problems with the questionnaire, it will need to be redrafted in order to address these problems. If they are of a major nature, it is usual to repeat the pilot phase. If they are minor, the researcher may make the necessary changes and then proceed to administration of the questionnaire to the full sample of respondents.

5. *Administration of the questionnaire*. After the questionnaire has been developed, it is administered to the full sample of respondents. The responses are then analysed in terms of the researcher's aims and objectives.

As with all research, the ethics of conducting surveys and designing questionnaires must be considered. For instance, respondents should not be misled concerning the aims of a survey. A blatant example of unethical conduct is if one is asked to respond to a general 'market survey' and then to find a high-pressure salesperson on the doorstep. If the survey is said to be anonymous, then it is questionable practice by the investigator to secretly code the forms. The follow-up of non-responders can cause a dilemma; people choosing not to participate in a survey should not be pestered. On the other hand, forms are sometimes mislaid or forgotten and it is necessary to follow these up to ensure a representative sample.

In clinical research, the ethical issues relating to the possible effect of the contents of the questionnaire on the respondent must be taken into account. As an example, one of the present authors was involved in a survey aimed at establishing levels of knowledge of Huntington's disease and certain attitudes of people at risk with the condition (Telsher & Polgar 1981). Before the survey was undertaken, a pilot study was carried out to establish whether or not the questions were upsetting to the subjects. The actual subjects were randomly selected from a 'pedigree chart'. However, the questionnaires could not be sent out before it was clearly established that each of the prospective subjects already knew that they were at risk of developing the condition. It would have been appalling if a person learned from receiving this questionnaire that they were at risk of a severe genetic disorder.

QUESTION AND QUESTIONNAIRE FORMATS

Questions and questionnaires come in a variety of formats. The researcher must decide which is the most appropriate for the purpose of the study. Let us first consider the issue of the questionnaire format.

In some instances, researchers will not prepare a formal questionnaire to be filled in by the respondent, but will design an interview schedule to guide the interviewer who asks the questions. (Interviews are discussed in Chapter 10.) There are costs and benefits in both approaches, as shown in Table 9.1.

The interview schedule approach requires expert interviewers to administer the questions and this is expensive and time-consuming. Further, interviewer bias has been shown to influence responses, as respondents modify their responses to fit in with what they perceive to be the opinions of the interviewer. It is important to note that the structure and content of a questionnaire conveys a lot of information about the researcher's agenda to the respondent. The

Table 9.1 Costs and benefits of interviews and questionnaires

	Costs	Benefits
Interview schedule administered by interviewer	Expensive to administer; requires expert help Responses much more susceptible to interviewer bias	Lower rejection rate More detailed responses can be elicited Greater control over filling out of response form
Self-administered questionnaire	Higher rejection rate Difficult to elicit detailed responses Less control over how response form is filled out	Cheap to administer Less susceptible to interviewer bias Can be administrated by mail

respondent generally has little opportunity to influence the agenda. A questionnaire is not a conversation but a monologue from the researcher to which the potential respondent may or may not respond.

However, the self administrated questionnaire approach is cheap, is less susceptible to interviewer bias, and can be administered by mail. The disadvantages of this approach include higher rejection or refusal rates and much less control over how the response forms are filled out. Anyone involved in self-administered questionnaire analysis will attest to the sometimes remarkable talents of respondents in returning incomplete questionnaire response forms.

Having decided whether the questionnaire will be self-administered or administered by interviewers, the researcher must then decide upon the format for the individual questions.

Open-ended and closed response formats

There are two major question formats, the open-ended and closed response types. The distinction between the two is best illustrated by example:

Question 1 is an open-ended question whereas the second question is a closed response question. In an open-ended question, there is no predetermined response

Table 9.2 Open-ended and closed response formats

Q1. How do you feel about the standard of the treatment you received while you were a patient at this hospital?

....
....
....

Q2. How would you rate the standard of the treatment you received while you were a patient at this hospital? (circle one number)

excellent	1
good	2
moderately good	3
fair	4
poor	5

schedule into which the respondent must fit his/her response. In a closed response question, the respondent is supplied with a predetermined list of response options.

The advantages and disadvantages of both question types are represented in Table 9.3.

Table 9.3 Costs and benefits of open-ended and closed response formats

	Costs	**Benefits**
Open-ended	Less structured Responses difficult to encode and analyse using powerful statistical methods Greater time taken by respondent to answer Respondent may find writing an essay more difficult than circling a number	More detailed answers elicited
Closed response	Less 'depth' in answers May frustrate respondents	Tightly structured Responses easily encoded and analysed Less time taken to collect responses

Although open-ended questions elicit more detailed responses, there are some possible disadvantages associated with this question type. The responses generated by such questions require a large amount of effort to encode for data analysis and tend to give rise to categorical scales. These scales necessitate the use of less powerful statistical methods. Further, some respondents may take a long time to answer this type of question.

Of course, to a researcher employing qualitative orientation, these 'disadvantages' may not be seen as such. The opportunity to study the respondent's interpretations expressed in their own words might lead a qualitative researcher to advocate extensive use of open-ended questions. It is more likely that interview techniques rather than a written questionnaire would be employed. Questionnaires, particularly of the self-administered variety, are generally for convenience and speed, not depth of analysis.

It is important that the lists of options for closed response questions are carefully designed by the questionnaire designer. It is very easy to bias responses by restricting the range of answers in this type of question.

This brings to mind a short questionnaire distributed by an insurance company to one of the authors. It read as follows:

Table 9.4

Why did you choose XYZ Insurance to insure your car?

❐ Newspaper advertisement
❐ TV advertisement
❐ Personal recommendation
❐ Previous insurance with us

Two features are remarkable about this question. First, it does not allow for any answers other than the ones listed. Second, the range of available answers is very limited. What we wanted to say was that the insurers were cheap and reliable, i.e. were likely to pay up in the event of a claim. Clearly, the survey designer was a marketing person who had not satisfactorily trialled the questions with a non-marketing audience. While the designers may well have obtained the answers they wanted, the answers may not have been the ones the respondents wished to give. In the health sciences, there are often large differences in the ways in which health professionals and consumers approach the same problems. In questionnaire design, it is vital that the researchers do not impose their own conceptualizations of the situations under investigation to the extent that validity is compromised.

A further example of this danger is provided by the results of a survey conducted at a major teaching children's hospital in Australia (Thomas McCoy & Smith 1989). The survey was designed to study why many parents chose to stay with their children in the hospital in order to plan better facilities and services. One of the questions asked of the respondents was 'Why did your child come to hospital today'? The investigators deliberately chose an open-ended response format for this question in order to tap into the parents' interpretations of the situation in their own words. What a treasure trove of answers! The answers provided considerable insight into the issues of importance to the parents, most of which we could not have predicted. Thus, the ways in which the questions are asked and the answers sought can have a major impact on the value of the information collected.

Likert and forced choice response formats

In attitudinal questions, two possible response formats may be chosen, the traditional five or seven point Likert-type format, or the four point forced choice format. These are best illustrated by examples as shown in Table 9.5.

Table 9.5 Likert and forced choice response formats

Q7. My medical practitioner always explains the chosen treatment to me (circle one number).

strongly agree	1
agree	2
undecided	3
disagree	4
strongly disagree	5

Q8. My medical practitioner always explains the chosen treatment to me (circle one number).

strongly agree	1
agree	2
disagree	3
strongly disagree	4

The first example is a conventional five point Likert-type scale. The second is a four point forced choice type. The advantages and disadvantages are summarized in Table 9.6.

The forced choice format does not allow respondents to give a 'middle of the road' or undecided answer. This is to guard against respondents using an **acquiescent response mode**. Acquiescent response mode refers to the phenomenon that occurs when respondents give middle responses all the time. **Extreme response mode** occurs when a respondent never selects an intermediate point on the rating scale.

Table 9.6 Advantages and disadvantages of response formats

Response format	Advantages	Disadvantages
Likert-type	Allows middle 'undecided' response	Acquiescent response mode
Forced choice	Respondent forced to give either a positive or a negative response	'Undecided' response not allowed

The wording and design of questions

The writing of good questions is an art, and a time consuming art at that. In order to obtain valid and reliable responses one needs well-worded questions. There are a number of pitfalls to be avoided:

Double-barrelled questions. This is where two questions are included in the one, 'Do you like maths or science?' for example. These questions should be separated so that it is perfectly clear to the respondent (and the researcher) which component is being answered.

Ambiguous questions. It is important to avoid vacuous words and terms that may mean different things to different people. For example, 'old people' may mean everyone above thirty to a teenager, but everyone above 60 to a 50-year-old.

Level of wording. It is important to tailor the level of wording of questions to accord with the intended respondents. Jargon is to be avoided, and it should be established in the pilot study that the respondents will understand the concepts. For instance, asking questions about 'Trisomy 21' might be inappropriate while 'mongolism' or 'Down syndrome' could be intelligible. Using double negatives should be avoided. In general, questions should be simple and concise.

Bias and leading questions. The wording of the question should not lead the respondent to feel committed to respond in a certain way. For example, the question 'How often do you go to church'?' may lead the respondent to respond in a way that is not entirely truthful if they in fact never go to church. Not only can the wording of a question be leading but the response format may also be leading. For example, if a 'never' response were excluded from the available answers to the above question, the respondent would be led to respond in an inaccurate way.

Bias might also arise from possible carry-over effects from answering a pattern of questions. For instance, a questionnaire on health workers' attitudes to abortion might include the questions 'Do you value human life?' followed by 'Do you think unborn babies should be murdered in their mothers' wombs?'. In this case, the respondent is being led both by the context in which the second question is asked and the bias involved in the emotional wording of the questions. Surely, one would have to be a monster to answer 'yes' to the second question, given the way it was asked.

Finally, it should be kept in mind that even a good questionnaire might be invalidly administered. For instance, a survey on 'Attitudes to migration' might be answered less than honestly by respondents if the interviewer is obviously of immigrant background.

THE STRUCTURE OF QUESTIONNAIRES

Questionnaires may be structured in different ways, but typically the following components are included.

1. Introductory statement. The introductory statement describes the purpose of the questionnaire, the information sought and how it is to be used. It also introduces the researchers and explains whether the information is confidential and/or anonymous.

2. Demographic questions. It is usual to collect information about the respondents, including details such as age, sex, education history and so on. It is best to position these questions first as they are easily answered and serve as a 'warm-up' to what follows.

3. Factual questions. It is generally easier for respondents to answer direct factual questions e.g. 'Do you have a driver's licence?' than to answer opinion questions. Often, this type of question is positioned early on in the questionnaire also to serve as a 'warm up'!

4. Opinion questions. Questions that require reflection on the part of the respondent are usually positioned after the demographic and factual questions.

5. Closing statements and return instructions. The closing statements in a questionnaire usually thank the respondent for their participation, invite the respondents to take up any issues they feel have not been satisfactorily addressed in the questionnaire and provide information on how to return the questionnaire.

It is best to avoid complicated structures involving, for example, many conditional questions such as 'If you answered yes to Question 6 and not to Question 9, please answer Question 10'. Conditional questions usually confuse respondents and ought be avoided where possible.

SUMMARY

Questionnaires are frequently used for data collection in health sciences research. This chapter has reviewed the principles of questionnaire design, including issues arising from the selection of appropriate questions and response formats.

SELF ASSESSMENT

Explain the meaning of the following terms:

acquiescent response mode   Likert-type scale
bias   open-ended format
closed response format   piloting
extreme response mode   questionnaire
forced response format

True or false

1. The aim of survey research is to manipulate the attitudes or beliefs of the respondents.
2. A questionnaire is a measuring instrument which can be employed across a variety of research strategies.
3. If the draft questionnaire is well constructed, there is no need for 'piloting'.
4. As a questionnaire can cause no illness or pain, there is no need to worry about ethical issues when using this instrument.
5. The advantage of an interview schedule over a self-administered questionnaire is that interviews are generally cheaper and less time-consuming to administer.
6. Open-ended questions are easier to analyse and interpret than closed response questions.
7. If we send out 100 copies of a well constructed self-administered questionnaire we can expect that at least 95 correctly filled-in forms will be returned.
8. A forced choice response format does not allow for 'undecided' responses.
9. 'Acquiescent response mode' refers to the phenomenon where respondents agree with only extreme points on a scale.
10. Survey research is more closely related to naturalistic designs than to true experimental designs.

Multiple choice

1. In which of the following ways is survey research similar to an experimental research design?
   a the selection of a representative sample from the population
   b the assignment of subjects into treatment groups
   c the manipulation of the independent variable by the investigator
   d *a* and *c*.

2. When a survey is employed as a research strategy:
   a the making of causal inferences from the data may be problematic
   b we must use a questionnaire for data collection
   c the respondents must be anonymous
   d the external validity of the investigation will be automatically assured.

3. Questionnaires:
   a might have ethical problems associated with their design and administration
   b are instruments for data collection
   c can be employed in experimental research
   d all of the above.

4. Redrafting a questionnaire involves:
   a eliminating questions which are not answered in the predicted direction
   b asking the 'pilot' subjects to write the questionnaire
   c rewriting the questionnaire on the basis of feedback from the 'pilot' administration
   d rewriting the questionnaire in such a way that 'pilot' subjects will select responses which are consistent with the investigator's predictions.

5. The question 'Do you attend gay parties?' is:
   a double-barrelled
   b leading
   c ambiguous
   d an acquiescent response.

6. The question 'Are you presently taking b-blockers?' is:
   a double-barrelled
   b ambiguous
   c biased
   d at the wrong level of difficulty.

7. The advantage(s) of an interview schedule approach over a self-administered questionnaire is that:
   a it is cheaper to administer
   b there is greater control over administration
   c observer bias is minimized
   d people who look a little odd need not be interviewed
   e all of the above.

Do you think it is important for undergraduate students in the health sciences to study statistics (circle one)?

Strongly agree
Agree
Undecided
Disagree
Strongly disagree.

8. The above is an example of:
   a an open-ended question
   b a Likert scale
   c a double-barrelled question
   d a leading question
   e none of the above.

9. The advantage of a closed response format over an open-ended response format is that:
   a more 'in depth' responses can be elicited
   b there is a lower response rate
   c the responses are easily encoded and analysed
   d it is more likely that the actual attitudes or feelings of the respondents will be revealed.

10

Interview techniques and the analysis of interview data

An interview may be defined as a conversation between interviewers and interviewees with the purpose of eliciting certain information.

Interviews are a key tool for the clinician and the health researcher as a means of collecting information. However, interviews may vary substantially in their structure, content and the way in which the data are elicited and analysed. This chapter is concerned with interviews and the analysis of interview data.

The specific aims of this chapter are to:

1. Distinguish between structured and unstructured interviews
2. Outline commonly used strategies for conducting interviews
3. Compare and contrast quantitative and qualitative strategies for conducting interviews.

Structured and unstructured interviews

Many researchers distinguish between structured and unstructured interviews. Sometimes the terms 'formal' and 'informal' or 'guided' and 'open-ended' are also used (see for example, Field & Morse 1985).

Denzin (1978, p. 113–116) distinguishes between three forms of the interview: the schedule standardized interview in which 'the wording and order of all questions are exactly the same for every respondent', the nonschedule standardized interview where 'certain types of information are desired from all respondents but the particular phrasing of questions and their order are redefined' and the nonstandardized interview in which 'no prescribed set of questions is employed'.

If one defines an interview as a conversation, then a schedule standardized interview is a very rigid form of conversation, almost like a play with a fixed script.

In its most structured form, a structured interview may involve the reading of a prepared questionnaire to a respondent and then filling in an answer form or response sheet for them on the basis of their answers. The questions are provided in a systematic order, with minimal or no deviation from the prepared script. In a structured interview, the role of the interviewer is to ask the questions and the role of the respondent is to provide the answers with minimal extraneous information. On the other hand, an unstructured interview may involve the interviewer in asking no direct questions, but simply prompting the respondent to reflect on their current interests and concerns. Clearly, between these extremes lies a variety of different types of interview strategies and degrees of structure. The extent of 'structure' or 'formality' is determined by a number of factors, including the following:

1. Whether there is a fixed set of questions or schedule. In a structured interview, the interviewer has a preplanned set of questions or schedule. These questions may or may not be presented in a fixed order. In an unstructured interview, there may be particular 'themes' to be explored without a specific order required nor specific question wordings.

2. The way in which the information is recorded. There are a number of ways in which interview information may be recorded. (This is discussed in detail in a later section of this chapter). Structured interviews tend to employ preplanned answer sheets or response schedules. Unstructured interviews have less expectations and restrictions on the answer formats of the respondents. The interviewer may record the interview or take free-form notes.

3. The types of questions. Structured interviews tend to employ more closed response questions, in which the valid answers have been preplanned, rather than open ended questions. As discussed in the survey chapter of this text, with open ended questions the respondents provide their answers in their own words, whereas closed response questions involve a choice of answers provided by the interviewer.

4. The extent of control by the interviewer. In a structured interview, the interviewer explicitly guides or directs the conversation (e.g. 'Now Mr. Smith, lets discuss how your family feels about your problem') rather than the respondent setting the agenda. In an unstructured interview, the respondent may assume a more active role in the conversation.

It is useful to consider some of the advantages and disadvantages of the different types of interview approaches. These are summarized in Table 10.1.

Table 10.1 Advantages and disadvantages of structured and unstructured interviews

	Advantages	**Disadvantages**
Structured interviews	May be less time consuming The same information is collected for all respondents	Responses may not be recorded in the respondents' own words
Unstructured interviews	Responses may be recorded in the 'own words' of the respondents, hence less bias through interpretation The respondent has some input into the research agenda	May be time consuming Not all the same information is collected for all respondents

The appropriateness of the different interview approaches is determined by the objectives of the researcher. If the researcher simply wished to collect some basic symptom data, an unstructured interview would be inefficient. However, if the researcher wished to study people's conceptualization and interpretation of their illness, an unstructured interview may be quite suitable.

Some clinical interviews such as history taking are highly structured whereas other clinical interviews such as those involving management of a long term problem may be less so.

Methods of conducting interviews

As an interview is a conversation, there exist several possible methods for conducting an interview. The interview may be conducted in person, 'face to face' so to speak, or by remote means such as by telephone. There are a number of advantages associated with face to face interview. (These are also discussed in the survey chapter of this text). Face-to-face interviews permit the non-verbal reactions of the respondent to be observed and perhaps the development of a closer rapport arising from the more 'natural' setting. The interviewer may use their observations of non-verbal cues to supplement the verbal information being provided and use their own non-verbal cues in a similar fashion. However, the face-to-face interview may require a substantial amount of participant travel time and hence higher costs than for a telephone interview. With certain interview objectives, however, telephone interviews may not be suitable. If the interviewer and their credentials are not well known to the interviewee, it is unlikely that participants in a telephone interview would provide valid and reliable personal information about personal topics. On the other hand, if the interviewer is trusted, some people find disclosure of sensitive information to be easier by telephone. The face to face interview may be too confronting or embarrassing for them.

The interview process

1. Selection of interviewees. One of the interviewer's first tasks is to select those people to be interviewed. In qualitative research, techniques such as random sampling are used infrequently. Rather, the interviewer selects those people who are most likely to provide the required insights into the situation or issue under study, i.e. the 'key informants'.

2. Recruitment of interviewees. The interviewer must then enlist the participation of the interviewees. Typically, the interviewer will contact the potential participant, explain the purposes of the interview and make a number of assurances. These assurances may include anonymity, the ability to vet materials based on the interview and the extent of time involvement of the interviewee. Often, the interviewer might write to the interviewee first and then contact them personally to be less 'confronting'.

3. The interview. The process of the interview varies substantially according to the methodology to be employed by the interviewer. The process of a structured interview is quite different from that of an unstructured interview. Some basic goals are shared however. The desirability of tapping the interviewee's views rather than reflecting those of the interviewer (i.e. maximization of validity) is paramount. To achieve this, interviewers need to be sensitive, non-evaluative, alert and skilled at delivering and sequencing their questions. In in-depth interviewing, multiple interviews may be required. In this type of approach, the emphasis is on depth of analysis with a smaller number of interviewees rather than the breadth of coverage of interviewees offered by a sample survey. Substantial practise and good interpersonal skills are required to achieve competence in interviewing.

4. Follow-up. Having completed the interviews, the interviewer may wish to follow-up the participants. Some interviewers undertake to give the interviewees copies of their findings and may offer the right of vetting the materials based on the interview.

Methods of recording interview information

Interviewers may use a number of different means of recording interview information, ranging from written summary notes of the interview to an actual video or audio taping of the live interview. These recording methods have a number of advantages and disadvantages, as discussed below.

1. Video recording. Video technology has reduced in cost and improved to such an extent that high quality video recordings of interviews are well within the budgets of many organizations and individuals. Video recordings provide a wealth of information about the interview. It is possible to observe non-verbal communication channels as well as to construct audio transcripts of the interaction between the participants. However, some interviewees find the presence of the camera to be threatening. This may have a number of effects; one may be to refuse to participate, another may be to alter the normal flow of the interview. Some respondents may be quite unwilling to commit personal information and/or controversial views to tape, if they believe there is a risk that the interviewer might disclose the interview to others. The interviewee would find it difficult to deny their views when they have been videotaped expressing them. This is why the police in some countries videotape their interviews with suspects!

2. Audio taping. Many interviewers use audio recording of interviews in order to be able to prepare transcripts for later study. Many of the same issues that pertain to video recording are also relevant to audio recording.

The use of audio recording may result in greater refusal rates and the 'sanitization' of the expressed views of participants for fear of reprisals arising from disclosure of the interview to others.

Both video and audio recording of interviews have one large advantage over other methods of recording interview information. This is that the interviewer's interpretation of the interviewee's answers is open to independent scrutiny, because the primary materials are available for study by others.

3. Use of response schedules/answer checklists. When conducting an interview, the interviewer may record the information provided by the interviewee on a predesigned response schedule/answer checklist. For example, the schedule may contain information such as the sex and age of the respondent and areas for recording their answers to particular questions. Typically, the response sheet is completed during the interview, although it can be completed at some time following the interview. Immediate recording is probably more valid and reliable, although, once again, the mere presence of a recording device may be of concern to the respondent. Unless the response sheet is well-designed, there is a major problem of handling novel or unexpected turns in the interview. The interviewer is interpreting, on the fly, the answers and information provided by the interviewee. If those do not conform to the assumptions designed into the response sheet, these interpretations may not be satisfactory or well considered. Telephone interviews may involve the use of computer assistance where the interviewer is prompted by, and records the responses on a computerised schedule.

4. Free form (unstructured) notes. This method of recording involves the interviewer making free form notes to record information they believe to be salient, either during or following the interview. This method of recording is used extensively by clinicians in case notes. There are a number of advantages and problems with such recording, basically resulting from the process whereby the interview is distilled into the notes. This process involves substantial judgment and interpretation on the part of the interviewer. Such distillations result in highly refined and reduced data, the validity of which, at least in terms of the interview, is inaccessible to scrutiny. Further, free form note-taking may not result in the recording of the same type of data across interviewees. Often, when case audits from records are being performed, it is not possible to derive the required data from clinical notes because of this problem. For example, it may be desirable to check whether the use of a particular medication is associated with particular symptoms or side effects. If the information is not recorded by the interviewer, this is an important loss.

Qualitative research methodologists have developed systematic methods in note-taking and coding of interview information. For an excellent treatment of these issues, the reader is referred to Minichiello et al (1991).

Advantages and disadvantages of interview recording methods

The advantages and disadvantages of the various recording methods may be summarized in Table 10.2. Thus, video recording is intrusive, requires substantial post-interview analysis, may result in less disclosure, yet provides very rich information that can be independently analysed. On the other hand, the use of a recording method such as a response sheet requires great trust in the judgment and recording abilities of the interviewer. There is a potential for bias arising from the interviewer 'adjusting' the information provided by the interviewee to fit the recording method and/or expectations of the interviewer. Further, there is no opportunity for re-analysis.

~~So which information recording method for interviews is the most appropriate?~~ The appropriateness of the method of recording interview information is determined by the needs of the person using the information. For example, if the information user simply wants some basic data such as the age, sex and symptom profile of a patient, it would be absurd to use video recording. This would be very time consuming. Each tape would have to be made then viewed again for analysis. In this instance, a simple response sheet or checklist would suffice. On the other hand, if the interviewer was interested in exploring reactions of interviewees to the death of a close relative, perhaps the use of audio or video recording would provide a richness of data suitable for that interest.

Table 10.2 Advantages and disadvantages of different ways of recording interview information

	Advantages	**Disadvantages**
Video recording	Full transcripts of interview possible Non-verbal data available Accessible to independent analysis	Intrusive Less disclosure Necessity for substantial, and costly, post interview analysis Potentially greater rates of refusal to participate
Audio recording	Full transcripts of interview possible Accessible to independent analysis	Intrusive (but probably less than video) Reduced disclosure Necessity for substantial, and costly, post interview analysis Potentially greater rates of refusal to participate
Response sheets	Same data recorded for all interviews Little post-interview analysis required reducing costs	Unexpected answers may not be well handled Interviewer may bias data in its recording Inaccessible to independent analysis
Unstructured notes	Cheap and simple	Interviewer may bias data in its recording some data may be omitted Inaccessible to independent analysis Necessity for some post interview analysis

Although most interviews are conducted with one interviewer and one interviewee present, sometimes group interviews with many participants are conducted. The focus group, which is a form of group interview, involves a discussion amongst a small group of people including a moderator or facilatator (Thomas et al 1992). The facilitators' role is to introduce the topics or questions for discussion and to facilitate the contributions of the group participants. Merton (1946) originally proposed the focussed interview, which was the forerunner for the focus group.

Focus groups differ fundamentally from the individual interview in that the researcher is outnumbered and the participants may interact with each other, modify each others responses and ask questions of each other. The researcher is no longer at the centre of the process. Focus groups are now widely used in health research because they provide rich sources of insights and interpretations from the participants.

The analysis of interview data

The manner in which interview data may be analysed is determined in part by how the data have been recorded and in part, by the theoretical orientation of the researcher. In the previous section, we have seen that these formats include videotapes, audiotapes, completed response sheets and free-form summary interviewer notes.

The basis for many analyses of interview data is the interview transcript. The transcript of an interview is a verbatim written version of the conversation that took place between the participants. To provide an example, an excerpt from an interview transcript produced by Janet Doyle at La Trobe University follows. The transcript is of an interview between a clinician and a client, concerning the client's hearing loss.

CLINICIAN:	Okay. So what are you noticing with your hearing?
CLIENT:	Well in a crowded area I can't you know understand the other people.
CLINICIAN:	Right, sound's a bit jumbled up.
CLIENT:	And when I am in the next room I can't even hear the phone.
CLINICIAN:	Right.
CLIENT:	I am not bad, it is like I am not that bad but still at times.
CLINICIAN:	Right.
CLIENT:	There is a lot of times I can't hear it.
CLINICIAN:	If people speak directly to you like this you are fairly good?
CLIENT:	Yes I am alright.
CLINICIAN:	But in a group have a bit of trouble?
CLIENT:	Have trouble.
CLINICIAN:	Right, does one ear seem better than the other ear?
CLIENT:	Yes, this one seems better than this.
CLINICIAN:	Right.
CLINICIAN:	How long have you been noticing your difficulty?
CLIENT:	Oh about 12 to 18 months I suppose.
CLINICIAN:	Just gradual was it?
CLIENT:	Yes.
CLINICIAN:	Okay. Do you get any ringing or buzzing in your ears?
CLIENT:	Oh now and again, very seldom though.
CLINICIAN:	It doesn't bother you?
CLIENT:	No.

CLINICIAN:	Okay. Have you had medical trouble with your ears like infection or anything?
CLIENT:	No, no.
CLINICIAN:	Do you know of any family history of hearing loss?
CLIENT:	No, only the older brother, he has got a hearing aid.
CLINICIAN:	Right.
CLIENT:	That's all.
CLINICIAN:	Have you been exposed to excessive noise?
CLIENT:	Yes.
CLINICIAN:	... machinery or?
CLIENT:	Yeah. I worked down the car plant you know with the heavy machinery.
CLINICIAN:	The assembly line?
CLIENT:	Right.
CLINICIAN:	Were you doing that sort of work for a long time?
CLIENT:	Oh yes, 30 years.
CLINICIAN:	Yeah, that's a fair...
CLIENT:	I wasn't on the line all the time but.
CLINICIAN:	Right.

And so the interview continued.

Let us consider some of the analysis options under the quantitative and qualitative headings.

Quantitative analysis of interview transcripts

A number of quantitative analyses possibilities are presented with interview transcripts. For example, the researcher might count the number of words spoken by each participant to obtain a quantitative measure of their relative contributions to the conversational process. Another possibility would be to count the number of questions asked by the clinician. These quantitative measures could then be used to test various hypotheses. Analyses of interview transcripts similar to the example shown above, in the study from which it was taken, have demonstrated substantial sex differences between the number of questions asked by male and female clients. It seems that the male clients asked many more questions than the females. Thus, the quantitative researcher might use interview transcripts to count and analyse certain features of the transcripts.

Qualitative analysis of interview transcripts

Under the qualitative heading there is a broad variety of approaches to the collection and analysis of interview data. Such approaches may, however, be broadly categorized as descriptive or theoretical.

A descriptive qualitative study is often termed an ethnography. They are often written from the perspective of the participant(s) in the first person. The purpose of the ethnography is to provide a detailed description of a particular set of circumstances and to encourage the reader to make their own interpretations.

A celebrated example of such an ethnography is found in Bogdan and Taylor's (1976) description of Ed Murphy's life. Ed Murphy was a former resident of a home for the intellectually disabled in the United States.

Many qualitative studies, however, are theoretical in nature. That is, they attempt to develop theories and concepts and, often, to verify these concepts and theories.

A key approach to theoretical qualitative research is provided by Glaser and Strauss' (1967) grounded theory (see also Strauss 1987). Glaser and Strauss advocate two methods for the development of grounded theory: the constant comparative method in which the researcher codes and analyses data to develop concepts and the theoretical sampling method in which cases are selected purposively to refine the 'theory' previously developed. Glaser and Strauss provide highly detailed examples of their analytic methods in the above references and the interested reader is referred to them for further detail.

Glaser and Strauss' approach is not universally accepted in that some qualitative researchers argue for the necessity to both develop and verify their theories. Taylor and Bogdan (1984) provide an extended discussion of these issues.

Notwithstanding these theoretical differences, many qualitative researchers share common analysis tools such as coding and thematic analysis.

Coding and thematic analysis

Coding is used to organize data collected in an interview, and for that matter in other types of documents such as field notes. Different qualitative researchers advocate different approaches to coding but it typically involves the following steps. The researchers first study their materials, in this case transcripts, and develop a close familiarity with the material. During this process, all the concepts, themes and ideas are noted to form major categories. For example, in interviews of nursing home residents, some theme might include personal safety, autonomy and decision making, personal hygiene and so on. Often the researcher will then attach a number or label to each category and record their positions in the transcript. Coding is an iterative process, with the researcher coding and recoding, as the scheme develops. Some computer programs are now available to assist with the coding analysis of machine-readable transcripts and these ease some of the clerical burden, although most qualitative researchers still employ manual coding methods. The researchers, having developed the codes and coded the transcripts, now attempt to interpret their meanings in the context in which they appeared. The reporting of this process typically involves 'thick' or detailed description of the categories and their context, with liberal use of examples from the original transcripts.

SUMMARY

Interviews may be defined as a conversation between interviewers and interviewees with the purpose of eliciting certain information. Structured interviews generally involve a fixed set of questions or schedule, the use of preplanned response sheets, a greater proportion of closed-response questions and direction from the interviewer. Unstructured interviews tend not to have these attributes, with less structure and control. Interviews may be conducted face to face or by telephone and both these methods have certain advantages and disadvantages. The focus group is a valuable alternative to the individual interview. Interview data may be recorded in a number of different ways, but the transcript is often used. Transcripts may be analysed using quantitative or qualitative techniques.

SELF ASSESSMENT

Explain the meaning of the terms:

interview	response schedule
structured interview	transcript
unstructured interview	grounded theory
coding	ethnography

True or false

1. A structured interview always involves a written questionnaire.
2. In an unstructured interview, the questions are asked in a fixed order.
3. In an interview, it is important for the interviewer to express their feelings.
4. In a response schedule, the interviewer records his/her interpretation of the interviewee's statements.
5. Coding is a method of qualitative analysis of interview transcripts.
6. An ethnography is generally written in the third person.
7. A transcript is a summary of the interviewer's interpretation of their questions.
8. Video recording of an interview may affect the honesty of the interviewee's answers.

Multiple choice

1. One of the problems with unstructured interviews is that:
   a the same questions may not be asked of all interviewees
   b the answers are recorded in the interviewee's own words
   c the questions are all asked in the same order
   d the interviews are often shorter in length.

2. One of the problems with structured interviews is that:
   a the same questions may not be asked of all interviewees
   b the answers are not recorded in the interviewee's own words
   c the questions are all asked in the same order
   d the interviews are often too long.

3. One of the advantages of a face to face interview is that:
   a the interviewer can take an audio recording of the interview
   b non-verbal cues can be ignored
   c the interviewer can minimise their influence on the answers
   d the interviewer has more credibility than a telephone interviewer.

4. A qualitative analysis of an interview transcript is likely to include:
   a counting the number of words spoken by each participant
   b the use of a checklist
   c coding of recurrent themes and ideas
   d checks on the quality of the interviewer's speech.

5. A quantitative analysis of an interview transcript is likely to include:
   a the use of unstructured field notes
   b coding of recurrent themes and ideas
   c counting the number of words spoken by each participant
   d checks on the quality of the interviewer's speech.

6. To record the age, sex, height and weight of a patient, it would be best:
   a to use a video recorder
   b to use an audio tape recorder
   c to use a transcript of the interview
   d to use a response checklist.

7. An ethnography is:
   a an interview with a non-English speaking person
   b an interview with a foreign-born but English-speaking person
   c a type of descriptive qualitative study of someone's experiences
   d a type of quantitative study.

8. Coding is:
   a a qualitative method of analysing interview data
   b a method of keeping interview data confidential
   c a quantitative method of analysing interview data
   d usually performed without a written transcript.

11

Observation

INTRODUCTION

Observation is a common method for data collection, both in scientific and health care research as well as in clinical practice. Observation involves being close to things, such that the observer is in a position to directly perceive and record specific aspects of the environment under study. The advantage of observational data collection over questionnaires and interviews in human research is that the researcher is in a position to see and hear how people actually act, rather than their perhaps biased reports and justification of their actions.

The specific aims of the present chapter are to:

1. Outline different approaches to conducting observations and examine their relative advantages
2. Discuss the different roles observers may adopt
3. Examine observation in the context of qualitative and quantitative approaches.

OVERVIEW OF DIFFERENT APPROACHES TO OBSERVATION

Depending on the phenomenon we are studying and the research questions being asked, one or more of a number of different observational approaches may be employed in the data collection. Each of these approaches have associated advantages and disadvantages. The basic issues are:

(i) who is to make the observations
(ii) the settings in which the observations are made
(iii) the use of instrumentation.

1. Self-observation or outside observer. When research involves the observation of human subjects, self-observation becomes possible and at times advantageous. As an example, consider the study of a phenomenon such as pain.

Here the patients themselves are particularly well positioned to provide subjective evidence concerning the intensity and location of pain over a period of time. Figure 11.1 shows a typical chart for guiding self-recorded pain observations in chronic pain patients, which is used in both research and clinical assessment.

	On average, what was your level of pain during today?
Monday	0 1 2 3 4 5 6 7 8 9 10 no pain very intense
Tuesday	0 1 2 3 4 5 6 7 8 9 10 no pain very intense
Wednesday	0 1 2 3 4 5 6 7 8 9 10 no pain very intense

Fig. 11.1 Typical chart for self recorded pain observations

The self-observations of the patients provide data for understanding how patients' pain experiences change over time, events correlating with the onset and offset of the pain and also evidence for evaluating the relative effectiveness of pain management strategies.

Given that the experience of pain may be expressed in the sufferer's overt behaviour, we may observe such pain related behaviours when assessing pain. For instance, in a study involving the comparison of pain behaviours of surgical patients with different cultural backgrounds, independent observers recorded pain related behaviours in patients at agreed upon time intervals during physiotherapy treatments. Figure 11.2 is based on whether the observers recorded a yes or no for each category for each time interval in which the behaviours were sampled.

	Time		
Behaviours	t_1	t_2	t_3
Verbal complaint			
Vocalisation			
Protective response			

Fig. 11.2 Observation guide for recording pain behaviours

There are probable relative advantages and disadvantages to using self-observation or outside observers, as shown in the Table 11.1.

Table 11.1 Advantages and disadvantages of using self-observation or outside observers

	Advantages	Disadvantages
Self-observation	Greater access to subjective experience (introspection) Less intrusive Less expensive	Greater bias Less likely to record accurately Less likely to carry out observation as agreed
Outside observer	Greater objectivity Less bias More likely to record accurately More likely to carry out observations as agreed	Cannot directly access subject's perceptions More intrusive More expensive and time consuming

2. Settings in which observation is conducted. Some disciplines, such as astronomy or geography, focus on phenomena which are best studied as they occur, in their natural settings. Other disciplines, such as anatomy or chemistry are more likely to be studied in a laboratory. In the broad range of health sciences research, phenomena are studied in either laboratory or natural settings, and observational data collection may be appropriate in both of these settings.

The general advantage of laboratory environments is that we can impose a considerable degree of control over extraneous variables which may systematically influence our observations. In addition, equipment for facilitating or recording observations is more readily available. For instance, in the 1960s, Masters and Johnson began a series of studies to examine the physiology of the human sexual response. The controlled laboratory setting and the use of appropriate instrumentation enabled these researchers to observe and record previously undiscovered aspects of human sexual functioning. This work was thought to be fundamental for developing clinically useful interventions aimed at helping people with sexual dysfunctioning.

The disadvantage with laboratory settings is that the phenomenon being observed may change in an artificial setting. This is particularly true for human behaviour, where the social contexts are a fundamental component of the behaviours and experiences. In other words, laboratory research sometimes has problematic ecological validity. Table 11.2 summarises some of the relative advantages and disadvantages of laboratory and natural settings for making observations.

3. Unaided observation or the use of instrumentation. The accurate observation of a variety of phenomena is possible through the unaided senses; for example, observing aspects of human behaviour or clinical symptoms such as abnormal postures, discolouration of the skin, or abnormalities in patients' eye movements.

Table 11.2 Advantages and disadvantages of laboratory and natural settings for making observations

	Advantages	Disadvantages
Laboratory setting	Better control over extraneous variables Observation aids and recording equipment available	Distortion of phenomena in artificial environments Problematic ecological validity
Natural setting	Increased ecological validity Observation of phenomenon as it occurs naturally	Little control over extraneous variables Observation aids and recording equipment may be more difficult to use

Other phenomena may be inaccessible to unaided observation such as, for instance, very small objects and events, where we might need to use a microscope for accurate observations. Also, some events are extremely complex and occur relatively quickly in relation to the observer. An example of this is human locomotion, and recording the event using a device such as a video camera greatly enhances the accuracy of the observation. A fundamental reason for the advancement of science and clinical practice has been the development of sophisticated instrumentation.

There are, however, certain disadvantages associated with using instrumentation. These issues are discussed further in Chapter 12, when we review instrumentation and measurement. We can note here, however, that the use of instruments may distort the event being observed: for instance, the preparation of tissue for electron microscopy changes to some extent the internal organelles of a cell being observed. It requires considerable expertise to use more complex instruments, and a strong theoretical background to separate the 'artifacts' from useful data and interpret the observations. Human subjects also react to being observed. The more intrusive the observer is with equipment and instruments the more likely that the subjects' behaviour will change.

The use and relative advantages and disadvantages of recording techniques were discussed in the context of interviewing techniques in Chapter 10.

Table 11.3 The advantages and disadvantages of using instruments for aiding observations

	Advantages	Disadvantages
Unaided observations	Less disruptive Best suited for observing human behaviour Relatively simple and inexpensive	Insufficient for observing some phenomena Insufficient accuracy and detail
Instrumentation	Access to events outside unaided human senses Increased accuracy and detail	May distort phenomena May be complex and expensive to use

Table 11.3 represents the relative advantages and disadvantages of using instruments for aiding observations.

OBSERVER ROLES

Whether or not instrumentation is used, observation involves a person perceiving and recording an event. There are various positions observers may take in relation to observing human behaviour in health care settings. The fundamental issue is the extent to which the observer becomes involved or participates in the events being observed.

There are four main roles: complete participant, participant as observer, observer as participant and complete observer.

The **complete participant** assumes the role of participant in the setting under investigation and does not normally disclose his or her intent to the other participants. Thus, the researcher actively participates in the setting without the knowledge or consent of the other participants. The purpose behind this approach is to minimize any changes in behaviour of the other participants as a result of their being observed. It can however, border on the edge of unethical practice, and is a technique that must be used with caution.

An example of the use of the complete participant method is provided by Rosenhan's (1975) study of 'pseudo-patients' in psychiatric hospitals. Here the observers posed as (and were admitted as) psychiatric patients in order to study the experiences of psychiatric patients. The pseudo-patients were not recognised as impostors by the staff or the institutions. In this way, they could make and record observations about the interpersonal interactions between the staff and patients. However, in order to be admitted, the observers deliberately misled the staff, who were in fact under study.

The **participant as observer** participates fully in the situation under study, but discloses his or her identity and purpose to the other participants. Example of this can be seen in anthropological studies, where the observer attempts to participate as an active member of a cultural group.

The **observer as participant** makes no pretence of participation but interacts with the other participants. When using this method in a health setting, the observer obtains permission to record events and observe patients, while interacting with the staff and the patients. An example of this method is provided by a study recently performed by a Ph.D. student with a nursing background, supervised by one of the authors. The student's objective was to investigate how psychiatric nurses working in the community make decisions to act in a crisis situation with a disturbed person. He accompanied the nurses on their crisis visits. While travelling to the crisis scene, he interviewed the nurses about their expectations. He observed the crisis scene and its participants and immediately following its conclusion interviewed the nurses about it.

The **complete observer** does not interact with the other participants at all and as with complete participation does not disclose his identity or purpose. As an example, one might investigate therapist-patient interactions by observing from behind a one-way mirror. Observers can, if they wish, use a structured schedule for making the observations.

~~The level of participation chosen involves a tension between the requirements~~ of objective and independent analysis, and the proximity from which the social and clinical phenomena can be studied. Clearly, the participation of the observer introduces changes in the phenomenon under study. It is a question of whether these changes are so large as to negate the benefits obtained by closer observation afforded by actual participation. This is a vexed question and one that has occupied much discussion in the social and clinical sciences.

OBSERVATION IN QUALITATIVE FIELD RESEARCH

Observation data collection in the context of qualitative field research is concerned with providing authentic pictures and reports of individuals functioning in their natural environments. Lofland (1971) outlined the following four features for approaching field research:

(i) The investigator should establish proximity with the subjects in both a physical and a social sense. It is desirable that this involvement should be long term, both to enable understanding and to reduce the subjects' reactivity to the presence of the investigator.

(ii) The report should be truthful. The reporter should not allow ideological biases to distort or censor their observations or deliberately lie to replace their subjects in a good or bad light.

(iii) The data should contain a large amount of 'pure description of action, people, activities and the like. The reality of the place should be conveyed through representation of its mundane aspects in a straightforward manner' (Lofland 1971, p.4).

(iv) The data should contain direct quotations from the participants. Note-taking, audio and video recordings are appropriate for conveying the actual situation. The obtrusiveness of the data collection methods is a major factor. It would not do to assume the role of a complete participant and turn up with a movie camera, while denying any other motives.

Lofland (1971) suggested that when observing subjects in the context of field research, the investigator might focus on the following categories:

1. Acts and activities. These are actions constituting brief or major involvements of an individual:

All pseudopatients took extensive notes publicly. Under ordinary circumstances, such behaviour would have raised questions in the minds of observers, as, in fact, it did among patients. Indeed, it seemed so certain that the notes would elicit suspicion that elaborate precautions were taken to remove them from the ward each day. But the precautions proved needless. The closest any staff member came to questioning these notes occurred when

one pseudo-patient asked his physician what kind of medication he was
receiving and began to write down the response. 'You needn't write it', he
was told gently. 'If you have trouble remembering, just ask me again.'

ROSENHAN (1975)

2. Meanings. These are verbal productions, defining or explaining the
subject's activities:

Holding her breath, standing still, sniffing, and coughing were all means of
countering what she felt as her mother's impingements.

MARY: I used to hold my breath because my mother used to go on so
quick and (pause).
INTERVIEWER: Moving you mean?
MARY: Yes.
INTERVIEWER: You mean your mother was moving about the house quickly?
MARY: Yes and everything.
INTERVIEWER: And what did you do?
MARY: Sort of stand like that.
INTERVIEWER: Can you demonstrate to me—sitting in a chair?
MARY: Yes. I just sort of (shows what she did).
INTERVIEWER: With your elbows?

LAING AND ESTERSON (1970)

3. Participation. This describes the subjects' involvement in a particular
setting:

the pseudopatient behaved afterward as he normally behaved. The
pseudopatient spoke to patients and staff as he might ordinarily. Because there
is uncommonly little to do on a psychiatric ward, he attempted to engage
others in conversation. When asked by staff how he was feeling, he indicated
that he was fine, that he no longer experienced symptoms. He responded to
instructions from attendants, to calls for medication (which was not
swallowed), and to dining-hall instructions. Beyond such activities as were
available to him on the admissions ward, he spent his time writing down his
observations about the ward, its patients, and the staff. Initially these notes
were written secretly, but as it soon became clear that no one much cared,
they were subsequently written on standard tablets of paper in such public
places as the day-room. No secret was made of these activities.

ROSENHAN (1973).

4. Relationships. These are descriptions of the nature of the interrelationships
among several people:

Her absence of social life, her withdrawal, appears to be an unwitting
invention of her parents that never seems to have been called into question.

RUTH:	Well the places I like to go to my parents don't like me to go to.
MOTHER:	Such as?
~~RUTH:~~	~~Eddie's club.~~
MOTHER:	Oh, goodness. You don't really—
FATHER:	?
RUTH:	I do.
INTERVIEWER:	What is 'Eddie's'?
MOTHER:	It's a drinking club. She doesn't really drink. It's just that she likes to meet different types.
INTERVIEWER:	She sounds as though the people that she does want to go out with are people she feels you disapprove of.
MOTHER:	Possibly.
FATHER:	Yes.
MOTHER:	Possibly.

Her parents' attitude to the life Ruth actually leads involves both the negation of its existence and the perception of mad or bad behaviour on Ruth's part. Thus, she is said to drink excessively, while, simultaneously, she is said not to drink at all.

LAING AND ESTERSON (1970)

5. *Settings.* These are descriptions of the entire setting for the investigation:

A stranger entering an ICU is at once bombarded with a massive array of sensory stimuli, some emotionally neutral but many highly charged. Initially, the greatest impact comes from the intricate machinery, with its flashing lights, buzzing and beeping monitors, gurgling suction pumps, and whooshing respirators. Simultaneously, one sees many people rushing around busily performing lifesaving tasks. The atmosphere is not unlike that of the tension-charged strategic bunker. With time, habituation occurs, but the ever-continuing stimuli decrease the overload threshold and contribute to stress at times of crisis.

As the newness and strangeness of the unit wears off, one increasingly becomes aware of a host of perceptions with specific stressful emotional significance. Desperately ill, sick, and injured human beings are hooked up to that machinery. And, in addition to mechanical stimuli, one can discern moaning, crying, screaming and the last gasps of life. Sights of blood, vomitus and excreta, exposed genitalia, mutilated wasting bodies, and unconscious and helpless people assault the sensibilities. unceasingly, the ICU nurse must face these affect-laden stimuli with all the distress and conflict that they engender.

HAY AND OKEN (1977)

Observations of the above classes of behaviours and settings will provide a report representing individuals' experiences and their interactions in a natural setting.

OBSERVATION IN QUANTITATIVE RESEARCH

Research involving human subjects may be conducted using either qualitative or quantitative approaches. With non-human phenomena, quantitative approaches are obviously more relevant. The following are common features of observations in the context of quantitative research.

(i) *Observer roles.* In quantitative research, the observer attempts to be as objective and detached as possible. Therefore, the observer as participant *or* the complete observer roles are most suited for quantitative approaches.

(ii) *Definition of relevant variables.* Considerable effort is made in quantitative research to specify precisely what aspect of an object, event or human behaviour the investigator intends to study and observe. In studies where several observers are involved in data collection, it is appropriate to discuss and demonstrate that there is a substantial degree of agreement among the observers. The above issues will be discussed in more detail in the context of operational definitions, validity and reliability in the following chapter.

(iii) *Observation and structure.* For quantitative studies, we prefer the maximum level of control and structure. Bailey (1987, p 243) suggested that there were two types of 'structures' relevant for observational data collection. The first is the degree of structure in the environment in which the observations are made. We have examined this point earlier, where we compared laboratory and natural settings, with laboratory settings having a higher degree of structure or predictability. The degree of structure for observation may be further increased by using explicit, previously prepared observation guides of protocols. This is quite similar to how degrees of 'structure' or 'formality' are determined in the context of interview techniques, as outlined in the previous chapters.

We have examined two different types of observation guides previously shown in Figures 11.1 and 11.2. If they are to be useful for conducting observational data collection, considerable effort must be made in the design of such guides; and in establishing their reliability and validity, as we shall see in the next chapter.

The advantages of an observation guide are that the recording of the observations is made simple, and the data are easily summarized and evaluated using descriptive and inferential statistics, as discussed in later chapters of the book. The disadvantage of highly structured observations (as with interview and questionnaire techniques) is that the spontaneity and uniqueness of certain events may be lost, to the extent that only predetermined categories are recorded.

CONCLUSION

Data collection based on observation is appropriate for a wide range of research designs, ranging from laboratory based experiments to qualitative field research.

A basic issue is the extent to which a structure is imposed on the observer. Highly structured observational frameworks are most suited for quantitative research while more loosely structured participant observation is better suited for qualitative research. In general, when making observations involving human subjects, researchers attempt to minimize subject reactivity and enhance the accuracy of recording the evidence. When appropriate, instrumentation may be used for enhancing or recording observations. It is worth noting that data collection using questionnaires, interviews and observations may well be used in combination in both research and clinical case work.

SELF ASSESSMENT

Explain the meaning of the following terms:

acts
complete observer
complete participant
meanings
natural setting
observer as participant
participation
relationships
settings

True or false

1. By 'meanings' Lofland was referring to verbal explanations of persons' behaviours.
2. Of the variety of observer roles, the 'complete participant' is the least likely to create ethical problems.
3. In a study involving changes in sleep patterns, self-observation would be an appropriate data collection strategy.
4. Detailed personal diaries of life events and their personal implications are suitable for qualitative research.
5. In the context of modern health sciences research, researchers must use instrumentation to facilitate and record their observations.
6. Anatomic research is well suited for the participant observer role.
7. 'Settings' refers to the physical and social environment in which field observations are conducted.
8. The 'observer as participant' attempts to create interesting, novel situations in the setting in which they carry out field research.
9. Laboratory settings require minimal structure for observational data collection.
10. Observational and interview data collection may be carried out simultaneously in clinical case work.

Multiple choice

1. The advantage of observation over interview as a data collection technique is that:
   - *a* observations may be recorded and scrutinized later
   - *b* observations enable the recording of actual behaviours, rather than subjects' interpretations
   - *c* observation is scientific, unlike interviews which necessarily involve personal interactions
   - *d* observations are unbiased and do not elicit reactions in human subjects.

2. You design an investigation to examine therapist-patient interaction in a hospital setting. Your suggested data collection involves a peep-hole and a hidden microphone for observing specific interactions unknown to the subjects. This study:
   - *a* may well be rejected on ethical grounds
   - *b* involves participant observation
   - *c* would probably maximise subject reactivity
   - *d* both *a* and *c*.

3. In order to reduce subjects' reactivity in the context of qualitative observational studies, the researcher should:
   - *a* use subjects who do not react to being observed
   - *b* inform the subjects of the detailed aims of the study, so as to reduce ambiguity
   - *c* carry out the observations over a prolonged period of time
   - *d* use video-recording equipment so as to minimize reactivity.

4. Participant observation may be defined as:
   - *a* the observation of participants in the study
   - *b* the observation of the researcher's input to a study
   - *c* participation in a group while studying it
   - *d* the study of observational and clinical techniques.

5. One of the major problems associated with the use of participant observation as a research strategy is that:
   - *a* it is more expensive than experimental approaches to implement
   - *b* it does not allow 'in-depth' study of any phenomena
   - *c* the results cannot be replicated
   - *d* participation may alter the phenomena under study.

6. Observation in the context of qualitative field research:
   - *a* involves the use of well designed and pre-defined observation guides
   - *b* depends on the precise definition of the variables being observed
   - *c* requires physical and social proximity with the subjects
   - *d* both *a* and *b*.

7. The advantage of observational data collection in laboratory settings is that:

   a extraneous events disrupting observations are more easily controlled

   b the ecological validity of the study as a whole is improved

   c there is less distortion of the phenomena because of the improved structure

   d there is no need to use expensive equipment for recording observations.

8. Which of the following would represent an 'observer as participant' role?

   a A researcher pretends to be a non English speaking migrant to observe doctors' responses to reports of low back pain

   b A physiotherapist carries out observations of patients while carrying out her normal clinical practice

   c A researcher is given permission to attend clinical sessions in order to observe doctor-patient interactions

   d A neurologist suffers a stroke and keeps detailed records of her observed cognitive and sensory changes.

12

Measurement and instrumentation

INTRODUCTION

The term **measurement** refers to the procedure of attributing qualities or quantities to specific characteristics of objects, persons or events. Measurement is a key process both in research and in clinical practice. If the measurement procedures in a study are poor, then the internal and external validity of the findings, and hence the usefulness of the study, will be severely limited. Similarly, the validity of diagnoses and treatment decisions can be compromised by inadequate measurement.

The specific aims of this chapter are to:

1. Discuss fundamental aspects of measurement procedures
2. Establish the features of 'good' measurement in both research and clinical settings
3. Evaluate and discuss the different types of measurement scales.

OPERATIONAL DEFINITIONS

Sometimes researchers start off with rather vague views of how to measure the variables included in a study. For instance, if researchers are interested in measuring 'levels of pain' experienced by patients, then the researchers must convert their notions of pain to a tightly defined statement of how this variable is to be measured. Depending on their theoretical interpretation of the concept of 'pain', and the practical requirements of the investigation, one of the many possible measures of pain is selected.

In general, the process of converting theoretical ideas to a tightly defined statement of how variables are to be measured is called **operationalization**. It is important that researchers give exact details of how the measures were taken in order that others may judge their adequacy and appropriateness. A study that is adequate in terms of design, sampling methods and sample size may have poor validity due to poor measurement techniques. Let us first consider the issue of operationalization.

The **operational definition** of a variable is a statement of how the researcher in a particular study chooses to measure the variable in question. It ought be unambiguous and have only one possible interpretation.

At the outset, let us note that there is no single best way of taking measurements, particularly in the case of social and clinical variables. For example, if a researcher claimed that her therapeutic techniques significantly increased 'motor control' in her sample of patients, the question that should immediately be asked is what was meant by 'motor control' and how it was measured. If our researcher replied that she was interested in motor control as measured by the Plunkett Motor Dexterity Task scores, she has, in fact, supplied her operational definition. Another researcher may challenge the adequacy of this definition and substitute her own, stating that patients' self ratings of control in various tracking tasks is a more appropriate definition.

A good operational definition will contain enough information to enable another investigator to replicate the measurement techniques if so desired. Similarly, a good operational definition of a clinically relevant variable will enable a fellow professional to replicate the diagnostic or assessment procedures. An operational definition can be an unambiguous description, a photograph or diagram, or the specification of a brand name. In describing a piece of research, one must include operational definitions of the measuring apparatus and all procedures, so that readers are quite clear as to what has been done and to whom.

OBJECTIVE AND SUBJECTIVE MEASURES

A distinction is commonly drawn between objective and subjective measures, often with overtones of suspicion directed towards subjective measures. Let us make a much less value-laden distinction and define them as follows: objective measurements involve the measurement of physical quantities and qualities using measurement equipment; subjective measures involve ratings or judgements by humans of quantities and qualities.

One should not confuse the distinction between objective and subjective measures as corresponding to good or bad measurement techniques. Equipment might be improperly calibrated, complicated to use, or become damaged during an investigation. For instance, a researcher might have an absolutely terrible weighing machine that gives results far at variance with the correct measures. With the sophistication and complexity of much current measurement equipment, it is often difficult to calibrate the equipment. One case recently involved the over-dosing of participants in a study with radioactive material due to the failure of the measurement equipment. This was not detected for some time after the trials. Just because a machine is involved in measurement does not mean that the results will be adequate. Furthermore, many quantities and qualities associated with persons and clinical phenomena are difficult to measure objectively, such as the personal attractiveness of individuals or aspects of patient-therapist relationships. In these instances, measurement of the variables might well call for subjective interpretations.

DESIRABLE PROPERTIES OF MEASUREMENT TOOLS

Measurement tools ought to yield measurements that are reproducible, accurate, applicable to the measurement task in hand and practical or easy to use. These properties correspond to reliability, validity, applicability and practicability. These properties will be reviewed in detail in the following sections. Test theory and method is concerned with the development of measurement tools that maximize these properties.

Before these specific test properties are reviewed, it is useful to review some basic concepts in test theory. In any measurement, we have three related concepts: the observed value or test score, the true value or test score and measurement error. Thus if I could be weighed on a completely accurate set of weighing scales, my true score might be 90 kg. However, the scales that I use in my bathroom might give me a reading of 85 kg. The difference between the observed score and my true score is the measurement error. This relationship can be expressed in the form of an equation such that:

Observed value = true value ± error

Thus, measurement tools are designed with a view to minimize measurement error.

RELIABILITY

Reliability is the property of reproducibility of the results of a measurement procedure or tool. There are several different ways in which reliability can be assessed. These include test–retest reliability, interobserver reliability and internal consistency. Let us examine each.

Test-retest reliability

A common way to assess test reliability is to administer the same test twice. The results obtained from the first test are then correlated with the second test. Reliability is generally measured by a correlation coefficient (see Ch. 16) which may vary from −1 to +1 in value. A test–retest reliability of +0.8 or above is generally considered to be quite sound, although the interpretation of this figure depends on the context in which the measures are to be applied. When the measurement process involves clinical ratings, e.g. a clinician's rating of the dependency level of a CVA patient, test–retest reliability is sometimes termed *intraobserver* reliability, i.e. the same observer rates the same patients twice and the results are correlated.

Interobserver reliability

A common issue in clinical assessment is the extent to which clinicians agree with each other in their assessments of patients. The extent of agreement is generally determined by having two or more clinicians independently assess the same patients and then comparing the results (also with a correlational statistical analysis). If the agreement is high then we have high *interobserver* reliability.

Table 12.1 illustrates examples of both high and low interobserver reliability on ratings of patients on a 5 point scale. Let's imagine that this scale measures the level of patient dependency and need for nursing support.

Table 12.1 Interobserver reliability

	Observers' ratings			
	Low reliability		High reliability	
Subjects	A	B	A	B
1	4	3	4	4
2	2	5	2	3
3	3	4	4	5
4	1	4	2	2
5	3	1	1	1
6	4	4	5	5

As we mentioned earlier, the degree of reliability is quantitatively expressed by correlation coefficients, which are examined in Chapter 16. However, by inspection you can see that in Table 12.1 there is a high degree of disagreement in the two observers' ratings in the 'Low reliability' column. Clearly, in this instance the clinical ratings would be unreliable, and inappropriate to use in the research project. On the other hand, the outcome shown in the 'High reliability' column in Table 12.1 shows a high level of agreement.

An example of a study of inter-rater and intra-rater reliability is provided by Coppleson et al (1970). Over an 11 month period, 29 biopsy slides with suspected Hodgkins disease were presented to 3 pathologists. The pathologists were asked to make a number of judgements about features of the specimens. The specimens were unlabelled and over the year of the study were presented on two occassions to each of the three observers. This permitted an assessment of the test–retest or intra-rater reliability of each observer. The three observers disagreed with themselves on 7, 8 and 9 occasions, respectively, out of the total number of specimens. Overall, inter-rater agreement was calculated at 76% or 54%, depending on the diagnostic classification system used by the observers.

Internal consistency

Measurement tools will often consist of multiple items. For example, a test of your knowledge of research methods might include 50 items or questions. Similarly, a checklist designed to measure activities of daily living might have 20 items. The internal consistency of a test is the extent to which the results on the different items correlate with each other. If they tend to be highly correlated with each other, then the test is said to be internally consistent. Internal consistency, is also measured by a form of correlation coefficient and is generally considered to be a desirable property for a test.

Thus, the reliability of an assessment or test can be determined in several different ways including the test–retest, intra-rater, inter-rater and internal consistency methods.

VALIDITY

However, just because one keeps getting the same result upon repeated administrations, or agreement among independent observers, doesn't mean that all is well. For example, an unscrupulous foreman might place a foot on his side of the scales, when fruit pickers come in to have their efforts weighed for payment. Although upon repeated weighings the same box of fruit would register the same result, the measurement error may be as large as, say, 20 kg.

Validity is concerned with the accuracy of a test or measure; in other words, the amount of measurement error. The concept of validity implies that we can know the true value of a test, that is, we have a 'gold standard'. In physical measurement, we usually do have gold standards and tests. For example, some sets of weighing scales such as beam balances have very high validity. We can time how long it takes people to walk 500 m to a very high degree of accuracy. However, in clinical measurement, we often do not have gold standards. What is the gold standard for the measurement of depression, for example? Fortunately, we have a number of types of procedures to assess validity that can cope without a gold standard.

A case study in clinical test validity

The early detection of breast cancer in women has been recognized as an important public health initiative in many countries. Common ways of detecting suspicious lumps include breast self-examination and mammography, an X-ray of the breasts. Mammography is a common screening procedure and some countries such as Australia have funded large-scale programs to promote it.

However, commendable as these initiatives may be, there are some doubts about the validity of mammography as a diagnostic tool. Walker and Langlands (1986) studied the mammography results of 218 women, who, through the use of a 'gold standard' diagnostic biopsy, were known to have breast cancer. Of the 218 women with cancer, 95 (43.6%) had recorded a (false) negative mammography test result. Of these patients, 47 had delayed further investigation and treatment for almost a year, no doubt relieved and reassured by their 'favourable' test results. The delays in treatment, in all likelihood, seriously compromised the health and ultimate survival of these women. In this instance, the accuracy (or lack of it) of the test results has very important consequences for the people concerned. Measurement theory might sometimes sound boring, but test design is of profound importance in research and clinical practice, as is demonstrated by this example.

Types of test validity

As with reliability, test validity may be assessed in a number of different ways. These include content validity, sensitivity and specificity and predictive validity.

Content validity. In many contexts it is difficult to find external measures to correlate with the measure to be validated. For example, an examination in a particular academic subject may be the sole measure of the student's performance available to determine grades. How can it be determined whether the tests administered will be valid or not? One way is to write down all the material covered in the course and then make sure that there is adequate sampling from the overall content. If this criterion is satisfied it can be said that the test has content validity.

Sensitivity and specificity. The concepts of sensitivity and specificity are most commonly applied to diagnostic tests, where the purpose of the test is to determine whether the patient has a particular problem or illness. There are four possible outcomes for a test result as shown in Table 12.2.

Table 12.2 Possible outcomes of test results

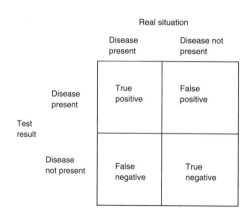

Sensitivity refers to the proportion of people who test as positive who really have the disease (i.e. the proportion of true positives out of all positives). Specificity refers to the proportion of individuals who test as negative who really do not have the disease (i.e. the proportion of true negatives out of all negative test results). If a diagnostic test has sensitivity of 1.0 and specificity of 1.0 it is a perfectly accurate or valid test.

Predictive validity. Predictive validity is concerned with the ability of a test to predict values of it or other tests in the future. Some tests are designed to assist with prognostic decisions.

Let us examine an example of predictive validity. Say a researcher devised a rating scale, X, for selecting patients to participate in a rehabilitation program. The effectiveness of the rehabilitation program is assessed with rating scale Y. Say that each rating scale involves assigning scores 1–10 to the patients' performance. Table 12.3 illustrates two outcomes: low predictive validity and high predictive validity.

Although the calculation of correlation coefficients is needed to indicate quantitatively the predictive validity of test X, it can be seen in Table 12.3 that in the 'Low predictive ability' column, the scores on X are not clearly related to the level of scores on Y. On the other hand, in the 'High predictive ability' column, scores on the two variables correspond quite closely. Within the limits of the fact that only six subjects were involved in this hypothetical study, it is clear that only the results in the 'High predictive ability' column are consistent with rating scale X being useful for predicting the outcome of the rehabilitation program, as measured on scale Y.

At this point we should again refer to the concepts of internal and external validity. The concepts of predictive and content validity apply to the specific tests and measures a researcher or clinician uses. Internal and external validity refer to characteristics of the total research project or program.

Test validity ought not be confused with other forms of research design validity such as external and internal validity.

Table 12.3 Predictive validity

	Low predictive validity		High predictive validity	
Subjects	Score on X	Score on Y	Score on X	Score on Y
1	4	3	3	3
2	4	8	4	3
3	5	2	5	5
4	5	7	5	5
5	6	4	6	6
6	8	5	8	7

External validity is concerned with the researcher's ability to generalize her or his findings to other samples and settings. It is affected by the sample size, the method of sampling, and the design characteristics and measures used in the study. If we say a study has high external validity, we mean that its findings generalize to other settings and samples outside the study. It does not make sense to talk about the external validity of a particular test.

Similarly, internal validity is concerned with the design characteristics of experimental studies. If a study is internally valid, any effects/changes or lack thereof in the dependent variable can be directly attributed to the manipulation of the independent variable. It is important not to confuse the meanings of these terms.

STANDARDIZED MEASURES AND TESTS

Because reliability and validity of measures are so important, many researchers have devoted considerable time and energy to the development of measuring instruments and procedures that have known levels of reliability and validity.

The development of measurement standards for physical dimensions, such as weight, length and time, has been fundamental for the growth of all areas of science. That is, we have standards for comparing our measurements of a variable, and we can meaningfully communicate our findings to colleagues living anywhere in the world. There are a variety of clinical measures, for instance the Apgar Tests for evaluating the viability of neonates, which represent internationally recognized standards for communicating information about attributes of persons or disease entities.

Furthermore, there are standards relevant to populations, in terms of which assessments of individuals become meaningful. For instance, there are standards for the stages of development of infants: levels of physical, emotional, intellectual and social development occurring as a function of age. The interpretation of these standards will be discussed further in Chapter 15.

Some tests have been trialled on large samples, and reliability and validity levels recorded. Tests which have been trialled in this way are known as standardized measures or tests. A large variety is available, particularly in the clinical and social areas. The classic book *Psychological Testing* (Anastasi 1976) is a very useful source of descriptions of such tests. Many American firms and co-operatives market standardized tests. However, many researchers use tests and measures that have not been standardized, and do not report levels of reliability in their literature. This is of particular concern in studies where subjective measures with incomplete operational definitions are employed.

MEASUREMENT SCALE TYPES

Measurement can produce different types of numbers, in the sense that some numbers are assigned different meanings and implications from others. For instance, when we speak of Ward 1 and Ward 2, we are using numbers in a different sense from when we speak of infant A being 1 month old, and infant B being 2 months old. In the first instance, we used numbers for naming, in the second instance the numbers indicate quantities. There are four scale types, distinguished by the types of numbers produced by the measurement of a specific variable.

1. Nominal scales

The 'lowest' level of the measurement scale types is the nominal scale, where the measurement of a variable involves the naming or categorization of possible values of the variable. The measurements produced are 'qualitative' in the sense that the categories are merely different from each other. If numbers are assigned to the categories they are merely labels and do not represent real quantities; for example Ward 1 and Ward 2 might be renamed St. Agatha's Ward and St. Martha's Ward without conveying any less information. Here are some other examples of nominal scaling:

Variable	Some possible values
Patients' admission numbers	3085001, 3085002
Sex	male, female
Religion	Catholic, Protestant, Jewish, Muslim, Hindu
Psychiatric diagnosis	manic-depressive, schizophrenic, neurotic
Blood type	A, B, AB, O
Cause of death	cardiac failure, neoplasm, trauma

The only mathematical relationship pertinent to nominal scales is equivalence or non-equivalence, that is, A = B or A ≠ B. A specific value of a variable either falls into a specific category, or it does not. Thus, there is no logical relationship between the numerical value assigned to its category and its size, quantity, or frequency of occurrence. The arbitrary values of a nominal scale can be changed without any loss of information.

2. Ordinal scales

The next level of measurement involves rank ordering values of a variable. For example, 1st, 2nd or 3rd in a foot race are values on an ordinal scale. The numbers assigned on an ordinal scale signify order or rank.

With ordinal scales, statements about ranks can be made. Where A and B are values of the variable, we can say A > B or B > A. For instance, we can say Mrs Smith is more co-operative than Mr Jones (A > B), or Mr Jones is more co-operative than Mr Krax (B > C). We cannot, however, make any statements about the relative sizes of these differences. Examples of ordinal scales are:

Variable	Possible values
Severity of condition	mild = 1, moderate = 2, severe = 3, critical = 4
Patient's satisfaction with treatment	satisfied = 1, undecided = 2, dissatisfied = 3
Age group	baby, infant, child, adult, geriatric
Co-operativeness with nurse or patients in a ward	(in decreasing order) Mrs Smith, Mr Jones, Ms Krax

3. Interval scales

Examples of interval scales are shown below. For these scales, there is no absolute zero point, rather, an arbitrary zero point is assigned. For instance, 0°C does not represent the point at which there is no heat, but the freezing point of water. An IQ of zero would not mean no intelligence at all, but a serious intellectual or perceptual problem in using the materials of the test. Some examples of internal scales include:

Variable	Possible values
~~Heat (Celsius or Fahrenheit)~~	~~-10°C, +20°C, +5°C, 10°F~~
Intelligence (IQ)	45, 100, 185

The use of an interval scale enables identification of equal intervals between any two values of measurements: we can say A–B = B–C. For example, if A, B, and C are taken as IQ scores, and A = 150, B = 100, and C = 50 then it is true that:

A–B = B–C

However, we cannot say that A = 3C (that A is three times as intelligent as C).

4. Ratio scales

The zero is not arbitrary in ratio scales. For example, in the Kelvin temperature scale, 0 K represents an absence of heat, in that the molecules have stopped vibrating completely; whereas 0°C is simply the freezing point of water. Thus K is a ratio scale and °C is an interval scale. Examples of variables measured on ratio scales are:

Variable	Possible values
Weight	10 kg, 20 kg, 100 kg
Height	50 cm, 150 cm, 200 cm
Blood pressure	110 mmHg, 120 mmHg, 160 mmHg
Heart Beats	10 per minute, 30 per minute, 50 per minute
Rate of firing of a neurone	10 per millisec, 20 per millisec, 30 per millisec
Protein per blood volume	2 mg/cc, 5 mg/cc, 10 mg/cc
Vocabulary	100 words, 1000 words, 30 000 words

Table 12.4 Characteristics of levels of measurement

Characteristic	Level of measurement			
	Nominal	**Ordinal**	**Interval**	**Ratio**
Distinctiveness	•	•	•	•
Ordering in magnitude		•	•	•
Equal intervals			•	•
Absolute zero				•

Distinctiveness: different numbers assigned to different values of property
Ordering in magnitude: larger values represent more of the property
Equal intervals: same distance between points on a scale
Absolute zero: zero value represents absence of property

Table 12.4 compares the characteristics of different scales or levels of measurement.

Interval and ratio scales produce quantitative measurements. A ratio scale is the 'highest' scale of measurement, in the sense that it involves all the characteristics of the other scales, as well as having an absolute zero. A measurement on a higher scale can be transformed into one on a lower level, but not vice versa, because the higher scale measurement contains more information, and the values can be put to more use by permitting more mathematical operations than those on a lower scale.

Also, a given variable might be measured on one of several types of scales, depending on the needs of the investigator. Consider, for instance, the variable 'height'. This variable could be measured on any of the four scales, as follows:

Ratio scale. The height of individuals above the ground, for example, 180 cm

Interval scale. The height of individuals above an *arbitrary* surface; for example 100 cm above the surface of a bench

Ordinal scale. The comparative heights of individuals, for example, rank ordered from tallest to shortest

Nominal scale. Categorising individuals as, for example, 'Normal' or 'Abnormal' (giant or dwarf).

The different types of measurement scales are important when considering statistical analysis of data. Statistics are numbers with special properties from data. The type of measurement scale determines the type of statistic that is appropriate for its analysis. This issue is taken up later in this book in Chapter 19.

SUMMARY

In previous chapters we examined how some measuring instruments such as questionnaires are constructed, and ways of collecting evidence in field research. This section extends issues in data collection by defining what constitutes good measurement and by examining and comparing types of numbers which measurement can produce.

The first step in measurement is to define concepts operationally, so that other investigators can also carry out or assess the measurement procedure. Secondly, using correlations we can establish the reliability and validity of our measurements. A high degree of reliability and validity is necessary for minimizing measurement error. It was pointed out that subjective measures are not necessarily unreliable or invalid. However, tests are available for clinical measurement which have the advantage of known validity and reliability.

Four different scale types were discussed: nominal, ordinal, interval, and ratio. These scales have different characteristics, particularly in relation to the permissible mathematical operations. In subsequent sections, we shall see that the scale type involved in our measurements determines the descriptive and inferential statistics appropriate for describing and analysing the data.

SELF ASSESSMENT

Explain the meaning of the terms:

> content validity
> interval scale
> interobserver reliability
> measurement
> nominal scale
> objective measures
> operational definition
> ordinal scale
> predictive validity
> ratio scale
> standardized measures
> standardized tests
> subjective measures
> test–retest reliability

True or false

1. The term 'measurement' refers to the assignment of qualities or quantities to specific aspects of objects or events.
2. An operational definition of a variable entails an explicit statement of how the variable is to be measured.
3. An objective measure is produced by the use of a measuring instrument.
4. A reliable test or measure will tend to produce accurate results.
5. A test–retest reliability as indicated by a correlation coefficient of 0.9 indicates a rather low reliability.
6. When an instrument is valid, we mean that it is measuring the characteristic which it is supposed to be measuring.
7. To establish the predictive validity of a test, we correlate the scores of individuals on the test with scores on other relevant measures.
8. A high correlation for scores between a college entrance examination and the subsequent examination results of students indicates that the entrance examination lacks predictive validity.
9. One of the advantages of using a standardized test is that its validity and reliability are already known.
10. Ordinal measures involve rank-ordering the values of a variable.
11. An interval scale has an absolute zero.
12. All arithmetical operations are permissible with measurements based on interval scales.
13. The levels of measurement which have the properties of distinctiveness, ordering of magnitude, and equal intervals are the ordinal and nominal scales.

14. The statement 'Anxiety is a feeling of impending injury' is an example of an operational definition.
15. 'Operationalization' is defined as a statement specifying how a variable should be measured.
16. For a general concept like 'intelligence' only one operational definition is possible.
17. Subjective measures are necessarily unreliable.
18. Objective measures can be invalid and unreliable.
19. A correlation coefficient of 1.0 indicates an excellent test–retest reliability.
20. If a measurement is valid, then it is necessarily reliable.
21. A test may be highly reliable but invalid.
22. A low interobserver reliability implies that the observed scores for a set of subjects on repeated tests tend to be unrelated to one another.
23. High predictive validity necessarily implies high content validity.
24. With a nominal scale, we can only make statements about the distinctiveness of scores.
25. The mathematical statement A–B = B–C is in correct form, given an ordinal scale.
26. Nominal scales do not have the characteristic of 'distinctiveness'.
27. The variable motor functioning' could be measured on either an ordinal or a nominal scale.
28. The variable 'blood sugar level' could be measured on either an ordinal or a ratio scale.
29. Ordinal scales are generally preferable to interval scales.
30. Statements such as y = zx can be made validly with ratio measures.

Multiple choice

1. Which of the following does not include an operational definition?
   a Patients were encouraged to eat healthy food.
   b Males under 60 who were currently in full-time employment were the population for study.
   c Anxiety was measured by the Spielberger Anxiety Scale.
   d Patients who did not return for a scheduled follow up appointment four weeks after initial treatment were classified as dropouts.
   e Students who get over half the test items correct will be classified as having passed.

2. Subjective measures:
   a are not operationally defined
   b are always less valid than objective measures
   c involve measuring physical attributes
   d are not reliable because everybody's subjective experience is different
   e none of the above.

3. Which of the following statements does not include an operational definition of the dependent variable?
   a In the present study, intelligence was measured on the Stanford Binet IQ test.
   b In the present study, intelligence was measured in terms of the level of subjects' knowledge of their cultures.
   c In the present study, intelligence was measured by the number of hairs on the subjects' heads.
   d b and c
   e a and c.

4. Objective measures:
   a are always more valid and reliable than subjective measures
   b involve extensive human intuition for interpretation
   c are always more reliable, but not necessarily more valid, than subjective measures
   d are used in experimental, but not in non-experimental, investigations
   e involve the measurement of physical qualities and quantities using measuring equipment.

5. A test is assessed for its reliability and its predictive validity. Both these measures are expressed as correlation coefficients, with the reliability coefficient being 0.9 and the predictive validity coefficient being 0.2. This indicates that:
   a the test is not reliable
   b the test has face validity
   c the test is reliable but does not appear to measure the variable of interest
   d the test is reliable, so it must measure the variable of interest
   e the test is a good one.

6. If the test–retest reliability of a measure is low, then it follows that:
   a the scores for different people tend to be different
   b the validity must be high
   c the scores for different people tend to be the same
   d the same person measured twice tends to produce different results.

7. If a test is valid then:
   a it might be reliable
   b it must be reliable
   c the reliability is unaffected
   d it must be unreliable.

8. The reading '64 kilograms' is a value on a(n):
   a ratio scale
   b interval scale
   c ordinal scale
   d nominal scale.

9. In a study of weight problems in a sample of pre-adolescent children, the relevant variable was expressed as 'percentage overweight' or 'underweight', given the child's height. This is an example of a(n):
   a ordinal scale
   b ratio scale
   c nominal scale
   d interval scale.

10. The gender of patients is an example of a(n):
    a ratio scale
    b nominal scale
    c ordinal scale
    d interval scale.

11. Which of the following variables has been labelled with an incorrect measuring scale?
    a The number of heart beats per minute: interval
    b Platform numbers at a railway station: nominal
    c Finishing order in a horse race: ordinal
    d Self-rating of anxiety levels on a five point scale: ordinal.

12. '10th' is a value on a(n):
    a ratio scale
    b interval scale
    c ordinal scale
    d nominal scale.

13. Response delay in milliseconds is an example of a(n):
    a ratio scale
    b ordinal scale
    c interval scale
    d nominal scale.

14. In a patient records system, patients are randomly assigned a unique identification number. These numbers represent a(n):
    a nominal scale
    b ratio scale
    c interval scale
    d ordinal scale.

Therapists assess levels of clients' 'independence' using the following scale:

0: Totally dependent on assistance from other/s for the activity

1: Maximum assistance from other/s; can assist in a limited way

2: Minimum assistance from 1 person; contributes significantly in carrying out the activity

3: Supervised by another person due to mental/physical limitations and/or to ensure safety

4: Independent with aids. Safe and consistent; would need assistance/supervision without aids

5: Independent. Safe and consistent without aids, supervision or assistance.

Questions 15–17 refer to this scale.

15. The above scale is:

   a ratio

   b interval

   c nominal

   d ordinal.

16. If the subjects are assigned scores by the therapist's clinical judgement, then the measurement process is:

   a subjective

   b objective

   c unreliable

   d invalid

   e *a* and *b.*

17. Given the following three independence scores for three clients A, B, and C:

     A 4

     B 2

     C 0

which of the following statements is (are) true?

   a Client A is twice as independent as B

   b The difference in independence between clients A and B is the same as that between clients B and C

   c Client A is more independent than either B or C

   d *b* and *c.*

18. Which of the following measures of the variable 'weight' is nominal?

   a Weight in kg

   b Weight as percentage overweight in relation to 'healthy' weight

   c Weight as obese/overweight/normal/underweight/grossly underweight

   d Weight as 'normal against pathological' (obese or grossly underweight).

19. If a variable is not defined operationally, then:
    a   the investigation of the variable might be difficult to replicate
    b   it might be difficult to explain how the variable was measured
    c   *a* and *b*
    d   neither *a* nor *b*.

20. The terms 'external' and 'internal' validity refer to:
    a   complete investigations
    b   specific measurements
    c   measurement scales, as a whole
    d   characteristics of standardized, objective measures.

DISCUSSION, QUESTIONS AND ANSWERS

The same research questions may be answered by the use of a variety of different research methodologies. There is no single 'correct' research method to answer a research question. Indeed the 'triangulation' of methods is sometimes used to try and answer the same research question, so that the answer can be demonstrated not to be an artefact of the method used. Just as in land surveying, in which several reference points are used to better fix the position of the object being surveyed, researchers may study the same question or phenomenon using a variety of research techniques. The results may then be compared to get a better 'fix' on the question. The use of a single reference point or methodology gives one perspective of the object under study.

To illustrate this point it is proposed to consider a research issue of some importance and much contention in modern health care: the allocation of donated organs to transplant recipients. Despite the advances in transplantation techniques, there is a chronic worldwide under supply of donor organs, to the extent that, in some countries, over one third of patients accepted for transplantation die while on the waiting list due to the unavailability of suitable organs. A consequence of the chronic under supply of donor organs is the necessity for transplantation teams to choose the most 'worthy' candidate to receive the donated organ from a panel of potential recipients. How these decisions are made and how they ought be made has been the subject of substantial research.

Many transplantation units around the world use a points system to assist with decisions concerning the priority of their people on the waiting lists. The points are typically based on tissue and blood type match (methods of measuring donor–recipient compatibility), time on the waiting list, 'urgency' (the extent to which the patient can wait) and prognosis (the quality of the expected outcome). This is in addition to certain technical requirements that vary with the organ system being replaced. For example, the size of the donor's and recipient's organ systems is a factor in heart–lung transplants. However, in recent years many commentators have presented data that indicate that 'social' criteria (such as the age, sex, education, race and wealth of the potential recipient) as well as 'medical' criteria are highly influential in the allocation of organs to recipients. These findings have generated considerable controversy.

How might one discover what criteria are used in the allocation of organs? One method might be to conduct a survey of those people involved in the decisions. The survey could take the form of an individual or group interview, or a written questionnaire. Alternatively, one could examine the written policies of various transplantation units or examine the medical records of the potential recipients for transplantation in the units and follow up the actual outcomes for each candidate.

179

Let us consider the questions we may wish to ask of people involved in the organ transplant decisions. They might include:

'In your opinion, what criteria *should be used* in deciding who should receive an organ transplant?'

'In your opinion, what criteria *are actually used* in deciding who should receive an organ transplant?'

These questions could be asked directly of the respondents in person and their comments recorded on tape and/or in the form of notes for subsequent analysis. In other words, the respondents could be interviewed. Excerpts of typical responses to these questions when the authors have asked them of members of transplant teams include:

We have an unwritten policy that we won't transplant into patients over 60. We think they have had their turn. Also their prognosis is often poorer than younger patients.

A consequence of the HLA emphasis is that people with unusual tissue types never get a transplant. I have a problem with this. In my area, there is only slim evidence that it makes much difference. Fifteen per cent max (sic) between best and worst case match. Most people fall in the middle so the actual difference would be even smaller. This means a lot of people miss out. I think it should be a strict queue.

Another method of collecting the data would involve getting people to use a structured response question in a questionnaire. The following might be an example:

In your opinion, what criteria *should be used* in deciding who should receive an organ transplant'. Please circle as many as you like.

Age	Urgency of need
Sex	Prognosis
Education level	Whether recipient is a parent
Race	Citizenship status
Occupation	Other, please specify
Wealth	

Blood type match between donor and recipient

HLA match between donor and recipient tissues

A follow-up question might include something like:

When you have selected the criteria you consider should be used in allocating organs to recipients, please write a number alongside each one to indicate your opinion of its importance in the decision. For example, the one you consider the most important should have a '1' placed alongside it, the second a '2' and so on until you have exhausted all the ones you selected.

In this type of exploratory study, the use of fixed response questions may send a clear signal to the respondent as to what the researcher considers to be acceptable criteria. Therefore, the respondent may not be inclined to reveal their true answer if it is not included in the list of available answers, because of fear of disapproval or perhaps disinclination for the effort to do so. Thus, before a structured response question is used, the clinical researcher needs to ensure that all possible and likely answers are included. The current authors advocate the use of unstructured questions with a small sample prior to the use of structured questions in a large scale survey.

It is interesting to note that in a study of 310 Australian people from the community recently conducted by the authors the respondents consistently nominated the age of the recipient, their prognosis, the length of time they spent on the waiting list and whether they had children as the four factors they considered ought be used to determine recipient priority in transplantation decisions.

Thus, the clinical researcher could use interview or questionnaire approaches in the conduct of their survey. A further approach would involve the auditing of potential recipient medical files over a period in the various transplantation units in order to check whether those who actually received the transplants were representative of the potential recipient pool. For example, if it were found that women were less likely to receive transplants than men, taking into account their relative proportions in the recipient pool, then this would be of major concern. Unfortunately, as mentioned above, there is strong evidence in the United States (where most such research has been performed) that social factors have an important impact upon the actual transplantation decisions. These findings reflect the situation in the delivery of health care in areas other than transplantation.

Questions

1. What are some of the possible disadvantages of using structured response questions when the researcher is unsure as to what answers respondents may want to use?
2. When are structured response questions best used?
3. If you wanted to study the outcomes of transplant patients at a hospital, how would you go about gaining access to the records?
4. In the case where a researcher uses a structured questionnaire, to what extent does the respondent have the opportunity to contribute to the research agenda?
5. How can a researcher avoid bias in designing a questionnaire?

Answers

1. If the researcher is unsure as to what answers the respondents wish to give, structured response questions will probably not do the job required. In fact, even an open ended response written question will not do the job, if the answer is complicated, because people are often are lot more fluent in their speech.

2. If the questions being asked are straightforward, e.g. what is your sex? or what is your age? or how often did you go to the doctor last month? then structured response questions will give structured data cheaply and quickly.

3. Access to confidential data requires a lot of work, although you may find that some of the data you require may be published in the annual report for the hospital or agency. Typically, one starts by contacting the head of the unit concerned and then progressing through the ethics committees and procedures laid down by the agency. If access is granted at all, it can be many months before permission is given, as the rights of the patients to their data are now strictly enforced in most countries.

4. Most structured research questionnaires are designed wholly by the researcher, without input from the respondents to be studied. What questions are asked, how these are asked and what is not asked can send clear messages to the respondents about the researcher's agenda and assumptions. In this context, it is rare that respondents challenge the researcher, even if they believe that the researcher has missed the point. The typically low level of respondent input avoids anarchy (imagine every single respondent to a survey questionnaire designing their own questions!). However, if the researcher has a totally different understanding of the situation under study from the respondents, then she may ask the 'wrong' questions. The data may then be invalid because they do not reflect the true positions of the respondents.

5. It depends upon the type of bias. With adherence to principles of question design, problems such as the use of leading questions should be avoided. However, since the researcher selects their questions, which may number thirty or so, from a range of several billion possible, selection bias is unavoidable. Every study is not a study of the universe. Focus and selectivity is unavoidable and is inherent to the reductionist scientific process. A problem of 'bias' may arise when the researcher does not ask the questions the respondents believe they should be answering.

Descriptive statistics

Depending on the complexity of the research design and the number of measurements obtained during data collection in the conduct of the project, we will have generated a set of scores which we call the 'raw data'. Section 5 is concerned with the principles of descriptive statistics, which include mathematical principles for organizing and summarizing the raw data.

In Chapter 13 we outline strategies used for tabulating and graphing data. These techniques enable us to visualize trends, and identify differences among the various groups. When the data is organized, we may calculate simple statistics, such as the percentages and proportions of scores found within the groups being studied.

Another important use for descriptive statistics is to 'crunch' or condense data into typical values for representing the distribution of scores. The statistics discussed in Chapter 14 include 'measures of central tendency' (mode, median and mean) and also measures of dispersal (including range, semi-interquartile range and standard deviation). Using these statistics enables us to condense the data and convey to the reader a large amount of information using only two numbers (e.g. the mean and the standard deviation).

Statistics such as the mean and the standard deviation can be applied also to the calculation of standard scores. Standard scores are used to establish the position of a particular score relative to a population.

In Chapter 15 we examine how the standardized normal distribution can be used to calculate the position of any specific score within a population and how to interpret the clinical implications of these scores.

In Chapter 16 we examine another important class of statistics called correlation coefficients. The correlation coefficient is used to express the degree and direction of association between two or more variables. For example, we could use correlation coefficients to demonstrate if there is an association between 'level of exercise' (variable X) and 'body weight' (variable Y). The closer the calculated correlation coefficient is to 1.0 (the maximum value), the more precisely we may predict from one variable to the other. Although correlation coefficients are extremely important for showing how different variables are associated, they do not necessarily indicate causal relationships between the variables. Showing causal effects requires appropriate research designs, as we argue in Section 3.

13

Organization and presentation of data

INTRODUCTION

The summary and interpretation of data from quantitative research entails the use of statistics. By statistics, we mean the way of organizing and interpreting observations and measurements. However, when we speak of a statistic, we mean a particular number obtained by the mathematical treatment of specific data.

Descriptive statistics describe specific characteristics of data, such as how many cases fall into a particular category of measurement, typical values and the degree of interrelationship or correlation among measurements.

In previous chapters we examined how interviews, observations and measurement should be employed to produce data in clinical or scientific investigations. It can be extremely difficult, however, to make sense of raw data when it consists of a large number of varied measurements. That is, before we can interpret or communicate the information provided by an investigation, the raw data must be organized and presented in a clear and intelligible fashion. The aim of this chapter is to outline methods used in descriptive statistics for the organization, tabulation and graphic presentation of data. Also we will examine the use of some simple statistics directly derived from the tabulation of the data into frequency and cumulative frequency distributions.

The specific aims of this chapter are to:

1. Outline methods for organizing and representing data as in the form of frequency distributions tables or graphs
2. Demonstrate how the scaling of the data influences organization and presentation
3. Discuss the calculation and use of some simple descriptive statistics, including percentages, ratios and rates.

THE ORGANIZATION AND PRESENTATION OF NOMINAL OR ORDINAL DATA

A fundamental consideration in selecting appropriate statistics is the question of whether the data are discrete or continuous. Nominal and ordinal data are necessarily discrete, so that the organization of the data involves counting the number (frequency) of cases falling into each category of measurement. Let us examine two simple examples as an illustration.

Organization of discrete data

Example 1: Nominal data

Say we are interested in the sex of patients (nominal data) undergoing gall bladder surgery (cholecystectomy) at a public hospital over a period of one year. The raw data, indicating the sex (M or F) of the patients is simply read off the patients' records, as follows:

F, M, M, F, F, F, M, F, M, F, M, F, F, F, F, F, F, F, F, F, F, M, F, F, F, M, M, F, M, F, M

Grouping the above nominal data involves counting the number of cases (or measurements) falling into each category. The tally is: M = 10; F = 20. The data can be presented in tabular form:

Table 13.1 Frequency distribution of gender of patients undergoing cholecystectomy at a hospital over a period of one year

Gender	f
Males (M)	10
Females (F)	20
	n = 30

Table 13.1 shows the following conventions in tabulating data:

1. Tables must be clearly and fully labelled; both the table as a whole, and the categories; so that the readers can interpret unambiguously what they are observing.
2. 'f' represents frequency of cases or measurements falling into a given category.
3. 'n' represents the total number of cases or measurements in a *sample*.
4. N represents the number of cases in a population. (See Section 3 for difference between samples and populations.)

Example 2: Ordinal data

Ordinal data are presented by counting the number of cases (frequency) of each ordered rank making up the scale.

An investigator intends to evaluate the effectiveness of a new analgesic versus placebo treatment. A post-test only control group design is used: the experimental group receives the analgesic and the control group the placebo. Twenty patients are randomly assigned into each of the two groups. Pain intensity is assessed by the patients' pain reports five hours after minor surgery, on the following scale:

5—Excruciating pain
4—Severe pain
3—Moderate pain
2—Mild pain
1—No pain

The raw data is:

- Experimental group
  3,4,5,3,3,3,4,2,1,3,2,1,3,4,5,2,3,3,3,3
- Control group
  5,4,4,4,5,3,4,3,2,4,4,2,4,5,3,4,4,4,5,5

After tallying the results, the above data can be presented as a frequency distribution, as shown in Table 13.2. This demonstrates that when the data have been tabulated, we can see the outcome of the investigation. Here, the pain reported by the experimental group is less than that of the control group.

Table 13.2 Reported pain intensity of patients following placebo and analgesic treatments

Pain intensity	Experimental group (analgesic) f	Control group (placebo) f
1	2	
2	3	2
3	10	3
4	3	10
5	2	5
	n = 20	n = 20

Graphing discrete data

Once a frequency distribution of the raw data has been tabulated, a variety of techniques is available for the pictorial or graphical presentation of a given set of measurements. Frequency distributions of qualitative data are often plotted as bar graphs (also termed 'column' graphs), or shown pictorially as pie diagrams.

A bar graph involves plotting the frequency of each category and drawing a bar, the height of which represents the frequency of a given category. Figure 13.1 graphs the data given in Table 13.1.

Figure 13.1 demonstrates conventions in plotting bar graphs:

1. The Y axis, also called the ordinate, is used to plot frequencies.
2. The X axis, also called the abscissa, is used to indicate the categories.
3. The bars do not touch each other, reflecting the discontinuity of the measurement categories.

It should be noted that considerable attention must be given to interpreting graphs, as the axes may be translated or compressed, causing a false visual

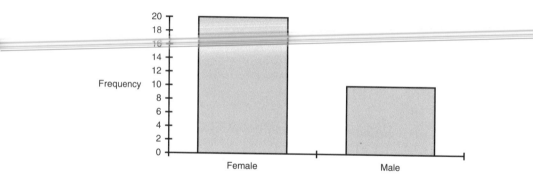

Fig. 13.1 Bar (column) graph of patients undergoing cholecystectomy

impression of the data. Make sure that you inspect the values along the axes, so that you are not mislead.

It is also acceptable to calculate the percentage of scores falling into each category and to plot the percentages instead of the frequencies. For instance, graphing Table 13.2 as percentages will produce the graph shown in Figure 13.2.

It can be seen in Figure 13.2 that by presenting the data for the experimental and control groups on the same graph, the reader gains a visual impression of the possible effectiveness of the analgesic treatment, in contrast to that of the control treatment.

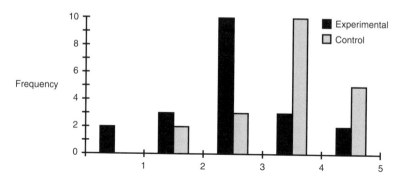

Fig. 13.2 Bar (column) graph of patients' pain intensity

Nominal data can also be meaningfully presented as a pie diagram, where the percentage of each category is converted into a proportional part of a circle or 'pie'. For instance; in a given hospital we have the hypothetical spending patterns shown below:

Item	Cost ($)	Percentage of total
Wages and salaries	1 500 000	50.00%
Medical supplies	500 000	16.67%
Food and provisions	500 000	16.67%
Administrative costs	500 000	16.67%
Total	$3 000 000	100.00%

Figure 13.3 represents a pie diagram of the information. In constructing Figure 13.3, we converted the numbers into percentages and then into degrees (out of a total of 100% = 360°), that is each 1% of the total is represented by 3.6° in the circle.

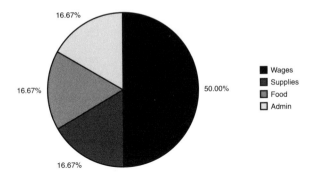

Fig. 13.3 Pie diagram of a hospital's spending pattern

ORGANIZATION AND PRESENTATION OF INTERVAL OR RATIO DATA

As we have discussed in Chapter 12, interval and ratio scales of measurement produce real numbers, which can be processed according to the rules of arithmetic. Interval and ratio measurements often produce continuous data (such as weight, length, time, IQ), implying that any values of the variable, depending on the sensitivity of the measurement, are possible.

Grouped frequency distributions

Often, when the continuous data are made up of a large number of varied measurements, it is useful to present the data as a grouped frequency distribution.

When drawing up a grouped frequency distribution, the following conventions should be taken into account:

1. The table of grouped frequency distributions should have no more than 9 groups of values, otherwise it is too difficult to inspect. However, if too few groups are used, the meaning of the data is obscured, as varied measurements are combined into too few equivalent categories.
2. There should be equally sized class intervals, the *width* of which is represented by i.
3. Individual scores within a given class interval 'lose' their precise identity. The midpoint of each class interval is taken to represent the class interval.

Example 1

On admission to hospital, patients are routinely weighed. You are asked to summarize the weights of 50 male patients who were admitted in your ward over a period of time. The weights (raw data) are as follows (to nearest kg):

75, 67, 76, 71, 73, 86, 2, 77, 80, 75, 80, 96, 93, 75, 73, 83, 81, 82, 73, 92, 81, 87, 76, 84, 78, 79, 99, 100, 88, 77, 71, 76, 75, 83, 66, 79, 95, 85, 77, 87, 90, 73, 72, 68, 84, 69, 78, 77, 84, 94

The steps in constructing a grouped frequency distribution are:

1. Organize data into an **ordered array,** and find the frequency of each score:

Score	f	Score	f	Score	f	Score	f
100	1	91	0	82	1	73	4
99	1	90	1	81	1	72	2
98	0	89	0	80	2	71	2
97	0	88	1	79	2	70	0
96	1	87	2	78	2	69	1
95	1	86	1	77	4	68	1
94	1	85	1	76	3	67	1
93	1	84	3	75	4	66	1
92	1	83	2	74	0		

2. Find the **range** of scores. The range is the difference between the highest and lowest score plus one. We add *one* to include the *real* limits for continous data (Figure 13.4). In this case the range is 100–66 + 1= 35.
3. Decide on the width (i) of the class intervals. i can be approximated by dividing the range by the number of groups or **class intervals**. In this instance, if we decide on 7 classes, i will be 35/7 = 5.0. When i is a decimal, it should be rounded up to the nearest whole number; here, $i = 5$. As stated earlier, the number of class intervals is arbitrary and will be chosen by the researcher, depending on the properties of the data. By convention, more than 9 class intervals are rarely employed.
4. The next step is to determine the lowest class interval, and then list the limits of each class interval. Clearly, the lowest class interval must include the lowest score in the distribution.
5. Then, the frequency of scores is determined from each class interval and tabulated, as in Table 13.3.

Table 13.3 Grouped frequency distribution of patients' weight in a given ward

Class interval	f
66-70	4
71-75	12
76-80	13
81-85	9
86-90	5
91-95	4
96-100	3
	n = 50

It is far easier to understand the data by inspecting Table 13.3 than by looking at the raw data. However, some precision in the data has been lost as somewhat different scores have been assigned into the same class intervals.

Graphing frequency distributions

The two common types of graphs used to graph frequency distribution of quantitative data are histograms and frequency polygons.

Histograms. A histogram resembles a bar graph but the bars are drawn to touch each other. The fact that the bars touch each other reflects the underlying continuity of the data. The height of the bars along the Y axis represents the frequency of each score or class interval plotted along the X axis. With grouped data, the midpoint of each class interval becomes the midpoint of each bar, and the width of the bar corresponds to the real limits of each class interval.

For instance, consider the lowest class interval 66–70 on Table 13.3. Because the data is *continuous*, the real upper and lower limits of the class interval are 65.5 and 70.4. Although all the weights are given as whole numbers of kilograms, these will in most cases be the result of rounding off by the nursing staff to the nearest whole number. Thus, someone who actually weighed 70.2 kg would have been recorded as weighing 70 kg and would fall into the 66–70 class. As Figure 13.4 shows, $i = 5$, and the midpoint of the class interval is 68.

Frequency polygons. Any data which can be represented by a histogram can also be graphed as a frequency polygon. For this type of graph, a point is plotted over the midpoint of each class interval, at a height representing the frequency of the scores. Figure 13.5 represents a histogram and a frequency polygon for the data in Table 13.3.

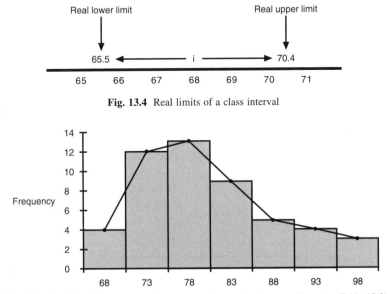

Fig. 13.4 Real limits of a class interval

Fig. 13.5 Combined histogram and frequency polygon for the same data (see Table 13.3)

Frequency polygons allow the reader to interpolate, that is, to estimate the frequency of values in between those actually measured or graphed. Of course, interpolation cannot be done for discrete data (for example, Fig. 13.1), as values between categories have no meaning. When a frequency polygon is plotted, it can take on a variety of shapes. The shapes which are of particular importance for frequency polygons are shown in Figure 13.6.

Figure 13.6A represents a bell shaped or normal distribution. It is symmetrical, in the sense that one half is the same as the other. The curve indicates

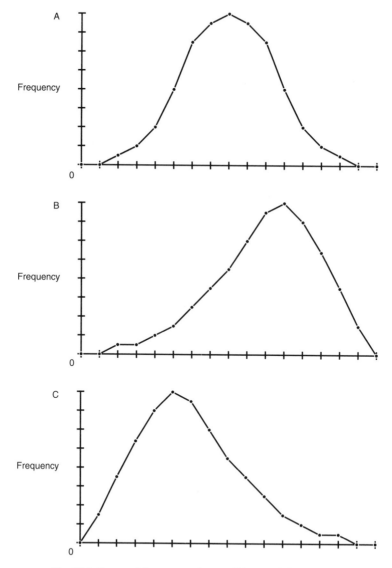

Fig. 13.6 Shapes of frequency polygons: (A) normal distribution; (B) negative skewing; (C) positive skewing

that most of the scores fell in the middle, with a relatively few scores towards either 'tail'. Figure 13.6B represented a negatively skewed distribution, with most of the scores being high and spreading out toward the lower end of the distribution. Figure 13.6C represents a positively skewed distribution, with most of the scores being low, but with some scores spreading out towards the upper end of the distribution.

An easy way to remember the direction of the skew is to consider the region where the 'tail' or portion of the graph with lower frequencies falls. For example, if it is toward the negative side of the X axis, the graph is negatively skewed.

The significance of the skew or normality of a distribution will be discussed in subsequent sections.

SIMPLE DESCRIPTIVE STATISTICS

Once the data have been summarized in a frequency distribution, it is often useful to make comparisons concerning the relative frequencies of scores falling into specific categories. The following statistics are useful for understanding comparative trends in the data, and can be used for measurements on any scale; nominal, ordinal, interval, or ratio. A **statistic** is a number resulting from the manipulation of the raw data. The calculation of statistics is essential for 'crunching' the raw data into single numbers, which summarize the data.

Ratios

Ratios are statistics which express the relative frequency of one set of frequencies, A, in relation to another, B. The formula for ratios is:

$$\text{Ratio} = \frac{A}{B}$$

Therefore, the ratio of males to females for the data presented in Table 13.1 (p. 186) is:

$$\text{Ratio (males to females)} = \frac{10}{20} = 0.5$$

or

$$\text{Ratio (female to males)} = \frac{20}{10} = 2.0$$

Ratios are useful in the health sciences when we are interested in the distribution of illnesses or symptoms or the categories of subjects requiring or benefiting from treatment. The ratio calculated above tells us about the relative frequency of gall bladder surgery for males and females.

Proportions

Proportions are statistics which are calculated by putting the frequency of one category over that of the total numbers in the sample or the population:

$$\text{Proportion of } A = \frac{A}{A + B}$$

Therefore, the proportion of males in the sample represented in Table 13.1 (p. 186) is:

$$\text{Proportion of males} = \frac{f(males)}{n}$$

$$= \frac{10}{30}$$

$$= 0.33$$

Percentages

Proportions can be transformed into percentages, by multiplying by 100. Of course, this is how we obtained the values of the Y axis for Figure13.2 (p. 188). To illustrate, patients scoring 5 (excruciating pain) in the Control group:

$$\% \text{ scoring } 5 = 5/20 \text{ x } 100$$

$$= 25\%$$

The calculations for the values of the pie chart (Fig. 13.3, p. 189), also involved such calculations.

Rates

When summarizing the results of epidemiological investigations (Ch. 5), it is often useful to use this statistic to represent the level at which a disorder is present in a given population. The two rates which are commonly used in the health sciences are:

Incidence rates, which represent the number of new cases of a disorder reported within a time period

Prevalence rates, which represent the total number of cases suffering from a disorder.

$$\text{Incidence rate} = \frac{\text{number of new cases of a disorder}}{\text{total population at risk of the disorder}} \times \text{base}$$

$$\text{Prevalence rate} = \frac{\text{number of existing cases of a disorder}}{\text{total population at risk of the disorder}} \times \text{base}$$

Let us illustrate the above equation by applying it to hypothetical data. Let us consider the condition herpes simplex. Say an epidemiologist is interested in the spread of the condition in a given community.

1. Assume that all the population above the age of 15 years ($N = 1\ 000\ 000$) is at risk of herpes.
2. In 1983, 5000 new cases were reported.
3. In 1983, there was a total (old and new active cases) of 15 000 known cases.

Here, substituting into the equation, incidence rate for herpes = 5000/ 1 000 000 × base = 0.005 × base

The statistic '0.005' is not seen as the best way to represent a rate.

Often, epidemiologists select a base to make the statistic more understandable. The base represents a number for transforming the rate. The base selected depends on the magnitude of the rate; conventionally a multiple of 10, such as 1000, 10 000 or 100 000 is selected. In this instance we select 1000 as the base. Therefore, substituting into the equation, we obtain:

Incidence rate for herpes simplex:

$$= 0.005 \times \frac{1000}{1}$$
$$= 5 \text{ per } 1000$$

Prevalence rate for herpes simplex:

$$= \frac{15000}{1000000} \times \frac{1000}{1}$$
$$= 15 \text{ per } 1000$$

The above statistics can be graphed. For instance, we may wish to represent pictorially the incidence of herpes simplex in the community over a period of five years. The evidence (fictitious) is:

Year	Incidence of herpes (per 1000)
1982	8
1983	15
1984	17
1985	16
1986	10

The graph of the time-series (Fig. 13.7) gives us a visual impression of the incidence rate of the problem in question.

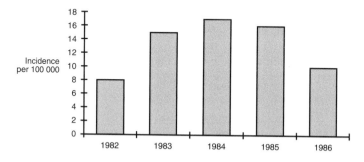

Fig. 13.7 Incidence rate of genital herpes 1982-1986

SUMMARY

We outlined several techniques for organizing, tabulating and graphically presenting both discontinuous (nominal, ordinal) and continuous (interval, ratio) data. It was shown that raw data can be organized and tabulated as a frequency distribution, by counting the number of cases falling into specific categories or class intervals. Data composed of a large number of highly varied measurements were shown to be best presented by grouping the scores into class intervals.

Several techniques of graphing data were discussed: bar graphs and pie charts for discontinuous data, and histograms and frequency polygons for continuous data. The possible shapes of frequency polygons were also examined. It was shown that data grouped in frequency distributions could be also represented as ratios, proportions, percentages or rates.

These statistics were obtained by the mathematical manipulation of the raw data, and were shown to be useful for summarizing the raw data. In the next section, we will examine further techniques of 'crunching' or condensing data by using appropriate descriptive statistics.

SELF ASSESSMENT

Explain the meaning of the terms:

bar graph	cumulative frequency
bell-shaped curve	discontinuous data
continuous data	frequency polygon

frequency distribution
histogram
incidence rate
negative skew
ordered array
pie diagram

positive skew
proportion
rate
ratio
real limit

True or false

1. The organization of nominal or ordinal data involves counting the number of scores falling into discrete categories.
2. Nominal and ordinal data are best graphed as histograms.
3. It is useful to organize interval or ratio data into ordered arrays before constructing frequency distributions.
4. Given a large number of varied scores, we can construct a grouped frequency distribution, usually with about seven class intervals.
5. The midpoint of a given class interval is i.
6. Frequency distributions of continuous data can be presented graphically as histograms or frequency polygons.
7. In a negatively skewed distribution most of the scores are low, with a few high scores spread along the x axis.
8. With a bell-shaped or normal distribution, most of the scores are located at the two extreme ends of the distribution.
9. 'Incidence rates' are statistics which represent the number of active cases of a disorder within a specific time period.
10. For a chronic condition like arthritis, we would expect the prevalence rates to be smaller than the incidence rates.
11. A 'base' represents a number for transforming a rate into a more easily understandable statistic.
12. The wider i, the more specific information is lost about the actual data.
13. A frequency polygon is appropriate for graphing continuously distributed variables.
14. The percentile rank of a score is equal to the frequency of the scores falling up to and including the score.
15. If a curve is negatively skewed, the distribution of the scores has a 'tail' towards the lower values of the variable.
16. The height of a bar (column) represents the frequency, rather than the value, of a variable.
17. A pie diagram is inappropriate for representing nominally scaled data.
18. Incidence rates represent the number of new cases of a disorder reported within a time period.
19. The 'base' for calculating incidence rates is always 10 000.
20. We cannot construct frequency tables for nominally or ordinally scaled data.
21. Ratios are the same as proportions.
22. We can only calculate proportions for nominally scaled data.

Multiple choice

1. Patients indicate their satisfaction with treatment by responding to a question with four options:
   (1) very dissatisfied
   (2) dissatisfied
   (3) satisfied
   (4) very satisfied.

This is an example of a(n) (i) scale, and the resulting frequency distribution should be plotted as a (ii)
   a   (i) nominal (ii) bar graph
   b   (i) ordinal (ii) bar graph
   c   (i) interval (ii) histogram
   d   (i) ordinal (ii) histogram
   e   none of the above.

2. Interval or ratio data should be graphed as a:
   a   histogram
   b   bar graph
   c   frequency polygon
   d   *a* and *b*
   e   *a* and *c*.

3. Your class is asked to do an exam in theoretical physics. Given that only a few students know anything about this subject, the distribution of scores would be:
   a   symmetrical
   b   negatively skewed
   c   positively skewed
   d   bell-shaped
   e   both *a* and *d*.

4. If a curve is symmetrical:
   a   most of the scores fall at the higher values of the *x* axis
   b   most of the scores fall at the lower end of the *x* axis
   c   most of the scores fall at the higher end of the *y* axis
   d   most of the scores fall at the lower end of the *y* axis
   e   if folded in half, the two sides of the curves will coincide.

5. The percentile rank of a person's score on a test is 35. This means that:
   a   the person got 35% of the items correct
   b   the person performed better than 65% of the sample doing the test
   c   both *a* and *b*
   d   the person's score was equal to or better than 35% of the sample doing the test.

6. You are interested in calculating the incidence rate for Huntington's Disease, which is a *very rare* disorder. Which of the following numbers would be your best 'base'?
   a   10
   b   100
   c   1000
   d   10 000

7. A continuous scale of measurement is different from a discrete scale in that a continuous scale:
   a   is an interval scale, not a ratio scale
   b   never provides exact measurements
   c   can take an infinite number of intermediate possible values
   d   never uses decimal numbers
   e   b and c.

A researcher wished to study the effectiveness of a new treatment, A, upon the severity of migraine. A random sample of 50 subjects ($n = 50$) was selected from a group of migraine sufferers attending a pain clinic. Patients were randomly allocated to be treated either with A, or with a currently available biofeedback treatment, B. A pre-test/post-test experimental design was used. Level of pain was assessed using a standardized pain questionnaire, measuring pain responses on a scale between 1–100.
Questions 8–14 refer to the above information.

8. The independent variable in this study was:
   a   the new treatment A
   b   the type of treatment used
   c   the migraine
   d   the patients' scores on the pain questionnaire.

9. The dependent variable in the above study was:
   a   the new treatment A
   b   the type of treatment used
   c   the migraine
   d   the patients' scores on the pain questionnaire.

10. The scale of measurement used to assess the pain responses was:
    a   nominal
    b   ordinal
    c   interval
    d   ratio.

The data for the post-test pain scores for the two groups are summarized in the following table.
Questions 11–14 refer to the table.

Pain ratings	Treatment A	Treatment B
31–40	1	1
41–50	2	2
51–60	3	–
61–70	10	3
71–80	4	4
81–90	3	10
91–100	2	5

11. What would be an appropriate way for this information to be graphed?
    a   frequency polygon
    b   histogram
    c   bar graph
    d   either a or b.

12. What are the real limits of the lowest category?
    a   31–40
    b   31.5–40.4
    c   30.5–40.4
    d   30.5–39.5

13. Which of the following statements is (are) true?
    a   The post-test scores for Treatment B are skewed.
    b   i is equal to 9.
    c   6% of Treatment A post-test scores are under 50.5.
    d   All of the above statements are true.

14. Which of the following statements is supported by the data, assuming that the pre-test scores were equivalent for the two groups?
    a   Treatment A appears to be more effective than B.
    b   Treatment B appears to be more effective than A.
    c   The two treatments appear to be equivalent.
    d   Treatment B appears to be harmful.
    e   a and d.

   The total number of deaths reported in a hypothetical country for a given year was 120 000. The following lists deaths by cause as a percentage of all deaths:

Heart disease	35%
Cancer	25%
Cerebro-vascular disease	15%
Trauma	10%
Respiratory illness	5%
Infections	5%
Other causes	5%

Questions 15–20 refer to this data.

15. Data such as the above are compiled by asking hospitals, physicians, etc. to report deaths to a central agency. This type of information collection is best described as:
    a a survey
    b an experiment
    c a mathematical model
    d field research.

16. The variable 'cause of death' is measured on a(n):
    a nominal scale
    b ordinal scale
    c interval scale
    d ratio scale.

17. The above table should be graphed as a:
    a frequency polygon
    b histogram
    c bar graph
    d *a* and *b*.

18. The number of people who died of either heart disease or cancer is:
    a 35 000
    b 60 000
    c 72 000
    d 90 000.

19. Which of the following statements is false?
    a The proportion of all deaths caused by cancer is 0.25.
    b 5 000 persons died of respiratory illnesses.
    c Twice as many persons died of trauma than infections.
    d 18 000 persons died of cerebro-vascular disease.

20. Of the people who died of trauma, the male:female ratio was 2:1. How many females died of trauma?
    a 4000
    b 8000
    c 12 000
    d Insufficient information to calculate answer.

21. Which of the following statements is true?
    a A graph of continuous data enables the reader to interpolate.
    b When constructing a frequency distribution for grouped scores, *i* should be equal to the number of class intervals.
    c A histogram is like a bar graph, except that with a histogram the bars do not touch each other.
    d A bell-shaped curve is an example of a skewed distribution.

22. Descriptive statistics:
    a are used to make inferences about populations from small samples
    b are only appropriate in non-experimental designs
    c summarize data about samples or populations
    d are derived from probability theory.

A researcher has collected data concerning the amount of time in seconds that it took a group of normal and a group of brain-damaged subjects to complete a standard motor task. The data is shown below arranged in a grouped frequency distribution.

Class interval	Time in seconds	
	Normals	**Brain-damaged**
12–14	1	0
15–17	2	0
18–20	5	1
21–23	10	2
24–27	4	4
28–30	3	10
31–33	1	3

23. The total number of subjects used in this study was:
    a 7
    b 26
    c 46
    d 50.

24. The class interval width *i* is:
    a 2
    b 3
    c 4
    d 7.

25. The real limits for the class interval 15-17 are:
    a 14.5–17.4
    b 15 + 0.5
    c 14–18
    d 2.

26. The scale of measurement used for the dependent variable was:
    a nominal
    b ordinal
    c interval
    d ratio.

27. Which of the following statements is true?
    a   The distribution of scores for the normals approximates a normal distribution.
    b   The scores for the brain-damaged subjects was highly skewed.
    c   The above investigation should not be classified as an experiment.
    d   All the above are true.

28. On the basis of previous evidence, the score of 27.4 is taken as demonstrating adequate motor function, while longer times for completing the task demonstrate some motor impairment. The proportion of normals who scored under 27.4 is___while the proportion of brain-damaged who scored under this score was___.
    a   4, 13
    b   0.85, 0.35
    c   0.80, 0.17
    d   0.26, 0.20.

29. Assuming external validity, which of the following statements is supported by the evidence?
    a   Brain-damaged subjects take longer to complete the standard task.
    b   The greater the degree of brain damage, the slower the task completion.
    c   The task is valid for discriminating subjects with brain damage.
    d   a and c.

14

Measures of central tendency and dispersion

INTRODUCTION

In the previous section we examined how raw data can be organized and represented as frequency distributions in order to be easily communicated and understood. We might need to further condense our data, so that we can represent our finding in terms of only a few numbers (or statistics). The two statistics necessary for representing a frequency distribution are measures of central tendency and dispersion.

Measures of central tendency are statistics or numbers expressing (numerically) the most typical or average scores in a distribution. Measures of dispersion (or variability) are statistics or numbers expressing the extent to which scores are dispersed (or spread out) numerically.

The overall aim of this Chapter is to examine the use of several types of measures of central tendency and dispersal commonly used in the health sciences. As quantitative evidence arising from investigations is commonly presented in terms of these statistics, it is absolutely essential for the student to understand these concepts.

The specific aims of this Chapter are to:

1. Discuss the selection and use of measures for central tendency
2. Discuss the selection and use of measures for dispersal
3. Outline the relationship between the shapes of frequency distributions and the selection of appropriate descriptive statistics.

MEASURES OF CENTRAL TENDENCY

The mode

When the data are nominal, the appropriate measure of central tendency is the mode. The mode is the most frequently occurring score in a distribution.

Therefore, for the data shown in Table 13.1 (p. 186), the mode is the 'females' category. The mode can be obtained by inspection. It is the category with the largest frequency on a frequency table, the highest bar on a bar chart, or the largest segment of a pie graph.

The median

With ordinal, interval, or ratio data, central tendency can also be represented by the median. The median is the score which divides the distribution into half; half of the scores fall under the median, and half above the median. That is, if scores are arranged in an ordered array, the median would be the middle score. With a large number of cases, it may not be feasible to locate the middle score simply by inspection. To calculate which is the middle score, we can use the formula $(n + 1)/2$, where n is the total number of cases in a sample. This formula gives us the number of the middle score. We can then count that number from either end of an ordered array.

In general, if n is odd, the median is the middle score; if n is even, then the median falls between the two centre scores. The formula $(n + 1)/2$ is again used to tell us which score in an ordered array will be the median. For example:

5, 8, 9, 10, 28.	Median = 9 (n is odd)
6, 17, 19, 20, 21, 27.	Median = 19.5 (n is even)

For a grouped frequency distribution, the calculation of the median might be a little more complicated. If we assume that the variable is continuous, (for example, time, height, weight, or level of pain) we can use a formula for calculating the median. This formula (explained in detail below) can be applied to ordinal data, provided the variable being measured has an underlying continuity. For instance, in a study of the measurement of pain reports we obtain the following data, where $n = 17$:

1, 1, 2, 2, 2, 2, 2, 3, 3, 3, 3, 4, 4, 4, 5, 5, 5

The above data can be represented by a bar graph. (Fig. 14.1).

Here we can obtain the mode simply by inspection. The mode = 2 (the most frequent score).

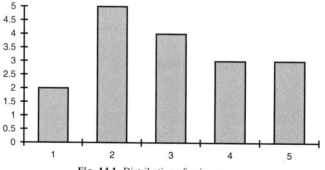

Fig. 14.1 Distribution of pain scores

For the median, we need the 9th score, as this will divide the distribution into 2 equal halves. By inspection, we can see that the median will fall into category '3'. Assuming underlying continuity, and applying the previously discussed formula, we have:

Score	Real class interval	f	$cum\ f$
1	0.5–1.4	2	2
2	1.5–2.4	5	7
3	2.5–3.4	4	11*
4	3.5–4.4	3	14
5	4.5–5.4	3	17
		$n = 17$	*class interval containing median

$$Mdn\ \text{(median)} = x_L + i\ \frac{(n/2) - cum\ f_L}{fi}$$

Where:

x_L = real lower limit of the class interval containing the median
i = width of the class interval
n = number of cases
$cum\ f_L$ = cumulative frequency at the real lower limit of the interval
fi = frequency of cases in the interval containing the median.

Substituting into the above equation:

$$Mdn = 2.5 + 1 \left[\frac{17/2 - 7}{4} \right]$$

$$= 2.5 + 1 \left[\frac{1.5}{4} \right]$$

$$= 2.875$$

The mean

The mean, $\overline{X}$ or μ, is defined as the sum of all the scores divided by the number of scores. The mean is, in fact, the arithmetic average for a distribution. The mean is calculated by the following equations:

$$\overline{X} = \frac{\Sigma x}{n} \quad \text{(for a sample)}$$

$$\mu = \frac{\Sigma x}{N} \quad \text{(for a population)}$$

Σx — the sum of the scores

$\overline{X}$ — the mean of a sample

μ — the mean of a population

x — the values of the variable, that is the different elements in a sample or population

n or N — the number of scores in a sample or population

Therefore, given the following sample scores:

2, 3, 5, 6, 7

To calculate the mean:

$$\overline{X} = \frac{\Sigma x}{n} = \frac{23}{5} = 4.6$$

When n or N are very large, the average is calculated with the formula above but usually with the assistance of computers.

COMPARISON OF THE MODE, MEDIAN, AND MEAN

The mode can be used as a measure of central tendency for any level of scaling. However, as it only takes into account the most frequent scores it is not a generally satisfactory way of presenting central tendency. For instance, consider the following two sets of scores, A and B:

A		B	
x	f	x	f
1	16	1	8
2	1	2	7
3	1	3	6
4	7	4	4
	$n = 25$		$n = 25$

You can see, either by inspection or by sketching a graph, that the two distributions A and B are quite different. Yet the modes are the same i.e.1.

The median divides distributions into two equal halves, and is appropriate for ordinal, interval or ratio data. For interval or ratio data, however, the mean is the most appropriate measure of central tendency for interval or ratio data. The reason for this is that in calculating this statistic, we take into account all the values of the variable. In this way, it gives the best representation of the average score. Clearly, it is inappropriate to use the mean with nominal data, as the concept of 'average' doesn't apply to discrete categories. What would be the 'average' of 10 males and 20 females?

There is some justification for using the median as a measure of central tendency when the variable being measured is continuous. However this is controversial, and the mean should be preferred. On the other hand, when a distribution is highly skewed, the median might be more appropriate than the mean for representing the 'typical' score. Consider the distribution:

2, 2, 2, 5, 7, 8, 9

mode   = 2

median   = 5

$\overline{X}$ = 5

Let's change the '9' to '44':

2, 2, 2, 5, 7, 8, 44

mode   = 2

median   = 5

$\overline{X}$ = 10

Clearly, the median and the mode are less sensitive to extreme scores, while the mean is pulled towards extreme scores. This might be a disadvantage. For example, there are 7 people working in a small factory, with the following incomes per week:

$100; $200; $200; $300; $400; $400; $1900

median   = $300

$\overline{X}$ = $500

The distribution of wages is highly skewed, by the high income of the owner of the factory ($1900). The mean, $500, is higher than six of the seven scores; it is in no way typical of the distribution. In cases like this the median is more representative of the distribution.

Figures 14.2 A, B, and C illustrate the relationships between the skew of frequency distributions and the three measures of central tendency discussed in this chapter. We should remember that the mode will always be at the highest point, the median will divide the area under the curve into halves, and the mean is the average of all the scores in the distribution. Also, the greater the skew in a distribution, the more the measures of central tendency are likely to differ.

MEASURES OF DISPERSAL

We have seen that a single statistic can be used to describe the central tendency of a frequency distribution. This information is insufficient to characterize a distribution; we also need a measure of how much the scores are dispersed or spread out. The dispersal of discrete data is of little relevance, as the degree of dispersal will be limited by the number of categories defined by the investigator at the beginning of measurement.

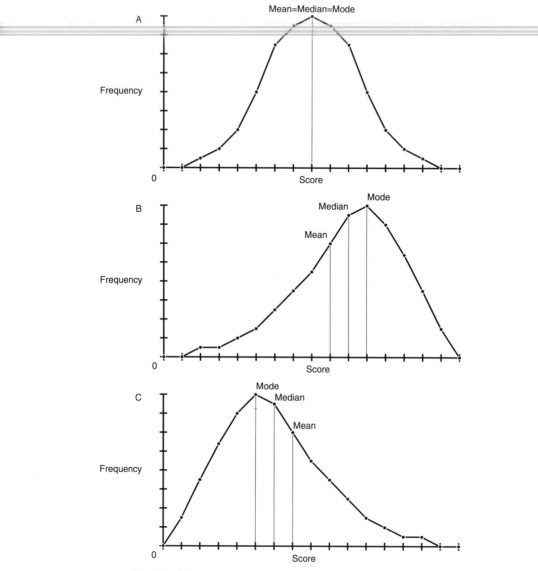

Fig. 14.2 Measures of central tendency in (A) normal distribution;
(B) negative skewing; (C) positive skewing

Consider the following two hypothetical distributions representing the IQs of two groups of intellectually disabled children:

Group A: 45, 50, 55, 60, 60, 70, 80

Group B: 57, 58, 59, 60, 61, 62, 63

It is evident that although $\overline{X}_A = \overline{X}_B = 60$, the variability (or dispersal) of the scores of Group A is greater than that of Group B. In so far as IQ is related to the activities appropriate for these children, Group A will provide a greater challenge to the therapist working with the children.

The three statistics commonly used to indicate the numerical value of dispersal are the range, the variance and the standard deviation.

The range

The range is the difference between the highest and lowest scores in a distribution. As we mentioned given the IQ data above, the ranges are:

Group A: $80 - 45 + 1 = 36$

Group B: $63 - 57 + 1 = 7$

Although the range is easy to calculate, it is dependent only on the two extreme scores. In this way, we are not representing the typical dispersal of the scores. That is, the range might be distorted by a small number of atypical scores or 'outliers'. Consider, for instance, the differences in the range for the data given. The example on page 209 shows that just one outlying score in a distribution has an enormous impact on the range ($1900 - $100 = 1800). Obviously, some measure of average dispersal would be a preferable index of dispersal.

Average deviation

A convenient measure of variability might be average deviation about the mean. Consider Group B shown previously. Here $\overline{X} = 60$. To calculate average dispersal about the mean, we subtract the mean from each score, sum the individual deviations, and divide by n, the number of measurements.

$$\text{Average deviation} = \frac{\Sigma(x - \overline{X})}{n}$$

x	$x - \overline{X}$
57	−3
58	−2
59	−1
60	0
61	+1
62	+2
63	+3

Therefore: $\Sigma(x - \overline{X}) = (-3) + (-2) + (-1) + (0) + (1) + (2) + (3) = 0$

This is a general result; the sum of the average deviations about the mean is always zero. You can demonstrate this for the average deviation of Group A. The problem can be solved by squaring the deviations, as the square of negative numbers is always positive. This statistic is called the sums of squares (SS) and is always a positive number. This leads to a new statistic called the variance.

The variance

The variance (σ^2 or S^2) is defined as the sum of the squared deviations about the mean divided by the number of cases.

$$\sigma^2 = \frac{\Sigma(x - \mu)^2}{N} \quad \text{(for a population)}$$

$$S^2 = \frac{\Sigma(x - \overline{X})^2}{n - 1} \quad \text{(for a sample)}$$

Divide by $n - 1$ when calculating the variance for a sample, when we use S^2 as an estimate of population variance. Dividing by n results in an estimate which is too small, given that a degree of freedom has been lost calculating $\overline{X}$.

For the IQ example shown above, the variance is calculated as follows:

x	$x - \overline{X}$	$(x - \overline{X})^2$
57	-3	9
58	-2	4
59	-1	1
60	0	0
61	1	1
62	2	4
63	3	9
$\overline{X} = 60$		$\Sigma(x - \overline{X})^2 = 28$

Substituting into the formula:

$$\sigma^2 = \frac{\Sigma(x - \overline{X})^2}{n - 1} = \frac{28}{6} = 4.67$$

The problem with variability as a measure of dispersal is that the deviations were squared. In this sense, we are overstating the spread of the scores. In taking the square root of the variance, we arrive at the most commonly used measure of dispersal for continuous data: the standard deviation.

The standard deviation

The standard deviation (σ or s) is defined as the square root of the variance:

$$\sigma = \sqrt{\sigma^2} = \sqrt{\frac{\Sigma(X-\mu)^2}{N}}$$

$$s = \sqrt{s^2} = \sqrt{\frac{\Sigma(x-\overline{X})^2}{n-1}}$$

Therefore, the standard deviation for Group B is:

$$s = \sqrt{s^2} = 4.67 = 2.16$$

The size of the standard deviation reflects the shape of the frequency distribution representative of the data. Clearly, the larger σ or s, the relatively more spread out the scores are about the mean in a distribution. Calculation of the variance or the standard deviation is extremely tedious for large n using the method shown above. Statistics texts provide a variety of calculational formulae to derive these statistics. However, the common use of computers in research and administration makes it superfluous to discuss these formulae in detail.

The semi-interquartile range

We have seen previously that if we are summarizing ordinal data, or interval or ratio data which is highly skewed, then the median is the appropriate measure of central tendency. The statistic called interquartile and semi-interquartile range is used as the measure of dispersion when the median is the appropriate measure of central tendency for a distribution.

The interquartile range is the distance between the scores representing the 25th (Q1) and 75th (Q3) percentile ranks in a distribution.

It is appropriate to define what we mean by percentiles (sometimes called centiles). The percentile or centile rank of a given score specifies the percentage of scores in a distribution falling up to and including the score. As an illustration, consider Figure 14.3, in which:

- 25% of cases fall up to and including Q1.
- 50% of cases fall up to and including the median.
- 75% of cases or scores fall up to and including Q3.
- 25% of cases or scores fall above Q3.

The distances A and B represent the distances between the median and Q1 and Q3. When a distribution is symetrical or normal, the distances A and B will be equal. However, when a distribution is skewed, the two distances will be quite different.

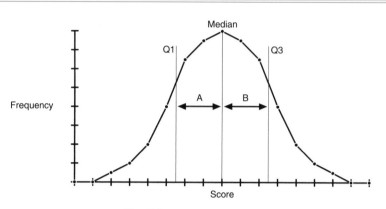

Fig. 14.3 Interquartile ranges

The semi-interquartile range (sometimes called the quartile deviation) is half of the distance between the scores representing the 25th (Q1) and 75th (Q3) percentile ranks in a distribution. Let us look at an example. Say we have a sample where $n = 16$ and the values of the variable are 1, 5, 7, 7, 8, 9, 9, 10, 11, 12, 13, 15, 19, 20, 20, 20. Clearly, a frequency distribution of this data is not even close to normal as the distribution is not symmetrical and the mode is at the maximum value. Therefore, the median is selected as the appropriate measure for central tendency, and we should use the interquartile range as the measure of dispersion.

Looking at the data, we find that:

1	5	7	7	*	8	9	9	10	†	11	12	13	15	‡	19	20	20	20

* 25th centile (first quartile, Q1)
† 50th centile: median (second quartile, Q2)
‡ 75th centile (third quartile, Q3)

The score which cuts off the first 25% of scores (25th centile) is the first quartile (Q1). As we have $n = 16$, Q1 will cut off the first 4 scores (25% of 16 is 4).

$$\text{Thus: } Q1 = \frac{7+8}{2} = 7.5$$

The third quartile (Q3) is the score which cuts off 75% of the scores. As $n = 16$, Q3 will cut off 12 scores (75% of 16 is 12).

$$Q3 = \frac{15+19}{2} = 17.0$$

Therefore, the semi-interquartile range is:

$$\frac{Q3 - Q1}{2} = \frac{17.0 - 7.5}{2} = 4.75$$

The larger the semi-interquartile range, the more the scores are spread out about the median.

SUMMARY

In this section we discussed two essential statistics for representing frequency distributions: measures of central tendency and dispersal. The measures of central tendency outlined were the mode and median for discrete data, and the mean for continuous data. Measures of dispersal or variability were shown to be the range, average deviation, variance, and standard deviation. These statistics are appropriate for 'crunching' the data together to the point that a distribution of raw data can be meaningfully represented by only two statistics. That is, the raw data representing the outcome of investigations or clinical measurements are expressed in this manner. We have seen that the mean and the standard deviation are most appropriate for interval or ratio data. The median and semi-interquartile range are used when the data was measured on an ordinal scale, or when interval or ratio data is found to have a highly skewed distribution. The mode represents the most frequent scores.

The contents of the section focused on the use and meaning of these concepts, rather than stressing involved calculations. These calculations are nowadays made by computers. In Chapter 15, we discuss the application of the mean and standard deviation for relating specific scores to an overall distribution.

SELF ASSESSMENT

Explain the meaning of the following terms:

central tendency	range
descriptive statistics	semi-interquartile range
dispersion	standard deviation
mean	statistic
median	variability
mode	variance

True or false

1. Inferential statistics are used to describe specific characteristics of the data.
2. With nominal data, the mean should be used as a measure of central tendency.
3. The mode represents the most frequently occurring score in a distribution.
4. With ordinal data, we can use both the mode and the mean as a measure of central tendency.

5. When the data are interval or ratio, we can use the mean as a measure of central tendency.
6. With continuous data, the median is the most appropriate measure of central tendency.
7. If a continuous distribution is highly skewed, the median might be the appropriate measure of central tendency.
8. When a frequency distribution is positively skewed, the mean is greater than the median or the mode.
9. Given a normal distribution, the three measures of central tendency are equivalent.
10. The range is the simplest indicator of variability.
11. The range is calculated by adding the lowest score to the highest score in a distribution.
12. Given nominal or ordinal data, we should use the standard deviation as a measure of dispersion.
13. The square root of the variance is called the standard deviation.
14. s and α indicate the extent to which scores are distributed about the mean.
15. When a distribution consists of very different scores, s or σ will be relatively large.
16. It is possible to have data with three different values for measures of central tendency.
17. The 50th percentile score and the median will always be the same value.
18. The median is less affected than the mean by extreme scores at one end of a distribution.
19. Central tendency describes the 'typical' value of a set of scores.
20. We use $n - 1$ in the denominator of the equation for calculating the sample standard deviation, because it provides us with an accurate estimate of the population standard deviation.
21. If the number of raw scores is odd, the median is the score in the middle position.
22. The mean must have a value equal to one of the scores in the distribution.
23. 25% of the scores fall between Q1 and the median.
24. The distance between Q1 and the median is always different to the distance between Q3 and the median.
25. The semi-interquartile range is inappropriate to use with skewed distributions.

Multiple choice

1. Given a set of nominally scaled scores, the most appropriate measure of central tendency is the:
   a   mean
   b   mode
   c   standard deviation
   d   range.

2. Which of the following statements is true?
   a   The mode is the most useful measure of central tendency.
   b   The variance is the square root of the standard deviation.
   c   The median and the 50th percentile rank have different values.
   d   The mean is more affected by extreme scores than the median.

Questions 3-5 refer to the following data:
   2, 2, 3, 4, 6, 6, 7.

3. Σx is equal to:
   a   30
   b   40
   c   50
   d   none of the above.

4. $(\Sigma x)^2$ is equal to:
   a   124
   b   128
   c   130
   d   900

5. The median is equal to:
   a   6
   b   5
   c   4
   d   3

6. The range for the above set of scores is:
   a   7
   b   5
   c   2
   d   1

A clinic had 50 patients attending in a month. The number of times each patient visited the clinic is given below in the form of frequency distribution.

No. of visits (X)	No. of patients (f)
7	3
6	6
5	6
4	10
3	21
2	0
1	4

Questions 7-9 refer to this information.

7. The total number of visits by the patients was:
   a   194
   b   28
   c   50
   d   none of the above.

8. The mean number of visits by patients was:
   a   3.89
   b   3.50
   c   1.00
   d   3.88

9. The median number of visits per patient was:
   a   3.88
   b   3.50
   c   3.00
   d   4.00

10. The more dispersed, or spread out, a set of scores is:
    a   the greater the difference between the mean and the median
    b   the greater the value of the mode
    c   the greater the standard deviation
    d   the smaller the interquartile range.

11. The measure of central tendency which is most strongly influenced by extreme values in the 'tail' of the distribution is:
    a   the mean
    b   the median
    c   the mode
    d   the standard deviation
    e   none of the above.

12. The mean height of a student group is 167 cm. Assuming height is normally distributed this enables us to deduce that:
    a   approximately half of all students are taller than 167 cm
    b   being a student stunts your growth
    c   approximately half of all students are shorter than 167 cm
    d   a and c
    e   none of these.

13. If we subtract the value of the mean from every score in a set of scores the sum of the remaining values will be:
    a   impossible to determine
    b   equal to the mean
    c   a measure of the dispersion around the mean
    d   zero
    e   none of the above.

14. Given a normally distributed continuous variable the best measure of central tendency is the:
    a   mode
    b   median
    c   mean
    d   standard deviation
    e   none of the above.

15. If a distribution is negatively skewed, then:
    a   the median is greater than the mean
    b   the mode is greater than the median
    c   the mean is greater than the median
    d   both a and b are true
    e   none of the above are true.

16. In a normal distribution, the mean, the median and the mode:
    a   always have the same value
    b   the mean has the higher value
    c   the mean has the lower value
    d   have no particular relationship
    e   cannot take the same value.

17. The measure of central tendency which is the most frequently occurring score is:
    a   the mean
    b   the median
    c   the mode
    d   the standard deviation
    e   none of these.

18. Given the group of scores 1, 4, 4, 4 and 7, it can be said of the mean, the median, and the mode that:
    a   the mean is larger than either the median or the mode
    b   all are the same
    c   the median is larger than either the mean or the mode
    d   all are different
    e   the mode is larger than either the median or the mean.

A nurse recorded the number of analgesic preparations taken by patients in a surgical ward. The resulting data were: 5, 2, 8, 2, 3, 2, 4, 12.
    Questions 19-23 refer to this data.

19. The mode for this distribution is:
    a   2
    b   3
    c   8
    d   there is no mode.

20. The median is:
    a 2.00
    b 3.50
    c 3.00
    d 3.25

21. The mean is:
    a 3.52
    b 5.43
    c 4.75
    d 4.15

22. The range is:
    a 9
    b 10
    c 12
    d 2

23. The standard deviation is:
    a 3.04
    b 5.81
    c 2.28
    d 3.58

Questions 24-28 refer to this data: 3, 3, 4, 5, 6, 7, 8, 9, 9, 10, 38, 60.

24. The median is:
    a 7.0
    b 7.5
    c 8.0
    d 3 or 9

25. Q1 is:
    a 4.5
    b 5.5
    c 8.0
    d 9.5

26. Q3 is:
    a 4.5
    b 6.0
    c 7.5
    d 9.5

27. The semi-interquartile range is:
    a 2.5
    b 4.5
    c 6.0
    d 9.0

28. The semi-interquartile range is preferred to the standard deviation as a measure of dispersal when:
   a   the sample size is small
   b   the distribution is standardized
   c   the distribution is highly skewed
   d   the range is small.

15

Standard scores and the normal curve

INTRODUCTION

In the present chapter we discuss the use of the mean and standard deviation for standardizing distributions. Standard distributions are useful for comparing different sets of measurements. Also, standard scores can specify the position of a score or measurement in relation to a population. In this way, standard scores can be applied to producing and understanding 'norms' in the health sciences.

That is, specific measurements are intelligible only against a background of how the population of scores are distributed.

The specific aims of this chapter are to:

1. Define 'standard' scores.
2. Describe the characteristics of normal and standard normal curves
3. Show how standard normal curves can be used for calculating percentile ranks
4. Show how standard normal curves can be used to compare scores from different distributions.

STANDARD SCORES (z SCORES)

Consider this example: infant A walked unaided at the age of 40 weeks, while infant B is 65 weeks old but still cannot walk. What sense can we make of these measurements? Could infant B need further clinical investigation, in case of some neurological abnormality? The fact that the infant B is unable to walk at the age of 65 weeks is not very informative in the absence of additional information as to how this compares with norms for other children. However, say that it is known that the distribution of walking ages is such that $\mu = 50$ weeks, and $\sigma = 5$. Given that the frequency distribution is normal, the frequency polygon representing the population would look something like that shown in Figure 15.1.

In this instance, infant B's score is clearly above the mean. In fact, by inspection, we can see the infant's score at this point of time was three standard deviations $(+3)$ above the mean $(65 = 50 + (3 \times 5))$. In contrast infant A began walking earlier than the mean, his score of 40 being two standard deviations (−2) below the mean. In general, any 'raw' score in a frequency distribution can be described in terms of its distance from the mean. The process of transforming a score into a measurement based on its distance from the mean in standard deviations is called **standardizing** the score. Such 'transformed' scores are called z scores or standard scores.

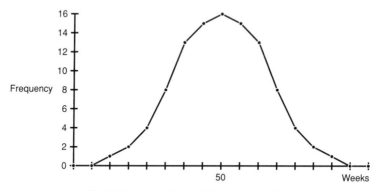

Fig. 15.1 Age at which children walk unaided

A z score represents how many standard deviations a given raw score is above the mean. The equation for transforming specific raw scores into z scores is given as:

$$z = \frac{x - \mu}{\sigma}$$

$$z = \frac{x - \overline{X}}{s}$$

Where x is the raw score, $\overline{X}$ or μ is the mean of the distribution from which the score was drawn, s or σ is the standard deviation of the distribution. That is, when we know the mean and standard deviation of a distribution, we can transform any raw score into a z score. Conversely, when the z score is known, we can use the above equations to calculate the corresponding raw scores.

In the above example, the z scores corresponding to the infants' raw scores are:

$$\text{Infant A: } z = \frac{x - \mu}{\sigma}$$
$$= \frac{40 - 50}{5}$$
$$= -2$$

$$\text{Infant B: } z = \frac{x - \mu}{\sigma}$$

$$= \frac{65 - 50}{5}$$

$$= +3$$

These calculations correspond to our previous observations that A's score was 2 standard deviations below the mean and B's score was 3 standard deviations above the mean. In other words, A walked very early and B was a very late starter. The particular value of standardizing scores for understanding clinical or research evidence will be discussed in the context of the concepts of normal and standard normal distributions.

NORMAL DISTRIBUTIONS

Many variables measured in the biological, behavioural and clinical sciences are approximately 'normally' distributed. What is meant by a normal distribution is illustrated by the normal curve (Fig. 15.2 below) which is a frequency polygon representing the theoretical distribution of population scores. We assume here that the variable x has been measured on an interval or ratio scale and that it is a continuous variable such as weight, height or blood pressure.

The normal curve has the following characteristics:

1. It is symmetrical about the mean, so that equal numbers of cases fall above and below the mean (mean = median = mode).
2. Relatively few cases fall into the high or low values of x. Most of the cases fall close to the mean. (For the theoretical normal distribution, the arms of the curve do not intersect with the X axis, allowing for a very few extreme scores).
3. The precise equation for the normal curve has been worked out by the mathematician Gauss, so that it is sometimes referred to as a Gaussian curve.

We need not worry about the actual formula. Rather, the point is that given that the functional relationship between f and x is known, integral calculus can be used to calculate areas under the curve for any value of x. All normal curves have the same general shape; whether we are graphing IQ or weight the same bell shape will appear. The only differences between the curves are the mean value and the amount of variation. This is why the mean and the standard deviation provide us with important information about any particular normal distribution. Note that it is unlikely that any real data are precisely normally distributed. Rather, the normal distribution is a mathematical model which is useful for *representing* real distributions.

The standard normal curve

If we transform the raw scores of a variable into z scores, and then plot the frequency polygon for the distribution we will have a standard curve. If the original distribution was normal, then the frequency polygon will be a standard normal curve. Standard normal curves are identical.

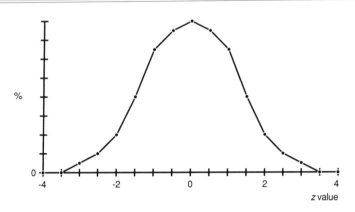

Fig. 15.2 Standard normal distribution

By transforming raw scores into z scores, we are getting rid of differences in means and standard deviations, which are the only things which distinguish between non-standardized normal curves (Fig. 15.2).

The standard normal curve has the following additional properties:

1. The mean is always 0 (zero). For example, the z score corresponding to $\mu = 50$ (as in the 'infants' walking age' example) is:

$$z = \frac{50 - 50}{5} = 0$$

2. The mean = median = mode.
3. The standard deviation of z scores is always 1 (one). For instance, the z score for 55 (which is clearly one standard deviation above the mean) is:

$$z = \frac{55 - 50}{5} = 1$$

4. It is assumed that the total area under the curve adds up to 1.00. Since the normal curve is symmetrical, 0.5 of the area falls above $z = 0$ and 0.5 falls below $z = 0$. This is another way of saying that 50% of the total cases fall below the mean, and 50% of the cases fall above the mean (which is equal to the median).
5. More generally, we can use appropriate tables to estimate the area under the standard normal curve for any given z scores. These areas are available in table form (see Appendix A) so that for any value of z we can read off the corresponding area.
6. The area under the curve between any two points is directly proportional to the percentage of cases falling between those two points. We can use

the standard normal curve to calculate the percentage of scores falling between any specified two scores.

In the next subsection, we will examine the use of the table of areas under the standard normal curve to understand the meaning of measurements in relation to distributions.

CALCULATIONS OF AREAS UNDER THE NORMAL CURVE

We have already examined the concept of percentile ranks (page 213). The normal curve is useful for evaluating the percentile rank of scores in normal distributions. Appendix A gives the proportion of areas under the standard normal curve which lies:

1. between the mean and a given z score
2. beyond the z score

Since normal distributions are symmetrical, the same proportions are true also for the area between the mean and any negative z score. Only the positive values are given in Appendix A.

Let us see how we can use this information to estimate the percentile ranks of the two infants' walking ages. We have shown previously that for infant A, $z = -2$. Let us now turn to Appendix A. In going down the column of z scores, we find that the area corresponding to $z = 2.0$ is 0.4772 (between) and 0.0229 (beyond).

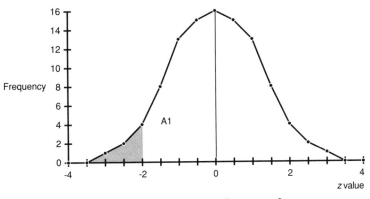

Fig. 15.3 Area (A1) corresponding to $z = -2$

Also, we know that the area A1 under the curve in Figure 15.3 must be:

Shaded portion = 0.5000 − 0.4772
= 0.0228 (as half the scores fall under the mean)

This proportion can be expressed as a percentage, so that 2.28% of the cases in the distribution fall below $z = -2$. We have defined percentile rank for a score as the percentage of cases in a distribution falling up to and including a specific score. Therefore, the percentile rank for infant A's walking is 2.28%. Of all children, only 2.28% learn to walk as early as or earlier than infant A. Clearly, he is doing well.

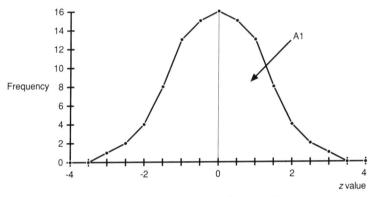

Fig. 15.4   Area (A1) corresponding to $z = 3$

What then is the percentile rank for infant B's performance? As you remember, $z = +3$. Looking up the area corresponding to $z = 3$ in Appendix A we find the area (A1 in Fig. 15.4) is equal to 0.4987. Therefore, the proportion of scores falling up to and including $z = +3$ is $0.5 + 0.4987 = 0.9987$.

Expressing this finding as a percentage, we find that 99.87% of children learn to walk by the age of 65 weeks. As we said earlier, infant B still isn't walking. Perhaps further clinical tests are indicated, although we should keep in mind that an unusual or extreme score is not necessarily indicative of pathological states.

Critical values

Of course, we can work the other way by determining the raw scores corresponding to areas under the normal curve in Appendix A. For example, say

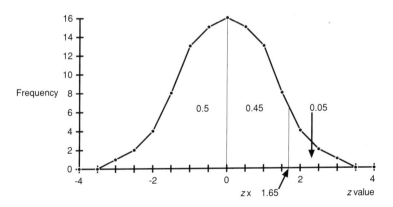

Fig. 15.5   Determining z score of 95th percentile

that the slowest 5% of infants are offered some special exercises in learning to walk. What would be the age at which the exercises should be offered, should the child not be walking? The question here is determining the score that corresponds to the 95th percentile of the distribution. This can be represented as shown in Figure 15.5.

From Figure 15.5 we can see that we need to discover the z score that corresponds to an area of 0.45 above the mean. By consulting the normal distribution table (see Appendix A), it can be seen that the corresponding z score is $z = 1.65$.

This is a critical value for the statistic in defining an area.

Given the z score, we can calculate the corresponding raw score from the formula:

$$z = \frac{(x - \mu)}{\sigma}$$

$$\textit{Therefore:} \quad 1.65 = \frac{x - 50}{5}$$

$$x = (5 \times 1.65) + 50$$

$$= 58.25$$

That is, if the slowest 5% are thought to be in need of help, then children somewhat over 58 weeks old and not still walking would be recommended for the remedial exercises.

STANDARD NORMAL CURVES FOR THE COMPARISON OF DISTRIBUTIONS

One of the uses of standard distributions is that we can compare scores from entirely different distributions.

For example, if a student scored 63 on test A, and 52 on test B, on which test did the student do better? If we define 'better' as solely in terms of raw scores, then clearly the student did better on test A. However, test A might have been easier than test B, so that if the overall performances of all students on the tests are taken into account, the student's relative performance might be better on test B.

Say test A, $\overline{X} = 65$ and $s = 8$
test B, $\overline{X} = 40$ and $s = 8$

Therefore, using the formula for calculating z scores, and looking up the corresponding areas in Appendix A (do this yourself) we find that:

Raw scores	z scores	Percentile ranks
$x = 63$	−0.25	40.1
$x = 52$	+1.50	93.3

Thus, the student performed better on test B, by scoring higher than 93% of other students sitting for the test.

This example illustrates that in some circumstances the meaning of specific scores have to be interpreted against 'standards'.

Another use of standard distributions is in interpreting the meaning of the results of investigations in the health sciences. Let us examine the following hypothetical example.

An investigator measured levels of blood cholesterol in a sample of 300 adults who are meat eaters, and 100 adults who are vegetarians. The results of the investigation are summarized below:

	Mean blood cholesterol (mg/cc)	**Standard deviation**
Meat eaters	0.6	0.15
Vegetarians	0.4	0.1

Now, say you are a clinician working with patients with cardiac disorders and you are interested in the following questions:

1. Approximately what per cent of vegetarians had blood cholesterol levels greater than the average meat eater?
2. Approximately what per cent of meat eaters had blood cholesterol levels lower than that of the average vegetarian?

The percentage of cases of vegetarians with blood cholesterol greater than 0.6 (the mean for the meat eaters) is represented by area A1 in Figure 15.6.

$$z = \frac{0.6 - 0.4}{0.1} = 2$$

$$\text{Area A1} = 0.0228$$

Therefore, approximately 2.3% of vegetarians had blood cholesterol levels higher than the average for meat eaters.

Figure 15.7 demonstrates the area (A1) corresponding to the percentage of meat eaters with lower blood cholesterol than the average vegetarian.

$$z = \frac{0.4 - 0.6}{0.15} = 1.33$$

$$\text{Area A1} = 0.0918$$

Therefore, approximately 9.2% of meat eaters had lower blood cholesterol levels than the average vegetarian.

SUMMARY

We found that if the mean and standard deviation for a given distribution have been calculated, then we can transform any raw score into a standard (or z) score.

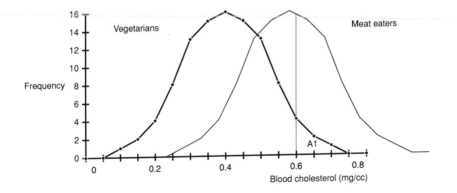

Fig. 15.6 Area A1 corresponds to the percentage of vegetarians
with blood cholesterol higher than 0.6 mg/cc

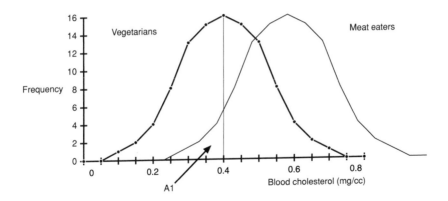

Fig. 15.7 Area A1 corresponds to the percentage of meat eaters
with lower blood cholesterol than the mean for vegetarians

The z score represents how many standard deviations a specific score is above
or below the mean. We described how to calculate this transformed score for a
population or a sample. Also, we outlined the essential characteristics of the
normal and the standard normal curves.

It was pointed out that if the original frequency distribution was approximately
normal, then the table of normal curves (Appendix A) could be used to calculate
percentile ranks of raw scores, or the percentage of scores falling between
specified scores. Also, z scores were shown to be useful in comparing scores
arising from two or more different normal distributions.

The above information is applicable to clinical practice, for instance in
interpreting the significance of an individual's assessment in relation to known
population norms.

SELF ASSESSMENT

Explain the meaning of the following terms:

normal curve	standard normal curve
probability	transformed score
standard score	z score

True or false

1. z scores express how many standard deviations a particular score is from the mean.
2. Negative z scores are further from the mean than positive z scores.
3. Even when the distribution of raw scores is skewed, the standardized distribution will be normal.
4. The mean of a standard normal distribution is always 1.0.
5. The total area under the standard normal curve is 1.0.
6. The area of a normal curve between any two designated z scores expresses the proportion or percentage of cases falling between the two points.
7. The greater the value of $\overline{X}$ and s the greater the value of the z scores in corresponding standard distributions.
8. About 10% of scores fall 3 standard deviations above the mean.
9. A standardized distribution has the same shape as the distribution from which it was derived.
10. Notwithstanding the level of skewness in a distribution, the standard normal curve is useful for determining the percentile rank of a score.
11. In a normal distribution, the higher the z score, the higher will be the frequency of the corresponding raw score.
12. 50% of scores fall between $z = 0.5$ and $z = -0.5$.
13. In a normal curve, approximately 34% of the scores fall between $z = 0$ and $z = -1$.
14. A percentile rank represents the number of cases falling above a particular score.
15. Given a bimodal distribution of raw scores, the standard normal curve is inappropriate for calculating percentile ranks.
16. $z = -2.58$ has a percentile rank of 98 in a normal distribution.
17. $z = 1.28$ cuts off the highest 10% of scores in a normal distribution.
18. Numerous human characteristics are distributed approximately as a normal curve.
19. If 20% of scores fall into a given class interval, then the percentile rank of the upper real limit of the class interval is 20.
20. The percentile rank of $z = 0$ is always 50.

Multiple choice

1. Which of the following statements is true?
   a A z score indicates how many standard units or deviations a raw score is above or below the mean.
   b The mean of a standard normal distribution is always 0 (zero).
   c The distribution of z scores takes the same shape as that of the raw scores from which they have been derived.
   d All the above statements are true.

2. In an anatomy test, your result is equivalent to a standard or z score of 0.2. What does this z score imply?
   a You performed poorly when compared to others.
   b You performed very well when compared to others.
   c Your result was slightly above average.
   d Your result was slightly below average.

3. The z scores of three persons X, Y and Z in a statistical methods test were +2.0, +1.0 and 0.0, respectively. In term of the original raw scores, which of the following statements is true?
   a The raw score difference between X and Y is greater than the raw score difference between Y and Z.
   b The raw score difference between X and Y is less than the raw score difference between Y and Z.
   c The raw score difference between X and Y is equal to the raw score difference between Y and Z.
   d No precise statement can be made about the relationships between the differences of the raw scores of X and Y and of Y and Z.

A group of patients has a mean weight of 80 kg, with a standard deviation of 10 kg. Questions 4–5 refer to this data.

4. What is the standard score (z) for a patient whose weight is 50 kg?
   a $z = +3$
   b $z = +2$
   c $z = -2$
   d $z = -3$

5. You are told that a patient's weight is two standard deviations below the mean. What is his weight?
   a 60 kg
   b 55 kg
   c 50 kg
   d 45 kg

6. We develop a new method of treating spastic hemiplegia by giving weekly ultrasound massages to the affected muscles. In a consecutive study of 200 children treated by this method we find that the average number of weeks to full recovery is 8, with a standard deviation of 2 weeks. Therefore we conclude that (given a normal distribution):

    a treatment may be stopped after 8 weeks
    b half of all children will need treatment for longer than 8 weeks
    c 90% of children will be fully recovered after 12 weeks of treatment
    d a and c.

7. A percentile rank:

    a represents the frequency of occurrence of a particular category
    b tells you whether or not a distribution is skewed
    c can be used to estimate the range of distribution
    d tells you what percentage of scores fall at or below a particular score.

Use this information in answering questions 8–12:

A normally distributed set of scores has a mean of 40 and a standard deviation of 8.

8. A raw score of 24 corresponds to a z score of:

    a 3.0
    b −3.0
    c 1.5
    d −1.5
    e −2.0

9. A z score of 1.25 corresponds to a raw score of:

    a 50
    b 10
    c 30
    d 56.4
    e 40

10. The percentile rank of a raw score of 48 is

    a 34.13
    b 15.87
    c 84.13
    d 65.87
    e incalculable from information given.

11. The percentage of scores between 32–44 is:

    a 68.26
    b 53.28
    c 46.82
    d 32.74
    e 43.32

12. The raw score which cuts off the lowest 5% of the population (rounded to the nearest whole number) is:
    a 38
    b 13
    c 27
    d 53
    e 42

Questions 13–16 refer to a standard normal distribution.

13. The percentage of cases falling above $z = 0.35$ is:
    a 16.8%
    b 34.1%
    c 84.1%
    d 36.3%

14. The percentage of cases falling between $z = -1$ and $z = +1$ is:
    a 16.8%
    b 33.6%
    c 34.1%
    d 68.3%

15. The percentage of cases falling between $z = -0.5$ and $z = +2$ is:
    a 85.0%
    b 66.9%
    c 28.6%
    d 68.2%

16. The percentage of cases falling either below $z = -2$ or above $z = +2$ is:
    a 95.5%
    b 68.2%
    c 47.7%
    d 4.6 %

The following information should be used in answering questions 17–20:
    A test of reaction times has a mean of 10 and a standard deviation of 4 in the normal adult population.

17. A person scores 8. That person's z score is:
    a 2
    b −2
    c −0.5
    d −1

18. What percentage of the population would have scores up to and including 14 on this test?
    a 84.13
    b 15.87
    c 65.87
    d 34.13

19. What is the percentile rank of a score of 8 on this test?
    a 19.15
    b 30.85
    c 80.85
    d 53.28

20. What score (to the nearest whole number) would cut off the highest 10% of scores?
    a 1
    b 14
    c 15
    d 18

Questions 21–25 refer to the following data:
   The mean for a population is 500, with a standard deviation of 90. The scores are normally distributed.

21. The percentile rank of a score of 667 is:
    a 4.14
    b 92.7
    c 3.22
    d 96.86

22. The proportion of scores which lie above 650 is:
    a 0.4535
    b 0.9535
    c 0.0475
    d 0.885

23. The proportion of scores which lie between 460 and 600 is:
    a 0.4394
    b 0.5365
    c 0.4406
    d 0.4635

24. The raw score which lies at the 90th percentile is:
    a 615.20
    b 384.80
    c 616.10
    d 383.90

25. The proportion of scores between 300–400 is:
    a 0.3665
    b 0.4868
    c 0.8533
    d 0.1203

16

Correlation

INTRODUCTION

A fundamental aim of scientific and clinical research is to establish relationships between two or more sets of observations or variables. Finding such relationships or covariations is often a fundamental initial step for identifying causal relationships.

The topic of correlation is concerned with expressing quantitatively the degree and direction of the relationship between variables. Correlations are useful in the health sciences in areas such as determining the validity and reliability of clinical measures or in expressing how health problems are related to crucial biological, behavioural or environmental factors.

The specific aims of this chapter are to:

1. Define correlation and correlation coefficients
2. Discuss the selection and calculation of correlation coefficients
3. Outline some of the uses of correlation coefficients
4. Discuss the relationship between correlation and causality.

CORRELATION

Consider the following two statements:

1. There is a positive relationship between cigarette smoking and lung damage.
2. There is a negative relationship between being overweight and life expectancy.

Unquestionably, you have a fair idea what the above two statements mean. The first statement is implying that there is evidence that if you score high on one variable (cigarette smoking) you are likely to score high on the other variable (lung damage). The second statement describes the finding that scoring high on the variable 'overweight' tends to be associated with low scores on the variable 'life expectancy'. The information missing from each of the statements is the numerical value for degree or magnitude of the association between the variables.

A **correlation coefficient** is a descriptive statistic or number that expresses the magnitude and direction of the association between two variables.

In order to demonstrate that two variables are correlated, we must obtain measures on both variables for the same set of subjects or events. Let us look at an example to illustrate this point.

Let's say we are interested to see whether scores for Anatomy examinations are correlated with scores for Physiology. To keep the example simple, assume that there are only five ($n = 5$) students who sat for both examinations:

Student	Score (out of 10)	
	Anatomy (X)	Physiology (Y)
1	3	2.5
2	4	3.5
3	1	0
4	8	6
5	2	1

For a visual representation of the relationship between the two variables, we can plot the above data on a **scattergram**. A scattergram is a graph of the paired scores for each subject on the two variables. By convention, we call one of the variables x, and the other one y. It is clear from Figure 16.1 that there is a positive relationship between the two variables. That is, students who have high scores for Anatomy (variable x) tend to have high scores for Physiology (variable y). Also, we can see that we can fit a straight line in close approximation of the points on the scattergram. In general, a variety of relationships is possible between two variables; the scattergrams on Figure 16.2 illustrate some of these.

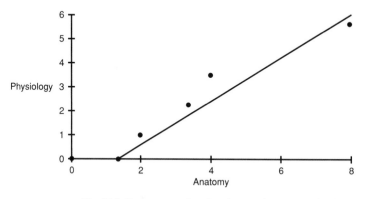

Fig. 16.1 Scattergram of students' scores in two examinations

Figures 16.2A and 16.2B represent a linear correlation between the variables x and y. That is, a straight line is the most appropriate representation of the relationship between x and y. Figure 16.2C represents a non-linear correlation, where a curve best represents the relationship between x and y.

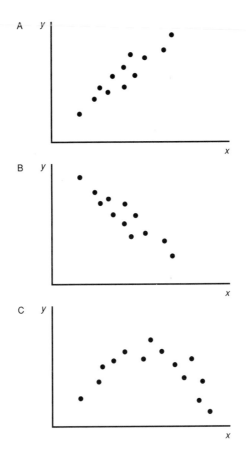

Fig. 16.2 Scattergrams showing relationships between two variables: (A) positive linear correlation; (B) negative linear correlation; (C) non-linear correlation

Figure 16.2A represents a *positive* correlation, indicating that high scores on x are related to high scores on y. For instance, the relationship between cigarette smoking and lung damage is a positive correlation. Figure 16.2B represents a *negative* correlation, where high scores on x are associated with low scores on y. For instance, the correlation between the variables 'being overweight' and 'life expectancy' is negative, meaning that the more you are overweight, the lower your life expectancy.

CORRELATION COEFFICIENTS

When we need to know or express the numerical value of the correlation between x and y, we calculate a statistic called the correlation coefficient. The correlation coefficient expresses quantitatively the magnitude and direction of the correlation.

Selection of correlation coefficient

There are several types of correlation coefficients used in statistics. Table 16.1 shows some of these correlation coefficients, and the conditions under which they are used.

Table 16.1 Correlation coefficient

Coefficient	Conditions where appropriate
ϕ (phi)	Both x and y measured on a nominal scale
ρ (rho)	Both x and y measured on, or transformed to, ordinal scales
r	Both x and y measured on an interval or ratio scale

All of the correlation coefficients shown in Table 16.1 are appropriate for quantifying *linear* relationships between variables. There are other correlation coefficients, such as η (eta) which are used for quantifying non-linear relationships. However, the discussion of the use and calculation of all correlation coefficients is beyond the scope of this text. Rather, we will examine only the commonly used Pearson's *r*, and Spearman's ρ (the Greek letter 'rho').

Regardless of which correlation coefficient we employ, these statistics share the following characteristics:

1. Correlation coefficients are calculated from pairs of measurements on variables *x* and *y* for the same group of individuals.
2. A positive correlation is denoted by + (plus sign) and a negative correlation by – (minus sign).
3. The values of the correlation coefficient range from + 1 to –1; where +1 means a perfect positive correlation, 0 means no correlation at all, and –1 a perfect negative correlation.
4. The square of the correlation coefficient represents the **coefficient of determination** (see p. 246).

CALCULATION OF CORRELATION COEFFICIENTS: PEARSON'S *r*

We have already stated that Pearson's *r* is the appropriate correlation coefficient when both variables *x* and *y* are measured on an interval or a ratio scale. Further assumptions in using *r* are that both variables *x* and *y* are normally distributed, and that we are describing a linear (rather than curvilinear) relationship.

Pearson's *r* is a measure of the extent to which paired scores are correlated. To calculate *r*, we need to represent the position of each paired score within its own distribution, so we convert each raw score to a *z* score. This transformation corrects for the two distributions *x* and *y* having different means and standard deviations. The formula for calculating Pearson's *r* is:

$$r = \frac{\Sigma z_x z_y}{n}$$

z_x = standard score corresponding to any raw x score
z_y = standard score corresponding to any raw y score
Σ = sum of standard score products
n = numbers of paired measurements.

Let's calculate the correlation coefficient for the data given in the example on page 238:

Student	Raw scores				z scores
	x	y	z_x	z_y	$z_x z_y$
1	3	2.5	-0.22	-0.04	+0.01
2	4	3.5	+0.15	+0.39	+0.06
3	1	0	-0.96	-1.12	+1.08
4	8	6	+1.63	+1.46	+2.38
5	2	1	-0.59	-0.69	+0.41
	$\overline{X} = 3.6$	$\overline{Y} = 2.6$			$\Sigma z_x z_y = 3.94$
	$S_x = 2.7$	$S_y = 2.33$			

$$\text{Therefore: } r = \frac{\Sigma z_x z_y}{n}$$
$$= \frac{3.94}{5}$$
$$= 0.79$$

(The z scores are calculated as discussed in Chapter 15.)

This is a quite high correlation, indicating that the paired z scores fall roughly on a straight line. In general, the closer the relationship between the two variables approximates a straight line, the more r approaches +1. Note that in social and biological sciences correlations this high do not usually occur. In general, we consider anything over 0.7 to be quite high, 0.3 to 0.7 to be moderate, and less than 0.3 to be weak. Let us examine some scattergrams to illustrate this point (Fig. 16.3).

When n is very large, the above equation is inconvenient to use to calculate r. Here we are not concerned with calculating r with a large n, although appropriate formulae and computer programs are available. Note that the degree of correlation is independent of the specific group means, so that we can have very different means for the two groups but still find a high correlation. For example, scores before and after treatment for the same person could be quite different but still highly correlated.

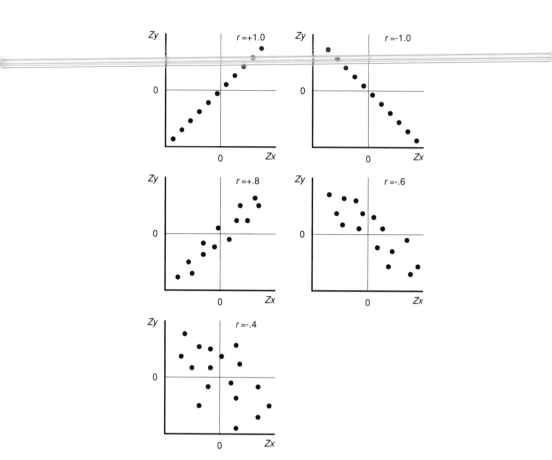

Fig. 16.3 Scattergrams and corresponding approximate r values

Assumptions for using r

It was pointed out earlier that r is used when two variables are scaled on interval or ratio scales and when it is shown that they are linearly associated.

If any of the above assumptions is violated, then the correlation coefficient might be spuriously low. Therefore, other correlation coefficients should be used to represent association between two variables. A further problem may arise from the truncation of the range of values in one or both of the variables. This occurs when the distributions greatly deviate from normal shapes. The higher scale can be readily reduced to an ordinal scale.

Say we measure the correlation between examination scores and IQs of a group of health science students. We might find a low correlation, because by the time students present themselves to tertiary courses, most students with low IQs are eliminated. In this way, the distribution of IQs would not be normal but rather negatively skewed. In effect, the question of appropriate sampling is also relevant to correlations, as it was outlined in Chapter 3.

CALCULATION OF CORRELATION COEFFICIENTS: SPEARMAN'S ρ (rho)

When the obtained data are such that at least one of the variables x or y was measured on an ordinal scale and the other on an ordinal scale or higher, we use ρ to calculate the correlation between the two variables. The higher scale can be readily reduced to an ordinal scale.

If one or both variables were measured on a nominal scale, ρ is no longer appropriate as a statistic.

$$\rho = 1 - \frac{6\Sigma d^2}{n^3 - n}$$

d = difference in a pair of ranks
n = number of pairs

The derivation of this formula will not be discussed here. The '6' is placed in the formula as a scaling device; it ensures that the possible range of ρ is from −1 to +1 and thus enables ρ and r to be compared. Let us consider an example to illustrate the use of ρ.

An investigator is interested in the correlation between socioeconomic status and severity of respiratory illness. Assuming that both variables were measured on, or transformed to, an ordinal scale, the investigator rank-orders the scores from highest to lowest on each variable:

Patient	Socioeconomic status (rank)	Severity of illness (rank)	d (difference between ranks)	d^2
1	6	5	1	1
2	7	8	−1	1
3	2	4	−2	4
4	3	3	0	0
5	5	7	−2	4
6	4	1	3	9
7	1	2	−1	1
8	8	6	2	4
				$\Sigma d^2 = 24$

$$\text{Therefore, } \rho = 1 - \frac{6\Sigma d^2}{n^3 - n}$$

$$= 1 - \frac{6 \infty 24}{8^3 - 8}$$

$$= 0.71$$

Clearly, the closer the association among the ranks for the paired scores on the two variables, the more ρ approaches +1. If the ranks tend to be inverse, then ρ approaches −1.

USES OF CORRELATION IN THE HEALTH SCIENCES

Prediction

When the correlation coefficient has been calculated it may be used to predict the value of one variable (y) given the value of the other variable (x). For instance, take a hypothetical example that the correlation between cigarette smoking and lung damage is $r = +1$.

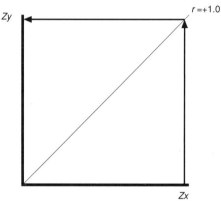

Fig. 16.4 Hypothetical relationship between cigarette smoking and lung damage. $r = +1.0$

We can see from Figure 16.4 that given any score on x, we can transform this into a z score (z_x) and then using the graph we can read off the corresponding z score on y (z_y). Of course it is extremely rare that there should be a perfect ($r = +1$) correlation between two variables. In this case, the smaller the correlation coefficient, the greater the probability of making an error in prediction. For example, consider Figure 16.5, where the scattergram shown represents a hypothetical correlation of approximately $r = 0.7$.

Here for any transformed value on variable x (say z_x) there is a range of values of z_y that correspond. Our best guess is z_y the *average value*, but clearly a range of scores is possible, as shown on the figure.

That is, as the correlation coefficient approaches 0 the range of error in prediction increases. A more appropriate and precise way of making predictions is in terms of regression analysis, but this topic is not covered in this introductory book.

Reliability and predictive validity of assessment

As you will recall, reliability refers to measurements using instruments or to subjective judgements remaining relatively the same on repeated administration (Ch.12). This is called test–retest reliability and its degree is measured by a correlation coefficient. The correlation coefficient can be used also to determine the degree of interobserver reliability.

As an example, say we are interested in the interobserver reliability for two neurologists who are assessing patients for degrees of functional disability

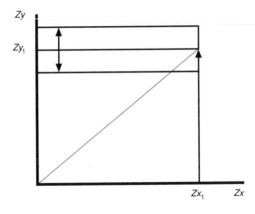

Fig. 16.5 Hypothetical relationship between cigarette smoking and lung damage. $r = {}^{+}0.7$.
With a correlation of <1.0 the data points will cluster around rather than exactly on
the line and may vary between the range of values shown for any given values of
X or Y and their corresponding z scores

following spinal cord damage. Table 16.2 represents a set of hypothetical results
of their independent assessment of the same set of five patients.

Table 16.2 Assessment of disability (%) by observers X and Y

Patient	Observer X	Observer Y	Rank X	Rank Y
1	85%	98%	1	1
2	75%	86%	2	2
3	74%	80%	3	3
4	72%	79%	4	4
5	69%	70%	5	5

Observer Y clearly attributes greater degrees of disability to the patients than
observer X. However, as stated earlier, this need not affect the correlation
coefficient. If we treat the measurement as an ordinal scale, we can see from
Table 16.2 that the ranks given to the patients by the two observers correspond,
so that it can be shown that $\rho = +1$.

Clearly, the higher the correlation, the greater the reliability. If we had treated
the measurement as representing interval or ratio data, we would have calculated
Pearson's r to represent quantitatively the reliability of the measurement.

Predictive validity is also expressed as a correlation coefficient. For instance,
say that you devise an assessment procedure to predict how much people will
benefit from a rehabilitation program. If the correlation between the assessment
and a measure of the success of the rehabilitation program is high (say 0.7 or
0.8), the assessment procedure has high predictive validity. If, however, the
correlation is low (say 0.3 or 0.4), the predictive validity of the assessment is
low, and it would be unwise to use the assessment as a screening procedure for
the entry of patients into the rehabilitation program.

Estimating shared variance

A useful statistic is the square of the correlation coefficient (r^2) which represents the proportion of variance in one variable accounted for by the other. This is called the **coefficient of determination**.

Say, for instance, the correlation between variable x (height) and variable y (weight) is $r = 0.7$. Here, the coefficient of determination is:

$r^2 = 0.49$ or 49%

This means that 49% of the variability of weight can be accounted for in terms of height. You might ask, what about the other 51% of the variability? This would be accounted for by other factors, say for instance, tendency to eat fatty foods. The point here is that even a relatively high correlation coefficient $(r = 0.7)$ accounts for less than 50% of the variability.

This is a difficult concept, so it might be worth remembering that 'variability' (see Ch. 15) refers to how scores are spread out about the mean. That is, as in the above example, some people will be heavy, some average, some light. So we can account for 49% of the total variability of weight (x) in terms of height (y) if $r = 0.7$. The greater the correlation coefficient, the greater the coefficient of determination, and the more of the variability in y can be accounted for in terms of x.

CORRELATION AND CAUSATION

In Chapter 4, we pointed out that there were at least three criteria for establishing causal relationship. Correlation or covariation is only one of these criteria. We have already discussed in Chapter 6 that even a high correlation between two variables doesn't necessarily imply a causal relationship. That is, there are a variety of plausible explanations for finding a correlation. As an example, let's take cigarette smoking (x) and lung damage (y). A high positive correlation could result from any of the following circumstances:

(a) x causes y
(b) y causes x
(c) There is a third variable, which causes both x and y
(d) The correlation represents a spurious or chance association.

For the example above, (a) would imply that cigarette smoking causes lung damage, (b) that lung damage causes cigarette smoking, and (c) that there was a variable (e.g. stress) which caused both increased smoking and lung damage.

Some associations between variables are completely spurious (d). For instance, there might be a correlation between the amount of margarine consumed and the number of cases of influenza over a period of time in a community. But each of the two events might have entirely different, unrelated causes. Also, some correlation coefficients do not reach statistical significance, that is, they may be due to chance (see Chs 18 and 19).

Also, if we are using a sample to estimate the correlation in a population, we must be certain that the outcome is not due to biased sampling or sampling error. That is, the investigator needs to show that a correlation coefficient is statistically significant and not just due to random sampling error. We will look at the concept of statistical significance in the following chapter.

While demonstrating correlation doesn't establish causality, we can use correlations as a source for subsequent hypotheses. For instance, in this example, work on carcinogens in cigarette tars and the causes of emphysema has confirmed that it is probably true that smoking does, in fact, cause lung damage (*x* causes *y*). However, given that there is often multiple causation of health problems, option (c) cannot be ruled out.

There are some statistical techniques available which can, under favourable conditions, enable investigators to use correlations as a basis for distinguishing between competing plausible hypotheses. One such technique, called 'path analysis' involves postulating the probable temporal sequence of events and then establishing a correlation between them. This technique was borrowed from systems theory, and has been applied in areas of clinical research, such as epidemiology.

SUMMARY

In this chapter we outlined how the degree and direction between two variables can be quantified, using statistics called correlation coefficients. Of the correlation coefficients, the use of two were outlined: Pearson's *r* and Spearman's ρ. Definitional formulae and simple calculations were presented, with the understanding that more complex calculations of correlation coefficients are done with computers.

Several uses for *r* and ρ were discussed: for prediction, for quantifying the reliability and validity of measurements, and by using r^2 in estimating amount of shared variability. Finally, we discussed the caution necessary in causal interpretation of correlation coefficients. Showing a strong association between variables is an important step towards establishing causal links and, although not sufficient without control, can help to discount plausible alternative hypotheses.

As with other descriptive statistics, caution is necessary when correlation coefficients are calculated for a sample and then generalized to a population. The question of generalization from a sample statistic to a population parameter will be discussed in the following chapters.

SELF ASSESSMENT

Explain the meaning of the following terms:

correlation	positive correlation
correlation coefficient	shared variance
curvilinear correlation	zero correlation
negative correlation	

True or false

1. ~~Correlation is defined as the relative difference between two variables.~~
2. The association between two variables can be plotted on a scattergram.
3. If the distribution of paired scores is best represented by a curve, the relationship is non-linear.
4. When we speak of a positive (+) relationship, we mean that high scores on one variable are associated with high scores on the other variable.
5. In a negative (–) relationship, low scores on one variable are associated with low scores on the other.
6. There are several types of correlation coefficients, the selection of which is determined by the level of scaling of the two variables.
7. When both variables are measured on an interval or ratio scale, Pearson's r is the most appropriate correlation coefficient.
8. When both variables are measured on, or converted to, ordinal scales, we must use ø (phi) to express correlation.
9. For two variables measured on nominal scales, we use ρ (rho) to express correlation.
10. Pearson's r is calculated by a formula where $\Sigma z_x z_y$ stands for the sum of the z score pairs multiplied together.
11. When calculating Spearman's ρ, Σd^2 is the sum of the square of the differences between the means.
12. When we use Pearson's r, we assume that both variables are continuous and normally distributed.
13. The calculated values of correlation coefficients range between 0 and -1.
14. When there is no linear association between two variables, r or ρ will be close to zero.
15. A correlation coefficient of –1 represents a very low linear correlation.
16. Where there is a correlation of $r = +1$ between two variables, then the z scores of variable x will be equal to the z scores of variable y.
17. The coefficient of determination is the square of the correlation coefficient.
18. If $r = 0.3$, then the coefficient of determination will be 9.0.
19. Say $r^2 = 0.36$ for a set of data. This implies that 36 percent of the variability of y is explained in terms of x.
20. As the correlation coefficient approaches zero, the possible error in linear prediction increases.
21. The closer the correlation coefficient is to zero, the greater the predictive validity of a test.
22. If a correlation coefficient for the test–retest reliability of a test is close to 1, then the test is unreliable.
23. Given a –1.00 correlation coefficient for two variables, a raw score of 50 on the first variable must be accompanied by a score of –50 on the second variable, for a given case.

24. Even a high correlation is not necessarily indicative of a causal relationship between two variables.
25. As the value of r increases, the proportion of variability of y that can be accounted for by x, decreases.
26. Eta (η) is the appropriate correlation coefficient to use when two variables are nominally scaled.
27. If the relationship between two variables is non-linear, the value of the correlation coefficient must be negative.
28. Spearman's ρ is used where one or both variables are at least of interval scaling.
29. A scattergram is used to help to decide if the relationship between two variables is linear or curvilinear.

Multiple choice

1. Which of the following statements about correlations is false?
   a Spearman's ρ (rho) is appropriate to use when the relationship between two variables is non-linear.
   b A correlation coefficient of –0.8 represents a higher degree of association between two variables than a correlation coefficient of +0.6.
   c The construction of a scattergram is useful for evaluating whether a relationship between two variables is linear or curvilinear.
   d In a perfect positive correlation between two quantitatively measured variables, each individual obtains the same z scores on each variable.
   e Negative correlation implies that high scores on one variable are related to low scores on another variable.

2. A scattergram:
   a is a statistical test
   b must be linear
   c must be curvilinear
   d is a graph of x and y scores
   e is none of the above.

3. If the relationship between variables x and y is linear, then the points on the scattergram:
   a will fall exactly on a straight line
   b will fall on a curve
   c must represent population parameters
   d are independent of the variance
   e are best represented by a straight line.

4. If the relationship between x and y is positive, as variable y decreases, variable x :
   a   increases
   b   decreases
   c   remains the same
   d   changes linearly
   e   varies.

5. In a 'negative' relationship:
   a   as x increases, y increases
   b   as x decreases, y decreases
   c   as x increases, y decreases
   d   both a and b
   e   none of the above.

6. The lowest strength of association is reflected by which of the following correlation coefficients?
   a   0.95
   b   −0.60
   c   −0.33
   d   0.29
   e   none of the above, as it cannot be determined.

7. The highest strength of association is reflected by which of the following correlation coefficients:
   a   −1.0
   b   −0.95
   c   0.1
   d   0.85
   e   none of the above, as it cannot be determined.

8. Which of the following statements is false?
   a   In a perfect positive correlation, each individual obtains the same z score on each variable.
   b   Spearman's ρ is used when one or both variables are at least of interval scaling.
   c   The range of the correlation coefficient is from -1 to +1.
   d   A correlation of $r = 0.85$ implies a stronger association than $r = -0.70$.

9. We can calculate the correlation coefficient if given:
   a   the top scores from one test and lowest scores from another test
   b   at least two scores from the same tests
   c   two sets of measurements for the same subjects
   d   either a or b.

10. The correlation between two variables x and y is -1.00. A given individual has a z score of $z_x = 1.4$ on variable x. We predict his z score on y is:
    a   1.4 above the mean
    b -1.4
    c   between 1.4 and -1.4
    d -1.00

11. Professor Shnook demonstrated a correlation of -0.85 between body weight and IQ. This means that:
    a   obesity decreases intelligence
    b   heavy people have higher IQs than light people
    c   people with high IQs are likely to be light
    d   malnutrition damages the brain
    e   none of the above.

12. A correlation coefficient of $+0.5$ was found between exposure to stressful life events and incidence of stress-induced disorders. A correlation of this direction and magnitude indicates that:
    a   a high level of exposure to stressful life events causes a high level of stress-induced disorders.
    b   a high level of stress-induced disorders causes a high likelihood of exposure to stressful life events.
    c   either or both of a and b may be correct—we can't be sure.
    d   the levels of stress-induced disorders and of exposure to stressful life events are not causally related in any way.

13. You are told that there is a high inverse association between the variables 'amount of exercise' and 'incidence of heart disease'. A correlation coefficient consistent with the above statement is:
    a $r = 0.8$
    b $r = 0.2$
    c $r = -0.2$
    d $r = -0.8$

14. Of the following measurement levels, which is at a minimum required for the valid calculation of a Pearson correlation coefficient?
    a   nominal
    b   ordinal
    c   interval
    d   ratio

15. Of the following measurement levels, which is required for the valid calculation of the Spearman correlation coefficient?
    a   nominal
    b   ordinal
    c   interval
    d   ratio

16. You are told that there is a high, positive correlation between measures of 'fitness' and 'hours of exercise'. The correlation coefficient consistent with the above statement is:
    a   0.3
    b   0.2
    c   −0.8
    d   −0.3
    e   none of these.

You are interested in selecting a test suitable for client assessment in a clinical situation. You find 4 tests in the literature, tests P, Q. R, and S. Each of these tests has been validated against a clinically relevant variable. The test–retest and predictive validity of the four hypothetical tests are:

	Test-retest reliability (*r*)	Validity *r*
P	0.8	0.50
Q	0.9	0.18
R	0.5	0.40
S	0.2	0.03

Questions 17–18 refer to the above information.

17. Which test would you choose for clinical assessment?
    a   P
    b   Q
    c   R
    d   S

18. Which test has the best test–retest reliability?
    a   P
    b   Q
    c   R
    d   S

An investigation aims to establish for a sample of subjects the relationship between blood cholesterol levels (in mg/cc) and blood pressure (in mmHg). Questions 19–20 refer to this investigation.

19. The correlation coefficient appropriate for establishing the degree of correlation between the two variables (assuming a linear relationship):
    a   is determined by the sample size
    b   depends on the direction of the causality
    c   is Spearman's ρ (rho)
    d   is Pearson's *r*
    e   both *b* and *c*.

20. Say that the correlation coefficient is calculated to be +0.7. A correlation of this direction and magnitude indicates that:
    a high blood pressure causes high blood cholesterol
    b high blood cholesterol causes high blood pressure
    c there might be a third variable which causes both high blood pressure and high blood cholesterol
    d none of the statements a, b or c is consistent with the evidence
    e any of the statements a, b, or c might be correct; we can't be sure from the available evidence.

21. When deciding which measure of correlation to employ with a specific set of data, you should consider:
    a whether the relationship is linear or nonlinear
    b the type of scale of measurement for each variable
    c *a* and *b*
    d neither *a* nor *b*.

22. The proportion of variance accounted for by the level of correlation between two variables is calculated by a:
    a $\overline{X}$
    b r^2
    c Σx
    d you cannot calculate this proportion under any circumstances.

23. If the correlation between two variables A and B is 0.36, then the proportion of variance accounted for is:
    a 0.13
    b 0.06
    c 0.60
    d 0.64

DISCUSSION, QUESTIONS AND ANSWERS

Descriptive statistics are an integral part of everyday life and an important part of clinical practice. They are used to describe the essential characteristics of measurements for a sample of cases. Some descriptive statistics are quite familiar to the lay person. The mean or average is frequently used in discussions of public policy. For example, the question 'What has happened to the average household income in the United Kingdom over the last year?' uses this concept. So does a question like 'What is the average length of stay in hospital for an orthopaedic patient with a fractured neck of femur in this ward?'. Descriptive statistics are shorthand ways of conveying information about a sample of cases.

In recent years in the United Kingdom, Australia, Canada and the United States, there has been a growing preoccupation with the effectiveness and efficiency of health services, in particular, and government services in general. Economic conditions have resulted in the reduced availability of tax revenues and this has led to increased scrutiny of spending. Hospital services are an expensive component of health services in these countries. Much statistical information is collected concerning stays in hospital. The use of statistical information concerning case costs is used heavily to determine funding of hospitals by agencies such as government and insurers.

A key component of hospital costs is the length of time spent by the patient in the hospital. Each 'bed day' is very costly and most hospital services are under pressure to reduce the length of stay for their patients. However, one cannot reduce the length of stay for each patient too far, as this might be dangerous. Patients can come back unexpectedly because they require further hospitalization following discharge. This is termed an 'unplanned' re-admission. Thus the goal is to reduce lengths of stay but not increase unplanned readmissions.

Obviously the expected length of stay for a woman giving birth ought be much shorter than a man recovering from serious internal injuries and multiple compound fractures following a motor vehicle accident. How can these cases be compared without some adjustment for their differences? There is a large literature concerning how different types of patients might be compared. Comparability of types of patients is often achieved by the use of Diagnosis Related Groups (DRG) where patients of the same type are categorized together. This grouping enables hospitals and their funding agencies to compare how efficient and effective different hospitals are in treating the same types of patient.

The table below shows some data for patients admitted to an orthopaedics ward in a hospital. All the cases with the same diagnostic category have been included.

Table D16.1 Details of patients admitted to an orthopaedics ward

Patient name	Diagnostic group	Length of stay in hospital(days)	Unplanned re-admission within 14 days?
Jones	Fractured neck of femur	15	No
Ng	Fractured neck of femur	10	Yes
Thomas	Fractured neck of femur	19	No
Evans	Fractured neck of femur	12	No
Valperri	Fractured neck of femur	14	No
Hart	Fractured neck of femur	14	No
Elmahdy	Fractured neck of femur	13	No
Smith	Fractured neck of femur	11	Yes
Cairns	Fractured neck of femur	12	No
Eisenberg	Fractured neck of femur	12	No

For this sample of cases, the average length of stay was 13.2 days (standard deviation 2.5). The minimum stay was 10 days and the maximum stay was 19 days. The rate of unplanned re-admissions within 14 days was 2 in 10 or 20%.

If one was to take larger samples of cases from a variety of hospitals (say a consecutive series of 30 cases for each, then it would be possible to compare their lengths of stay and the rate of readmissions. This has been done in the following table with data from five hospitals.

Table D16.2 Lengths of stay and readmission rates for 30 consecutive patients with a fractured neck of femur at 5 hospitals

Hospital	Number of cases (n)	Length of stay in hospital		Rate of unplanned readmissions per 100
		Average $\bar{x}$	Standard deviation (s)	
A	30	13.0	2.6	6.7
B	30	12.3	2.4	10.0
C	30	13.4	2.8	6.7
D	30	14.4	3.3	3.3
E	30	14.8	3.0	3.3

Although the differences in average numbers of days spent in hospital between the five hospitals may not seem to be great, a difference of 2.5 days for example, between hospital B and E may represent over $1000 or over

£500 for each case. In a busy hospital department, this would soon run into large sums of money. However, it is worrying that the hospital with the shortest period of stay also seems to be the one with the highest rate of readmissions within 14 days. Perhaps they are discharging some of their patients too soon? With such a small sample of hospitals, (i.e. only five) and such a small number of readmissions (only three out of the 30 in the worst case), it would be difficult to conclude whether there is such a relationship. However, if these data were collected from a large number of hospitals with a larger number of cases, it would be possible to correlate these two variables to study the size of the relationship between them.

Correlation coefficients measure the size and direction of the statistical relationship between two variables. Following on from the above discussion, we might hypothesize that there is a negative correlation between the average length of stay and rate of readmission to hospital. In other words, we might expect that a shorter average stay in a hospital could result in a greater rate of readmission. The graph below (Fig. D16.1) shows the association between length of stay and rate of readmission for 30 hospitals, based on their 1993/ 1994 discharges for all their patients with a fractured neck of femur.

Each of the dots in the graph represents a different hospital. The graph shows that there is a tendency towards those hospitals with longer average lengths of stays for their patients to have lower readmission rates.

The Pearson correlation between these variables is –0.52, which indicates a moderately sized negative correlation between average length of stay and readmission rate for the thirty hospitals.

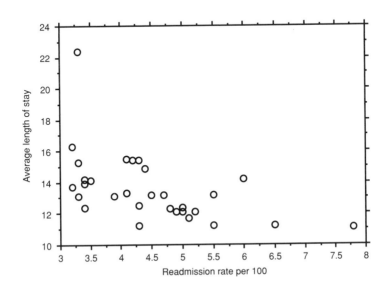

Fig. D16.1 Relationship between average lengths of stay and readmission rates for patients with fractured neck of femur at 30 hospitals

Questions

1. In Table D16.1, how many patients had a length of stay in hospital that was above the average of 13.2 days?
2. If a patient had a length of stay of 14 days, given that the sample mean was 13.2 days and the standard deviation 2.5, what would be their standard or z score?
3. Is it appropriate to compare hospital lengths of stay for patients with different diagnoses?
4. From Figure D16.1, what is the longest average length of stay for this sample of hospitals? What is the shortest?
5. Why is the correlation between average length of stay and readmission rate negative in sign?

Answers

1. Four: Jones, Thomas, Valperri and Hart
2. The standard score is calculated using the following formula:

$$z = \frac{x - \bar{x}}{s}$$

Substituting into the equation, we find that:

$$z = \frac{14 - 13.2}{2.5} = 0.32$$

3. It is like comparing apples with oranges. It is quite reasonable to expect that an uncomplicated birth may involve a hospital stay of 3–4 days, whereas this would be quite unreasonable for a heart transplant. Thus it does not make sense to compare the lengths of stays of different types of patients, because the averages or means are quite different. However, it would make sense to compare standard scores for different types of patients.
4. About 22.5 days; About 11 days
5. Because an increase in average length of stay is associated with a decrease in readmission rate.

Inferential statistics

The statistical analysis of the data is an essential stage in the process of quantitative research. The principles of inferential statistics as introduced in this section, must be applied to data analysis, before we can decide if the data obtained shows the differences and patterns we set out to demonstrate. This is true for descriptive, predictive and causal research, if we are using sample data to make inferences concerning populations.

Quantitative research in the health sciences mostly involves working with samples drawn from populations. In order to generalize our findings, we must draw inferences from sample statistics (e.g. $\bar{X}$, s) concerning the population parameters (e.g. μ, σ). Inferences are always probabilistic, because even with random samples there is always the chance of sampling error. This implies that the differences or patterns which we identified in our sample data represent random variations or chance patterns, rather than 'real' ones which are true for the population as a whole.

As an illustration, say we have collected data in a study aimed at identifying age related differences in the use of sedatives and tranquillisers in a given population. Say that our participants ($n = 200$) kept diaries over a period of a year, recording each time they had taken a sedative or tranquilliser. Assume that the following hypothetical data was obtained:

Age Group	Sedative and tranquilliser consumption		
	n	$\bar{X}$	s
20–39	100	20	5
40–59	100	30	5

Two important and interrelated issues are raised in Section 6 concerning sample data such as shown in the above table.

1. Even if we used an adequate sampling procedure (see Ch. 3) how confident are we to infer that the true population parameters (μ) are the same as, or are at least close to $\bar{X}$? For example, is it true that the mean tranquilliser intake for the 20–39 age group is $\mu = 20$?

2. It appears that there is a large difference between the two sample means; but is this difference also true for the populations? In other words, is this difference 'real' or significant, or is it simply due to sampling error?

We cannot eliminate sampling error, even with large and well chosen samples but, as outlined in Section 6, we can apply the principles of inferential statistics to calculate the probability of error. We then use this information to minimize the probability of making errors when we generalize from sample statistics to population parameters.

In Chapter 17 we examine how sampling distributions are derived and used for calculating the probability of obtaining a given sample statistic. This information can be applied to the calculation of confidence intervals, which represents a range of scores which contains, the true population parameter (at a given level or probability).

In Chapter 18 we outline the logic of hypothesis testing, using single sample 'z' and 't' tests as exemplars. Hypothesis testing is a procedure used to decide if a difference or pattern identified in our sample data is statistically significant. If the outcome of our analysis is significant, then we are in a position to decide that the patterns or differences found in our data may be generalized to the populations from which the samples were obtained.

There are numerous statistical tests available for analysing the significance of our data. In Chapter 19, we will discuss basic criteria for selecting an appropriate statistical test, including (i) scale of measurement used to collect the data, (ii) the number of groups being compared and (iii) the dependence or independence of measurements. We will use the χ^2(chi squared) test to demonstrate how statistical tests are selected and used to analyse the data.

Ultimately, statistical decision making is probabilistic, implying that the possibility of making decision errors can not be eliminated. Decisions may be correct, or involve what are called Type I and Type II errors. In Chapter 20, we examine how these errors may influence our interpretation of the obtained data in relation to the aims or hypotheses guiding our research, and we will examine strategies which can be employed to reduce the probability of making such errors.

17

Probability and sampling distributions

INTRODUCTION

Sample statistics (such as $\overline{X}$, s) must be seen as estimates of the actual population parameters. Even where adequate sampling procedures are adopted, there is no guarantee that the sample statistics are the exact representations of the parameters of the population from which the samples were drawn. Therefore, inferences from sample statistics to population parameters necessarily involve the possibility of sampling error. As stated in Chapter 3, sampling errors represent the discrepancy between sample statistics and population parameters. Given that investigators usually have no knowledge of the true population parameters, inferential statistics are employed to estimate the probable sampling errors. That is, while sampling error cannot be eliminated completely; its probable magnitude can be calculated using **inferential statistics**. In this way, investigators are in a position to calculate the probability level at which their estimations of population parameters are acceptable.

The aim of this chapter is to examine how probability theory is applied to generating sampling distributions and how sampling distributions are used for relating sample statistics to population parameters. Sampling distributions can be used for specifying confidence intervals, as discussed in this chapter, as well as for testing hypotheses, as demonstrated in Chapter 18.

PROBABILITY

The concept of probability is central to the understanding of inferential statistics. Probability is expressed as a proportion between 0 and 1, where 0 means an event is certain not to occur, and 1 means an event is certain to occur. The probability of any event (say event A) occurring is given by the formula:

$$p(\text{A}) = \frac{\text{number of occurrences of A}}{\text{total number of possible occurrences}}$$

Sometimes the probability of an event can be calculated *a priori* (before the event) by reasoning alone. For instance, we can predict that the probability of throwing a head (H) with a fair coin is:

$$p(\text{H}) = \frac{\text{number of occurrences of H}}{\text{total number of possible occurrences}}$$

$$= \frac{\text{H}}{\text{H} + \text{T(tails)}} = \frac{1}{2} = 0.5$$

Or, if we buy a lottery ticket in a draw where there are 100 000 tickets, the probability of winning first prize is:

$$p(\text{1st prize}) = \frac{1}{100\ 000} = 0.00001$$

This is true only if the lottery is fair; if all tickets have an equal chance of being drawn by random selection.

In some situations, there is no model which we can apply to calculate the occurrence of an event *a priori*. For instance, how can we calculate the probability of an individual dying of a specific condition? In such instances, we use previously obtained empirical evidence to calculate probabilities *a posteriori* (after the event).

For instance, if it is known that the percentages (or proportions) for causes of death are distributed in a particular way, then the probability of a particular cause of death for a given individual can be predicted. Table 17.1 represents a set of hypothetical statistics for a community.

Table 17.1 Cause of death for persons over 65

Cause of death	Percentage of deaths
Coronary heart disease	50
Cancer	25
Stroke	10
Accidents	5
Infections	5
Other causes	5

Given the data in Table 17.1, we are in a position to calculate the probability of a selected individual of over 65 dying of any of the specified causes.

For instance, the probability of a given individual dying of coronary heart disease is:

$$p(\text{dying of heart disease}) = \frac{\text{percentage of cases dying of heart disease}}{100\%}$$

$$= \frac{50\%}{100\%} = 0.5$$

This approach ignores individual risk factors and assumes that the conditions under which the empirical data were obtained are still pertinent. However, the example illustrates the principle that once we have organized the data into a frequency distribution, we can calculate the probability of selecting any of the tabulated values. This is so whether the variable was measured on a nominal, ordinal, interval or ratio scale. Here we will examine how to calculate the probability of values for normally distributed, continuous variables.

We can use the normal curve model, as outlined in Chapter 15, to determine the proportion or percentage of cases up to, or between, any specified scores. In this instance, probability is defined as the proportion of the total area cut off by the specified scores under the normal curve. The greater the proportion, the higher the probability of selecting the specified values.

For example, say that on the basis of previous evidence, we can specify the frequency distribution of neonates' weight. Let us assume that the distribution is approximately normal, with the mean ($\overline{X}$) of 5.0 kg and a standard deviation (s) of 1.5. Now, say that we are interested in the probability of a randomly selected neonate having a birth weight of 2.0 kg or under. Figure 17.1 illustrates the above situation.

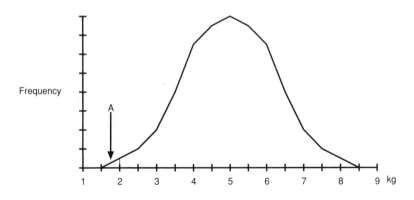

Fig. 17.1 Frequency distribution of neonate birth weights. Area A corresponds to $z \leq -2$

The area A under the curve in Figure 17.1 corresponds to the probability of obtaining a score of 2 or under. Using the principles outlined in Chapter 15 to calculate proportions or areas under the normal curve, we firstly translate the raw score of 2 into a z score.

$$z = \frac{x - \overline{X}}{s}$$

$$= \frac{2 - 5}{1.5}$$

$$= -2$$

Now we look up the area under the normal curve corresponding to $z = -2$ (Appendix A). Here we find that A is 0.0228. This area corresponds to a probability, and we can say that 'The probability of a neonate having a birth weight of 2 kg or less is 0.0228'. Another way of stating this outcome is that the chances are 2 in 100, or 2%, for a child having such birth weight.

We can also use the normal curve model to calculate the probability of selecting scores between any given values of a normally distributed continuous variable.

For instance, if we are interested in the probability of birth weights being between 6 and 8 kg, then this can be represented on the normal curve. (Area A2 on Figure 17.2). To determine this area, we proceed as outlined in Chapter 15. Let $s = 1.5$.

$$z_1 = \frac{6-5}{1.5} = 0.67$$

$$z_2 = \frac{8-5}{1.5} = 2.0$$

Therefore: the area between z_1 and $\overline{X}$ is 0.2486 (from Appendix A) and area between z_2 and $\overline{X} = 0.4772$ (from Appendix A). Therefore, the required area A2 (Figure 17.2) is:

$$A2 = 0.47720 - 0.2486 = 0.2286$$

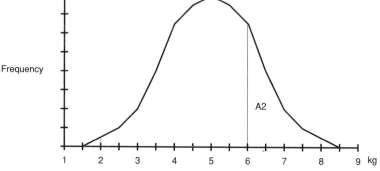

Fig. 17.2 Frequency distribution of neonate birth weights. Area A2 corresponds to probability of weight being between 6–8 kg

It can be concluded that the probability of a randomly selected child having a birth weight between 6 and 8 kg is $p = 0.2286$. Another way of saying this is that there is a chance of 23 in 100 or a 23% chance that the birth weight will be between 6 and 8 kg.

The above examples demonstrate that if the mean and standard deviation are known for a normally distributed continuous variable, this information can be applied to calculating the probability of any set of events related to this distribution. Of course, probabilities can be calculated for scores not in a normal continuous distribution, but this requires integral calculus which is beyond the scope of this text. In general, regardless of the shape or scaling of a distribution, scores occurring within ranges of a high level of frequency are more likely to be selected than scores occurring within ranges of a low level of frequency. Obviously, scores which are common or 'average' are more likely to be selected then scores which are unusually high or low.

SAMPLING DISTRIBUTIONS

Probability theory can be applied also to calculate the probability of obtaining specific samples from populations.

Consider a container with a very large number of identically sized marbles. Say that there are two kinds of marbles present, black (B) and white (W). Say that these colours are present in equal proportions, so that $p(B) = p(W) = 0.5$.

Given the above population, say that samples of marbles are drawn randomly and with replacement. (By 'replacement' we mean the samples are put back into the population, in order to maintain as a constant the proportion of $B = W = 0.5$.) If we draw samples of four (that is, $n = 4$) then the possible proportions of black and white marbles in the samples can be deduced *a priori* as shown in Figure 17.3.

Possible outcomes	Number black	Number white	Proportion black
● ● ● ●	4	0	1.00
● ● ● ○	3	1	0.75
● ● ○ ○	2	2	0.50
● ○ ○ ○	1	3	0.25
○ ○ ○ ○	0	4	0.00

Fig. 17.3 Characteristics of possible samples of $n = 4$, drawn from a population of black and white marbles

Ignoring the order in which marbles are chosen, Figure 17.3 demonstrates all the possible outcomes for the composition of samples of $n = 4$. It is logically possible to draw any of the samples shown in Figure 17.3. However, only one of the samples, (2B) is representative of the true population parameter. The other samples would generate incorrect inferences concerning the state of the population. In general, if we know or assume (hypothesize) the true population parameters, we can generate distributions of the probability of obtaining samples of a given characteristic.

In this instance, when attempting to predict the probability of specific samples drawn from a population with two discrete elements, the binomial theorem can be applied. The expansion of the binomial expression, $(P + Q)^n$, generates the probability of all the possible samples which can be drawn from a given population. The general equation for expanding the binomial expression is:

$$(P + Q)^n = P^n + \frac{n}{1} P^{n-1}Q + \frac{n(n-1)}{2} P^{n-2}Q^2 + \ldots Q^n$$

P is the probability of the first outcome
Q is the probability of the second outcome
n is the number of trials (or the sample size)

In this instance, P = proportion black (B) = 0.5; Q = proportion white (W) = 0.5; n = 4 (sample size).

Therefore, substituting into the binomial expression:

$$(B + W)^4 = B^4 + 4B^3W + 6B^2W^2 + 4BW^3 + W^4$$

Note that each part of the expansion stands for a probability of obtaining a specific sample. For the present case:

Sample 1 p(4B0W)	= B^4	= $(0.5)^4$	= 0.0625
Sample 2 p(3B1W)	= $4B^3W$	= 4 x $(0.5)^3(0.5)$	= 0.2500
Sample 3 p(2B2W)	= $6B^2W^2$	= 6 x $(0.5)^2(0.5)^2$	= 0.3750
Sample 4 p(1B3W)	= $4BW^3$	= 4 x $(0.5)^3(0.5)$	= 0.2500
Sample 5 p(0B4W)	= W^4	= $(0.5)^4$	= 0.0625

Note that the calculated probabilities add up to 1, indicating that all the possible sample outcomes have been accounted for. However, the important issue here is not so much the mathematical details, but the general principle being illustrated by the example. For a given sample size (n) we can employ a mathematical formula to calculate the probability of obtaining all the possible samples from a population with known parameters. The relationship between the possible samples and their probabilities can be graphed, as shown in Figure 17.4.

Taking the statistic 'number of black marbles in sample' the graph in Figure 17.4 shows the probability of obtaining any of the outcomes. The distribution shown is called a 'sampling distribution'. In general, a **sampling distribution** for a statistic indicates the probability of obtaining any of the possible values of a statistic.

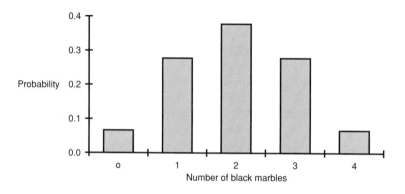

Fig. 17.4 Sampling distribution of black marbles. n = 4

Therefore, having obtained our sampling distribution, we can see that some sample outcomes are quite improbable while others are highly likely. Although there is a finite chance of obtaining a sample such as 'all blacks', the probability of this happening is rather small ($p = 0.0625$). On the other hand a sample of 2B2W, which is equal to the true population proportions, is far more probable ($p = 0.375$). Generating sampling distributions for calculating the probability of given sample statistics is a basic practice in inferential statistics. The sampling distributions enable researchers to infer (with a determined level of confidence) the population parameters from the sample statistics.

SAMPLING DISTRIBUTION OF THE MEAN

The binomial theorem is appropriate for generating sampling distributions for discontinuous, nominal data. However, when measurements are continuous, the mean and standard deviations are appropriate as sample statistics. Therefore, with variables measured on interval or ratio scales, sampling distributions represent the probability of obtaining sample means from the population.

The sampling distribution of the mean represents the frequency distribution of sample means obtained from random samples drawn from the population. The sampling distribution of the mean enables the calculation of the probability of obtaining any given sample mean ($\overline{X}$). This may seem pointless but, as we shall see in Chapter 18, it is essential for hypothesis testing.

In order to generate the sampling distribution of the mean, we use a mathematical theorem called the **central limit theorem**. This theorem provides a set of rules which relate the parameters (μ, σ) of the population from which samples are drawn to the distribution of sample means ($\overline{X}$).

The central limit theorem states that if random samples of a fixed n are drawn from any population, as n becomes large the distribution of sample means approaches a normal distribution, with the mean of the sample means ($\overline{X}_{\bar{x}}$ or, $\mu_{\bar{x}}$) being equal to the population mean (μ) and the standard error of estimate ($s_{\bar{x}}$ or $\sigma_{\bar{x}}$) being equal to $\sigma / \sqrt{n}$. The standard error of the estimate is the standard deviation of the distribution of sample means.

What does this theorem imply? Let us follow the meaning step by step.

1. Say we have a population of continuous scores or measurements with a mean of μ and a standard deviation of σ. These two parameters are crucial for describing a population.
2. Now we select a very large number of random samples, each sample being of a size n.
3. Having obtained our samples, for each sample we calculate the sample mean ($\overline{X}_1$, $\overline{X}_2$, ...and so on).
4. Each sample mean, $\overline{X}$, is of course a number. The sampling distribution of the mean is a frequency distribution produced from the large number of sample means.
5. The central limit theorem predicts theoretically the shape (normal for large n), mean ($\overline{X}_{\bar{x}}$ or $\mu_{\bar{x}}$) and standard deviation ($s_{\bar{x}}$ or $\sigma_{\bar{x}}$) of a large number of sample means.

It should be noted that:

1. The sampling distribution of the mean is a frequency distribution of a large number of sample means of size n drawn from a given population. When n increases, the sampling distributions approach normal.
2. The mean of the sample means ($\mu_{\bar{x}}$ or $\bar{X}_{\bar{x}}$) is the mean of the distribution of sample means. $\bar{X}_{\bar{x}}$ and, $\mu_{\bar{x}}$ are equal to μ the population mean.
3. The standard error of the mean ($s_{\bar{x}}$ or $\sigma_{\bar{x}}$) is the standard deviation of the frequency distribution of sample means drawn from a population. The magnitude of $s_{\bar{x}}$ or $\sigma_{\bar{x}}$ is equal to $\sigma / \sqrt{n}$; the population standard deviation divided by the square root of the sample size.
4. $\mu_{\bar{x}}$ and $\sigma_{\bar{x}}$ are used in reference to a sampling distribution based on all the possible samples drawn from a population (a population of samples, would you believe?); while $\bar{X}_{\bar{x}}$ and $s_{\bar{x}}$ are used when the sampling distribution is based on a 'sample' of samples.

Let us have a look at an example.

Say for a hypothetical test of motor function $\mu = 50$, and $\sigma = 10$. What is the probability of drawing a random sample from this population with $\bar{X} = 52$ or greater (i.e. $\bar{X} \geq 52$) given that $n = 100$? The central limit theorem predicts that when we draw samples of $n = 100$ from the above population, the sampling distribution of the means will be as follows:

The shape of the sampling distribution will be approximately normal.

The mean of the sampling distribution will be equal to μ

$$\mu_{\bar{x}} = \mu = 50$$

The standard error of estimate ($\sigma_{\bar{x}}$) will be:

$$\sigma_{\bar{x}} = \frac{\sigma}{\sqrt{n}} = \frac{10}{\sqrt{100}} = 1$$

(We can show this as in Figure 17.5.)

Previously, we saw how we can use normal frequency distributions for estimating probabilities. Using the same principles as in Chapter 15, we can calculate the z score corresponding to $\bar{X} = 52$, and look up Appendix A to find out the area representing the probability in question:

$$z = \frac{\bar{X} - \mu_{\bar{x}}}{\sigma_{\bar{x}}} = \frac{52 - 50}{1} = 2$$

That is, $\bar{X} = 52$ is two standard error units above the population mean.

Using Appendix A for establishing the probability, we find that the area representing $p(\bar{X} \geq 52)$, that is area A1 in Figure 17.5B, is

$$p(\bar{X} \geq 52) = 0.5000 - 0.4772 = 0.0228$$

Therefore the probability of drawing a sample of $\bar{X} \geq 52$ is 0.0228). We will apply this notion to hypothesis testing in Chapter 18.

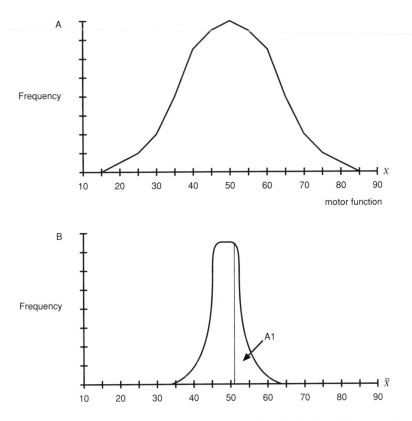

Fig. 17.5 Relationship between original population and sampling distribution of the mean, where $\mu = 50$ and $\sigma = 10$; (A) original population; (B) sampling distribution of the mean

APPLICATION OF THE CENTRAL LIMIT THEOREM TO CALCULATING CONFIDENCE INTERVALS

Let us say that you are asked to estimate the weight of a newborn baby. If you are experienced in working with neonates, you should be able to make a reasonable guess. You might say 'The baby is 6 kg'. Someone might ask 'How certain are you that the baby is exactly 6 kg?' You might then say 'Well, the baby might not be exactly 6 kg, but I'm very confident that it weighs somewhere between 5.5 and 6.5 kg'. This statement expresses a confidence interval; a range of values which probably include the true value. Of course, the more certain or confident you want to be of including the true value, the bigger the range of values you might give: you are unlikely to be wrong if you guess that the baby weighs between 4 and 8 kgs.

We have seen previously that if we know the population parameters we can estimate the probability of selecting from that population a sample mean of a given magnitude. Conversely, if we know the sample mean we can estimate the population parameters from which the sample might have come, at a given level of probability. Let us take an example to illustrate this point.

A researcher is interested in the systolic blood pressure (BP) levels of smokers of more than 10 cigarettes per day. She takes a random sample of 100 10+ smokers in her district and finds that the mean BP = 148 for the sample, with a standard deviation of $s = 10$.

She wants to generalize to the population of smokers of more than 10 cig./ day in her district. Her best estimate of μ (the population parameter) is 148. But it is possible that, because of sampling error, 148 is not the exact population parameter. However she can calculate a confidence interval: a range of blood pressures that will include the true population mean at a given level of probability.

A confidence interval is a range of scores which includes the true population parameter at a specified level of probability. The precise probability is decided by the researcher and indicates how certain he/she can be that the population mean is actually within the calculated range. Common confidence intervals used in statistics are 95% confidence intervals, which offer a probability of $p = 0.95$ for including true population mean, and 99% confidence intervals, which include the true population mean at a probability of $p = 0.99$.

Calculating the confidence interval requires the use of the following formula:

$$\overline{X} - zs_{\overline{x}} \leq \mu \leq \overline{X} + zs_{\overline{x}}$$

(lower confidence limit)   (upper confidence limit)

$\overline{X}$ is the sample mean

z is the z score obtained from the normal curve table, such that it cuts off the appropriate area of the normal curve corresponding to the required probability of the confidence interval.

$s_{\overline{x}}$ is the sample standard error. It is equal to s (the sample standard deviation) divided by $\sqrt{n}$; that is $s_{\overline{x}} = s / \sqrt{n}$.

Let us turn to the previous example to illustrate the use of the above equation. Here $\overline{X} = 148$, and $s_{\overline{x}} = 10\sqrt{100}$. Say we want to calculate a 95% confidence interval. We are looking for a pair of z scores which have 95% of the standard normal curve between them. In this case, 1.96 is the value for z which cuts off 95% of a normal distribution. That is, we looked up the value of z corresponding to an area (probability) of 0.4750, as the 0.05 has to be divided among the two *tails* of the distribution, given 0.025 at either end.

Substituting into the equation above we have:

$$148 - (1.96)\,(10 / \sqrt{100}) \leq \mu \leq 148 + (1.96)\,(10 / \sqrt{100})$$
$$= \; 146.04 \leq \mu \leq 149.96$$

That is, the investigator is 95% confident that the true population mean, the true mean BP of smokers, lies between 146.04 and 149.96. There is only a 5% or 0.05 probability that it lies outside this range.

If we chose a 99% confidence interval, then using the formula as above, we have:

$$148 - (2.58)\left(10 / \sqrt{100}\right) \leq \mu \leq 148 + (2.58)\left(10 / \sqrt{100}\right)$$
$$= 145.42 \leq \mu \leq 150.58$$

Here, the 2.58 is the value of z which cuts off 99% of a normal distribution (Fig. 17.6). That is, the investigator is 99% confident that the true population mean lies somewhere between 145.42 and 150.58. Clearly the 99% interval is wider than the 95% interval; after all, here the probability of including the true mean is greater than for the 95% interval.

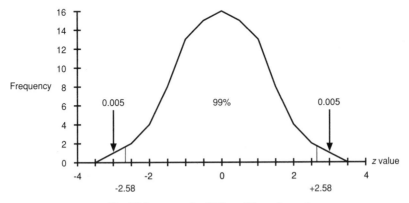

Fig. 17.6 z scores for 99% confidence interval

CONFIDENCE INTERVALS WHERE n IS SMALL: THE t DISTRIBUTION

It was previously stated that: 'as n becomes large, the distribution of sample means approaches a normal distribution' (central limit theorem). The questions left to explain are:

How large must be the sample size, n, before the sampling distribution of the mean can be considered a normal curve? What are the implications for the sampling distribution if n is small?

It has been shown by mathematicians that the sample size, n, for which the sampling distribution of the mean can be considered an approximation of a normal distribution is $n \geq 30$. That is, if n is 30 or more, we can use the standard normal curve (Appendix A) to describe the sampling distribution of the mean.

However when $n < 30$, the sampling distribution of the mean is a rather rough approximation to the normal distribution. Instead of using the normal distribution, we use the 't' distribution, which takes into account the variability of the shape of the sampling distribution due to low n.

The t **distributions** is a family of curves, representing the sampling distributions of means drawn from a population when sample size, n, is small ($n < 30$). A 'family of curves' means that the shape of t distribution varies with sample size. It has been found that the distribution is determined by the 'degrees of freedom' of the statistic.

The **degrees of freedom** (*df*) for a statistic represents the number of scores which are free to vary when calculating the statistic. Since the statistic we are calculating in this case is the mean, all but one of the scores could vary. That is, if you were inventing scores in a sample with a known mean, you would have a free hand until the very last score. For the *t* distribution, *df* is equal to *n* − 1 (the sample size, minus one). Each *row* of figures shown in Appendix B represents the critical values of '*t*' for a given distribution.

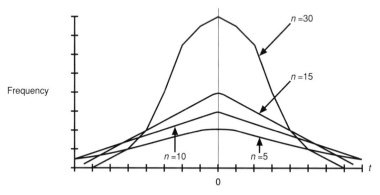

Fig. 17.7 *t* distributions

1. The *t* distribution is symmetrical about the mean.
2. The values of *t* along the *x* axis cut off specific areas under the curve, just as for *z*. These areas are given at the top of the page, under 'Directional' and 'Non Directional' probabilities.
3. The *t* distribution approaches a normal distribution as *n* becomes larger. As we stated earlier, when *n* ≥ 30, for all practical purposes the *t* and *z* distributions coincide.

The *t* distribution, just as the *z* distribution, can be used to approximate the probability of drawing sample means of a given magnitude from a population. Also, *t* can be used for calculating confidence intervals. Let us re-examine the example presented on page 270. Here, let us assume that *n* = 25, with the other statistics remaining the same: $\overline{X}$ = 148; *s* = 10.

The general formula for calculating the confidence intervals for small samples is:

$$\overline{X} - ts_{\overline{x}} \leq \mu \leq \overline{X} + ts_{\overline{x}}$$

You will notice the similarity to the equation on page 270; here '*t*' replaces '*z*'. If we want to show the 95% confidence interval, then we use the same logic as for *z* distributions (Fig. 17.8).

To look up the '*t*' values from the tables (Appendix B) consider (i) direction (ii) probabilities (iii) degrees of freedom.

We are looking at a 'non-directional' or 'two-tail' probability in the sense that the *t* values cut off 95% of the area of the *t* curve between them, leaving 5% distributed at the two tails of the *t* distribution.

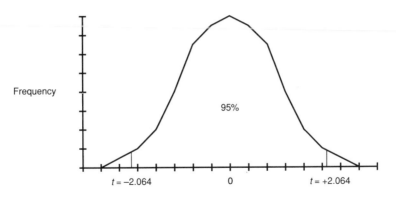

Fig. 17.8 95% confidence interval for sample size of 25

$p = 0.05$ (see Figure 17.8)
$df = 25 - 1 = 24$

Therefore $t = 2.064$ (from tables in Appendix B). Substituting into the equation for calculating confidence intervals:

$$148 - (2.1)(10/\sqrt{25}) \leq \mu \leq 148 + (2.1)(10/\sqrt{25})$$

(Note $s_{\bar{x}} = s/\sqrt{n}$)
$148 - 4.2 \leq \mu \leq 148 + 4.2$
$143.8 \leq \mu \leq 152.2$

Note that this is a wider interval than that which we obtained when n was 100. As sample size, n, becomes smaller, our confidence interval becomes wider, reflecting a greater probability of sampling error.

To calculate the 99% confidence interval (Fig. 17.9), we need to look up $p = 0.01$, non-directional, $df = 24$; in Appendix B to obtain the critical value of t, which is 2.797.

$$148 - (2.8)(10/\sqrt{25}) \leq \mu \leq 148 + (2.8)(10\sqrt{25})$$
$142.4 \leq \mu \leq 153.6$

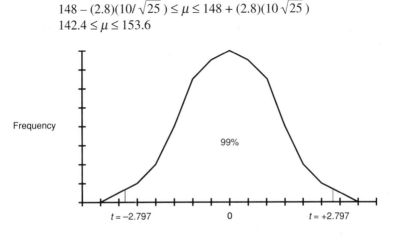

Fig. 17.9 99% confidence interval for sample size of 25

As for the 95% confidence interval, and for the same reasons, we can see that when $n = 25$, the 99% confidence interval was wider than for $n = 100$. That is, the bigger our sample size, the narrower (more precise) becomes our estimate of the range of values which includes the true population parameter.

SUMMARY

It was argued in this chapter that even with randomly selected samples, the possibility of sampling error must be taken into account when making inferences from sample statistics to population parameters. It was shown that probability theory can be applied to generating sampling distributions, which express the probability of obtaining a given sample from a population. With discontinuous, nominal data, the binomial theorem provides an adequate mathematical distribution for estimating the probability for obtaining possible samples. However, with continuous data, the central limit theorem is applied to generate the sampling distributions of the mean. The standard distribution of the mean enables the calculation of the probable specified sample mean by random selection from a population. The sampling error of the mean ($s_{\bar{x}}$ or $\sigma_{\bar{x}}$), which expresses statistically the range of the sampling error, depends inversely on the sample size, such that the larger n the smaller $s_{\bar{x}}$ or $\sigma_{\bar{x}}$.

One of the applications of sampling distributions is for calculating confidence intervals for continuous data. Confidence intervals represent a range of scores which specify, from sample data, the probability of capturing the true population parameters. When sample sizes are small ($n < 30$), the t distribution is appropriate for representing the sampling distribution of the mean. With large sample sizes, the two distributions merge together. As the next chapter will demonstrate, sampling distributions are essential for testing hypotheses, a procedure which uses inferential statistics to calculate the level of probability at which sample statistics support the predictions of hypotheses.

SELF ASSESSMENT

Explain the meaning of the following terms:

confidence interval	sampling error
sampling distribution	population parameter
sampling distribution of the mean	probability
standard error of the mean	t distribution

True or false

1. If death and taxes are an absolute certainty, then the probability of their occurrence is infinite.
2. Probability values fall between 0 and 1.

3. When a score occurs at a relatively high level of frequency the probability of randomly selecting it from a distribution is $p = 1$.
4. The higher the corresponding z score, the lower the probability of randomly selecting the score from a distribution.
5. For a normal distribution, σ is the score which has the highest probability of random selection.
6. It is possible to have a negative z scores but not a negative probability.
7. For a continuous normal distribution, the probability of selecting a score up to and including the mode is $p = 0.5$.
8. The probability of randomly selecting a score 2 standard deviations above the mean is $p = 0.2$.
9. We can generate appropriate sampling distributions for statistics derived from nominal or ordinal data.
10. Statistical inference involves the estimation of population parameters from sample statistics.
11. Statistical inference depends on knowing the true population parameters before beginning research.
12. The sampling distribution of the mean is a frequency polygon of mean scores.
13. Using the sample mean as an estimate for the population mean is an example of statistical inference.
14. The sampling distribution of the mean is always normally distributed.
15. As n increases, the variability of the sampling distribution of the mean increases .
16. $\mu_{\bar{x}} = \mu$ regardless of the shape of the sampling distribution of the mean.
17. The characteristics of the sampling distribution of the mean vary with the size of the sample.
18. If a random selection method is used, sampling error will be zero.
19. The bigger the sampling error the smaller the confidence interval.
20. Generally speaking, the higher level of confidence we have that an interval contains the population mean, the larger is that interval.

Multiple choice

1. The mean age of the Canadian population is known to be 31 years. A small randomly selected sample of Canadians is found to have a mean age of 32. This discrepancy is an example of:
   a   a sampling error
   b   a measurement error
   c   a problem in ecological validity
   d   failure to control for the effects of maturation.

At a large maternity hospital the following hypothetical data are compiled concerning the birth weights and survival of neonates.

Table M17.1 Birthweight and survival of neonates

Weight of neonates (g)	Numbers (n)	Percentage of neonates surviving
0–499	25	40
500–999	50	60
1 000–1499	75	80
1 500–1999	150	90
2000–2499	250	95
2500 +	450	98

Questions 2–5 refer to this table.

2. What is the probability that a randomly selected neonate will weigh under 500 g?
   a   0.4000
   b   0.1700
   c   0.0250
   d   0.0025

3. What is the probability that a randomly selected neonate will have a birth weight of 2000 g or over?
   a   0.7000
   b   0.9638
   c   0.3000
   d   0.9500

4. What is the probability that a neonate weighing 499 g or under will survive?
   a   0.4000
   b   0.1700
   c   0.040
   d   0.025

5. What is the probability that a neonate weighing 2500 g or over will not survive?
   a   0.400
   b   0.300
   c   0.006
   d   0.020

A test of reaction times has a mean of 10 and a standard deviation of 4 in the normal adult population with a normal distribution. Questions 6–12 refer to this information.

6. A person scores 8. That persons's z score is:
   a   2
   b   −2
   c   −0.5
   d   −1

7. What percentage of the population would have scores up to and including 14 on this test?
   a 84.13
   b 15.87
   c 65.87
   d 34.13

8. What is the percentile rank of a score of 8 on this test?
   a 19.15
   b 30.85
   c 80.85
   d 53.28

9. What score (to the nearest whole number) would cut off the highest 10% of scores?
   a 1
   b 14
   c 15
   d 18

10. What is the probability that a randomly selected individual will score greater than 6 on this test?
   a 0.4987
   b 0.3413
   c 0.8413
   d 0.6587

11. What is the probability that a randomly selected individual will score between 8 and 14 on this test?
   a 0.1498
   b 0.5328
   c 0.6816
   d 0.4671

12. What is the probability that a randomly selected individual will score either more than 14 or less than 10 on this test?
   a 0.6587
   b 0.6816
   c 0.3184
   d 0.8184

13. Sampling error of the mean:
   a occurs because of poor sampling techniques
   b decreases as sample size increases
   c is independent of the standard deviation
   d is always equal to 1.

14. Samples of 100 are drawn from a normally distributed population with a mean of 50 and a standard deviation of 10. The distribution of sample means will:
    a have a mean of 50
    b have a standard deviation of 1
    c be normally distributed
    d all of the above.

15. Increasing the sample size, in '*n*':
    a decreases sampling error
    b increases sampling error
    c has no effect on standard error of the mean
    d requires increasing correction of sample estimates of population parameters
    e none of these.

16. If the dispersion of the raw score population increases while *n* is held constant $\sigma_{\bar{x}}$:
    a decreases
    b increases
    c remains the same
    d need more information.

17. The sampling distribution of the mean:
    a is always positively skewed for continuous data
    b is normally distributed if the population raw scores are not normally distributed
    c is approximately normally distributed if sample size is large
    d all of the above.

18. As the degrees of freedom decrease, the similarity between the *t* and *z* distributions:
    a increases
    b decreases
    c remains the same
    d approaches infinity.

19. The theoretical sampling distributions of the *t* statistics depend on:
    a *p*
    b *r*
    c $s_{\bar{x}}$
    d *df.*

A normally distributed population has a mean of 80 and a standard deviation of 12.
    Questions 20–24 refer to the above information.

20. For samples of $n = 36$, what is the standard error of the mean?
    a 12
    b 0.33
    c 2
    d 3

21. A sample of 64 cases is found to have a mean of 83. What is the z score of this mean?
    a 2
    b 0.25
    c 4
    d 1.5

22. A sample of $n = 144$ has a mean of 77. What is the probability that a mean this low would occur by chance?
    a 0.0300
    b 0.0013
    c 0.4989
    d 0.9987

23. A sample of 36 cases is selected. What is the probability that its mean falls outside the range of 79–81?
    a 0.6813
    b 0.8085
    c 0.3085
    d 0.6170

24. Which is more likely, that a randomly selected sample of $n = 36$ will have a mean greater than 82 or that it will have a mean less than 77?
    a Greater than 82
    b Less than 77
    c Both are equally probable
    d Impossible to tell.

25. The t distribution differs from the z distribution in which of these ways?
    a Its mean is not exactly equal to 0.
    b It is not quite symmetrical.
    c It is somewhat wider and flatter.
    d All of the above.

26. The 95% confidence interval arrived at from a particular experiment is 72–79. Therefore:
    a the probability is 0.05 that μ falls between 72–79
    b the probability is 0.95 that the interval 72–79 contains $\overline{X}$
    c the probability is 0.95 that the interval 72–79 contains μ
    d *a* and *c*.

27. Compared to a 99% confidence interval, a 95% confidence interval is:
    a larger
    b smaller
    c more likely to contain the population mean
    d less likely to contain the sample mean.

The following information should be used in answering questions 28–31:
    A random sample of 25 clients is selected, and their systolic blood pressures measured. The mean BP is 115 mmHg, with a standard deviation of 10.

28. This is an example of:
    a an experiment
    b a natural comparison study
    c a survey
    d field research.

29. What is the standard error of the mean for a sample of this size?
    a 10
    b 20
    c 2
    d 2.5

30. In order to calculate the 99% confidence interval of the mean, what t score will be used?
    a 2.492
    b 2.787
    c 2.797
    d 1.711

31. What is the 99% confidence interval of the mean in this example?
    a $110.0 \leq \mu \leq 120.0$
    b $109.4 \leq \mu \leq 120.6$
    c $111.6 \leq \mu \leq 118.4$
    d $113.0 \leq \mu \leq 117.0$

32. A random sample of 25 University students is found to have a mean IQ of 110, with a standard deviation of 10. Between what two possible scores can we be 99% confident that the true mean IQ for the students at the university lies?
    a 95.5–112.5
    b 85–135
    c 102.4–117.6
    d 104.1–115.9

In order to establish the mean weight of newborn babies at a large maternity hospital, a random sample of 64 babies is weighed. Their mean weight is 2500 g, with a standard deviation of 80 g.

Questions 33–35 require this information.

33. What is the standard error of the mean?
    a   80
    b   10
    c   1.25
    d   0.1

34. In calculating the 95% confidence interval of the mean, what z value is used?
    a   1.96
    b   2.33
    c   2.58
    d   1.64

35. What is the 95% confidence interval of the mean in this example (to the nearest whole number)?
    a $2480 \leq \mu \leq 2520$
    b $2477 \leq \mu \leq 2523$
    c $2474 \leq \mu \leq 2526$
    d $2484 \leq \mu \leq 2516$

18

Hypothesis testing

INTRODUCTION

In the previous section, we examined the use of inferential statistics for estimating population parameters from sample statistics. In the case of some non-experimental research strategies, such as surveys (see Section Three), parameter estimation is adequate for analysing the data. After all, these investigations aim at describing the characteristics of specific populations. However, other research strategies involve data collection for the purpose of testing hypotheses such as whether two therapeutic techniques have different effectiveness. Here, the investigator has to establish if the data support or refute the hypotheses being investigated.

The aim of this chapter is to introduce the logical steps involved in hypothesis testing in quantitative research. Given that hypothesis testing is probabilistic, special attention must be paid to the possibility or making erroneous decisions, and to the implications of making such errors.

The specific aims of the chapter are to:

1. Examine the logic of hypotheses testing in relation to retaining or rejecting null hypotheses.
2. Outline how decisions are made involving directional and non-directional alternative hypotheses.
3. Introduce the use of the single sample z and t test for analysing the statistical significance of the data.
4. Outline the probability and implications of making Type 1 and Type II decision errors.

A SIMPLE ILLUSTRATION OF HYPOTHESIS TESTING

One of the simplest forms of gambling is betting on the fall of a coin. Let us play a little game. We, the authors, will toss a coin. If it comes out heads (H) you will give us $1; if tails (T) we will give you $1. To make things interesting, let us have 10 tosses. O.K., here we go. The results are:

Toss	1	2	3	4	5	6	7	8	9	10
Outcome	H	H	H	H	H	H	H	H	H	H

Oh dear. You seem to have lost. Never mind, we were just lucky, so send along your cheque for $10. What's that? You are a little hesitant? Are you saying that we 'fixed' the game? As a matter of fact, there is a systematic procedure for demonstrating the probable truth of your allegations:

1. We can state the hypotheses concerning the outcome of the game:
   (a) The authors fixed the game; that is, the outcome does not reflect the fair throwing of a coin. Let us call this statement the 'alternative hypotheses', H_A. In effect, the H_A claims that the sample of 10 heads came from a population other than P (probability of heads) = Q (probability of tails) = 0.5
   (b) The authors did not fix the game; that is, the outcome is due to the tossing of a fair coin. Let us call this statement the 'null hypothesis', or H_0. H_0 suggests that the sample of 10 heads was a random sample from a population where $P = Q = 0.5$
2. It can be shown that the probability of tossing 10 consecutive heads with a fair coin is $p = 0.001$, as we discussed previously (see Ch. 15). That is, the probability of obtaining such a sample from a population where $P = Q = 0.5$ is extremely low.
3. Now we can decide between H_0 and H_A. It was shown that the probability of H_0 being true was $p = 0.001$ (one in a thousand). Therefore, in the balance of probabilities, we can reject it as being true and accept H_A, which is the logical alternative. In other words, it is likely that the game was fixed and no $10 cheque needs to be posted.

The probability of calculating the truth of H_0 depended on the number of tosses (n = the sample size). For instance, the probabilities of obtaining all heads with up to 5 tosses, according to the binomial theorem (Ch. 17) are:

n (number of tosses)	p (all heads)
1	0.5000
2	0.2500
3	0.1250
4	0.0625
5	0.0313

Clearly, the above table shows that as the sample size (n) becomes larger, the probability at which it is possible to reject H_0 becomes smaller. With only a few tosses we really cannot be sure if the game is fixed or not: it becomes hard to reject H_0 at a reasonable level of probability.

A question emerges: 'What is a reasonable level of probability for rejecting H_0?' As we shall see, there are conventions for specifying these probabilities.

One way to proceed, however, is to set the appropriate probability for rejecting H_0 on the basis of the implications of erroneous decisions.

Obviously, any decision made on a probabilistic basis might be erroneous. Two types of elementary decision errors can be identified, Type I and Type II. Type I error involves mistakenly rejecting H_0, while Type II error involves mistakenly retaining H_0.

In the above example, Type I error would involve deciding that the outcome was not due to chance, when in fact it was. The practical outcome of this would be to falsely accuse the authors of fixing the game. A Type II error would represent the decision that the outcome was due to chance, when in fact it was due to a fix. The practical outcome of this would be to send your hard earned $10 to a couple of crooks. Clearly, in a situation like this, a Type II error would be more odious than a Type I error, and you would set a fairly high probability for rejecting H_0. However, if you were gambling with Wild Bill Hickock, who had a loaded revolver handy, you would tend to set a very low probability for rejecting H_0. We will examine these ideas more formally in subsequent parts of this chapter.

THE LOGIC OF HYPOTHESIS TESTING

Hypothesis testing is the process of deciding statistically whether the findings of an investigation reflect chance or 'real' effects at a given level of probability.

The mathematical procedures for hypothesis testing are based on the application of probability theory and sampling, as discussed previously. Because of the probabilistic nature of the process, decision errors in hypothesis testing cannot be entirely eliminated. However, the procedures outlined in this section enable us to specify the probability level at which we can claim that the data obtained in an investigation support experimental hypotheses. This procedure is fundamental for analysing data, as well as being relevant to the logic of clinical decision making.

Steps in hypothesis testing

The following steps are conventionally followed in hypothesis testing:

1. State the alternative hypothesis (H_A), which is the prediction intended for evaluation. The H_A claims that the results are 'real' or 'significant': that the independent variable influenced the dependent variable, or that there is a real difference among groups.
2. State the null hypothesis (H_0), which is the logical opposite of the H_A. The H_0 claims that any differences in the data were just due to chance: that the independent variable had no effect on the dependent variable, or that any difference among groups is due to random effects.
3. Set decision level, α (alpha). There are two mutually exclusive hypotheses (H_A and H_0) competing to explain the results of an investigation. Hypothesis testing, or statistical decision making, involves establishing

the probability of H_0 being true. If this probability is very small, we are in a position to reject the H_0. You might ask 'how small should be the probability (α) for rejecting H_0?' By convention, we use the probability of $\alpha = 0.05$. That is, if the H_0 being true is less than 0.05 we can reject H_0. We can choose an α of < 0.05, but not more, That is, by convention among researchers results are *not significant* if $p > 0.05$.

4. Calculate the probability of H_0 being true. That is, we assume H_0 is true and calculate the probability of the outcome of the investigation being due to chance alone, that is, due to random effects. We must use an appropriate sampling distribution for this calculation.

5. Make decision concerning H_0. If the probability of H_0 being true is less than α, then we reject H_0, at the level of significance set by α. However, if the probability of H_0 is greater than α, then we must retain H_0. In other words, if:

p (H_0 is true) $\leq \alpha$; reject H_0

p (H_0 is true) $> \alpha$; retain H_0

It follows that if we reject H_0, we are in a position to accept H_A, its logical alternative. If we reject H_0, we conclude that the H_A is probably true.

Let us look at an example. A rehabilitation therapist devises an exercise program which is expected to reduce the time taken for people to leave hospital following orthopaedic surgery. Previous records show that the recovery time for patients has been $\mu = 30$ days, with $\sigma = 8$ days. A sample of 64 patients are treated with the exercise program, and their mean recovery time is found to be $\overline{X} = 24$ days. Do these results show that patients who had the treatment recovered significantly faster than previous patients?

We can apply the steps for hypothesis testing to make our decision.

1. State H_A:
   The exercise program reduces the time taken for patients to recover from orthopaedic surgery.
   That is, the researcher claims that the independent variable (the treatment) had a 'real' or 'generalizable' effect on the dependent variable (time to recover).

2. State H_0:
   The exercise program does not reduce the time taken for patients to recover from orthopaedic surgery.
   That is, the statement claims that the independent variable had no effect on the dependent variable. The statement implies that the treated sample with $\overline{X} = 24$, and $n = 64$ is in fact a random sample from the population $\mu = 30$;
   $\sigma = 8$. Any difference between $\overline{X}$ and μ can be attributed to sampling error.

3. Decision level, α, is set before the results are analysed. The probability of α depends on how certain the investigator wants to be that the results

show real differences. If she sets $\alpha = 0.01$, then the probability of falsely rejecting a true H_0 is less than or equal to 0.01 (1/100). If she sets $\alpha = 0.05$, then the probability of falsely rejecting a true H_0 is less than or equal to 0.05 or (1/20). That is, the smaller α, the more confident the researcher is that the results support the alternative hypothesis. We also call α the level of *significance*. The smaller α, the more significant the findings for a study, if we can reject H_0. In this case, say that the researcher sets $\alpha = 0.01$.

Note: by convention, α *cannot* be greater than 0.05!

4. Calculate the probability of H_0 being true. As stated above, the H_0 implies that the sample with $\overline{X} = 24$ is a random sample from the population with $\mu = 30$, $\sigma = 8$. How probable is it that this statement is true? To calculate this probability, we must generate an appropriate sampling distribution. As we have seen in Chapter 17, the sampling distribution of the mean will enable us to calculate the probability of obtaining a sample mean of $\overline{X} = 24$ or more extreme from a population with known parameters.

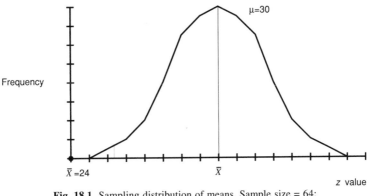

Fig. 18.1 Sampling distribution of means. Sample size = 64; population mean = 30; standard deviation = 8

As shown in Figure 18.1, we can calculate the probability of drawing a sample mean of $\overline{X} = 24$ or less. Using the table of normal curves (Appendix A) as outlined previously, we find that the probability of randomly selecting a sample mean of $\overline{X} = 24$ (or less) is extremely small. In terms of our table, which only shows the exact probability of up to $z = 4.00$, we can see that the present probability is less than 0.00003. Therefore, the probability that H_0 is true is less than 0.00003.

5. Make a decision. We have set $\alpha = 0.01$.
    The calculated probability was less than 0.0001. Clearly, the calculated probability is far less than α.
    Therefore, the investigator can reject the statement that H_0 is true, and accept H_A: that patients treated with the exercise program recover earlier than the population of untreated patients.

DIRECTIONAL AND NON-DIRECTIONAL HYPOTHESES, AND CORRESPONDING CRITICAL VALUES OF STATISTICS

In the previous example, H_A was *directional*, in that we asserted that the difference between the mean of the treated sample and the population mean was expected to be in a particular direction. If we state that there was some effect due to the dependent variable, but do *not* specify which way, then H_A is called *non-directional*. In the previous example, if the investigator stated the H_A as:

The exercise program *changes* the time taken to recover following surgery

then H_A would have been non-directional.

In general, an alternative hypothesis is directional if it predicts a specific outcome concerning the direction of the findings by stating that one group mean will be higher or lower than the other(s). An alternative hypothesis is non-directional if it predicts a difference, without specifying which group mean is expected to be higher or lower than the others.

If we propose a directional H_A, it is understood that we have reasonable information on the basis of pilot studies or previously published research for predicting the direction of the outcome. The advantage of a directional H_A is that it increases the probability of rejecting H_0. However, the decision of the directionality of H_A must be decided *before* the data are collected and analysed.

Let us now examine the concept of the 'critical' value of a statistic. The critical value of a statistic is the value of the statistic which bounds the proportion of the sampling distribution specified by α. The critical value of the statistic is influenced by whether H_A is directional or non-directional.

Figures 18.2 and 18.3 represent the sampling distributions of the mean where n is large; that is, the sampling distribution for the statistic $\overline{X}$. As we have seen in Chapter 17, these are the sampling distributions for $\overline{X}$ we would expect by the random selection of samples, as specified by H_0. Therefore, we can estimate from the distributions the probability of selecting any sample mean, $\overline{X}$, by chance alone (Ch. 17). Alpha (α, the level of significance) specifies the criterion for rejecting H_0. We can see that the critical value for the statistic (in this case z_{crit}) cuts off an area of the distribution corresponding to α ($p = 0.05$ or $p = 0.01$).

In Figure 18.2, we can see that $z_{crit} = 1.65$ (for $\alpha = 0.05$) and $z_{crit} = 2.33$ (for $\alpha = 0.01$). (These values are obtained from Appendix A.) Therefore, for any sample mean, $\overline{X}$, where the transformed (z) value is greater than or equal to z_{crit}, we will reject H_0 (that the sample mean was a random sample). However, if the absolute value of the transformed statistic is less than z_{crit}, then we must retain H_0. Note that when $\alpha = 0.01$, the z_{crit} is greater than when $\alpha = 0.05$. Clearly, the higher the level of significance set for rejecting H_0, the greater the absolute critical value of the statistic. Figure 18.2 shows statistical decision making with a directional H_A, where the probabilities associated with only one of the tails of the distribution are used.

Figure 18.3 shows the critical values for z with a non-directional H_A. Here, the probabilities associated α (0.05 or 0.01) are divided between the two tails of the distribution. That is, where $\alpha = 0.05$, half (0.025) goes into each tail and where $\alpha = 0.01$, half (0.005) also goes into each tail. This changes the values of

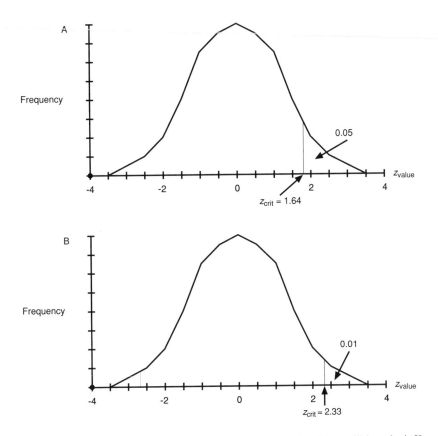

Fig. 18.2 Two examples of statistical decision-making with directional (one tail) hypothesis H_A

z_{crit}, which becomes ± 1.96 or ± 2.58, respectively, as shown in Figure 18.3. Here, we reject H_0 if the calculated transformed z value of $\overline{X}$ falls beyond the values of z_{crit}. When we compare the values of z_{crit} for the one-tail and two-tailed decisions, we find that the critical values are greater for the two-tail decisions. This implies that it is more difficult to reject H_0 if we are making two-tail decisions on the basis of a non-directional H_A.

Decision rules

In general, Figures 18.2 and 18.3 illustrate the decision rules for statistical decision making for hypotheses concerning sample means. These rules are:

$$|z_{obt}| \geq |z_{crit}|; \text{ reject } H_0$$

$$|z_{obt}| < |z_{crit}|; \text{ retain } H_0$$

The same decision rules hold for the t distributions associated with the sampling distribution of the mean when n (the sample size) is small (see Chapter 16).

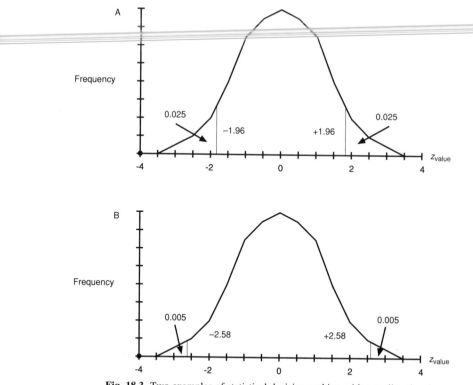

Fig. 18.3 Two examples of statistical decision-making with non-directional (two tail) hypothesis H_A

$$|t_{obt}| \geq |t_{crit}|; \text{ reject } H_0$$
$$|t_{obt}| < |t_{crit}|; \text{ retain } H_0$$

z_{obt}, t_{obt} refer to the calculated value of the statistic, based on the data:

$$z_{obt} = \frac{\bar{X} - \mu}{s_{\bar{x}}}$$

$$t_{obt} = \frac{\bar{X} - \mu}{s_{\bar{x}}}$$

z_{crit}, t_{crit} are the critical values of the statistic obtained from the tables in Appendices A and B. As we have seen, the values of these depend on α and the directionality of H_A.

$| \, |$ is the symbol for 'modulus', implying that we should look at the absolute value of a statistic. That is, we can ignore the sign (+ or –).

In effect, the greater z_{obt} or t_{obt}, the more deviant or improbable the particular sample mean, $\bar{X}$ is under the sampling distribution specified by H_0.

STATISTICAL DECISIONS WITH SINGLE SAMPLE MEANS

The following examples illustrate the use of statistical decision making concerning a single sample mean, $\overline{X}$. Such decisions are relevant when our data consists of a single sample and we are to decide if the $\overline{X}$ of the sample is significantly different to a given population, with a mean of μ.

A *statistical test* is a procedure appropriate for making statistical decisions concerning the significance of the data. The z test and the t test are procedures appropriate for making decisions concerning sample means. (As shown in Chapter 19, there is a variety of statistical tests available for hypothesis testing.)

Example 1

A researcher hypothesizes that males nowadays weigh more than in previous years. To investigate this hypothesis he randomly selects 100 adult males and records their weights. The measurements for the sample have a mean of $\overline{X} = 70$ kg. In a census taken several years ago, the mean weight of males was $\mu = 68$ kg, with a standard deviation of 8 kg.

1. Directional H_A: Males are heavier. That is, $\overline{X} = 70$ is not a random sample from population $\mu = 68$.
2. H_0: Males are not heavier. That is, $\overline{X} = 70$ is a random sample from population with $\mu = 68$.
3. Decision level: $\alpha = 0.01$
4. Calculate probability of H_0 being true. Here, $\alpha = 0.01$, one-tail.
   We can find from the tables (Appendix A) z_{crit}, the z score which cuts off an area of 0.01 of the total curve.

$$z_{crit} = +2.33 \ (\alpha = 0.01; \text{one-tail})$$

Calculating the z score (z_{obt}) representing the probability of the sample being drawn from the population under H_0 ($\mu = 68$) we use the formula:

$$z_{obt} = \frac{\overline{X} - \mu}{s_{\overline{x}}}$$

$$where \ s_{\overline{x}} = \frac{s}{\sqrt{n}}$$

$$z_{obt} = \frac{70 - 68}{8 / \sqrt{100}}$$

$$= 2.5$$

$$\text{Here, } z_{crit} = 2.33$$

5. The decision rule is that if:

$|z_{obt}| \geq |z_{crit}|$; reject H_0

$|z_{obt}| < |z_{crit}|$; retain H_0

$2.5 > 2.33$, so the z_{obt} falls into the area of rejection, as shown in Figure 18.4. Therefore, the researcher can reject H_0, and accept H_A at a 0.01 level of significance. That is, the results of the investigation indicated that the mean weight of males has increased (consistently with the predictions of the research hypothesis).

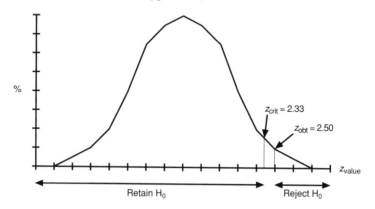

Fig. 18.4 Hypothesis testing: directional

Example 2

A researcher hypothesized that men today have different weights (either more or less) than in previous years. (Assume the same information as for Example 1.)

1. Non-directional H_A: Males are of different weight, that is,
   $\overline{X} = 70$ is not a random sample from population $\mu = 68$.
2. H_0: Males are not different, that is $\overline{X}$ is a random sample from $\mu = 68$.
3. Decision level: $\alpha = 0.01$
4. Calculate the probability of H_0 being true. Here, $\alpha = 0.01$ (two-tail).
   The value of $|z_{crit}| = 2.58$ (from Appendix A)
   The value of $|z_{obt}| = 2.5$ (as calculated in Example 1).
5. Decision:
   Applying the decision rule as outlined in Example 1:
   $|z_{obt}| < |z_{crit}|$; as $2.5 < 2.58$

z_{obt} falls into the area of acceptance, as shown in Figure 18.5. Therefore, the researcher must retain the H_0, and conclude that the study did not support H_A at a 0.01 level of significance. Therefore, the investigation has not provided evidence that the mean weight of males has increased.

The above examples involved sample sizes of $n > 30$. However, as we saw in Chapter 17 if $n < 30$, the distribution of sample means is not a normal, but a t distribution. This point must be taken into account when we calculate the probability of H_0 being true (Example 3). That is, for small samples, we use the 't' test to evaluate the significance of our data.

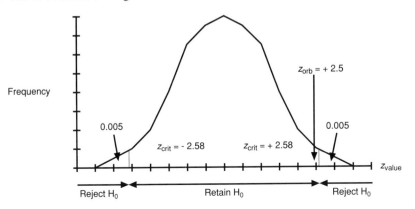

Fig. 18.5 Hypothesis testing: non-directional

Example 3

Assume exactly the same information as in Example 1; except that sample size is $n = 16$.

1. Directional H_A: as in Example 1
2. H_0: as in Example 1
3. $\alpha = 0.01$, one-tail
4. We can find from the t table (Appendix B) the value for t_{crit}. To look up t_{crit} we must have the following information:
    a α, the level of significance (0.05 or 0.01)
    b   direction of H_A (directional or non-directional)
    c   the degrees of freedom, (df)

In this instance:
a $\alpha = 0.01$
b H_A is directional, therefore we must look up a one-tail probability.
c $df = n - 1 = 16 - 1 = 15$

Looking up the appropriate value for t; $t_{crit} = 2.602$. Calculating the t score (t_{obt}) representing the probability of the sample being drawn from the population under H_0, we use the formula:

$$t_{obt} = \frac{\overline{X} - \mu}{s_{\overline{x}}}$$

$$= \frac{70 - 68}{8 / \sqrt{16}}$$

$$= 1.0$$

5. As we stated earlier, the decision rule is identical to that of the z-test:

$$|t_{obt}| \geq |t_{crit}|; \text{ reject } H_0$$
$$|t_{obt}| < |t_{crit}|; \text{ retain } H_0$$

Here, $1.0 < 2.602$, such that t_{obt} falls into the area of retention. Therefore, we must retain H_0 at a 0.01 level of significance. Clearly, when $n = 16$, the investigation did not show a significant weight increase for the males.

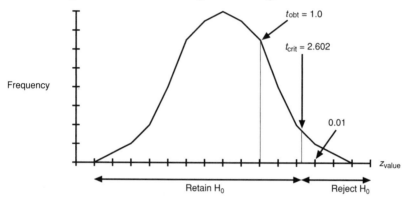

Fig. 18.6 Hypothesis testing: directional

The above examples demonstrate the following points about statistical decision making:

- We are more likely to reject H_0 if we use a one-tail test (directional H_A) than a two-tail test (non-directional H_A). In effect, we are using the prediction of which way the differences will go to increase the probability of rejecting H_0, and therefore accepting H_A. Examples 1 and 2 demonstrate this point; in Example 1 we rejected H_0 with a directional H_A, while we retained H_0 in Example 2, with exactly the same data.
- The larger the sample size, n, the more likely we are to reject H_0 for a given set of data. Comparing Examples 1 and 3 demonstrates this; although μ, σ, and $\overline{X}$ were the same, where n was small, we had to retain H_0. Also, when n is small, $(n < 30)$, we must use the t test to analyse the significance of our sample mean being different.
- The more demanding the decision level (that is, if α is small) the less likely we are to reject H_0. To illustrate this point, repeat Example 2, but set $\alpha = 0.05$. Here $z_{crit} = 1.96$ so that z_{obt} is greater than z_{crit}. Therefore, we can reject H_0, and accept H_A at a 0.05 level of significance. That is, with exactly the same data, we have rejected or accepted H_0, depending on the level of significance, α.

ERRORS IN INFERENCE

It should be evident from the previous discussion that statistical decision making might result in incorrect decisions. There are two main types of inferential error; Type I and Type II.

Type I error occurs when we mistakenly reject H_0; that is when we claim that our experimental hypothesis was supported when it is, in fact, false. The probability of a Type I error occurring is less than or equal to α. For instance, in the previous Example 1 we set $\alpha = 0.01$. The probability of making a Type 1 error is less than or equal to 0.01; the chances are equal to or less than 1/100 that our decision in rejecting H_0 was mistaken. Therefore, the smaller α, the less the chance of making a Type I error.

Type II error occurs when we mistakenly retain H_0; that is , when we falsely conclude that the experimental hypothesis was not supported by our data. The probability of a Type II error occurring is denoted by β (beta). In Example 3 we retained H_0, perhaps falsely. If n were larger, we might well have rejected H_0, as in Example 1. Type 1 errors represent a 'false alarm' and Type II errors a 'miss'. Table 18.1 illustrates this.

Table 18.1 illustrates that if we reject H_0, we are making either a correct decision or a Type I error. If we retain H_0, we are making either a correct decision or a Type II error. While we cannot, in principle, eliminate these from scientific decision making, we can take steps to minimize their occurrence.

Table 18.1 Decision outcomes

Reality	Decision: Reject H_0	Decision: Retain H_0
H_0 correct (no difference or effect)	'False alarm' Type I error	Correct decision
H_0 incorrect (real difference or effect)	Correct decision	'Miss' Type II error

We minimize the occurrence of Type I error by setting an acceptable level for α. In scientific research, editors of most scientific journals require that α should be set at 0.05 or less. This convention helps to reduce 'false alarms' to a rate of less than 1/20. Replication of the findings by other independent investigators provides important evidence that the original decision to reject H_0 was correct.

How do we minimize Type II error rate?

1. Increase sample size, n.
2. Reduce the variability of measurements ($s_{\bar{x}}$, either by increasing accuracy (Ch. 12) or by using samples which are not highly variable for the measurement producing the data).
3. Use of a directional H_A, on the basis of previous evidence about the nature of the effect.
4. Set a less demanding α, Type I error rate. There is a relationship between a and b, such that the smaller α, the greater β. This relationship is illustrated in Figure 18.7.

Figure 18.7 shows that as α decreases, β increases. Inevitably, as we decrease Type I error rate, we increase the probability of Type II error. This is the reason why we don't normally set α at lower than $p = 0.01$. Although a significance level such as say $\alpha = 0.001$ would reduce 'false alarms' it would also increase the probability of a 'miss'.

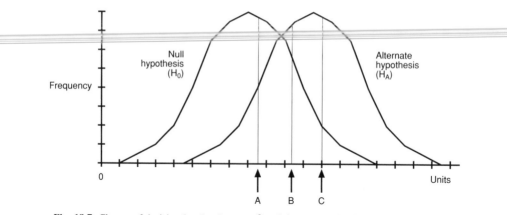

Fig. 18.7 Change of decision level to increase β and decrease α. As the decision criterion is moved from A to B to C, the relative frequency of Type I and Type II errors alters

SUMMARY

It was argued in this chapter that once the data have been collected and summarized, the investigator must analyse the evidence to demonstrate its statistical significance. Significant results for an investigation mean that differences or changes demonstrated were 'real', rather than just the outcome of random sampling error.

The general steps in using tests of significance were explained, and several illustrative examples using the z and t tests for single sample designs were presented. A critical value is set for the statistic (in this case z_{crit}, t_{crit}) as specified by α. If the magnitude of the obtained value of the statistic (z_{obt}, t_{obt}) exceeds the critical value, H_0 is rejected. In this case, the investigator concludes that the data supported the differences predicted by the alternative hypothesis (at the level of significance specified by α). However, if the obtained value of the statistic is calculated to be less than the critical value, then the investigator must conclude that the data did not support the hypothesis. It was noted that following these steps doesn't guarantee the absolute truth of decisions made about the rejection or acceptance of the alternative hypotheses, but rather specifies the probability of the decisions being correct.

Two types of erroneous decisions were specified, Type I and Type II errors. Type I error involves falsely concluding that differences or changes found in a study were real, that is concluding that the data supported a hypothesis (which is, in fact, false). Type II error involves falsely concluding that no differences or changes exist, that is concluding that the data did not support a hypothesis (which is, in fact, true). It was demonstrated that the probability of these errors depended on factors such as the size of n, the directionality of H_A and the variability of the data.

The procedures of hypothesis testing and error were related to the logic of clinical decision making. The probabilities (α and β) of making Type I and Type II errors are interrelated. In this way, both researchers and clinicians must take into account the implications of possible error when setting levels of significance for interpreting the data.

SELF ASSESSMENT

Explain the meaning of the following terms:

alternative hypothesis
critical value of a statistic
decision rule
directional or non-directional alternative hypothesis
null hypothesis
one tail or two tail test of significance
region of acceptance
region of rejection
significance (level of)
Type I and Type II error
z test or t test

True or false

1. The alternative hypothesis states that there is an effect or difference in the results.
2. If the probability of H_0 being true is greater than α, we can reject H_0.
3. Sampling distributions are used to enable the calculation of H_0 being true.
4. The critical value of a statistic is the value which cuts off the region for the rejection of H_0.
5. If the critical value of a statistic is less than the obtained or calculated value, we can reject H_0.
6. α is a probability, usually set at 0.01 or 0.05.
7. The t test requires that the sampling distribution of t should be normally distributed.
8. Hypothesis testing involves choosing between two mutually exclusive hypotheses, H_0 and H_A.
9. If α is set at 0.01 instead of 0.05, then the probability of making a Type I error decreases.
10. If we retain H_0, then we must conclude that the investigation did not produce significant results.
11. If n is greater than 30, the t test is more appropriate than the z test.
12. If results are statistically significant, the independent variable must have had a very large effect.
13. A directional H_A should be used when there is theoretical justification for the existence of a directional effect in the data.
14. When the results are statistically significant, they are unlikely to reflect sampling error.
15. It is impossible to prove the truth of H_A when using sample data as opposed to population data.
16. If we reject H_0 then we are in a position to accept H_A.
17. If alpha decreases (is made more stringent) then beta increases.

18. If H_0 is true and we reject it, we have made a Type I error.
19. If H_0 is false and we reject it, we have made a Type II error.
20. If H_0 is false, and we fail to reject it, we have made a Type II error.

Multiple choice

1. Hypothesis testing involves:
   a deciding between two mutually exclusive hypotheses H_0 and H_A
   b deciding if the investigation was internally and externally valid
   c deciding if the differences between groups was large or small
   d none of the above.

2. An alpha level of 0.01 indicates that:
   a the probability of falsely rejecting H_0 is limited to 0.05
   b the probability of Type II error is 0.01
   c the probability of a correct decision is 0.01
   d none of the above.

3. If alpha is changed from 0.01 to 0.001:
   a the probability of making a Type II error decreases
   b the probability of a Type I error increases
   c the error probabilities stay the same
   d the probability of Type I error decreases.

4. If we reject the null hypothesis, we might be making:
   a a Type II error
   b a Type I error
   c a correct decision
   d a or c
   e b or c.

5. Statistical tests are used:
   a only when the investigation involves a true experimental design
   b to increase the internal validity of experiments
   c to establish the probability of the outcome of an investigation being due to chance alone
   d a and b.

6. The outcome of a statistical analysis is found to be $p = 0.02$. This means that:
   a the alternative hypothesis was directional
   b we can reject H_0 at $\alpha = 0.05$
   c we must conclude that H_A must be true
   d a and c.

7. When the results of an experiment are non-significant, the proper conclusion is:
   a the experiment fails to show a real effect for the independent variable
   b chance alone is at work
   c accept H_0
   d accept H_A.

8. It is important to know the possible errors (Type I or Type II) we might make when rejecting or failing to reject H_0:
   a to minimize these errors when designing the experiment
   b to be aware of the fallacy of accepting H_0
   c to maximize the probability of making a correct decision by proper design
   d all of the above.

9. An α level of 0.05 indicates that:
   a if H_0 is true, the probability of falsely rejecting it is limited to 0.05
   b 95% of the time, chance is operating
   c the probability of a Type II error is 0.05
   d the probability of a correct decision is 0.05.

10. A directional alternative hypothesis asserts that:
    a the independent variable has no effect on the dependent variable
    b a random effect is responsible for the differences between conditions
    c the independent variable does not have an effect
    d there are differences in the data in a given direction.

11. If alpha is changed from 0.05 to 0.01:
    a the probability of a Type II error decreases
    b the probability of a Type I error increases
    c the error probabilities stay the same
    d the probability of Type II error increases.

12. If the null hypothesis is retained, you may be making:
    a a correct decision about the data
    b a Type I error
    c a Type II error
    d a or c
    e a or b.

13. When the results are statistically significant, this means:
    a the obtained probability is equal to or less than α.
    b the independent variable has had a large effect
    c we can reject H_0
    d all of the above
    e a and c.

14. 'Beta' refers to:

    a ~~the probability of making a Type I error~~

    b the probability of the $(1 - \alpha)$

    c the inverse of the probability of sampling error

    d the probability of making a Type II error.

15. Setting $\alpha = 0.0001$ would reduce the probability of Type I error. However, it would:

    a increase Type II error probability

    b increase the standard error of variance

    c reduce external validity

    d all of the above.

16. We retain H_0 if:

    a $|t_{obt}| \leq |t_{crit}|$

    b $|t_{obt}| > |t_{crit}|$

    c $|t_{obt}| < |t_{crit}|$

    d none of the above.

17. If α is changed from 0.01 to 0.001:

    a the probability of a Type II error decreases

    b the probability of a Type I error increases

    c the error probabilities stay the same

    d none of the above.

The researcher believes that the average age of unemployed persons has changed. To test this hypothesis, the ages of 150 randomly selected unemployed are determined. This mean age is 23.5 years. A complete census taken a few years before showed a mean age of 22.4 years, with a standard deviation of 7.6.

Questions 18–22 refer to this data.

18. The alternative hypothesis should be:

    a $\bar{X}_A = \bar{X}_B$

    b $\mu_A = \mu_B$

    c $\mu_A \neq \mu_B$

    d $\bar{X}_A \neq \bar{X}_B$

19. z_{crit} where $\alpha = 0.01$ is:

    a +2.58

    b +1.64

    c +2.33

    d −1.64

20. The obtained value of the appropriate statistic for testing H_0 is:

    a 2.88

    b 2.35

    c 1.84

    d 1.77

21. What do you decide, using $\alpha = 0.01$?

    a retain H_0
    b reject H_0
    c it is not possible to decide
    d *a* and *b*.

22. Therefore, the researcher should conclude that:

    a unemployed persons are getting older on the average
    b there is no evidence supporting the hypothesis that the average age of unemployed people has changed
    c too many young people are unemployed
    d *b* and *c*.

23. When the results are not statistically significant, this means that:

    a the experimental hypothesis was not supported by the data at a given level of probability
    b the null hypothesis was retained at a given level of probability
    c the alternative hypothesis must have been directional
    d the investigation was internally valid
    e *a* and *b*.

24. If $\alpha = 0.05$ and the probability of the statistic calculated from the data is $p = 0.02$, then:

    a we should retain H_0
    b we should reject H_A
    c we should reject H_0 at $\alpha = 0.05$
    d we should restate H_0 so that the findings will become significant at the 0.05 level.

19

Selection and use
of statistical tests

INTRODUCTION

In the previous chapter, we examined the logic of hypothesis testing and the use of z and t tests for testing hypotheses about single sample means. There are, in fact, numerous statistical tests which are used in a conceptually similar fashion in order to analyse the statistical significance of the data. That is, all statistical tests involve setting up the relevant hypotheses H_0, H_A, and then, on the basis of the appropriate inferential statistics, computing the probability of the obtained sample statistics occurring by chance alone. This probability is used to determine whether the experimental hypothesis has been supported by the data. We are not going to examine all of the various available statistical tests. These are available in various statistics text books. Rather, we will examine the criteria used for selecting tests appropriate for the analysis of the data obtained in specific investigations. To illustrate the use of statistical tests we will examine the use of the chi-square test (χ^2). This is a statistical test commonly employed to analyse nominally scaled data.

The aims of this chapter are to:

1. Discuss the criteria by which a statistical test is selected for analysing the data for a specific study
2. Use chi-square to illustrate the use of statistical tests.

THE RELATIONSHIP BETWEEN DESCRIPTIVE
AND INFERENTIAL STATISTICS

As we have seen, statistics may be divided into two classes: descriptive and inferential. Descriptive statistics are concerned with issues such as 'What is the average length of hospitalization of a group of patients?' Inferential statistics are used to address issues such as whether the differences in average lengths of hospitalization of patients in two groups are statistically significantly different. Thus descriptive statistics describe aspects of the data such as frequencies, the most common, the average, or the range of values for groups of cases; whereas when using inferential statistics, one attempts to infer whether differences between groups, or relationships between variables, represent persistent and reproducible trends.

In Section Five we saw that the selection of appropriate descriptive statistics depends on the nature of the data being described. For example, in a variable such as incomes of patients, the best statistics to represent the typical income would be the mean and/or the median. If you had a millionaire in the group of patients, the mean would give a distorted impression of the central tendency. In this situation the median would be most appropriate. The mode is most commonly used when the data being described are categorical. For example, if in a questionnaire respondents were asked to indicate their sex and 65 said they were male and 32 selected the female category, 'male' is the modal response. It is quite unusual to use the mode only with data that are not nominal. Therefore, the scale of measurement used to obtain the data and its distribution determine which descriptive statistics are selected.

In the same way, the appropriate inferential statistics are determined by the nature of the data being analysed. For instance, where the mean is the appropriate descriptive statistic, the inferential statistics will determine if the differences between the means are statistically significant. In the case of ordinal data, the appropriate inferential statistics will make it possible to decide if either medians or rank orders are significantly different. With nominal data, the appropriate inferential statistic will decide if proportions of cases falling into specific categories are significantly different.

Thus, when the data have been adequately described, the appropriate inferential statistic will be closely related. However, in selecting an appropriate statistical test, the design of the investigation must also be taken into account.

SELECTION OF THE APPROPRIATE INFERENTIAL STATISTICAL TEST

Before addressing the issue of the selection of the appropriate inferential statistical test, it is useful to reiterate the reason why a statistical test should be employed.

In many studies, inferential statistical tests are not required. For example, if a health care needs-assessment survey is conducted in a particular community, using a full population, the investigator might not be overly concerned with generalizing the results to other communities, or demonstrating that certain relationships between variables are reliable. It may be enough to be able to say, for example, that '35% of the respondents indicated that they were dissatisfied with the existing level of medical services.' In this instance, descriptive statistics are all that the investigator requires.

If, however, the investigator wishes to argue that certain differences between groups or that certain correlations between variables for a sample are generalizable to the population, then inferential statistical tests are necessary.

The inferential statistic provides the investigator with a means of determining how reproducible the obtained results are, by enabling access to a probability.

The probability associated with the value of an inferential statistic informs the investigator of the likelihood that the obtained results were due to chance factors, or if they are significant at a given level of probability.

Please note that we are not going to examine all of the numerous statistical tests available for decision making. Rather, the aim of this chapter is to examine the criteria investigators use for selecting tests appropriate for the analysis of data obtained in investigations. To illustrate the use of statistical tests we will look at the χ^2 (chi-square) test, commonly employed for analysing nominal data. We examine the interpretation of findings which do not reach statistical significance, and the relationship between statistical and clinical significance. In Chapter 20 we will consider some of the personal and social values implicit in making decisions concerning the actual adoption and use of treatments and diagnostic tests in clinical settings.

There is a variety of statistical tests some of which are named in Table 19.1. The selection of the appropriate statistical test is determined by the following considerations:

1. The scale of measurement used to obtain the data (nominal, ordinal, interval, or ratio).
2. The number of groups used in an investigation (one or more).
3. Whether the measurements were obtained from independent subjects or from related samples, such as those involving repeated measurements of the same subjects.
4. The assumptions involved in using a statistical test, such as the distribution of the scores or the minimum required sample size.

Table 19.1 Selection of tests of significance

| | Two groups | | Three or more groups | |
Scale	Independent	Dependent	Independent	Dependent
Nominal	Chi-square (χ^2) test	McNemar test	Chi-square (χ^2) test	Cochran's Q test
Ordinal	Mann-Whitney U test	Sign test	Kruskal-Wallis H test	Friedman two way analysis of variance
Interval or ratio	t test (independent groups)	t test (dependent groups)	ANOVA (F) (independent groups)	ANOVA (F) (dependent groups)

Table 19.1 offers a sample of statistical tests in order to illustrate how statistical tests are selected for analysing data. Several points are worth noting.

1. It can be seen that tests are selected on the basis of the criteria outlined above. When we have determined these four criteria for a given investigation, the cell containing the appropriate test can be readily selected. We might need additional criteria for deciding between two tests within a cell. For instance, we saw in the previous section that if n < 30, we use the t test rather than z test.

2. The tests appropriate for analysing ordinal and nominal data are called **non-parametric** or **distribution free.** The tests for analysing interval or ratio data are called **parametric** tests. The parametric tests (for example, z, t, or F) require that certain assumptions (such as normality or equal variance) be valid concerning the populations from which the samples were drawn. The non-parametric tests (e.g. χ^2, Mann-Whitney U) require few, if any, assumptions about the underlying population distributions.
3. Even before the data are collected, an investigator should have a good idea which statistical test is appropriate for analysing the data. Sometimes, however, the distribution of the data is such that the test which was initially selected is found to be inappropriate.

Let us have a look at some examples to illustrate how statistical tests are selected.

An investigator wishes to evaluate the effectiveness of a new treatment in contrast to a conventionally used treatment. Say that the outcome (dependent variable) is measured on a five point ordinal scale. Each subject is assigned to one of the two treatment groups. Which test would the investigator use to analyse the data?

1. The measurement was ordinal.
2. There were two groups (new treatment, conventional treatment).
3. Subjects were independently assigned to a specific group.

By inspection of Table 19.1 the investigator would select the Mann-Whitney U test to analyse the significance of the data.

If we change the above example by stating that the dependent variable was measured on an interval scale, the appropriate test would now be a t test (for independent groups).

Let us say that three groups were used (by the inclusion of a placebo group) by the investigator. Now, if the outcome measurement remained ordinal, the appropriate test for analysing the data is the Kruskal-Wallis H test. If, however, the outcome measures were interval, it follows from Table 19.1 that the appropriate test for analysing the results would be ANOVA (Analysis of Variance).

Finally, say that in the original example *each* of the subjects was treated with both the new and old treatments. Now, the data would have been obtained from the repeated measurement of the same subjects, and the appropriate statistical test would be the Sign test (ordinal, two groups, dependent).

Table 19.1 does not include all the available statistical tests and their uses. In fact, mathematical statisticians can generate inferential tests appropriate for a whole variety of designs. The basic idea is to use probability theory to generate appropriate sampling distributions in terms of which the probability of H_0 being true can be calculated, and the *statistical significance* of the findings evaluated.

Rather than examining all the tests and their underlying assumptions, we will look at the use of the χ^2 test in some detail. As well as being a very useful test for analysing nominal data, it will (along with the z and t) illustrate how statistical tests are carried out to test hypotheses.

THE χ^2 (CHI-SQUARE) TEST

As shown in Table 19.1, χ^2 is appropriate for statistical analysis when:

1. Variables were measured on a nominal scale.
2. Measurements were of independent subjects.

The χ^2 test is appropriate for deciding if proportions of cases falling into categories are different at a given level of significance.

The statistic, χ^2, is given by the formula:

$$X^2 = \sum \frac{\left(f_o - f_e\right)^2}{f_e}$$

f_o = observed frequency for a given category

f_e = expected frequency for a given category

The sampling distribution for χ^2 is a family of curves, which, like t, vary with degrees of freedom. The use of this inferential statistic is best illustrated by an example.

Suppose that an investigator is interested in finding out whether there is a difference in the relative frequency of different kinds of treatments currently offered to extremely depressed patients. A random sample of 150 patients is selected from a population of patients in Australia, and the type of treatment offered to them is determined from their medical records, as shown below.

Psychotherapy	Drugs	Electroconvulsive therapy
$n = 45$	$n = 40$	$n = 65$

The entries in each cell represent the frequency with which patients were given the various treatments. Thus, 45 patients were offered psychotherapy, 40 drugs and 65 electroconvulsive therapy. Chi-square is the appropriate test for analysing these data. Let us follow the steps involved in hypothesis testing, as outlined in Chapter 18.

1. H_A: there is a difference in the population proportions for the three treatments. H_A is non-directional when we use χ^2.
2. H_0: there is no difference in the population proportions of the three treatments. The frequencies shown in each cell in the table occurred through random sampling from a population where there is an equal frequency of the three treatments.
3. Decision level, α: Say the investigator sets a significance level of 0.05 for rejecting H_A. $\alpha = 0.05$

4. Calculation of the statistic: χ^2_{obt} is the value of χ^2 calculated from the obtained data.

To calculate χ^2_{obt}, we must determine f_e for each cell (f_o is, of course, determined by the data). If the null hypothesis is true, then our expectation is that the frequencies in each cell should be the same. In this case, $n = 150$, so that f_e should be $150/3 = 50$, given that there are three cells. Let us show this in tabular form (f_e shown in parentheses):

Psychotherapy	Drugs	Electroconvulsive therapy
45	40	65
(50)	(50)	(50)

We can now calculate χ^2_{obt}, by calculating $(f_o - f_e)^2/f_e$ for each cell, and then summing the values.

$$X^2_{obt} = \sum \frac{(f_o - f_e)^2}{f_e}$$

$$= \frac{(45-50)^2}{50} + \frac{(45-50)^2}{50} + \frac{(65-50)^2}{50}$$

$$= 0.5 + 2.0 + 4.5$$

$$= 7.0$$

The greater the discrepancy between f_e and f_o, the greater the calculated value of the chi-square statistic (χ^2_{obt}). The direction of the difference is of no account as the difference between fe and f_o is squared.

5. Making decisions concerning H_0: The decision rule for χ^2 is similar to that of the z and t test, as shown in the previous section:

$$\chi^2_{obt} \geq \chi^2_{crit}, \text{ reject } H_0$$

$$\chi^2_{obt} < \chi^2_{crit}, \text{ retain } H_0$$

Here, χ^2_{crit} is the critical value of the statistic χ^2, which cuts off a proportion of the sampling distribution equal to α. The value of χ^2_{crit} is obtained from the tables in Appendix C. To look up this statistic, we need to know:

(a) α, which was set at 0.05 for this example
(b) the degrees of freedom, df.

Note that with χ^2 the degrees of freedom with one variable is $k - 1$, where k stands for the number of categories or groups. In this instance, we have

$k = 3$ (three treatments) so that $df = 3 - 1 = 2$. Now we can look up the tables in Appendix C. In this case, $\alpha = 0.05$ and $df = 2$, therefore:

$$\chi^2_{crit} = 5.99$$

Here, since $\chi^2_{obt} > \chi^2_{crit}$ we can reject H_0 at a 0.05 level of significance. The investigator is in a position to accept H_A (that the three treatments are offered at *different* frequencies to depressed patients). Clearly, electro-convulsive therapy is given most frequently for the condition (in this hypothetical example).

χ^2 AND CONTINGENCY TABLES

In the previous example, we discussed the use of χ^2 where we had clear expectations concerning the expected frequencies (f_e), and were dealing with only one variable. The χ^2 test is also relevant for analysing nominal data where f_e is not known, and where we are interested in the effects of more than one variable. Thus, χ^2 is a statistical test appropriate for deciding whether two variables are significantly related.

For example an investigator wishes to compare the effectiveness of drug therapy with coronary artery surgery in males 55–60 years old, suffering from coronary heart disease. A sample of 40 patients consenting to the investigation is selected from this population, and randomly divided into the two treatment groups (drugs only or coronary artery surgery). The treatment outcome is measured in terms of survival over five years. The outcome of this hypothetical study is shown in Table 19.2.

Table 19.2 Contingency table showing obtained frequencies for a hypothetical study comparing survival after treatments

	Drugs	**Surgery**	**Row marginal**
Dead	11	8	19
Alive	9	12	21
Column marginal	20	20	$n = 40$

Table 19.2 is called a contingency table. A **contingency table** is a two-way table showing the relationship between two or more variables. Note that the variables have been classified into mutually exclusive categories ('drug or surgery' for the independent variable, and 'dead or alive' for the dependent variable, in this instance). The cells in the contingency table show the frequency of cases falling into each joint category (for example, 11 people who had 'drugs only' died during the 5 years). The row and column marginal scores are the sums of the frequencies. The row and column marginals necessarily add up to n, the sample size ($n = 40$ for this example).

The above table is called a two-by-two (2×2) contingency table. Depending on the number of categories (or levels) in each of the two variables, we might have 3×2 tables, 3×3 tables, or whatever. Let us now turn to analysing the data.

1. H_A: there is a difference in the proportion of patients surviving for 5 years following the two types of treatment

2. H_0: there is no difference in the frequency of survival rates; any difference between observed and expected frequencies is due to chance

3. Decision level: $\alpha = 0.05$

4. Calculation of the statistic χ^2_{obt}

$$\chi^2_{obt} = \Sigma \frac{\left(f_o - f_e\right)^2}{f_e}$$

To make our explanation of the calculation easier, let us label the cells and the marginal values, as shown in Table 19.3.

Table 19.3 General format for 2 × 2 contingency table

A	B	j
C	D	k
l	m	n

We calculate χ^2_{obt} by calculating f_e for each of the cells and then substituting this value into the equation for χ^2_{obt}.

In order to calculate the expected frequencies, f_e for each of the cells, we use the formula:

$$\frac{\text{row total} \times \text{column total}}{n}$$

Substituting into the above formula for each of the cells:

$$f_{eA} = \frac{j \times l}{n} \quad f_{eB} = \frac{j \times m}{n} \quad f_{eC} = \frac{k \times l}{n} \quad f_{eD} = \frac{k \times m}{n}$$

Now f_o are the observed frequencies as in the data, summarized in the contingency table above. Substituting the values for f_e and f_o for each cell is shown below.

	f_o	f_e	$(f_o - f_e)^2$	$(f_o - f_e)^2/f_e$
A	11	9.5	2.25	0.236
B	8	9.5	2.25	0.236
C	9	10.5	2.25	0.214
D	12	10.5	2.25	0.214
n	40			$\chi^2 = 0.90$

5. Making decisions concerning H_0: the degrees of freedom for a contingency table are calculated by the following formula:

$$df = (r - 1)(c - 1)$$

where r stands for the number of rows
and c stands for the number of columns.
In this instance, given a 2×2 contingency table

$$df = (2 - 1) \, (2 - 1) = 1$$

Now we can look up χ^2_{crit}, for $\alpha = 0.05$ and $df = 1$. From tables in
Appendix C,

$$\chi^2_{crit} = 3.84$$

Therefore, as $\chi^2_{obt} < \chi^2_{crit}$ we must retain H_0: there is no difference in the
frequencies of survival over five years following the two kinds of
treatments. Our data shows that either there is no difference in the
outcomes of the two treatments or we made a Type II error.

The χ^2 test can be used to analyze the statistical significance of nominal data
arising from experimental or non-experimental investigations. This non-
parametric test can be used provided two simple assumptions are met:

1. Each subject has provided only one entry into the χ^2 table; that is, each of
   the entries are independent.
2. The expected frequency (f_e) in each cell is at least five. Therefore, if the
   sample size is too small, χ^2 may not be used.

If either of these assumptions is violated, the use of χ^2 is inappropriate for
statistical decision making.

SUMMARY

There is a variety of statistical tests available for analysing the significance of
the obtained data. The statistical test appropriate for analysing a given set of data
is selected on the basis of (1) the scaling of the data, (2) the dependence/
independence of the measurements, (3) the number of groups being studied, as
well as (4) specific requirements for using a statistical test. Generally, parametric
and non-parametric statistical tests were distinguished on the grounds of the
scaling of the data and the assumptions underlying the sampling distributions.

None of the individual statistical tests was discussed in detail, except the χ^2
test which was presented as an example. Together with the discussion on the z
and t tests in Chapter 18, the χ^2 test illustrates the principle that theoretical
sampling distributions can be generated, and the probability of obtaining specific
obtained outcomes can be calculated. If the obtained value of the inferential
statistic is greater than or equal to the critical value, the null hypothesis can be
rejected at the level of significance specified by the Type 1 error rate (α). This
is the case regardless of which particular statistical test is being used.

The retention of H_0 might reflect a correct decision, or a Type II error. Sample
size is a factor which contributes to Type II error rate, as shown in both
Chapters 18 and 20.

SELF ASSESSMENT

Explain the meanings of the following terms:

chi-square	non-parametric test
contingency table	observed frequency
expected frequency	parametric test

True or false

1. Inferential statistics are used to decide if differences obtained in sample data are persistent, 'real' trends.
2. The selection of descriptive and inferential statistics is independent of the scaling of the data.
3. Inferential statistics must be used, regardless of the nature and aims of an investigation.
4. Parametric tests are used to analyse the significance of interval or ratio data.
5. The use of non-parametric tests depends on the normal distribution of the underlying population.
6. Each statistical test entails the use of sampling distributions for calculating the probability of the obtained sample outcomes.
7. It is impossible to select an appropriate statistical test before the data is collected.
8. The number of groups being compared in an investigation influences the selection of the appropriate statistical test.
9. A basic assumption for using t is that the samples were drawn from a normally distributed population. A basic assumption of χ^2 is that the scores in each cell are independent.
10. When using χ^2, the closer the observed frequency for each cell is to the expected frequency, the higher the probability of rejecting H_0.
11. In order to reject the null hypothesis, $\chi^2_{obt} > \chi^2_{crit}$.
12. The χ^2 sampling distribution is a family of curves, the distribution of which varies with the degrees of freedom.
13. The χ^2 test is appropriate for testing hypotheses about proportions.
14. Each entry in a χ^2 table is a frequency.
15. The value of f_e is looked up in the appropriate χ^2 table.
16. If the f_e and f_o values are the same for each cell, χ^2_{obt} will not be statistically significant.
17. The decision level, α is generally set at 0.05 or 0.01 with χ^2.
18. If we use sample data to calculate the values of f_e, then we use contingency tables for calculating χ^2_{obt}.
19. A 2×2 contingency table shows the relationship between two variables.
20. 'rc' stands for the degrees of freedom for a 2×2 contingency table.

Multiple choice

1. In a study, three independent samples are compared and the dependent variable is measured on a ratio scale. A statistical test appropriate for analysing these findings is:
   a χ^2
   b Mann-Whitney U
   c t
   d ANOVA (analysis of variance).

2. In a study two independent samples are compared and the dependent variable is measured on an ordinal scale. A statistical test appropriate for analysing these findings is:
   a χ^2
   b Mann-Whitney U
   c t
   d Wilcoxon.

3. Which of the following is a 'non-parametric' test?
   a ANOVA (analysis of variance)
   b t
   c z
   d Kruskal-Wallis H

4. Which of the following is a 'parametric test'?
   a Median test
   b McNemar's test
   c z
   d Cochran's Q

5. Which of the following tests is appropriate for analysing data where 3 or more groups were used?
   a z
   b t
   c χ^2
   d sign test

6. The larger the discrepancy between f_o and f_e for each cell in a contingency table:
   a the more likely it is that the results will not be significant
   b the more likely it is that H_0 will be rejected
   c the more likely it is that the population proportions are the same
   d the more likely it is that the population proportions are different
   e a and c
   f b and d.

7. For any given level of significance, $\chi^2_{crit:}$
   a increases with increases in sample size
   b decreases with increases in degrees of freedom
   c increases with increases in degrees of freedom
   d decreases with increases in sample size.

8. A contingency table:
   a always involves two degrees of freedom
   b always involves two dependent frequencies
   c always involves two variables
   d all of the above
   e a and b.

9. Entries into the cells of a contingency table should be:
   a frequencies
   b means
   c percentages
   d degrees of freedom.

10. The degrees of freedom for a contingency table:
    a equal $n - 1$
    b equal rc $- 1$
    c cannot be determined if r = c
    d equal $(r - 1)(c - 1)$.

11. Chi-square should not be used with a 2×2 contingency table if:
    a $df > 1$
    b f_e is below 5 in any cell
    c f_o is below 5 in any cell
    d $f_e = f_o$
    e b and c.

An investigator is interested in determining whether there is a relationship between gender and susceptibility to a substance known to trigger an allergic response. 'Susceptibility' is measured as 'yes' or 'no'.

Questions 12–15 refer to this example. The raw data are presented in the contingency table below.

	Not susceptible	Susceptible	
Female	90	110	200
Male	60	140	200
	150	250	400

12. The value of χ^2_{obt} is:
    a 2.50
    b 8.09
    c 9.60
    d 11.05

13. The value of *df* is:
    a 2
    b 1
    c 3
    d need more information.

14. Using $\alpha = 0.05$, χ^2_{crit} is:
    a 3.841
    b 5.412
    c 2.706
    d −3.841

15. Using $\alpha = 0.05$, what is your conclusion?
    a Accept H_0: there is no relationship between gender and susceptibility
    b Reject H_0: there is a significant relationship between gender and susceptibility
    c Fail to reject H_0: the study does not show a significant relationship between gender and susceptibility
    d Fail to reject H_0: this study shows a significant relationship between gender and susceptibility.

16. In selecting an appropriate statistical test:
    a *z* should be used as it is most powerful
    b *t* should be used as it takes the sample size into account
    c the choice depends on the design of the study
    d χ^2 should be avoided.

17. The χ^2 test requires that:
    a data be measured on a nominal scale
    b data conform to a normal distribution
    c expected frequencies are equal in all cells
    d all of the above occur.

The following information should be used in answering questions 18–25:

Aerobics classes are conducted by the student union of a tertiary institution. Although there are equal numbers of male and female students enrolled at the institution, it is observed that far more female than male students attend. A test is performed to see whether the proportions of the two sexes at the class is representative of the proportions of the two sexes enrolled at the institution as a whole. Of the 50 students who attend the classes, 10 are male. A χ^2 is conducted on these data.

18. What type of χ^2 will be conducted?
    a one-way
    b two-way
    c contingency analysis
    d a parametric chi-square.

19. How many cells will there be in the χ^2 table?
    a 1
    b 2
    c 3
    d 4

20. What is the expected frequency of male students at the aerobic classes?
    a 10
    b 40
    c 25
    d 8

21. What is the obtained value of χ^2?
    a 4.5
    b 2.5
    c 18.0
    d 9.0

22. What are the degrees of freedom?
    a 1
    b 2
    c 49
    d 48

23. If α is set at 0.01, what is the critical value of χ^2?
    a 0.0201
    b 4.605
    c 9.210
    d 6.635

24. What statistical decision should be made on the basis of these data?
    a Reject null hypothesis
    b Retain null hypothesis
    c Increase α
    d Increase size of sample.

25. What conclusion can be drawn on the basis of these data?
    a Overall, the tendency for more females than males to attend the classes is not statistically significant.
    b There is a statistically significant tendency for more females than males to attend the classes ($\alpha = 0.01$)
    c The aerobics classes should have their format changed to attract more male students.
    d There is a statistically significant trend ($\alpha = 0.01$) for differential attendance by the two sexes, but it is impossible to state the direction of this trend.

The following information should be used in answering questions 26–31:

In a test of the effectiveness of phenothiazine in treating schizophrenia, 60 patients are randomly assigned to receive either the drug or a placebo. After two weeks of daily treatment, each patient is assessed by the chief psychiatrist as 'improved' or 'not improved'. A 2 × 2 table is constructed to indicate improved number of patients falling into each category:

	Treatment	
Assessment	Phenothiazine	Placebo
Improved	20	10
Not improved	10	20

26. The degrees of freedom in this table are:
    a 1
    b 2
    c 3
    d 4

27. The obtained χ^2 is:
    a 1.33
    b 13.5
    c 8.71
    d 6.67

28. With α set at 0.05, the critical value of χ^2 is:
    a 3.841
    b 5.991
    c 6.635
    d 0.013

29. The correct statistical decision in this case is to:
    a reject H_0
    b retain H_0
    c decrease α
    d decrease α.

30. The appropriate conclusion to be drawn from these data is:
    a Patients receiving the active drug are not significantly more likely to get an 'improved' rating than those receiving the placebo.
    b Those receiving the active drug are significantly more likely to be rated as 'improved' ($\alpha= 0.05$).
    c The drug cures schizophrenia.
    d The improvements cannot be due to the drug, as some people received the drug and didn't improve.

31. Following the publication of this study, it is revealed that the psychiatrist who did the ratings of improvement was also the person who had assigned the patients to phenothiazine or placebo groups. What type of problem could have invalidated these findings?

    a   Rosenthal effects
    b   Placebo effects
    c   Instrumentation effects
    d   All of the above.

20

The interpretation of statistical tests

INTRODUCTION

At the outset, it is important to recognize the distinction between establishing the statistical significance of an outcome in a study, and the process of interpreting the importance and implications of the results.

As we have discussed earlier, in the process of data analysis, the investigator assembles the data, chooses an appropriate statistic, calculates the value of the statistic and then consults a table relating the values of the statistics to probabilities to find whether the results are *statistically significant*. Statistical significance is agreed to be reached when the probability value is lower than a predefined value (1 in 20 or 0.05 is a popular value). Unfortunately many researchers stop at this point, believing that if they have established statistical significance, no further analysis or interpretation is required. Nothing could be further from the truth.

It is necessary to consider, in addition to statistical significance of the results, a set of further issues, including:

1. Effect size, that is, how large are the relationships or differences observed in the data
2. The social and clinical significance of factors such as cost effectiveness and quality of life issues.

EFFECT SIZE

The effect size in a study refers to the actual size of the differences observed between groups or the strength of relationships between variables, as opposed to the statistical significance of these effects.

It is important to recognize that although statistical significance may be reached, the effect size in a study may not be clinically significant, or may be of such minimal size as to be theoretically uninteresting. Many students new to the research process believe that the reaching of statistical significance implies that the results in question necessarily illustrate important or 'significant' trends. This is not the case.

This situation can be illustrated by results from two student research projects supervised by the authors.

Study 1—Test–retest reliability of a force measurement machine

In the first study, the student was concerned with demonstrating the test–retest reliability of a device designed to measure maximum voluntary forces being produced by patients' leg muscles under two conditions (flexion and extension).

Twenty-one patients took part and the reliability of the measurement process was tested by calculating the Pearson correlation between the readings obtained from the machine in question during two trials separated by an hour for each patient. The results were:

Pearson correlations between trials 1 and 2

Flexion	Extension
0.56	0.54

Both results reach the 0.01 level of significance

The student was ecstatic when the computer data analysis program informed her that the correlations were statistically significant at the 0.01 level (indicating that there was less than a 1 in 100 chance that the correlations were illusory or actually zero.) We were somewhat less ecstatic because, in fact, the results indicated that approximately 69% ($1-0.56^2$) and 71% ($1-0.54^2$) of the variation was not shared between the measurements of the first and second trial. In other words, the measures were all over the place, despite statistical significance being reached. Thus, far from being an endorsement of the measurement process, these results were somewhat of a condemnation. This is a classic example of the need for careful interpretation of effect size in conjunction with statistical significance.

Study 2—A comparative study of improvement in two treatment groups

The second project was a comparative study of two groups; one group suffering from suspected repetition strain injuries (RSI) induced by computer keyboard input and a group of 'normals'. An Activities of Daily Living (ADLs) assessment scale was used and yielded a 'disability' index of between 0 and 50. There were 60 people in each group. The results were:

Mean ADL disability scores

	RSI group	Normals
Mean	33.2	30.4
Standard deviation	1.6	1.2

The appropriate statistic for analysing these data happens to be the independent groups t test, although this is not important to the understanding of this example. The t value for these data was significant at the 0.05 level. However, if one inspects the means, the differences are slight, notwithstanding the statistical significance of the results. This example, further illustrates the problems of interpretation that may arise from focusing on the level of statistical significance and not on the effect sizes shown by the data.

When we say that the findings are **clinically significant** we mean that the effect is sufficiently large to influence clinical practices.

HOW TO INTERPRET NULL RESULTS

Often, the researcher will analyse data that show no relationships or effects according to the chosen statistical test and criteria. In other words, the researcher cannot reject the null hypothesis. There are several reasons why the researcher may obtain a null result.

1. There really isn't the trend that researcher believes exists.
2. The sample of cases and observations included in the analysis is biased.
3. There are insufficient cases in the sample to detect the trend; this is especially a problem if the trends are subtle.
4. The measurements chosen have very high or very low inherent variability.

Therefore, if the researcher obtains a null result, it is difficult, if not impossible, to determine which one or more of the above explanations is appropriate. There are, however, measures that can be taken to minimize the chance of missing real effects. In order to understand these measures, it is necessary to again invoke the table illustrating the possible outcomes of a statistical decision (Table 20.1 similar to Table 18.1).

There are four possible outcomes. On the basis of the statistical evidence you may (a) correctly conclude there is an effect when there is indeed an effect; (b) you may decide that there is an effect when there is not (false alarm); (c) you may decide statistically that there is not an effect when there really is (miss); or (d) correctly decide there is not an effect when indeed there is not. The probability that researchers consult in their statistical tables is in fact the probability of a false alarm. Thus, if I decide that any time my obtained statistical probability value is below 0.05 I will assume that there is an effect, only one time out of twenty will I be wrong in the sense of making a false alarm error. How many times, however, will I miss an effect? The probability of making this type of error is affected by the size of the effect and number of cases, amongst other things. In other words, if you have large effects and large samples the number of misses will be small. If the effect is small, larger samples are needed to detect it.

Table 20.1 Statistical decision outcomes

Reality	Decision: Effect	Decision: No effect
Effect	Correct	'Miss' Type II error
No effect	'False alarm' Type I error	Correct

STATISTICAL POWER ANALYSIS

For any analysis, it is often useful to know how likely a miss is to occur. We can do this by calculating the **statistical power** of a design. The statistical power for a given effect size is defined as:

1 – probability of a miss (Type II error or β)

Thus, if the power of a particular analysis is 0.95, for a given effect size we will correctly detect the existence of the effect 95 times out of 100. Power is an important concept in the interpretation of null results. For example, if a researcher compared the improvements of two groups of only five patients under different treatment circumstances, the power of the analysis would almost certainly be low, say 0.1. Thus 9 times out of 10, even with an effect really present, the researcher would be unable to detect it.

It is well to be careful in the interpretation of null results where they are used to demonstrate a lack of superiority of one treatment method over another, especially when there is a low number of cases. This may be purely a function of low statistical power than lack of superiority.

Unfortunately the calculation of statistical power is a complicated business and beyond the scope of this text. There are books of tables available to look up the power of various analyses. The best defence against low power is a good sized sample.

CLINICAL DECISION MAKING

It should be noted that decision procedures confronting a clinician making a diagnosis on the basis of uncertain information is exactly analogous to the scientist's hypothesis testing procedure.

Imagine that a clinician wishes to decide whether a patient has heart disease, on the basis of the cholesterol concentration in a sample of patient's blood.

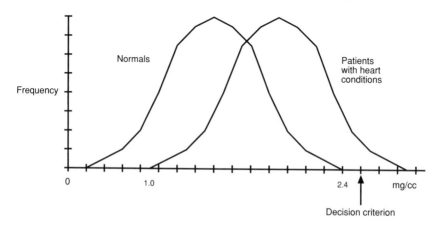

Fig. 20.1 Decision criterion: risk of Type II error (miss)

Previous research of patients with heart disease and 'normals' has shown that, indeed, heart patients tend to have a higher level of cholesterol than normals.

When the frequency distributions of cholesterol concentrations of a large group of heart patients and a group of normals are graphed, they appear as shown in Figure 20.1. You will notice that if a patient presents with a cholesterol concentration between 1.0 and 2.4 mg/cc, it is not possible to determine with complete certainty whether they are normal or have a heart disease, due to the overlap of the normal and heart disease groups in the cholesterol distribution.

Therefore, the clinician, like the scientist, has to make a decision under uncertainty: to diagnose pathology (that is, reject the null hypothesis) or normality (that is retain the null hypothesis). The clinician risks the same errors as the scientist, as shown in Table 20.2.

Table 20.2 Clinical decision outcomes

Reality	Decision: Pathology	Decision: No pathology
No pathology	'False alarm' Type 1 error	Correct decision
Pathology	Correct decision	'Miss' Type II error

The relative frequency of the type of errors made by the clinician can be altered by moving the point above which the clinician will decide that pathology is indicated (that is the decision criterion). For example, if the clinician were particularly keen not to bother his colleagues or patients with false alarms (Type I errors), he might shift the decision criterion to 2.5 mg/cc (Fig. 20.2). Any patient presenting with a cholesterol level below 2.5 mg/cc would be considered normal. In this particular case with a decision point of 2.5 mg/cc no 'false alarms' would occur. However, a huge number of people with real pathology would be 'missed' (Type II errors).

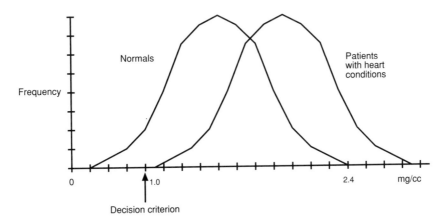

Fig. 20.2 Decision criterion: risk of Type I error (false alarm)

If the clinician values the sanctity of human life (and his bank balance after a successful malpractice suit) he will probably adjust the decision criterion to the points shown in Figure 20.1. In this case, there would be no misses but lots of false alarms.

Thus, most clinicians are rewarded for adopting a conservative decision rule, where misses are minimized, by receiving lots of false alarms. Unfortunately, this generates a lot of useless, expensive and sometimes even dangerous clinical interventions.

The scientist considers it more acceptable to make a Type II error (a miss) rather than a Type I error (a false alarm). This is even more so the case since the integrity of some medical researchers has been questioned because of 'irregularities' in their data. That is, claims of breakthroughs or novel findings have been made, but other researchers have been unable to replicate the results.

SUMMARY

In the interpretation of a statistical test, the researcher calculates the statistical value and then compares this value against the appropriate table to determine the probability level. If the probability is below a certain value (0.05 is a commonly chosen value), the researcher has established the statistical significance of the analysis in question.

The researcher must then interpret the implications of the results by determining the actual size of the effects observed. If these are small, the results may be statistically significant but clinically unimportant. Statistical significance does not imply clinical importance.

A null result (indicating no effects) must be carefully interpreted. It is possible that the researcher has missed an effect because of its small size and/or insufficient cases in the analysis. The statistical analysis measures the chance of correctly detecting a real effect of given size. Thus, a null result may be a function of low statistical power, rather than there being no real effect.

There are several criteria, beyond statistical significance, which need to be considered before making decisions concerning the clinical applications of investigations. These criteria are to a large extent influenced by values and economic limitations concerning the administration of health care in a given community.

SELF ASSESSMENT

Explain the meanings of the terms:

effect size
clinical significance
null result
power analysis
social significance
statistical significance

True or false

1. If the effect size is small, clinical significance will be large.
2. In order to establish statistical significance, clinical significance must first be established.
3. In order to establish clinical significance, statistical significance must first be established.
4. The effect size in an analysis is directly measured by the size of the p value associated with the statistic.
5. High inherent variability in measures will promote the detection of effects within data.
6. If a statistical analysis has high power, this means that β will be low.
7. A 'miss' is a correct rejection of the null hypothesis.
8. If a statistical analysis has low power, the null hypothesis will be accepted more frequently.
9. Power = $1 - \beta$ (Type II error).
10. It is more difficult to detect small effects in data where the statistical power is high.

Multiple choice

1. If $\beta = 0.80$ and $\alpha = 0.1$, the power of an analysis equals:
   a 0.9
   b 0.7
   c 0.2
   d 0.65

2. In a study there was a 1% difference in improvement of systolic blood pressure for two groups of patients receiving different treatments. This was statistically significant at $p = 0.05$. The results probably demonstrate:
   a clinical and statistical significance for the difference
   b clinical significance only
   c statistical significance only
   d neither clinical nor statistical significance.

3. A study of the relationship between family income and probability of occurrence of nutritionally related disorders demonstrated a correlation of 0.8 with $p < 0.001$. The results probably demonstrate:
   a clinical and statistical significance of the relationship.
   b clinical significance only
   c statistical significance only
   d neither clinical nor statistical significance.

4. If the effect size in a study is large, the results are likely to be:
   a clinical and statistical significance for the difference
   b clinical significance only
   c statistical significance only
   d neither clinical nor statistical significance.

5. If the power of the statistical analysis of a study is high there will be:
   a   less misses
   b   less correct rejections
   c   less correct acceptance
   d   more misses.

6. The effect of large sample sizes in a study upon statistical power is generally to:
   a   increase it
   b   decrease it
   c   not affect it.

7. In a study, the effect of larger sample sizes upon clinical significance is generally to:
   a   increase it
   b   decrease it
   c   not affect it.

8. In a study, the effect of a larger sample size upon obtained statistical significance as measured by *p* is generally to:
   a   increase it
   b   decrease it
   c   not affect it.

9. If a null result is obtained in an experimental clinical study, the clinical significance of any observed differences between treatment groups:
   a   cannot be supported
   b   can be supported if it is big
   c   can be supported if it is small
   d   should be determined by power analysis.

10. If a power analysis is not performed, is it sensible to accept a null result from a study at face value?
   a   Yes
   b   No.

DISCUSSION, QUESTIONS AND ANSWERS

Inferential statistical tests arise from the desire of the clinical researcher to generalize from the data they have collected in a sample to the population from which the sample has been drawn. 'Is what I have found in my sample a true representation of the population (and hence other samples)?' is the basic question to be answered through the use of inferential statistical tests.

Inferential statistical tests all have the same basic format. The data are processed using the appropriate calculation procedure (often with the support of a computer program) and the value of the statistic is calculated. This obtained value is then compared with a table of known values in order to interpret the outcome of the statistical test. This is very much like the application of clinical tests where, in order to interpret the value of the test result, it is compared with a known standard. As with the clinician, the clinical researcher needs to know which test to choose in which circumstance. It would not be appropriate to try and measure the weight of a patient by giving them an X-ray. Similarly, it is not appropriate to use a χ^2 test when the t test is required. It is beyond the scope of an introductory text to have an extended discussion of the various types of statistical tests and when they might be used (although it should be noted that there are many fewer statistical than clinical tests). However, it is essential that the student understands the basic use of inferential tests.

Consider the following analysis using χ^2. This statistic is designed to test the relationship between variables with nominal or categorical scales (i.e. the values are categories).

The clinical researcher is using the χ^2 test to examine the relationship between length of stay in hospital and the rate of unplanned readmissions. These data are described more fully in Section Five, Descriptive statistics. The goal is to determine whether there is a statistically significant association between the two variables. The raw data appear in Table D20.1.

As demonstrated in Section Five, we could use the Pearson correlation to analyse these data. However, to illustrate the use of χ^2 we will recode the data to categorical data and use this technique. We will recode the data using the averages for each variable to convert the data from ratio data to categorical data. For example, all those cases (hospitals) with a mean length of stay of 13.6 days or greater will considered as having an 'above average' length of stay. Those cases (hospitals) with a stay below 13.6 days will be considered as having a 'below average' length of stay. The same procedure will be followed for readmissions rates of 4.47 or greater. These are the respective means for the two variables shown in the table above. The recoded data appear as Table D20.2.

From these data we can construct a contingency table which shows the relationship between the two newly coded variables. We do this by counting the number of times the 30 cases fall into the appropriate categories.

327

Table D20.1 Average lengths of stay and readmission rates per 100 patients for patients with fractured neck of femur at 30 hospitals

Hospital	Average length of stay (days)	Unplanned readmission rates per 100 patients
1	11.100	7.800
2	11.200	6.500
3	11.200	4.300
4	11.200	5.500
5	11.700	5.100
6	12.100	5.200
7	12.100	5.000
8	12.100	4.900
9	12.300	4.800
10	12.400	3.400
11	12.400	5.000
12	12.500	4.300
13	13.100	3.900
14	13.100	3.300
15	13.200	4.700
16	13.200	4.500
17	13.200	5.500
18	13.300	4.100
19	13.700	3.200
20	13.900	3.400
21	14.100	3.500
22	14.200	3.400
23	14.200	6.000
24	14.900	4.400
25	15.300	3.300
26	15.400	4.200
27	15.400	4.300
28	15.500	4.100
29	16.300	3.200
30	22.400	3.300

As can be seen from Table D20.3, only one hospital with an above average length of stay had an above average readmission rate, while 11 hospitals with above average lengths of stay had below average readmission rates.

These data can be subjected to χ^2 analysis. If these calculations are performed, we obtain a χ^2 value of 9.98, $df = 1$, $p < .01$. In other words there is a statistically significant association between length of stay and readmission rates for the 30 hospitals. This confirms the analysis conducted in Section Five.

Questions

1. From Table D20.1, how many hospitals have a below average length of stay, if the average length of stay is 13.6 days? How many have an above average length of stay? Why is it not 15 above and below?

2. From Table D20.3, why is there one degree of freedom in this analysis?

Table D20.2 Recoded average lengths of stay and readmission rates per 100 patients for patients with fractured neck of femur at 30 hospitals

Hospital	Average length of stay (days)	Unplanned readmission rates per 100 patients
1	Below average	Above average
2	Below average	Above average
3	Below average	Below average
4	Below average	Above average
5	Below average	Above average
6	Below average	Above average
7	Below average	Above average
8	Below average	Above average
9	Below average	Above average
10	Below average	Below average
11	Below average	Above average
12	Below average	Below average
13	Below average	Below average
14	Below average	Below average
15	Below average	Above average
16	Below average	Above average
17	Below average	Above average
18	Below average	Below average
19	Above average	Below average
20	Above average	Below average
21	Above average	Below average
22	Above average	Below average
23	Above average	Above average
24	Above average	Below average
25	Above average	Below average
26	Above average	Below average
27	Above average	Below average
28	Above average	Below average
29	Above average	Below average
30	Above average	Below average

3. On the basis of this analysis, what would you conclude about the relationship between average length of stay in hospital and unplanned readmission rate for patients with fractured neck of femur at the 30 hospitals?

4. To what other groups of patients could these findings be generalized?

Table D20.3 Contingency table of relationship between average length of stay and readmission rates at 30 hospitals for patients with fractured neck of femur

	Unplanned readmission rate	
	Above average	**Below average**
Length of stay		
Above average	1	11
Below average	12	6

Answers

1. In this sample, 18 hospitals have a below average length of stay. 12 hospitals have an above average length of stay. Although that is how the median is defined, i.e. the score above which and below which half of the cases fall, the mean does not always fall at the exact half way point of the sample.
2. The number of degrees of freedom in a contingency table is calculated by the formula (rows − 1) multiplied by (columns − 1) = $(2 − 1) \times (2 − 1) = 1$.
3. There is a moderately sized statistical association between average length of stay in hospital and unplanned readmission rate. That is, those hospitals with shorter lengths of stay for patients with a fractured neck of femur tend to have higher unplanned readmission rates.
4. It is difficult to say. The current data include patients with one condition only, i.e. fractured neck of femur. These patients may be atypical of other acute/surgical patients; they are likely to be older and perhaps more debilitated. These analyses would need to be extended to other types of patients before the results could be generalized. The country in which the study has been performed also needs to be considered, as procedures and incentives may vary considerably from one country to the next.

Dissemination and critical evaluation of research

Having completed the analysis and interpretation of our data, we are now ready to communicate our results to the community of health scientists and professionals. Depending on the context in which our research was carried out, this entails the writing up of a report, a thesis or a 'paper' for a health sciences journal. The most common way of communicating research findings by established researchers is to first report the results at a professional conference and then to write a more formal paper for a relevant journal.

Each journal has its particular set of rules and requirements for how research projects should be written up for publication. In general, at least for quantitative research, the format for presenting our research follows the sequential stages of the research process outlined in the present book. This general format is outlined in Chapter 21, which includes a detailed discussion of the specific sections of a research paper and outlines some 'stylistic' considerations required by journal editors.

It is an ethical requirement that we report our results in an accurate and honest fashion. Before a paper is published in a reputable journal, it is critically evaluated by experts in the area (called referees) for errors or problems. However, sometimes problems remain unidentified. Ultimately it is our task, as health professionals, to read important publications in a critical fashion. We owe it to our patients and clients to be cautious and critical concerning recent developments in theories and practices. Being critical of course, does not imply the adoption of a cynical or derogatory approach towards the work of other health researchers. We are aware that ethical and economic constraints, and the complex nature of the subject matter as discussed in Section 2, make it difficult to ensure the external and internal validity of research projects.

The critical evaluation of a paper is not like judging a dog show; we don't simply award or subtract points for the strengths and weaknesses of a research project. Rather, if the information is relevant to advancing the effectiveness of our practices, we have a stake in the project (even as readers). In this way, we take an active role in trying to 'repair' the problems which might cloud or invalidate the evidence.

In Chapter 22, we outline some of the criteria which we generally apply to evaluate specific sections of a research paper. We also discuss the implications of finding serious problems with the design, data collection, and analysis and interpretations of a research project.

In effect, a single research project is rarely sufficient either to verify or falsify a theory, or to convincingly demonstrate the effectiveness of a treatment program. Rather, we need to evaluate and summarise the literature as a whole, that is produce a literature review. Conflicting findings or gaps in the knowledge for a given area of health care identified in our literature review provide the impetus for further research, as outlined in Section 2. In this way research is a circular process.

21

Presentation of health science research

INTRODUCTION

Knowledge in the health sciences is the sum of the individual efforts of investigators working all over the world. Professional journals in science and health care provide the dominant medium for disseminating information about the outcome of specific investigations. Investigators must report their procedures and results in an accurate and complete fashion. In this chapter, we outline the format and style generally followed for presenting the results of empirical investigations.

The specific aims of this chapter are to:

1. Describe the conventional way in which quantitative research is presented for publication
2. Discuss the style or language used to describe research
3. Outline briefly the way in which research papers are selected for publication.

THE STRUCTURE OF RESEARCH PUBLICATIONS

The format of a professional publication reporting empirical research reflects the stages of the research process discussed in this book. Table 21.1 represents the relationship between the stages of research and the commonly used publication format. This format is generally used to report quantitative empirical research, although you will find that some variations on this theme are adopted by some professional journals. This format is not necessarily followed for certain types or scholarly communications, such as for qualitative research, theoretical papers or literature reviews. In the sub-sections following, we examine in detail each of the components of a research report shown in Table 21.1.

Title and abstract

The Title is a descriptive sentence stating the exact topic of the report. Many titles of research reports take one of the following two forms:

- *Y* as a function of *x*
- The effect of *x* upon *y*

In causal research, such as experiments, *y* refers to the dependent variable being measured and *x* refers to the independent variable being manipulated. For example:

- The incidence of alcoholism in health professionals as a function of work related stress
- The effect of major tranquilizers on the cognitive functioning of persons with schizophrenia

For descriptive or qualitative research the title should inform the reader about the groups being studied and the characteristics being reported. For example:

- The attitudes of physicians to the professional functions of podiatrists

In general, titles should be concise and informative, enabling a prospective reader to identify the nature of the investigation. Immediately below the title should appear the name(s) of the investigator(s) and their affiliation.

The Abstract, is a short (not more than 250 words) description of the entire report. The purpose of this section is to provide the reader with a general overview of your communication. It should provide enough details to enable the reader to decide whether or not the article is of interest. This section can be difficult to write because of its precise nature. When writing an abstract you should include:

1. A brief statement about previous findings which led you to conduct your own research
2. The hypothesis and/or aim of your research
3. Methods, including subjects, apparatus and procedure
4. A short description of what you found and how you interpreted your results
5. What you concluded.

In some journals, this section may appear at the end of the manuscript in the form of a Summary. For our purposes, however, we will treat this section as an Abstract.

Table 21.1 Format of research publications and the research process

Publication format	Research process
Title	
Abstract	
Introduction	Research planning
Method:	Design
Subjects	
Apparatus	Measurement
Procedure	
Results	Descriptive statistics
	Inferential statistics
Discussion	Interpretation of the data
References	
Appendices	

The Title and the Abstract together are important for containing key words that enable the efficient retrieval of the information.

Introduction

The introduction is equivalent to the planning stages of research discussed in Section 2. A good introduction will set the stage for the hypotheses being tested. It should do this by discussing the theoretical background of the problem under consideration and evaluating the relevant research done previously. The introduction thus serves as a link between the past and the present.

Generally, all aspects of the literature cannot be covered in a relatively brief research paper, therefore, the review of past research is done with a bias towards only those aspects of the problem which are of direct relevance to your report. In this way the hypotheses being tested can be derived in a logical manner. For this reason, a good introduction starts out by making a few general statements about the field of research, leading logically to a narrow and specific set of statements which represent the aims or hypotheses. The last paragraph of the introduction should state the precise aims or the hypotheses being investigated.

Method

The purpose of this section is to inform the reader of how the investigation was carried out. It is important to remember that the Method Section should contain enough detail to enable another researcher to replicate your investigation. (Of course, replications may not be feasible for a unique event, such as a case study of a specific individual). Conventionally, three subsections are used: Subjects, Apparatus and Procedure.

Subjects. Three questions must be answered concerning the subjects: who were they, how many were there and how were they selected. Specific information must be given concerning your subjects, as results may vary from one sample to another.

Apparatus. A description of all equipment, including questionnaires, etc., used in your research must be provided. If it is commercially available, provide the reader with the manufacturer's name and the commercial identification of the equipment. On the other hand, if the equipment was privately made, provide the reader with enough information to allow replication. Measurements and perhaps a diagram will be necessary.

Procedure. Once again, this section should provide enough information for other researchers to replicate your investigation. Details of how research was carried out should include how subjects were assigned to groups, how many subjects per group, the experimental procedure and a description of how the data were collected.

In a sense, the Method section should read like a 'cookbook'. The Subjects subsection describes the 'ingredients'. The Apparatus subsection describes the equipment necessary for 'baking' (notice we did *not* say 'cooking' the experiment) and, finally, the Procedure subsection describes how the 'ingredients' were mixed for producing the final outcome: the Results section.

Results

This section presents the findings of the investigation and draws attention to points of interest. Raw data and statistical calculations are not presented in this section. Rather, we use the principles of descriptive and inferential statistics to present the summarized and analysed data: graphs, tables and the outcomes of statistical tests are presented in this section. It is essential that all the findings are presented and that the graphs and tables are correctly identified.

Discussion

This section restates the aim(s) of the investigation and discusses your results with reference to the aims or experimental hypothesis stated in the Introduction. Did you find what you expected? How do the present results relate to previous research?

It is important to remember that one experiment in isolation cannot make or break a theory or establish the effectiveness of a practice. Thus, the discussion should connect the findings with similar studies and especially with the theory underlying such studies. If unexpected results were obtained, possible reasons for the outcome (such as faulty design and controls) should be discussed. By this, the discussion will point the way to further problems which remain to be solved, Unconstructive, negative or unimportant criticism should be avoided, so that the report does not end with long discussions of possible reasons for the outcome. Brief, concise discussion is more appropriate.

In the Conclusion, usually the last paragraph of the Discussion section, you summarize your main findings and make suggestions for further research. For example, you may have demonstrated certain phenomena which may have implications for explaining broader concepts which can be empirically tested. You are therefore taking your findings and generalizing them to phenomena not directly tested in the present research.

References and appendices

It is expected that all the literature discussed in your paper is reported in the reference section. This enables your reader to evaluate your sources. You should refer to appropriate style manuals for information on how references should be listed. You must give sufficient information for an interested reader to be able to identify and retrieve your sources. In addition, a report may include labelled appendices. These might include a full description of questionnaires or other measuring instruments, raw data, or statistical calculations if required for some reason.

THE STYLE OF RESEARCH PUBLICATIONS

It is essential that you read research publications in your professional area to gain a 'feel' for the appropriate style of writing. In general, the following points should be kept in mind when writing reports:

1. Avoid long phrases or complicated sentences. Short, simple sentences are far more easily understood by your reader. In other words, try not to posture but to communicate.
2. Use quotations sparingly; put ideas in your own words. Quotations are only used when it is necessary to convey precisely the ideas of another researcher, for instance, while conducting a critique of a paper.
3. Use past tense when writing your research report.
4. Use an objective style, avoiding personal pronouns wherever possible.
5. Make sure you are writing to your audience; if the material is specialized or difficult, explain it clearly.
6. Make sure that you are concise and clear; don't introduce issues and concepts which are not strictly relevant to reporting your investigation. Raising interesting but superfluous issues might distract and confuse your reader.

In general, you should aim to improve your report writing and your ability to communicate your finding and ideas by seeking constructive criticism from your colleagues and supervisors.

THE PUBLICATION PROCESS

The formal knowledge representing the empirical and professional basis for your professional practice is in a large part stored in journals, books and conference reports, Journals are published by appropriate professional associations, government departments or private companies. Having completed a research project, how does one publish it in a professional journal? After all, the value of research is negligible if it is not made public.

In general, the prospective author will:

1. Select a professional or scientific journal appropriate for the material
2. Present the research report in a format required by the journal
3. Send the completed manuscript to the journal's editor.

The editor is a person of high standing in a given scientific or professional area. If the article is judged as being appropriate for the journal, the editor will send the article to two or more referees and, on the basis of the referees' report, publish or reject the manuscript. Sometimes the referees recommend certain additions or changes which have to be made by the author before the manuscript is judged to be publishable.

Therefore, when you read research publications in referred journals, you can be confident that the articles have been scrutinized by experts. However, as shown in the next sub-section, this doesn't necessarily guarantee the truth of either the evidence or the conclusions.

ETHICS OF PRESENTING RESEARCH

The health science researcher has an obligation to publish honest and accurate results that would not harm those people who participated in the research.

Most ethics committees in health care institutions and universities have the twin objectives to not only advance knowledge for the common good but also to prevent harm to those participating in the research. This is particularly so in the situation where the participants may have a diminished capacity to freely consent to their involvement (e.g. children or people who are unconscious or seriously ill). It is crucial to maintain the dignity and confidentiality of participants in health research.

Therefore, in the process of ethical evaluation of health science research, the researcher can expect to be closely questioned on these issues. If they cannot convince the ethics committee that the research will deliver knowledge for the common good and that it will not harm the participants, then the research will usually not proceed.

In research performed for a higher degree, many universities will not accept a thesis without an accompanying ethical clearance from the relevant ethics committee. Most hospitals and universities have strict ethical procedures that must be followed before any research work is commenced by their staff. Most, if not all, health research grant bodies require an ethical clearance before they will release the funds to successful applicants. Many journals also require certification from the researcher that the work complies with ethical principles. It is likely that this trend towards tightening of procedures will continue.

The ultimate unethical act is to manufacture data. Board and Wade (1982), in their book *Betrayers of the Truth* describe this problem. It would seem to be a growing problem that may be associated with the 'publish or perish' requirements placed upon health science researchers by granting bodies and employers.

In the health sciences, it is not only the participants in research who may be harmed or assisted by the research. If an erroneous research finding is widely applied, it may harm many thousands of people. Thus ethics are not simply concerned with whether the researcher has good intentions and treats the research participants well. There is also the issue of competence. Poorly designed research is unethical in that it may bring great harm to others. Thus the ethical researcher must also be a competent researcher.

SUMMARY

In this chapter we outlined the general format followed by researchers for publishing their results. The format is related to the logical steps of planning, conducting and interpreting research. The style involves clarity, accuracy and sufficient completeness for colleagues to understand or replicate the research project. Research is published in journals, which are edited by persons of high standing in the area. Every effort is made by editors to ensure the validity of the research published in their journals. The individual researcher is also ethically bound to report findings in an unbiased and truthful fashion.

Although the format and style outlined in this chapter might seem rather arduous, poor presentation may destroy the intrinsic value of a research project.

SELF ASSESSMENT

Explain the meaning of the following terms:

abstract
apparatus
discussion
method
plagiarism
procedure
refereed journal
subjects

True or false

1. As a rule, the title of a research investigation should not contain more than seven words.
2. Generally, the research hypothesis should be presented in the Introduction.
3. A research report should contain sufficient information so that the investigation can be replicated.
4. The Results section should contain all computational details for each statistic.
5. The Abstract should normally contain the key tables of the results.
6. The design of an investigation influences the content of the Method section.
7. All the names and addresses of your subjects must be published to enable replication of your investigation.
8. Quotations should be used sparingly in a research report.
9. A research report should be written in the past tense.
10. The outcomes of statistical analyses are reported in the Results section.
11. Scientists do not normally report the results of their investigations, in case their work is stolen or misrepresented.
12. Calculations are best presented in appendices.
13. The 'referees' are hired by the investigator in order to convince the editor that an investigation should be published.
14. The role of an editor for a scientific journal is to censor research publications for pornographic, blasphemous or politically undesirable material.

15. Good research is unique and cannot be replicated.
16. A researcher should report data even if it is inconsistent with the researcher's original preconceptions.
17. Scientific and professional journals are important for disseminating and storing knowledge.
18. Fortunately, there have been no major scandals concerning scientists publishing fabricated data.
19. Provided that the results are statistically significant, there is no need to present descriptive statistics.

Multiple choice

1. Scientific journals:
   a only publish empirical evidence
   b depend on the services of referees to comment on the validity of the research project
   c publish only true knowledge
   d b and c.

2. The literature review is normally found in which section of a research report?
   a Abstract
   b Introduction
   c Discussion
   d References

3. A literature review for a research report should:
   a contain a detailed review of all previously published reports
   b contain a selective review of evidence pertinent to the current research project
   c be at least 5 000 words in length
   d a and c
   e b and c.

4. Which of the following is most inadequate as title for a research report?
   a The effects of the twentieth century culture on being human: An empirical evaluation of personal functioning in declining cultures
   b Electrical stimulation of the limbic system: Effects on emotion and memory
   c A survey of the incidence of mental illness in the London metropolitan area
   d Popularity, friendship selection and specific peer interaction among children.

5. The Methods section of a research report:
    a informs the reader of the purpose of an investigation
    b informs the reader about the state of methodological advances in the subject area
    c informs the reader as to how the investigation was carried out
    d informs the reader as to how the hypothesis or aim of the investigation was formulated.

6. When writing a scientific report one should:
    a make sure the Introduction contains 250 words or less
    b use personal pronouns as much as possible
    c try to impress the readers by one's level of general knowledge
    d use the past tense.

7. In which part of a research report are the descriptive and inferential statistics normally reported?
    a Abstract
    b Results
    c Discussion
    d Appendices.

8. In writing a Discussion, one should:
    a relate the results to findings reported in previous publications
    b establish if the results of the investigation supported the hypothesis
    c neither *a* nor *b*
    d both *a* and *b*.

9. Which of the following statements is true?
    a The Discussion section should relate present findings to previous research.
    b The literature review should be conducted in a special appendix labelled References.
    c The Results section should contain only tables and graphs, but not any verbal descriptions of the data.
    d All the above statements are true.
    e None of the above statements is true.

10. Which of the following statements is false?
    a The Abstract should be a brief summary of the research.
    b It is unethical to fabricate data.
    c A refereed journal is one in which experts independently evaluate a research report before it is published.
    d A well designed research project need not have a Procedure section.

22

Critical evaluation of published research

INTRODUCTION

By the time a research report is published in a reputable journal, it has been critically scrutinized by several experts. Nevertheless, even this detailed evaluation procedure doesn't necessarily guarantee the validity of the design or the conclusions. Ultimately, you as a health professional must be responsible for judging the validity and relevance of published material.

The proper attitude to published material is hard-nosed scepticism. This attitude is based on our understanding of the probabilistic and provisional nature of scientific and professional knowledge. In addition, health researchers deal with the investigation of complex phenomena, where it is often impossible for ethical reasons to exercise desired levels of control. The aim of critical evaluation is to identify the strengths and weaknesses of a research publication, so as to ensure that patients receive assessment and treatment based on the best available evidence.

This is essentially a revision chapter. Its general aim is to demonstrate how select concepts in design, measurement and statistics can be applied to the critical evaluation of published research. The chapter is organized around the evaluation of specific sections of research publications.

The specific aims of this chapter are to:

1. Examine the criteria used for the critical evaluation of a quantitative research paper
2. Discuss the implications of identifying problems in design, measurement and analysis in a given publication
3. Outline briefly strategies for summarizing and analysing evidence from a set of papers
4. Discuss the implications of critical evaluation of research for health care practices.

CRITICAL EVALUATION OF THE INTRODUCTION

The Introduction of a paper essentially reflects the planning of the research. Inadequacies in this section might signal that the research project was erroneously conceived or poorly planned. The following issues are essential for evaluating this section.

Adequacy of the literature review

The literature review must be sufficiently complete so as to reflect the current state of knowledge in the area. Key papers should not be omitted, particularly when their results could have direct consequences for the research hypotheses or aims. Researchers must be unbiased in presenting evidence which is unfavourable to their points of view. A particular 'howler' occurs when a research project is undertaken in ignorance of the fact that the same research has been already conducted and published.

Clearly defined aims or hypotheses

As stated in Chapter 2, the aims or hypotheses of an investigation should be clearly and operationally stated. If this is lacking, how the evidence obtained in the investigation is to be used for conceptual advances in the area will be ambiguous.

Selection of an appropriate research strategy

In formulating the aims of the investigation, the researcher must have taken into account the appropriate research strategy. For instance, if the demonstration of causal effects is required, a survey may be inappropriate for satisfying the aims of the research.

Selection of appropriate variables

The operational definition of the variables being investigated calls for selecting appropriate measurement strategies. If the selection of the variables is inappropriate to the construct being investigated, then the investigation will not produce useful results.

CRITICAL EVALUATION OF THE METHODS SECTION

A well documented Methods section is a necessary condition for understanding, evaluating and perhaps replicating a research project. In general, the critical evaluation of this section will reveal the overall internal and external validity of the investigation.

Subjects

This section shows if the sample was representative of the target population and the adequacy of the sampling model used.

Sampling model used. In Chapter 3, we outlined a number of sampling models which can be employed to optimize the representativeness of a sample. If the sampling model is inappropriate, then the sample might be biased, raising questions concerning the external validity of the research findings.

Sample size. Use of a small sample is not necessarily a fatal flaw of an investigation, if the sample is representative. However, given a highly variable, heterogenous population, a small sample will not be adequate to ensure representativeness (Ch. 3). Also, a small sample size could decrease the power of the statistical analysis (Ch. 20).

Description of the sample. A clear description of key sample variables (for example, age, sex, type and severity of condition) should be provided. When necessary and possible, demographic information concerning the population should be provided. If not, the reader cannot judge the representativeness of the sample. Also, the reader might not be able to decide if the findings are applicable to the specific groups of patients being treated.

Instruments/apparatus

The validity and reliability of observations and measurements are fundamental characteristics of good research. In this section, the investigator must demonstrate the adequacy of the equipment used for data collection.

Validity and reliability. The investigator should use standardized apparatus, or establish the validity and reliability of new apparatus used. The lack of proven validity and reliability will raise questions about the adequacy of the empirical findings.

Description of instrumentation. Full description of the structure and use of novel instrumentation should be presented so that the instrument can be replicated by independent parties.

Procedure

Full description of how the investigation was carried out is necessary for both replication and for the evaluation of its internal and external validity.

Adequacy of the design. It was stated previously that a good design should control for alternative interpretations of the data. A poor design will result in uncontrolled influences by extraneous variables, negating the unequivocal evaluation of causal effects. In Section Three, we looked at a variety of threats to internal validity which must be considered when critically evaluating an investigation.

Control groups. A specific way of controlling for extraneous effects is the use of control groups (such as placebo, no treatment, conventional treatment). If control groups are not employed, then the internal validity of the investigation might be questioned. Also, if placebo or untreated groups are not present, the size of the effect due to the treatments might be difficult to estimate.

Subject assignment. When using an experimental design, care must be taken in the assignment of subjects so as to avoid significant initial differences between treatment groups (see Ch. 4). Even when quasi-experimental or natural comparison strategies are used, care must be taken to establish the equivalence of the groups (see Chs 5–6).

Treatment parameters. It is important to describe all the treatments given to the different groups. If the treatments differ in intensity or in the equality of the administering personnel, the internal validity of the project is threatened.

Rosenthal and Hawthorne effects. Whenever possible, studies should be double or single blind. If the subjects, experimentors or observers are aware of the aims and predicted outcomes of the investigation, then the validity of the investigation will be threatened through bias and expectancy effects (see Ch. 4)

Settings. The setting in which a study is carried out has implications for external (ecological) validity. An adequate description of the setting is necessary for evaluating the generalizability of the findings (see Ch. 3).

Times of treatments and observations. The sequence of treatments and observations must be clearly indicated, such that issues such as series and confounding effects can be detected. Identification of variability in treatment and observation times can influence the internal validity of experimental, quasi-experimental or $n = 1$ designs, resulting in, for instance, internal validity problems.

CRITICAL EVALUATION OF THE RESULTS

The results should represent a statistically correct summary and analysis of the data (Sections Five and Six). Inadequacies in this section could indicate that inferences drawn by the investigator were erroneous.

Tables and graphs. Data should be correctly tabulated or drawn and adequately labelled for interpretation. Complete summaries of all the relevant findings should be presented.

Selection of statistics. Both descriptive and inferential statistics must be selected according to specific rules outlined in Sections Five and Six. The selection of inappropriate statistics could distort the findings and lead to inappropriate inferences.

Calculation of statistics. Clearly, both descriptive and inferential statistics must be correctly calculated. The use of computers generally ensures this, although some attention must be paid to gross errors when evaluating the data.

CRITICAL EVALUATION OF THE DISCUSSION

In the discussion, the investigator draws inferences from the data in relation to the initial aims or hypotheses of the investigation. Unless the inferences are correctly made, the conclusions drawn might lead to useless and dangerous treatments being offered to clients.

Drawing correct inferences from the data. The inferences from the data must take account of the limitations of descriptive and inferential statistics. We have seen, for instance in Chapter 16, that correlations do not necessarily imply causation, or that a lack of significance in the analysis could imply a Type II error (see Ch. 20).

Logically correct interpretations of the findings. Interpretations of the findings must follow from the statistical inferences, without extraneous evidence being introduced. For instance, if the investigation used a $n = 1$ design, the conclusions should not claim that a procedure is generally useful.

Protocol deviations. In interpreting the data, the investigator must indicate, and take into account, unexpected deviations from the intended design. For instance, a placebo/active treatment code might be broken, or 'contamination' between control and experimental groups might be discovered. If such deviations are discovered by investigators, they are obliged to report these, so that the implications for the results might be taken into account.

Generalization from the findings. Strictly speaking, the data obtained from a given sample are generalizable only to the population from which the sample was drawn. This point is sometimes ignored by investigators and the findings are generalized to subjects or situations which were not considered in the original sampling (see Ch. 3).

Statistical and clinical significance. As was explained in Chapter 20, statistical significance does not necessarily imply that the results of an investigation are clinically applicable. In deciding on clinical significance factors such as the size of the effect, side effects and cost effectiveness, as well as value judgements concerning outcome, must be considered.

Theoretical significance. It is necessary to relate the results of an investigation to previous relevant findings which have been identified in the literature review. Unless, the results are logically related to the literature, the theoretical significance of the investigation remains unclear. The processes involved in comparing the findings of a set of related papers are introduced in the next sub-section.

Table 22.1 summarizes some of the potential problems and their implications, which might emerge in the context-critical evaluation of an investigation. A point which must be kept in mind is that even where an investigation is flawed, useful knowledge might be drawn from it. The aim of critical analysis is not to discredit or tear down published work, but to ensure that the reader understands its implications and limitations with respect to theory and practice.

CRITICAL EVALUATION OF THE LITERATURE: META-ANALYSIS

By 'literature' we mean publications relevant to a specific area of science or clinical practice. Given the complexity of health care problems, it is unusual when the results of a single research publication are adequate for making clinical decisions.

As stated before, in preparing literature reviews and evaluating research findings, a multiplicity of papers must be considered, according to the following steps:

Table 22.1 Checklist for evaluating published research

Problems which might be identified in a research article	Possible implications
1 Inadequate literature review	Misrepresentation of the conceptual basis for the research
2 Vague aims or hypothesis	Research might lack direction; interpretation of evidence might be ambiguous
3 Inappropriate research strategy	Findings might not be relevant to the problem being investigated
4 Inappropriate variables selected	Measurements might not be related to concepts being investigated
5 Inadequate sampling method	Sample might be biased, investigation could lack external validity
6 Inadequate sample size	Sample might be biased; statistical analysis might lack power
7 Inadequate description of sample	Application of findings to specific groups or individuals might be difficult
8 Instruments lack validity or reliability	Findings might represent measurement errors
9 Inadequate design	Investigation might lack internal validity; i.e. outcomes might be due to uncontrolled extraneous variables
10 Lack of adequate control groups	Investigation might lack internal validity; size of the effect difficult to estimate
11 Biased subject assignment	Investigation might lack internal validity
12 Variations or lack of control of treatment parameters	Investigation might lack internal validity
13 Observer bias not controlled (Rosenthal effects)	Investigation might lack internal and external validity
14 Subject expectations not controlled (Hawthorne effects)	Investigation might lack internal and external validity
15 Research carried out in inappropriate setting	Investigation might lack ecological validity
16 Confounding of times at which observations and treatments are carried out	Possible series effects; investigation might lack internal validity
17 Inadequate presentation of descriptive statistics	The nature of the empirical findings might not be comprehensible
18 Inappropriate statistics used to describe and/or analyse data	Distortion of decision process false inferences might be drawn
19 Erroneous calculation of statistics	False inferences might be drawn
20 Drawing incorrect inferences from the data analysis (e.g. Type II error)	False conclusions might be made concerning the outcome of an investigation
21 Protocol deviations	Investigation might lack external or internal validity
22 Overgeneralisation of findings	External validity might be threatened
23 Confusing statistical and clinical significance	Treatments lacking clinical usefulness might be encouraged
24 Findings not logically related to previous research findings	Theoretical significance of the investigation remains doubtful

1. Identify relevant literature (Section Two).
2. Evaluate critically the key papers, as discussed in this section. You might decide to discard some papers if irreparable problems are discovered.
3. Identify general patterns of findings in the literature. Tabulate findings.
4. Identify crucial disagreements and controversies.
5. Propose valid explanations for the disagreements. Such explanations provide a theoretical framework for resolving controversies and proposing future research.

Dooley (1984) discussed the availability of two general types of strategies for summarizing research findings from multiple papers:

1. *Qualitative.* A qualitative review involves the selection of key features of related publications, such as designs, subject characteristics or measures used in the studies. These features are presented in a table form, such that differences in the features of the research can be related to outcomes.
2. *Quantitative.* A quantitative review calls for the condensation of the results from several papers into a single statistic. This statistic represents an average effect size.

These procedures are also related to meta-analyses, which are systematic procedures for summarizing the overall implications of a set of research papers.

There are advantages and disadvantages in these two review approaches, but discussion of the quantitative approach is beyond the scope of the present text. To illustrate the qualitative method, consider a set of four hypothetical studies reporting on levels of compliance by diabetics to insulin administration. The results and key features of these hypothetical studies are tabulated in Table 22.2.

Table 22.2 Compliance to insulin use by diabetics (hypothetical reports)

Publication	Sample size	Average age of patients	Method of measuring compliance	Percentage of patients compliant
Smith (1980)	50	55	Self-report	85
Jones (1981)	60	58	Self-report	82
Brown (1980)	50	59	Blood sugar level	40
Miller (1981)	55	56	Blood sugar level	35

Table 22.2 represents how findings from several publications might be tabulated. Key information about each study, as well as the outcomes, is presented in the table, enabling the emergence and demonstration of an overall pattern.

Unfortunately, in some reviews no clear pattern will emerge from the tabulated findings. Even when controlling for the quality of the individual publications, a conflict might emerge concerning the nature and causes of the findings. In the rather simple, hypothetical example above, the percentage of compliance reported by Smith (1980) and Jones (1981) is over twice that reported by Brown (1980) and Miller (1981). A possible explanation for this discrepancy might emerge by the inspection of Table 22.1. Clearly, neither differences in sample size nor the average ages of the patients suggest an explanation of the difference. However, the method by which compliance was measured emerges as a plausible explanation. The investigators, Smith and Jones, who relied on the patients' self-reports might have overestimated compliance levels in contrast to Brown and Miller who used a more objective method. Of course, this explanation is not necessarily true, but is simply a hypothesis for guiding future investigations of the problem.

One should not underestimate the difficulty of writing adequate literature reviews on the basis of the above simple illustrative example. Writing an adequate literature review should bring into play your knowledge of research design, measurement and statistics as well as your understanding of health science issues.

SUMMARY

The critical evaluation of published material at a level of detail suggested by this chapter is a time consuming, even pedantic task. One undertakes such detailed analysis only when professional communications are of key importance, for example, when writing a formal literature review or when evaluating current evidence for adopting a new treatment. Nevertheless, it is a necessary process for an indepth understanding of the empirical and theoretical basis of your clinical practice.

Even when problems are identified with a given research report, it is likely that the report will provide some useful empirical knowledge. Given the problems of generalization, an individual research project is usually insufficient for deciding on the truth of a hypothesis or the usefulness of a clinical intervention. Rather, the reader needs to scrutinize the range of relevant research and summarize the evidence using qualitative and quantitative review methods. In this way, individual research results can be evaluated in the context of the research area. Disagreements or controversies are ultimately useful for generating hypotheses for guiding new research and for advancing theory and practice.

SELF ASSESSMENT

Explain the meaning of the following terms:

   critical evaluation
   meta-analysis
   protocol deviation
   qualitative review
   quantitative review

True or false

1. Critical analysis of a publication aims to identify the internal and external validity of the investigation.
2. If an investigation is published in a reputable journal by established investigators then the validity of the investigation can be taken for granted.

3. Random assignment of subjects to treatment groups ensures that the investigation uncovers casual effects.
4. The outcome of an investigation can be useful even with a small sample size.
5. If an investigation produces statistically significant results, its design must have been adequate.
6. Obtaining statistical significance in an investigation is a condition for the demonstration of the clinical significance of a quantitative study.
7. The replication of an investigation demonstrates the internal validity of the original investigation.
8. Without adequate controls the size of an effect might be difficult to estimate.
9. If a study is internally valid, the investigator is justified in generalizing the results to any other population.
10. Provided that the outcomes are statistically significant, it doesn't matter which statistical tests were chosen to analyse the data.
11. If the design of an investigation is inadequate, none of the empirical findings are of scientific or clinical use.
12. Controversies in an area of science usually reflect the presence of fraudulently published evidence.
13. One of the problems with using human subjects for research is the expectations of the subjects concerning the purpose of the investigation.
14. Even poorly planned research can provide some useful results.
15. The application of the scientific method ensures the validity of a researcher's conclusions.
16. Disagreements among researchers in an area are useful for generating new hypotheses.
17. A qualitative research review is useful for generating hypotheses concerning trends in the literature.
18. A quantitative research review is useful for estimating effect sizes.
19. To understand a clinical phenomenon we should review the range of relevant research findings.

Multiple choice

1. The aim of the critical analysis of a publication is to:
   - a identify the relevance of the results for clinical practice
   - b identify the internal and external validity of the investigation
   - c identify and attack incompetent researchers in one's area of interest
   - d a and b.

2. If the internal validity of a study is adequate, then:
   - a the results will be statistically significant
   - b the results will be clinically useful
   - c the investigation may demonstrate casual effects
   - d a and b.

3. Say that an investigation has generated some interesting findings. However, you find that the investigators selected an inappropriate statistical test to analyse their findings. You should:
   a regretfully discard the study as useless
   b re-analyse the data from the descriptive statistics provided
   c write to the investigators for their raw data, and re-analyse yourself
   d b or c.

4. The reason one should evaluate the 'literature' as a whole is to:
   a identify general patterns of findings in the area
   b condense results from related papers into a single statistic
   c identify and attempt to explain controversies in the area
   d all of the above.

5. In judging the clinical significance of a well designed investigation one should consider:
   a the cost effectiveness of the interventions
   b the size of the therapeutic effects
   c the possible undesirable side effects of the treatment
   d a, b and c.

An investigation was carried out in order to show that 'prepared childbirth' was an effective method for reducing pain during delivery. 90 women attending a large hospital constituted the sample. 60 of the women chose to participate in childbirth preparation, based on the Lamaze method, provided by trained instructors working at the hospital. This method encourages 'natural' (drug free) childbirth through teaching physical and mental strategies for coping with pain or discomfort occurring during childbirth. The other 30 women chose not to attend the childbirth preparation program. The level of pain experienced was assessed on the McGill pain questionnaire, which has been shown to be a valid and reliable interval scale for pain. It was administered following the childbirth. In addition the number of women seeking analgesia during childbirth was recorded as a measure of levels of discomfort experienced. The results for the investigation are as follows:

Groups	Mean pain scores
Women with no training ($n = 30$)	38
Women with childbirth preparation ($n = 60$)	32

The difference was statistically significant at $\alpha = 0.05$

Groups	Number given medication
Women with no training ($n = 30$)	24
Women with childbirth preparation ($n = 60$)	49

The difference was not statistically significant at $\alpha = 0.05$

Questions 6–14 refer to the above investigation.

6. The strategy for the investigation is best described as:
   a   an experiment
   b   a quasi-experiment
   c   a correlational study
   d   an $n = 90$ design.

7. One of the problems with the above investigation was that:
   a   the subjects could not be randomly assigned to treatment groups
   b   the dependent variable was irrelevant to the aims
   c   basic ethical issues were not considered
   d   the instructors teaching the Lamaze method were incompetent.

8. From the information given above, it is clear that the investigators controlled for:
   a   Hawthorne effect
   b   Rosenthal effects
   c   subject assignment
   d   none of the above.

9. If you wanted to calculate the proportion of women with no training who had greater McGill pain scores than women with childbirth preparation, then the required statistics are:
   a   the distribution of t for $n = 98$
   b   the normal distribution
   c   the indicies for reliability and validity
   d   the standard deviations for the two groups.

10. Which of the following statistical tests is most appropriate for analysing the significance of the data for the McGill pain scores?
   a   Mann-Whitney U
   b   sign test
   c z test for two means
   d χ^2 test.

11. Which of the following statistical tests is most appropriate for analysing the significance of the data for women requiring medication?
   a   Mann-Whitney U
   b   sign test
   c t test for two means
   d χ^2 test.

12. The lack of statistical significance for the data on medication implies that:
   a   the power for the test may have been too low
   b   equal sample sizes should have been used
   c   training has no effect
   d   both a and c.

13. The outcome of this investigation can be generalized to:
    a   women having children and undergoing Lamaze training
    b   women having children without Lamaze training
    c   women who chose the type of childbirth they undergo
    d   none of the above groups.

14. Considering the evidence provided, one concludes that:
    a   prepared childbirth is a waste of time
    b   there is evidence that Lamaze preparation at this hospital results in statistically significant reductions in pain during delivery
    c   that women undergoing childbirth find Lamaze preparation useless at this hospital
    d   a and c.

A decision is to be made concerning whether Treatment x or Treatment y is to be used to treat seriously ill cancer patients in a hospital. There are three published studies in the area, comparing the proportion of clients surviving up to five years with the treatments.
    The results for the three hypothetical studies are:

STUDY A		Number surviving	Number not surviving	Outcome
Treatment x	$n = 10$	5	5	Not significant $\alpha = 0.01$
Treatment y	$n = 15$	5	10	

STUDY B		Number surviving	Number not surviving	Outcome
Placebo control	$n = 100$	20	80	Significant at $\alpha = 0.01$
Treatment y	$n = 100$	40	60	

STUDY C		Number surviving	Number not surviving	Outcome
Treatment x	$n = 50$	40	10	Significant at $\alpha = 0.01$
Treatment y	$n = 60$	30	30	

Questions 15–18 refer to the above information.

15. Which of the following statements is true on the basis of the above?
    a   Study C must be fraudulent
    b   Study A is more powerful than Study B
    c   In Study A, subjects must have been assigned on the basis of matching
    d χ^2 test was appropriate for analysing the results.

16. Which of the above statements is false?
    a Treatment *y* appears more effective than placebo treatment
    b The scale of measurements used for the dependent variables was nominal in the three studies
    c None of the three studies controlled for the effects of 'history'
    d In Study A, 33.3% of patients followed Treatment *y*.

17. In Study A, 50% of patients survived for 5 years, following Treatment *x*, while in Study C, 80% of patients survived following the same treatment. Which of the following is a possible explanation?
    a The therapists in Study C were more effective in carrying out the treatment
    b There is a random sampling error
    c Either *a* or *b* is a possible explanation
    d Neither *a* nor *b* is a possible explanation.

18. On the basis of the combined results of the 3 studies what is the approximate probability that a client will survive for over 5 years following Treatment *y*?
    a less than 0.33
    b between 0.3 and 0.4
    c between 0.33 and 0.5
    d 0.5 or more.

19. On the basis of the evidence provided by the above three studies, one should adopt for the treatment of patients:
    a Treatment *x*
    b Treatment *y*
    c Neither Treatment *x* nor Treatment *y*
    d the less expensive treatment.

DISCUSSION, QUESTIONS AND ANSWERS

This question is based on a survey which was published in an Australian newspaper. Of course, such surveys do not represent research published in scientific journals, but they are important sources for public knowledge or/ and attitudes towards health sciences issues. The survey questioned a sample of adults concerning their smoking habits. Only one of the questions asked is discussed here and the results are hypothetical.

Survey characteristics

Sample:	1000 voters
Coverage:	Australia wide
Method:	Telephone
Question:	Do you smoke? (Yes or No)

Results

	Percentage of replies to the question in two major cities	
	Melbourne	Sydney
Yes	24	18
No	76	82

Questions

The following questions involve the critical analysis of the above survey.

1. If we assume that cigarette smoking is nowadays a 'stigmatized' behaviour, do you think the telephone survey produced valid answers?
2. 180 people were interviewed in Melbourne and 220 in Sydney. If the population of Australia is 17 million and the populations of Melbourne and Sydney are 2.5 and 3.2 million respectively, do the samples appear to be quota samples?
3. Which categories of smokers may not have been reached by this survey? What implications might this have for the external validity of the survey?
4. A journalist commented on the results, saying: 'This difference is ironic, given that anti-smoking lobbyists have applauded Melbourne as a pacesetter for smoking law reform, such as tobacco tax-funded health promotion.'

    Explain why this comment is inappropriate given the design of the survey?

What research design would be appropriate to show a causal effect on smoking due to health promotion on smoking? (Hint: see Ch. 6).

5. Explain why the comment quoted in question 4 is inappropriate, given that the statistical significance of the results was not calculated.

6. Which statistical test should be used to analyse the significance of the results concerning differences in smoking between the two cities? Justify your selection.

7. Setting $\alpha = 0.05$, calculate the statistic and decide if the results were significant (note that we gave the results in percentages).

8. Do you think the sample size ($n = 1000$) was adequate? Explain.

Answers

1. Although telephone interviews and mailed out questionnaires are a relatively cost-efficient strategy for collecting data, we have problems validating the responses. This is particularly true for conditions and behaviours which are socially stigmatized; why should the respondent disclose such information about themselves? In face-to-face interviews, we can explore issues; for example, if the respondents have nicotine-stained fingers or smell of cigarettes, we may pursue the issue further to establish the accuracy of the replies.

2. Given that $n = 1000$, 18% of the respondents were from Melbourne and 22% from Sydney. For a quota sample, the expected samples would be:

Melbourne: $\dfrac{2.5}{17} \times 100$ $= 14.7\%$

and

Sydney: $\dfrac{3.2}{17} \times 100$ $= 18.8\%$

Assuming that the information used to calculate the above figures is correct, it seems that the sample included more respondents from Melbourne. This may reflect the different proportion of 'voters' in the two cities, or a rather poor quota sample.

3. People who are not on the electoral roll, such as persons under 18 years of age, and people who do not have, or do not answer their telephones, would not have been contacted. In this way, the sample may not be representative of all the smokers in the city (e.g. young people, poor or itinerant people, people with unlisted telephone numbers). In this way, the survey may not be externally valid if we generalize to all persons in Australia who smoke.

4. The present surveys did not tell us how rates of smoking have changed over a period of time. We may use a quasi-experimental design and introduce the program in one city (A) but not in the other equivalent city

(B). If the reduction is greater over time in A than in B, we may argue that this difference could reflect the causal effect of health promotion.

5. Although results for the samples show a difference between the two cities, this may simply reflect sampling error. We must establish the significance of the results before we can draw inferences ('ironic' or otherwise) about populations.

6. χ^2 ; nominal data and independent measurements or samples.

7. Convert the data into frequencies (see Ch. 19) before entering obtained values into a 2 X 2 contingency table (values rounded to closest whole number).

	Melbourne	**Sydney**	**Total**
Smokers	43 Cell 1	40 Cell 2	83
Non-smokers	137 Cell 3	180 Cell 4	317
Total	180	220	400

Expected values: (for calculation procedure, see Ch. 19)

$$f_e \text{ (cell 1)} = \frac{83 \times 180}{400} = 37.4$$

$$fe \text{ (cell 2)} = \frac{83 \times 220}{400} = 45.7$$

$$f_e \text{ (cell 3)} = \frac{317 \times 180}{400} = 142.6$$

$$f_e \text{ (cell 4)} = \frac{317 \times 220}{400} = 174.3$$

Calculation of χ^2

Cell	f_o	f_e	$(f_o - f_e)^2$	$\dfrac{(f_o - f_e)^2}{f_e}$
1	43	37.4	31.36	.84
2	40	45.7	32.49	.71
3	137	142.6	31.36	.22
4	180	174.3	32.49	.19

$$\chi^2_{obt} = \sum \frac{(f_o - f_e)^2}{f_e} = 1.96$$

Critical value of χ^2; $\alpha = .05$ where (degrees of freedom) = 1
(Appendix C)

$$\chi^2_{crit} = 3.84$$

In this case we would retain H_0: there is no association between the variables 'city' (M or S) and smoking (Yes or No). (For details of decision making process, refer to Chapter 19).

It is apparent that the results are not significant, therefore we are not justified in drawing any inferences concerning the different proportions of smokers in Melbourne and Sydney.

8. Although a sample size of $n = 1000$ appears quite large, this was an Australia wide sample which was divided up to represent regions.

It may be that the null results obtained in question 7 are because there are, in reality, no differences in smoking rates between the two cities. But there are other possibilities (see Ch. 20).

Perhaps the sample size was inadequate and we made a Type II error in our decision. Replicating the study with larger sample sizes might enable us to show significant differences in smoking rates.

Glossary of research terms

AB design   A type of experimental design in which the participant is monitored during a baseline phase followed by an intervention phase.

ABAB design   A type of experimental design in which the participant is monitored during a baseline phase followed by an intervention phase which, in turn, is followed by further baseline and intervention phases.

Abstract   An abbreviated summary of a research report, generally found at the beginning of the report.

Acquiescent response mode   A style of answering questions which results in the respondent choosing the middle category in a response scale.

Alternative hypothesis   Sometimes also known as the experimental hypothesis. This is the hypothesis for which the researcher is trying to gain support in a statistical analysis, by rejecting the null hypothesis. The alternative hypothesis is represented by the symbol H_A or H_1.

Apparatus   Any equipment or special facilities used in a research project.

Area sample   A type of sampling procedure in which the units of the sample are where people live or work, rather than who they are. The researcher divides the target area into sections and then samples the sections.

Assignment   The process in an experiment where the researcher allocates subjects to the various groups. Matching and random assignment are the two most common methods. The goal of assignment is to achieve identical groups.

Assignment errors   A situation that arises in an experiment where the assignment or allocation of people to groups results in groups with different characteristics.

Authority   An appeal to authority argument is based on the proposition that someone of high status knows best, not whether the argument is soundly based.

Bar graph   A method of displaying data where the frequency of a particular category is reflected in the height of the bar in the graph.

Baseline   A phase in an intervention study where the participant is receiving no intervention.

Bell shaped curve   This is the characteristic shape of the normal distribution.

Bias   In a questionnaire, bias is introduced by inappropriately framed questions, such as leading questions.

Biased sample   A biased sample is one that is not representative. It does not reflect the composition of the population to which the researcher is attempting to generalize.

Causal explanation   An attempt to explain the occurrence of a particular phenomenon or event by identifying the cause(s).

Causality   An event or factor (A) is generally argued to have caused another one (B) if the following conditions are met: (i) if (A) occurs then (B) occurs; (ii) if (A) does not occur then (B) does not occur; (iii) if (A) precedes (B) in time.

Central tendency   The central tendency of a frequency distribution is the average, middle or most common score. Measures of central tendency include the mean, the median and the mode.

Chi-square   A statistical test often used with categorical data. It is based on a comparison of the frequencies observed and the frequencies expected in the various categories.

Clinical significance   The clinical significance of a research finding is the extent to which that finding is clinically meaningful.

Closed response format   A method of eliciting answers from people in a questionnaire in which the researcher provides fixed response categories e.g. Yes or No.

Coding   A qualitative method of analysis of materials such as interviews where categories are formed and their interrelationships examined.

Complete observer   A type of research strategy in which the researcher observes social interactions with no direct personal input; for example, observation via a one-way mirror or through the analysis of a video tape.

Complete participant   A research strategy in which the researcher completely participates in the research setting in order to experience its characteristics.

Confidence interval   The confidence interval of a sample statistic is the expected range in which the actual population value will be found, at a given level of confidence or probability.

Content validity   The extent to which a test or assessment matches the real requirements of the situation e.g. a living skills assessment would have high content validity if it measured cooking, self care etc.

Contingency table   A method of presenting the relationship between two categorical variables in the form of a table.

Continuous data   Data with values that do not fall into discrete categories. For example, measures of temperature and mass.

Control   In an experiment, the researcher attempts to control or eliminate the influence of extraneous variables so that any changes or differences may be attributed solely to the intervention.

Control group   In an experiment, a control group is generally a non-treatment group which is compared with the experimental group, to study the effects of the intervention.

Correlation coefficient   A statistic designed to measure the size and direction of the association between two variables. The values vary between 0 and ± 1.

Correlational studies   Studies that are concerned with investigating the associations between variables.

Critical theory   In qualitative research, critical theory explains how personal meanings and actions are influenced by the person's social environment.

Critical value of a statistic   The value of the statistic (obtained from appropriate tables) that the calculated value for a given result must exceed, in order to attain statistical significance.

Curvilinear correlation coefficient   A measure of association between variables designed to investigate curved rather than straight line relationships.

Data   The information collected by a researcher.

Deduction   A process where a general principle is applied to a particular case to explain it, e.g. all humans die; this is a human, therefore he or she will die.

Descriptive statistics   Statistics designed to describe characteristics of a sample. For example, the most common or typical value or the extent of variation amongst such values.

Determinism   The view that all events are caused by other events.

Directional hypothesis   A directional hypothesis is one that asserts that differences between groups in the data will occur in a particular direction. For example, the hypothesis 'smokers die younger than non-smokers' is a directional hypothesis.

Discontinuous data   Sometimes termed discrete data; variables that have discrete categories, for example male versus female.

Discussion   A section of a research report in which the research findings are discussed.

Dispersion   Sometimes known as variability; the extent to which scores in a group of scores vary. This may be measured by statistics such as the standard deviation, variance, range and semi-interquartile range.

Ecological validity   The extent to which the results of a study may be generalized to the real world.

Effect size   The amount of change created by an intervention, especially in an experimental study.

Empathy   In qualitative research, the ability to understand the perspectives of others.

Epidemiology   The study of the distribution and determinants of disease within a community.

Ethics   A project is ethical to the extent that its design and execution conforms to a set of standards or conventions guiding research.

Ethnomethodology   A qualitative approach to research which involves the study of social processes associated with the ways in which people perceive, describe and explain the world.

Ethnography   A descriptive qualitative study, often of an individual or situation, usually written from the perspective of the participant(s) in the first person.

Expected frequency   In the analysis of categorical data, the expected frequency is the one that would be expected in a particular category, under certain theoretical conditions. The expected frequency of women in a sample of 100 people would be 50, if equal proportions of sexes were assumed.

Experiment   A research design involving the random allocation of subjects to groups and the application of different interventions to these groups. A non-intervention control group is often employed in an experimental design. The aim of an experiment is to be able to validly conclude that differences in outcomes for the groups were caused by the different interventions.

External validity   The extent to which the results of the study may be generalized to the population.

Extreme response mode   A method of responding to questions in which the respondent chooses the most extreme available response categories.

Factorial design   A type of research design in which combinations of several independent variables are manipulated concurrently. A 2×2 factorial design involves the manipulation of two independent variables each with two levels.

False negative   The situation that occurs when a diagnostic test indicates that the person being assessed does not have a disease when they actually do.

False positive   The situation that occurs when a diagnostic test indicates the person being assessed has a disease when they actually do not.

Forced response format   A method of eliciting responses to a questionnaire in which there is no middle response category. This is sometimes done to avoid acquiescent response mode.

Frequency distribution The way in which scores within a given sample or population are distributed.

Frequency polygon A method of graphing frequency distributions.

Grounded theory A qualitative research approach that advocates the development of theories to explain social phenomena grounded in data, following a process of induction, deduction and verification.

Hawthorne effect An effect which results in the improvement of peoples' performances through being observed and/or social contact. An example of a placebo effect.

Histogram A method of graphing frequency distributions.

History A threat to the validity of studies in which unforeseen and uncontrolled events occur to the participants during the study that are outside the control of the researcher and which may be responsible for changes in the participants.

Hypothesis A proposition advanced by the researcher which is evaluated using the collected data.

Incidence rate The occurrence of new cases of a disease or condition within a specified time frame. *See also* prevalence.

Incidental sample A method of sampling in which the researcher takes the most conveniently available cases.

Independent variable In an experiment an independent variable is the variable or condition manipulated by the researcher.

Induction The process in which a set of observations is made and a general principle formed to explain them. For example, every human I have read about eventually dies; this is a human; therefore I expect him or her to die.

Informed consent The situation where a competent person, in possession of all the relevant facts, has agreed to participate in a research study.

Instrumentation In a study, instrumentation may be a threat to internal validity. It refers to the situation when the instrumentation changes over the period of the study, thus invalidating comparison of measured results.

Internal validity In a study, internal validity refers to the ability of the researcher to attribute differences in the groups or participants to the independent variable.

Interobserver reliability The extent to which observers rating a particular phenomenon agree with each other.

Interrupted time series A type of research design in which a case is repeatedly measured over time to produce a series of measurements. The series is interrupted by an intervention or event, the effects of which may then be monitored by continuing the measurement series.

Interval scale   A type of measurement scale with the following properties: (i) the values are distinguishable, (ii) they are ordered, (iii) the intervals between the points on the scale are equal, (iv) the zero point is not absolute, i.e. does not represent the absence of the quantity.

Interview   A conversation between one or more interviewers and interviewees with the purpose of eliciting certain information.

Intraobserver reliability   The extent to which an observer rating a particular phenomenon agrees with their own rating when presented with the same task on two different occasions.

Likert scale   A Likert scale is a five point response scale used in questionnaires, e.g. strongly agree, agree, undecided, disagree, strongly disagree.

Literature review   This is a section of a research report in which the previous research that has been done in the area is reviewed and related to the present problem being studied.

Matching   In a study, subjects may be assigned to their groups using matching or random assignment. In matching in a two group study, pairs of similar 'matched' subjects are formed and then one member of the pair is randomly assigned to one group and the other member to the other group. This ensures that the two groups have similar characteristics.

Maturation   The phenomenon where participants in a study change spontaneously over time due to natural maturational changes. For example, children may grow older or an infection may spontaneously clear up.

Mean   The average of a group of scores. For example, the mean of the scores 7, 8 and 9 is $(7+8+9) \div 3 = 8$. In statistical notation the mean of a sample is represented by the symbol $\overline{X}$. The mean of a population is represented by the symbol μ.

Measurement   A procedure where qualities or quantities are attributed to characteristics of objects, persons or events. Weighing a patient involves a measurement process as does a clinical judgment about whether a symptom is present or not.

Median   The 'middle' score of a group of scores. For example, the median of the scores, 7, 8 and 9 is 8. The median is the 50 percentile. The median is often used in preference to the mean when a group of scores contains a small number of extremely small or large scores because it is less sensitive to extreme values.

Mode   The mode is the most frequently occurring score in a group of scores. For example, the mode of the scores 7, 8, 8, 9, 10 is 8.

Mortality   Used to describe a situation where some participants in a study are unable to continue in a study. This might be because they died or because they refuse to continue. If there is high mortality in a group in a study this can jeopardise the internal validity of the study, because differences between the groups may be due to differential mortality.

Multiple group time series   A type of research design where two groups or cases are repeatedly measured over time to produce a series of measurements. One group or case receives an intervention and the other does not. The effects of intervention may then be studied by comparing the two series.

$n = 1$ design   A research design in which one subject rather than a group of subjects is studied.

n   The symbol used to represent the number of cases in a sample.

N   The symbol used to represent the number of cases in a population.

Natural setting   The normal setting of the phenomenon or people under study. Studies performed under laboratory conditions may sometimes have diminished external validity.

Natural comparison study   A type of study in which naturally occurring groups are compared with one another. For example, the health status of smokers versus non smokers may be studied in a natural comparison study. The researcher does not assign the participants to the groups. These are naturally occurring. Studies of gender differences are natural comparisons.

Negative correlation   A correlation is a measure of the strength and direction of the association between two variables. A negative correlation between two variables implies that as one variable gets bigger the value of the other variable becomes smaller.

Negative skew   A frequency distribution where there is a long tail towards the negative end of the X axis. The figure below represents both positively and negatively skewed samples.

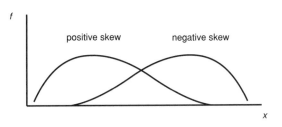

The position of 'tail' of the distribution determines whether the skew is positive or negative.

Nominal scale   Measurement scales may be either nominal, ordinal, interval or ratio. A nominal scale (often called a categorical scale) is one in which the values are distinct categories e.g. male or female, Catholic or Protestant or

Jewish or Muslim. It has the property of distinctiveness of values, but not ordering, equidistant intervals or an absolute zero.

Non-directional hypothesis   A non-directional hypothesis asserts that there are differences between groups in the data but with no direction specified. For example, the hypothesis 'smokers and non-smokers have different life expectancies' is a non-directional hypothesis.

Non-experimental study   A study in which the researcher observes a situation but does not systematically manipulate or experiment with it. This may also be called a descriptive design.

Non-parametric test   Statistical tests are chosen on the basis of the type of scales that are being analysed. Statistical tests that are suitable for the analysis of ordinal or nominal data are termed non-parametric.

Normal curve   A bell shaped curve as shown in the figure below.

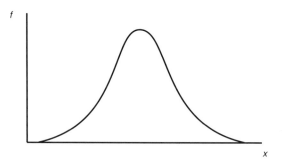

The normal curve is symmetrical and unimodal (has one peak).

Null hypothesis   The hypothesis in a study that asserts there is no difference between groups or relationship between variables. The statistician normally poses the null hypothesis and then tests it statistically. If it is rejected, the alternative hypothesis (that there is a difference between two groups or a relationship between variables) is accepted. The null hypothesis is re-presented by the symbol H_0.

Objective measures   Measures derived from a mechanical measuring process involving a minimum amount of human interpretation, e.g. weight measurements.

Observation   A situation where the researcher studies the phenomenon without deliberate intervention.

Observed frequency   The actual number of occurrences of an event observed by a researcher. For example, the observed frequency of females who passed the exam in a group of students might be 37 students. *See also* expected frequency.

Observer as participant   Where the researcher studies the behaviour of a group by actively participating in the group's activities and situation.

One tailed test   A statistical test where a difference between two groups is expected to occur in a particular direction. For example, it may be hypothesized that smokers will have more health problems than non-smokers. This would be tested by applying a one tailed test of significance.

Open ended question   If a question is asked without a pre-defined set of responses it is an open ended question. For example, the question, "What did you think about the program?" is an open ended question.

Operational definition   The specific way in which a concept or variable has been measured in a study. For example, the operational definition of anxiety in a study might be scores from the Spielberger State-Trait Anxiety Inventory scores or a self rating on a 1 to 10 scale.

Ordinal scale   Measurement scales may be either nominal, ordinal, interval or ratio. An ordinal scale has the following properties: (i) the values are distinguishable, (ii) they are ordered but the intervals between the points are not equidistant nor is there a meaningful zero point scale. The values of an ordinal scale are often ranked, e.g. 1st, 3rd.

Parametric test   Statistical tests are chosen on the basis of the type of data being analysed. Statistical tests that are suitable for the analysis of interval or ratio data are termed parametric.

Participation   A situation where the researcher studies the phenomenon by actively participating.

Phenomenology   In qualitative research, the study and understanding of human conscious experience.

Pie diagram   A graphical method of representing the frequency distribution of a set of categorical data in the shape of a pie.

Pilot study   A preliminary study where the procedures and protocols are tested or 'piloted'.

Placebo effect   The phenomenon where an otherwise worthless intervention in a study nevertheless induces an improvement in the patient's condition or perception of their condition, perhaps due to the expectations of the participants in the study.

Population   A group of people, institutions, cases or objects defined as that under study by the researcher. Samples are drawn from populations. Examples of populations are all coronary heart disease cases in the United Kingdom, all Australian men, all 'not for profit' hospitals in Canada.

Population parameter   A value derived from a population. For example, the average age of all the patients in a population defined by the researcher is a population parameter. In statistical notation, population parameters are represented by Greek letters.

Population validity   The extent to which a sample reflects the characteristics of a population from which it is drawn.

Positive correlation   A correlation is a measure of the strength and direction of the association between two variables. A positive correlation between two variables implies that as the values of one variable get bigger, so do the values of other variable.

Positive skew   A frequency distribution where there is a long tail towards the positive end of the x axis.

Post test only design   A type of experimental study in which measurements of the groups are taken only after an intervention has occurred. This is generally done to avoid the effects of measurement upon people's response to the interventions.

Power   The probability of rejecting the null hypothesis when the alternative hypothesis is true, i.e. correctly identifying an effect when it is there.

Pre-test/post-test design   A type of experimental study in which measurements of the groups are taken both prior to and following an intervention. This allows the direct comparison of pre-intervention and post-intervention results for individual subjects and groups of subjects.

Predictive validity   The extent to which a test or measure can validly predict a future event. For example, a clinical test may have high predictive validity with respect to 5 year mortality of people with cancer. It is often expressed in the form of a correlation coefficient.

Prevalence   The overall occurrence of a particular disease in a specific population at a specific point in time.

Probability   The chance or likelihood of an event. The probability of flipping a 'heads' with a fair coin is 0.5 or 1/2. Probabilities may vary in value from 0 ('no chance') to 1 (certain).

Procedure   A section in a research report that describes the protocol or procedure followed for the collection of data.

Proportion   The ratio of one value to another expressed as a fraction of one. For example, the proportion of women in the adult population is about .5.

Protocol deviation   A deviation from the ideal procedure described as having been followed in a study by the researcher.

Qualitative methods   An approach to research that emphasizes the non-numerical and interpretive analysis of social phenomena.

Quantitative methods   An approach to research that emphasizes the collection of numerical data and the statistical analysis of hypotheses proposed by the researcher.

Quasi experimental design   A structured research design that is experiment-like but does not involve its full characteristics such as a control group and random assignment of subjects to treatment groups.

Questionnaire   A means of collecting data from people where they provide written responses to a set of questions, either in their own words, or by selecting pre-defined answers.

Quota sample   The result of a sampling procedure in which the researcher sets quotas for the number of cases in particular categories to be included in the sample. For example, a sample of 100 might have quotas of 50 men and 50 women. The cases, however, are still selected on the basis of convenience rather than randomly. *See also* stratified random sample.

Random assignment   In an experiment, subjects are assigned to their groups by using a random assignment method. In random assignment, subjects are assigned to their groups using a random procedure. For example, in a two group study the tossing of a coin to assign subjects to groups would be a random assignment procedure.

Random sample   A group of cases drawn from a population such that each member of the population has had an equal chance of selection.

Random sampling   The process of selecting cases from a population such that each member of the population has had an equal chance of selection.

Range   In a group of scores the range is the difference between the maximum and minimum scores.

Ratio scale   Measurement scales may be either nominal, ordinal, interval or ratio. A ratio scale has the following properties: the values are distinctive, ordered, equidistant and the zero point represents an absence of the quantity rather than being an arbitrary zero. Metres and kilograms are examples of ratio scales.

Refereed journal   A journal in which the articles are vetted by independent referees for quality and interest. Refereed journals generally carry more highly regarded articles.

Regression to the mean   Refers to the phenomenon where an individual who is measured on a test and obtains an extreme (very high or low) score and then upon remeasurement tends to move towards (regress) the average score (mean). Regression to the mean may be misinterpreted as representing a real change in score.

Reliability   The extent to which a test or measurement result is reproducible.

Relationships   Associations between variables.

Repeated measures   The situation where a group of cases are measured on more than one occasion, for example prior to and following an intervention.

Representative sample   A sample that accurately reflects the characteristics of the population from which it is drawn. Sometimes termed an 'unbiased' sample.

Reversal   Reversal of the order of interventions is often used in experimental studies to control for the effects of order of administration. For example, intervention B, preceded by intervention A may have a different effect than B followed by A.

Risk factors   In epidemiology, a risk factor is an agent that is believed to increase the probability of a certain outcome or illness. For example, smoking may be a risk factor for the onset of coronary heart disease.

Rosenthal effect   The phenomenon where the expectations of the researchers in a study influence the outcome. For example, if an observer believes that a particular intervention is effective they may under-report or discount symptoms inconsistent with this belief.

Sample   A group of cases selected from a population.

Sampling error   Because a sample is smaller than the population from which it is drawn, there is often a discrepancy between the values obtained for the sample and those that apply to the population. For example the average age of a sample might be 22 years and the average age of the population might be 28 years. This discrepancy is termed the sampling error.

Sampling method   The method by which a sample is drawn from a population. Broadly, there are two approaches: random, in which every case in the population has an equal chance of selection and non-random in which cases have different chances of selection.

Scattergram   A graph displaying the relationship between two variables as shown in the following figure:

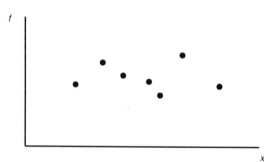

Sensitivity   The proportion of people who test as positive to a disease who really do have the disease *See also* true positive.

Shared variance   In the examination of relationships between variables, researchers are concerned about the extent to which when one variable changes the other also changes. Shared variance refers to the extent to which this occurs.

Skewness   A characteristic of the shape of a frequency distribution. *See also* negative skew.

Specificity   The proportion of people who test negative to a disease who really do not have the disease. *See also* true negative.

Standard deviation   A measure of the dispersion or variability of a group of scores. The standard deviation of a sample is represented by the symbol s and by the symbol σ for a population.

Standard error of the mean   If a number of samples were taken from the same population and the mean calculated for each sample, the standard deviation of this distribution of means is known as the standard error of the mean. The standard error of the mean is used in statistical inferences about population means.

Standard normal curve   An idealised normal or bell-shaped frequency distribution with a mean of 0 and a standard deviation of 1 unit.

Standardized test   A standardized test is one that has known characteristics, especially known levels of reliability and validity. Researchers use standardized tests, wherever possible, in preference to unstandardized tests.

Statistic   A statistic is a number with known properties derived from sample data. There are two types of statistics: inferential statistics which are used to apply statistical tests, descriptive statistics which are used to describe characteristics of the sample.

Statistical significance   When a researcher has demonstrated statistical significance through the application of a statistical test, they have demonstrated that the obtained result is probably not due to chance but is 'real'. This does not mean the result is 'important' or interesting'. *See also* clinical significance.

Stratified random sample   A type of sample in which the researcher wishes to ensure that important sub groups and their representation are preserved in the sample. For example, if a researcher randomly selected a sub sample of 50 men and then 50 women, the sample has been stratified with respect to gender. *See also* quota sample.

Structured interview   An interview in which the questions are generally predefined, i.e. asked in a fixed order with the answers recorded by the researcher on a response sheet.

Subjective measures   Measures derived from a measurement process involving a substantial degree of human interpretation, e.g. subjective ratings of pain, clinical ratings of social skills.

Subjects   Participants in a study.

Surveys   A type of research design in which characteristics of the cases under study are systematically recorded without the researcher attempting to actively change the situation. A non-experimental type of study.

Systematic sample   A method of drawing a sample from a population where say every tenth case is selected from a population list.

Test–retest reliability   When a test or assessment procedure is administered twice to the same group of people, the correlation between the first score and the second score is termed the test–retest reliability. This is a measure of the reproducibility of an assessment procedure.

Time series   A series of measurements taken repeatedly from the same person or group of people, over time.

Transcript   A verbatim written version of an interview.

Transformed score   A score that has been altered by an arithmetic manipulation, such as a z score.

True negative   The situation that occurs when a diagnostic test indicates the person being assessed does have a disease when they really do not.

True positive   The situation that occurs when a diagnostic test indicates the person being assessed does have a disease when they really do.

Two tailed test   A statistical test where a difference between two groups is tested without reference to the expected direction of the difference.

Type I error   When a researcher, on the basis of a statistical test applied to a sample of data, *wrongly* concludes that there is evidence of an association between variables or difference between groups in the population, they have committed a Type I error. The probability of a Type I error is represented by the symbol α.

Type II error   A 'miss'. When a researcher, on the basis of a statistical test applied to a sample of data, *wrongly* concludes that there is no evidence of an association between variables or difference between groups in the population, they have committed a Type II error. The probability of a Type II error is represented by the symbol β.

Unstructured interview   An interview in which there may be no preplanned questions or fixed agenda. The dialogue is usually recorded in a transcript or field notes which are subsequently analysed.

Validity   The extent to which a test measures what it is intended to measure.

Variability   The extent to which a group of scores varies or is spread out. This is usually measured by a descriptive statistic such as the standard deviation range or semi-interquartile range.

Variable   A property or attribute that varies. For example, gender, age, weight are all variables.

Variance   A measure of the dispersion or variability of a group of scores. The variance of a sample is represented by the symbol s^2 and the symbol σ^2 for a population. *See also* standard deviation.

z scores   Transformed scores which express how many standard deviations a specific score is above or below the mean. For instance, a corresponding z score of -2 implies that a given score is two standard deviations below the mean.

Zero correlation   Correlation is used to measure the strength and direction of an association between two variables. A zero correlation implies that two variables are unrelated to one another.

References and further reading

REFERENCES

Anastasi A 1976 Psychological testing, 4th edn. Macmillan, New York
Bailey K D 1987 Methods of social research. Free Press, New York
Beecher H K 1959 Measurement of subjective responses. Oxford University Press, Oxford
Bloch R 1987 Methodology in clinical pain trials. Spine 12:430–432
Broad W, Wade N 1982 Betrayers of the truth. Simon & Schuster, New York
Chalmers A F 1976 What is this thing called science? Queensland University Press, St Lucia
Cohen L, Manion L 1985 Research methods in education. Croom Helm, London
Cook T D, Campbell D T 1979 Quasi-experimentation: design and analysis issues for field
    settings. Rand McNally, Chicago
Coppleson L, Factor R, Strums S, Graff P, Rappaport H 1970 Observer disagreement in the
    classification and histology of Hodgkin's disease. Journal of the National Cancer Institute
    45:731–740
Denzin N K 1978 The research act: a theoretical introduction to sociological methods, 2nd edn.
    Aldine, Chicago
Dooley D 1984 Social research methods. Prentice Hall, New Jersey
Engel G 1977 The need for a new medical model: a challenge for biomedicine. Science
    196:129–136
Feyerabend P 1975 Against method. Verso, London
Field P A, Morse J M 1985 Nursing research: the application of qualitative approaches.
    Rockville, Aspen
Gardner H (ed) 1989 The politics of health: the Australian experience. Churchill Livingstone,
    Melbourne
Glaser B G, Strauss A 1967 The discovery of grounded theory: strategies for qualitative
    research. Aldine, New York
Grundy S 1987 Curriculum: product or praxis. Falmer Press, East Sussex
Guba E G, Lincoln Y S 1983 Epistemological and methodological bases of naturalistic enquiry.
    In: Madaus G F, Scriven M, Stufflebeam D L (eds) Evaluation models. Kluwer Nishoff,
    Boston, pp.311–339
Hay D, Oken D 1977 The psychological stress of intensive care unit nursing. In: Monat A,
    Lazarus R S (eds) Stress and coping. Columbia University Press, New York, pp.118–131
Hersen M, Barlow D H 1976 Single case experimental designs: strategies for studying behaviour
    change. Pergamon, New York
Huck S W, Cormier W H, Bounds W G 1974 Reading statistics and research. Harper & Row,
    New York
Jacobsen G, Thiele J E, McCune J H, Farrell L 1985 Handwashing: ring-wearing and number of
    micro organism. Nursing Research 34:186–188
Krzyzwoski J 1989 The historical development of electroconvulsive therapy. European Journal
    of Psychiatry 3(1):49-54
Kuhn T S 1970 The structure of scientific revolutions. Chicago University Press, Chicago

Laing R D, Esterson A 1970 Sanity, madness and the family. Penguin, London

Lakatos I 1970 Falsification and the methodology of scientific research programmes. In: Lakatos I, Musgrave A (eds) Criticism and the growth of knowledge p 91–196

Lofland J 1971 Analyzing social settings. Wadsworth, Belmont California

McGartland M, Polgar S 1994 Paradigm collapse in psychology: the necessity for a 'two methods' approach. Australian Psychologist 29(1): 21–28

Melzack R F, Wall P D 1965 Pain mechanisms: a new theory. Science 1250:971

Merton R K 1946 The focused interview. American Journal of Sociology 51:541–557

Minichiello V, Aroni R, Timewell E, Alexander L 1991 In depth interviewing. Longman Cheshire, Melbourne

Rosenhan D L 1975 On being sane in insane places. In: Krupat E (ed) Psychology is social. Scott Foresman, Glenview, Illinois, pp.189–200

Rosenthal R 1976 Experimenter effects in behavioural research. Irvington, New York

Schatzman L, Strauss A L 1973 Field research: strategies for a natural sociology. Prentice Hall, Englewood Cliffs, New Jersey

Strauss A L 1987 Qualitative analysis for social scientists. Cambridge University Press, New York

Taylor R 1979 Medicine out of control. Sun Books, Melbourne

Taylor S J, Bogdan R C 1984 Introduction to qualitative research methods: the search for personal meanings, 2nd edn. Wiley, New York

Teltscher B, Polgar S 1981 Objective knowledge about Huntington's disease and attitudes towards predictive tests of persons at risk. Journal of Medical Genetics 18(1):31–39

Thomas S A, Henry P, McCoy A, Smith J 1989 Why do parents stay overnight with children in hospitals? Australian Health Review 12(2) 39–49

Thomas S A, Wearing A, Bennett M 1991 Clinical decision making for nurses and health professionals. Harcourt Brace Jovanovich, Sydney

Thomas S A, Steven I, Browning C, Dickens E, Eckermann E, Carey L, Pollard S 1992 Focus groups in health research: a methodological review. Annual Review of Health Social Sciences 2:7–20

Thomas S A, Steven I, Browning C, Dickens E, Eckermann E, Carey L, Pollard S 1993 Patient knowledge, opinions, satisfaction and choices in primary health care provision: a progress report. In: Doessel D P (ed) The general practice evaluation program: the 1992 work-in progress conference. Australian Government Publishing Service, Canberra

Walker Q, Langlands A 1986 The nurse of mammography in the management of breast cancer. Medical Journal of Australia 1435:185–187

FURTHER READING

Babbie E 1979 The practice of social research, 2nd edn. Wadsworth, Belmont California
    This book offers a lucid theoretical account of social research methods.

Bailey K D 1978 Methods of social research. Free Press, New York
    This is an excellent book with a very good set of chapters on survey design and execution

Castle W M 1976 Statistics in small doses, 2nd edn. Churchill Livingstone, Edinburgh
    This is a good little book for extra computational examples in statistics.

Cook T D, Campbell D T: 1979 Quasi-experimentation: design and analysis issues for field settings. Rand McNally, Chicago
    Following on from Campbell's earlier book with Stanley, this text offers an excellent account of design and control issues in quasi-experimental research, with an excellent chapter on philosophy of science issues.

Hersen M, Barlow D H 1976 Single case experimental designs: strategies for studying behaviour change. Pergamon, New York
    This is a useful book for additional reading in the area of single case experimental approaches. It is, however, rather lengthy in its descriptions of the theory rather than the practicalities of carrying out such research.

Minichiello V. Aroni R, Timewell E, Alexander L 1991 In depth interviewing. Churchill Livingstone, Melbourne
    An excellent text for qualitative researchers who use interviews in their research.

Moser C, Kalton G 1971 Survey methods in social investigation, 2nd edn. Heinemann, London
    An excellent book on survey methods.

Answers to questions

Chapter 1

True or False

1. T
2. F
3. T
4. T
5. T
6. T
7. F
8. F
9. F
10. F
11. F
12. T
13. T
14. T
15. F
16. T
17. T
18. F
19. T
20. F

Multiple Choice

1. d
2. b
3. b
4. a
5. c
6. a
7. c
8. d
9. b
10. c
11. a
12. d
13. c
14. d
15. c
16. a

Chapter 2

True or False

1. F
2. F
3. F
4. F
5. T
6. F
7. T
8. F
9. T
10. F
11. F
12. T
13. F
14. T
15. F
16. T
17. T
18. F
19. F
20. T
21. T
22. F
23. T
24. F
25. F
26. F
27. F
28. T

Multiple Choice

1. e
2. d
3. b
4. a
5. b
6. b
7. c
8. b
9. d
10. d
11. c

Chapter 3

True or False

1. T
2. F
3. T
4. T
5. T
6. F
7. F
8. F
9. F
10. F
11. F
12. F
13. F
14. T
15. F
16. F
17. T
18. T
19. T
20. F
21. F
22. T
23. F

Multiple Choice

1. a
2. d
3. a
4. c
5. d
6. a
7. d
8. b
9. a
10. c
11. b
12. c
13. c

Chapter 4

True or False

1. F
2. F
3. T
4. F
5. F
6. T
7. F
8. F
9. T
10. T

Multiple Choice

1. a
2. b
3. c
4. d
5. c
6. a
7. a
8. d

Chapter 5

True or False

1. T
2. T
3. F
4. F
5. F
6. F
7. T
8. F

Multiple Choice

1. d
2. c
3. b
4. c
5. d
6. c
7. c
8. a
9. d
10. a
11. d
12. c
13. a
14. c
15. a
16. d
17. b
18. a
19. d
20. d

Chapter 6

True or False

1. T
2. F
3. T
4. T
5. T
6. F
7. T
8. T
9. T
10. T
11. F
12. T
13. F
14. F
15. F
16. T
17. T
18. F
19. T
20. F
21. F
22. T

Multiple Choice

1. d
2. b
3. d
4. a
5. d
6. d
7. a
8. b
9. d
10. b
11. d
12. a
13. c
14. d

Chapter 7

True or False

1. F
2. T
3. F
4. F
5. F
6. T
7. F
8. T
9. F
10. T
11. F
12. F
13. T
14. T
15. F
16. T

Multiple Choice

1. c
2. b
3. c
4. a
5. a
6. c
7. c
8. c
9. c
10. c

Chapter 8

True or False

1. T
2. F
3. T
4. F
5. F
6. F
7. F
8. T
9. T
10. T
11. F
12. T

Multiple Choice

1. b
2. d
3. d
4. b
5. a
6. a
7. c

Chapter 9

True or False

1. F
2. T
3. F
4. F
5. F
6. F
7. F
8. T
9. F
10. T

Multiple Choice

1. a
2. a
3. d
4. c
5. c
6. d
7. b
8. b
9. c

Chapter 10

True or False

1. F
2. F
3. F
4. T
5. T
6. F
7. F
8. T

Multiple Choice

1. a
2. b
3. d
4. c
5. c
6. d
7. c
8. a

Chapter 11

True or False

1. T
2. F
3. T
4. T
5. F
6. F
7. T
8. F
9. F
10. T

Multiple Choice

1. b
2. a
3. c
4. c
5. d
6. c
7. a
8. c

Chapter 12

True or False

1. T
2. T
3. T
4. F
5. F
6. T
7. T
8. F
9. T
10. T
11. F
12. F
13. F
14. F
15. T
16. F
17. F
18. T
19. T
20. T
21. T
22. F
23. F
24. T
25. F
26. F
27. T
28. T
29. F
30. T

Mutliple Choice

1. a
2. e
3. b
4. e
5. c
6. d
7. b
8. a
9. b
10. b
11. a
12. c
13. a
14. a
15. d
16. a
17. c
18. d
19. c
20. a

Chapter 13

True or False

1. T
2. F
3. T
4. T
5. F
6. T
7. F
8. F
9. F
10. F
11. T
12. T
13. T
14. F
15. T
16. T
17. F
18. T
19. F
20. F
21. F
22. F

Multiple Choice

1. b
2. e
3. c
4. e
5. d
6. d
7. c
8. b
9. d
10. c
11. d
12. c
13. a
14. a
15. a
16. a
17. c
18. c
19. b
20. a
21. a
22. c
23. c
24. b
25. a
26. d
27. d
28. b
29. d

Chapter 14

True or False

1. F
2. F
3. T
4. F
5. T
6. F
7. T
8. T
9. T
10. T
11. F
12. F
13. T
14. T
15. T
16. T
17. T
18. T
19. T
20. T
21. T
22. F
23. T
24. F
25. F

Multiple Choice

1. b
2. d
3. a
4. d
5. c
6. b
7. a
8. d
9. b
10. c
11. a
12. d
13. d
14. c
15. d
16. a
17. c
18. b
19. a
20. b
21. c
22. b
23. d
24. b
25. a
26. d
27. a
28. c

Chapter 15

True or False

1. T
2. F
3. F
4. F
5. T
6. T
7. F
8. F
9. T
10. F
11. F
12. F
13. T
14. F
15. T
16. F
17. T
18. T
19. F
20. T

Multiple Choice

1. d
2. c
3. c
4. d
5. a
6. b
7. d
8. e
9. a
10. c
11. b
12. c
13. d
14. d
15. b
16. d
17. c
18. a
19. b
20. c
21. d
22. c
23. b
24. a
25. d

Chapter 16

True or False

1. F
2. T
3. T
4. T
5. F
6. T
7. T
8. F
9. F
10. T
11. F
12. T
13. F
14. T
15. F
16. T
17. T
18. F
19. T
20. T
21. F
22. F
23. F
24. T
25. F
26. F
27. F
28. F
29. T

Multiple Choice

1. a
2. d
3. e
4. b
5. c
6. d
7. a
8. b
9. c
10. b
11. c
12. c
13. d
14. c
15. b
16. e
17. a
18. b
19. d
20. e
21. c
22. b
23. a

Chapter 17

True or False

1. F
2. T
3. F
4. T
5. F
6. T
7. T
8. F
9. T
10. T
11. F
12. T
13. T
14. F
15. F
16. T
17. T
18. F
19. F
20. T

Multiple Choice

1. a
2. c
3. a
4. a
5. d
6. c
7. a
8. b
9. c
10. c
11. b
12. a
13. b
14. d
15. a
16. b
17. c
18. b
19. d
20. c
21. a
22. b
23. d
24. a
25. c
26. c
27. b
28. c
29. c
30. c
31. b
32. d
33. b
34. a
35. a

Chapter 18

True or False

1. T
2. F
3. T
4. T
5. T
6. T
7. F
8. T
9. T
10. T
11. F
12. F
13. T
14. T
15. T
16. T
17. T
18. T
19. F
20. T

Multiple Choice

1. a
2. d
3. d
4. e
5. c
6. b
7. a
8. d
9. a
10. d
11. d
12. d
13. e
14. d
15. a
16. a
17. d
18. c
19. a
20. d
21. a
22. b
23. e
24. c

Chapter 19

True or False

1. T
2. F
3. F
4. T
5. F
6. T
7. F
8. T
9. T
10. F
11. T
12. T
13. T
14. T
15. F
16. T
17. T
18. T
19. T
20. F

Multiple Choice

1. d
2. b
3. d
4. c
5. c
6. f
7. c
8. c
9. a
10. d
11. b
12. c
13. b
14. a
15. b
16. c
17. a
18. a
19. b
20. c
21. c
22. a
23. d
24. a
25. b
26. a
27. d
28. a
29. a
30. b
31. a

Chapter 20

True or False

1. F
2. F
3. T
4. F
5. F
6. T
7. F
8. T
9. T
10. F

Multiple Choice

1. c
2. c
3. a
4. a
5. a
6. a
7. c
8. a
9. a
10. b

Chapter 21

True or False

1. F
2. T
3. T
4. F
5. F
6. T
7. F
8. T
9. T
10. T
11. F
12. T
13. F
14. F
15. F
16. T
17. T
18. F
19. F

Multiple Choice

1. b
2. b
3. b
4. a
5. c
6. d
7. b
8. d
9. a
10. d

Chapter 22

True or False

1. T
2. F
3. F
4. T
5. F
6. T
7. F
8. T
9. F
10. F
11. F
12. F
13. T
14. T
15. F
16. T
17. T
18. T
19. T

Multiple Choice

1. d
2. c
3. d
4. d
5. d
6. b
7. a
8. d
9. b
10. c
11. d
12. d
13. d
14. b
15. d
16. d
17. c
18. c
19. a

Appendix A — z scores and associated areas between z and mean and beyond

z	area between mean and z	area beyond z	z	area between mean and z	area beyond z	z	area between mean and z	area beyond z	z	area between mean and z	area beyond z	z	area between mean and z	area beyond z	z	area between mean and z	area beyond z
0.00	.0000	.5000	0.55	.2088	.2912	1.10	.3643	.1357	1.65	.4505	.0495	2.22	.4868	.0132	2.79	.4974	.0026
0.01	.0040	.4960	0.56	.2123	.2877	1.11	.3665	.1335	1.66	.4515	.0485	2.23	.4871	.0129	2.80	.4974	.0026
0.02	.0080	.4920	0.57	.2157	.2843	1.12	.3686	.1314	1.67	.4525	.0475	2.24	.4875	.0125	2.81	.4975	.0025
0.03	.0120	.4880	0.58	.2190	.2810	1.13	.3708	.1292	1.68	.4535	.0465	2.25	.4878	.0122	2.82	.4976	.0024
0.04	.0160	.4840	0.59	.2224	.2776	1.14	.3729	.1271	1.69	.4545	.0455	2.26	.4881	.0119	2.83	.4977	.0023
0.05	.0199	.4801	0.60	.2257	.2743	1.15	.3749	.1251	1.70	.4554	.0446	2.27	.4884	.0116	2.84	.4977	.0023
0.06	.0239	.4761	0.61	.2291	.2709	1.16	.3770	.1230	1.71	.4564	.0436	2.28	.4887	.0113	2.85	.4978	.0022
0.07	.0279	.4721	0.62	.2324	.2676	1.17	.3790	.1210	1.72	.4573	.0427	2.29	.4890	.0110	2.86	.4979	.0021
0.08	.0319	.4681	0.63	.2357	.2643	1.18	.3810	.1190	1.73	.4582	.0418	2.30	.4893	.0107	2.87	.4979	.0021
0.09	.0359	.4641	0.64	.2389	.2611	1.19	.3830	.1170	1.74	.4591	.0409	2.31	.4896	.0104	2.88	.4980	.0020
0.10	.0398	.4602	0.65	.2422	.2578	1.20	.3849	.1151	1.75	.4599	.0401	2.32	.4898	.0102	2.89	.4981	.0019
0.11	.0438	.4562	0.66	.2454	.2546	1.21	.3869	.1131	1.76	.4608	.0392	2.33	.4901	.0099	2.90	.4981	.0019
0.12	.0478	.4522	0.67	.2486	.2514	1.22	.3888	.1112	1.77	.4616	.0384	2.34	.4904	.0096	2.91	.4982	.0018
0.13	.0517	.4483	0.68	.2517	.2483	1.23	.3907	.1093	1.78	.4625	.0375	2.35	.4906	.0094	2.92	.4982	.0018
0.14	.0557	.4443	0.69	.2549	.2451	1.24	.3925	.1075	1.79	.4633	.0367	2.36	.4909	.0091	2.93	.4983	.0017
0.15	.0596	.4404	0.70	.2580	.2420	1.25	.3944	.1056	1.80	.4641	.0359	2.37	.4911	.0089	2.94	.4984	.0016
0.16	.0636	.4364	0.71	.2611	.2389	1.26	.3962	.1038	1.81	.4649	.0351	2.38	.4913	.0087	2.95	.4984	.0016
0.17	.0675	.4325	0.72	.2642	.2358	1.27	.3980	.1020	1.82	.4656	.0344	2.39	.4916	.0084	2.96	.4985	.0015
0.18	.0714	.4286	0.73	.2673	.2327	1.28	.3997	.1003	1.83	.4664	.0336	2.40	.4918	.0082	2.97	.4985	.0015
0.19	.0753	.4247	0.74	.2704	.2296	1.29	.4015	.0985	1.84	.4671	.0329	2.41	.4920	.0080	2.98	.4986	.0014
0.20	.0793	.4207	0.75	.2734	.2266	1.30	.4032	.0968	1.85	.4678	.0322	2.42	.4922	.0078	2.99	.4986	.0014
0.21	.0832	.4168	0.76	.2764	.2236	1.31	.4049	.0951	1.86	.4686	.0314	2.43	.4925	.0075	3.00	.4987	.0013
0.22	.0871	.4129	0.77	.2794	.2206	1.32	.4066	.0934	1.87	.4693	.0307	2.44	.4927	.0073	3.01	.4987	.0013
0.23	.0910	.4090	0.78	.2823	.2177	1.33	.4082	.0918	1.88	.4699	.0301	2.45	.4929	.0071	3.02	.4987	.0013
0.24	.0948	.4052	0.79	.2852	.2148	1.34	.4099	.0901	1.89	.4706	.0294	2.46	.4931	.0069	3.03	.4988	.0012

0.25	.0987	.4013	0.80	.2881	.2119	1.35	.4115	.0885	1.90	.4713	.0287	2.47	.4932	.0068	3.04	.4988	.0012
0.26	.1026	.3974	0.81	.2910	.2090	1.36	.4131	.0869	1.91	.4719	.0281	2.48	.4934	.0066	3.05	.4989	.0011
0.27	.1064	.3936	0.82	.2939	.2061	1.37	.4147	.0853	1.92	.4726	.0274	2.49	.4936	.0064	3.06	.4989	.0011
0.28	.1103	.3897	0.83	.2967	.2033	1.38	.4162	.0838	1.93	.4732	.0268	2.50	.4938	.0062	3.07	.4989	.0011
0.29	.1141	.3859	0.84	.2995	.2005	1.39	.4177	.0823	1.94	.4738	.0262	2.51	.4940	.0060	3.08	.4990	.0010
0.30	.1179	.3821	0.85	.3023	.1977	1.40	.4192	.0808	1.95	.4744	.0256	2.52	.4941	.0059	3.09	.4990	.0010
0.31	.1217	.3783	0.86	.3051	.1949	1.41	.4207	.0793	1.96	.4750	.0250	2.53	.4943	.0057	3.10	.4990	.0010
0.32	.1255	.3745	0.87	.3078	.1922	1.42	.4222	.0778	1.97	.4756	.0244	2.54	.4945	.0055	3.11	.4991	.0009
0.33	.1293	.3707	0.88	.3106	.1894	1.43	.4236	.0764	1.98	.4761	.0239	2.55	.4946	.0054	3.12	.4991	.0009
0.34	.1331	.3669	0.89	.3133	.1867	1.44	.4251	.0749	1.99	.4767	.0233	2.56	.4948	.0052	3.13	.4991	.0009
0.35	.1368	.3632	0.90	.3159	.1841	1.45	.4265	.0735	2.00	.4772	.0228	2.57	.4949	.0051	3.14	.4992	.0008
0.36	.1406	.3594	0.91	.3186	.1814	1.46	.4279	.0721	2.01	.4778	.0222	2.58	.4951	.0049	3.15	.4992	.0008
0.37	.1443	.3557	0.92	.3212	.1788	1.47	.4292	.0708	2.02	.4783	.0217	2.59	.4952	.0048	3.16	.4992	.0008
0.38	.1480	.3520	0.93	.3238	.1762	1.48	.4306	.0694	2.03	.4788	.0212	2.60	.4953	.0047	3.17	.4992	.0008
0.39	.1517	.3483	0.94	.3264	.1736	1.49	.4319	.0681	2.04	.4793	.0207	2.61	.4955	.0045	3.18	.4993	.0007
0.40	.1554	.3446	0.95	.3289	.1711	1.50	.4332	.0668	2.05	.4798	.0202	2.62	.4956	.0044	3.19	.4993	.0007
0.41	.1591	.3409	0.96	.3315	.1685	1.51	.4345	.0655	2.06	.4803	.0197	2.63	.4957	.0043	3.20	.4993	.0007
0.42	.1628	.3372	0.97	.3340	.1660	1.52	.4357	.0643	2.07	.4808	.0192	2.64	.4959	.0041	3.21	.4993	.0007
0.43	.1664	.3336	0.98	.3365	.1635	1.53	.4370	.0630	2.08	.4812	.0188	2.65	.4960	.0040	3.22	.4994	.0006
0.44	.1700	.3300	0.99	.3389	.1611	1.54	.4382	.0618	2.09	.4817	.0183	2.66	.4961	.0039	3.23	.4994	.0006
0.45	.1736	.3264	1.00	.3413	.1587	1.55	.4394	.0606	2.10	.4821	.0179	2.67	.4962	.0038	3.24	.4994	.0006
0.46	.1772	.3228	1.01	.3438	.1562	1.56	.4406	.0594	2.11	.4826	.0174	2.68	.4963	.0037	3.25	.4994	.0006
0.47	.1808	.3192	1.02	.3461	.1539	1.57	.4418	.0582	2.12	.4830	.0170	2.69	.4964	.0036	3.30	.4995	.0005
0.48	.1844	.3156	1.03	.3485	.1515	1.58	.4429	.0571	2.13	.4834	.0166	2.70	.4965	.0035	3.35	.4996	.0004
0.49	.1879	.3121	1.04	.3508	.1492	1.59	.4441	.0559	2.14	.4838	.0162	2.71	.4966	.0034	3.40	.4997	.0003
0.50	.1915	.3085	1.05	.3531	.1469	1.60	.4452	.0548	2.15	.4842	.0158	2.72	.4967	.0033	3.45	.4997	.0003
0.51	.1950	.3050	1.06	.3554	.1446	1.61	.4463	.0537	2.16	.4846	.0154	2.73	.4968	.0032	3.50	.4998	.0002
0.52	.1985	.3015	1.07	.3577	.1423	1.62	.4474	.0526	2.17	.4850	.0150	2.74	.4969	.0031	3.60	.4998	.0002
0.53	.2019	.2981	1.08	.3599	.1401	1.63	.4484	.0516	2.18	.4854	.0146	2.75	.4970	.0030	3.70	.4999	.0001
0.54	.2054	.2946	1.09	.3621	.1379	1.64	.4495	.0505	2.19	.4857	.0143	2.76	.4971	.0029	3.80	.4999	.0001
									2.20	.4861	.0139	2.77	.4972	.0028	3.90	.49995	.00005
									2.21	.4864	.0136	2.78	.4973	.0027	4.00	.49997	.00003

Appendix B —— t distribution

Directional p	0.4	0.25	0.1	0.05	0.025	0.01	0.005	0.001
Non-directional p	0.8	0.5	0.2	0.1	0.05	0.02	0.01	0.002
Degrees of freedom								
1	0.325	1.000	3.078	6.314	12.706	31.821	63.657	318.31
2	.289	0.816	1.886	2.920	4.303	6.965	9.925	22.326
3	.277	.765	1.638	2.353	3.182	4.541	5.841	10.213
4	.271	.741	1.533	2.132	2.776	3.747	4.604	7.173
5	0.267	0.727	1.476	2.015	2.571	3.365	4.032	5.893
6	.265	.718	1.440	1.943	2.447	3.143	3.707	5.208
7	.263	.711	1.415	1.895	2.365	2.998	3.499	4.785
8	.262	.706	1.397	1.860	2.306	2.896	3.355	4.501
9	.261	.703	1.383	1.833	2.262	2.821	3.250	4.297
10	0.260	0.700	1.372	1.812	2.228	2.764	3.169	4.144
11	.260	.697	1.363	1.796	2.201	2.718	3.106	4.025
12	.259	.695	1.356	1.782	2.179	2.681	3.055	3.930
13	.259	.694	1.350	1.771	2.160	2.650	3.012	3.852
14	.258	.692	1.345	1.761	2.145	2.624	2.977	3.787
15	0.258	0.691	1.341	1.753	2.131	2.602	2.947	3.733
16	.258	.690	1.337	1.746	2.120	2.583	2.921	3.686
17	.257	.689	1.333	1.740	2.110	2.567	2.898	3.646
18	.257	.688	1.330	1.734	2.101	2.552	2.878	3.610
19	.257	.688	1.328	1.729	2.093	2.539	2.861	3.579
20	0.257	0.687	1.325	1.725	2.086	2.528	2.845	3.552
21	.257	.686	1.323	1.721	2.080	2.518	2.831	3.527
22	.256	.686	1.321	1.717	2.074	2.508	2.819	3.505
23	.256	.685	1.319	1.714	2.069	2.500	2.807	3.485
24	.256	.685	1.318	1.711	2.064	2.492	2.797	3.467
25	0.256	0.684	1.316	1.708	2.060	2.485	2.787	3.450
26	.256	.684	1.315	1.706	2.056	2.479	2.779	3.435
27	.256	.684	1.314	1.703	2.052	2.473	2.771	3.421
28	.256	.683	1.313	1.701	2.048	2.467	2.763	3.408
29	.256	.683	1.311	1.699	2.045	2.462	2.756	3.396
30	0.256	0.683	1.310	1.697	2.042	2.457	2.750	3.385
40	.255	.681	1.303	1.684	2.021	2.423	2.704	3.307
60	.254	.679	1.296	1.671	2.000	2.390	2.660	3.232
120	.254	.677	1.289	1.658	1.980	2.358	2.617	3.160
∞	.253	.674	1.282	1.645	1.960	2.326	2.576	3.090

Appendix C — Chi-square

df	.99	.98	.95	.90	.80	.70	.50	.30	.20	.10	.05	.02	.01	.001
1	.00016	.00063	.0039	.016	.064	.15	.46	1.07	1.64	2.71	3.84	5.41	6.64	10.83
2	.02	.04	.10	.21	.45	.71	1.39	2.41	3.22	4.60	5.99	7.82	9.21	13.82
3	.12	.18	.35	.58	1.00	1.42	2.37	3.66	4.64	6.25	7.82	9.84	11.34	16.27
4	.30	.43	.71	1.06	1.65	2.20	3.36	4.88	5.99	7.78	9.49	11.67	13.28	18.46
5	.55	.75	1.14	1.61	2.34	3.00	4.35	6.06	7.29	9.24	11.07	13.39	15.09	20.52
6	.87	1.13	1.64	2.20	3.07	3.83	5.35	7.23	8.56	10.64	12.59	15.03	16.81	22.46
7	1.24	1.56	2.17	2.83	3.82	4.67	6.35	8.38	9.80	12.02	14.07	16.62	18.48	24.32
8	1.65	2.03	2.73	3.49	4.59	5.53	7.34	9.52	11.03	13.36	15.51	18.17	20.09	26.12
9	2.09	2.53	3.32	4.17	5.38	6.39	8.34	10.66	12.24	14.68	16.92	19.68	21.67	27.88
10	2.56	3.06	3.94	4.86	6.18	7.27	9.34	11.78	13.44	15.99	18.31	21.16	23.21	29.59
11	3.05	3.61	4.58	5.58	6.99	8.15	10.34	12.90	14.63	17.28	19.68	22.62	24.72	31.26
12	3.57	4.18	5.23	6.30	7.81	9.03	11.34	14.01	15.81	18.55	21.03	24.05	26.22	32.91
13	4.11	4.76	5.89	7.04	8.63	9.93	12.34	15.12	16.98	19.81	22.36	25.47	27.69	34.53
14	4.66	5.37	6.57	7.79	9.47	10.82	13.34	16.22	18.15	21.06	23.68	26.87	29.14	36.12
15	5.23	5.98	7.26	8.55	10.31	11.72	14.34	17.32	19.31	22.31	25.00	28.26	30.58	37.70
16	5.81	6.61	7.96	9.31	11.15	12.62	15.34	18.42	20.46	23.54	26.30	29.63	32.00	39.29
17	6.41	7.26	8.67	10.08	12.00	13.53	16.34	19.51	21.62	24.77	27.59	31.00	33.41	40.75
18	7.02	7.91	9.39	10.86	12.86	14.44	17.34	20.60	22.76	25.99	28.87	32.35	34.80	42.31
19	7.63	8.57	10.12	11.65	13.72	15.35	18.34	21.69	23.90	27.20	30.14	33.69	36.19	43.82
20	8.26	9.24	10.85	12.44	14.58	16.27	19.34	22.78	25.04	28.41	31.41	35.02	37.57	45.32
21	8.90	9.92	11.59	13.24	15.44	17.18	20.34	23.86	26.17	29.62	32.67	36.34	38.93	46.80
22	9.54	10.60	12.34	14.04	16.31	18.10	21.34	24.94	27.30	30.81	33.92	37.66	40.29	48.27
23	10.20	11.29	13.09	14.85	17.19	19.02	22.34	26.02	28.43	32.01	35.17	38.97	41.64	49.73
24	10.86	11.99	13.85	15.66	18.06	19.94	23.34	27.10	29.55	33.20	36.42	40.27	42.98	51.18
25	11.52	12.70	14.61	16.47	18.94	20.87	24.34	28.17	30.68	34.38	37.65	41.57	44.31	52.62
26	12.20	13.41	15.38	17.29	19.82	21.79	25.34	29.25	31.80	35.56	38.88	42.86	45.64	54.05
27	12.88	14.12	16.15	18.11	20.70	22.72	26.34	30.32	32.91	36.74	40.11	44.14	46.96	55.48
28	13.56	14.85	16.93	18.94	21.59	23.65	27.34	31.39	34.03	37.92	41.34	45.42	48.28	56.89
29	14.26	15.57	17.71	19.77	22.48	24.58	28.34	32.46	35.14	39.09	42.56	46.69	49.59	58.30
30	14.95	16.31	18.49	20.60	23.36	25.51	29.34	33.53	36.25	40.26	43.77	47.96	50.89	59.70

Index

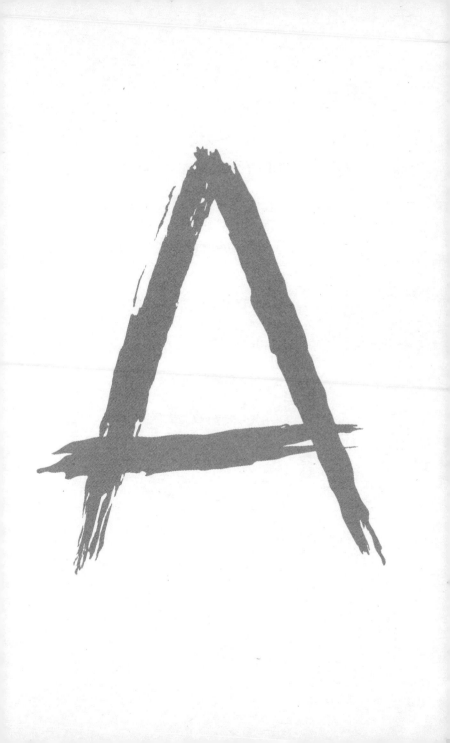

ALSO IN THE CHAOS WALKING TRILOGY

The Knife of Never Letting Go

Monsters of Men

ALSO BY PATRICK NESS

More Than This

The Crane Wife

A Monster Calls

Topics About Which I Know Nothing

The Crash of Hennington

CHAOS WALKING
BOOK TWO

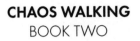

THE ASK AND THE ANSWER

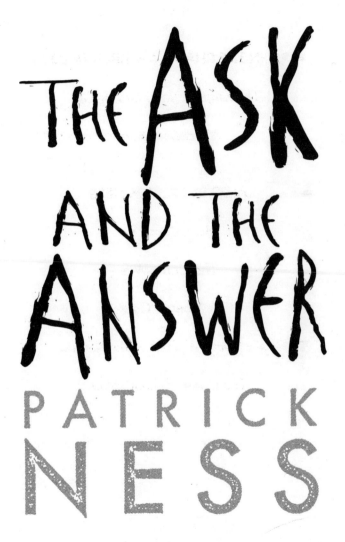

PATRICK NESS

WALKER
BOOKS

First published 2009 by Walker Books Ltd
87 Vauxhall Walk, London SE11 5HJ

This edition, including *The Wide, Wide Sea*, published 2014

6 8 10 9 7

Text © 2009, 2013 Patrick Ness

This book has been typeset in Fairfield, Tiepolo and Optima

Printed and bound in Great Britain by CPI Group (UK) Ltd, Croydon CR0 4YY

British Library Cataloguing in Publication Data:
a catalogue record for this book is available from the British Library

ISBN 978-1-4063-5799-8

www.walker.co.uk

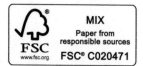

For Patrick Gale

Battle not with monsters
lest you become a monster
and if you gaze into the abyss
the abyss gazes into you.

Friedrich Nietzsche

THE END

"YOUR NOISE REVEALS YOU, TODD HEWITT."

A voice–

In the darkness–

I blink open my eyes. Everything is shadows and blur and it feels like the world's spinning and my blood is too hot and my brain is clogged and I can't think and it's dark–

I blink again.

Wait–

No, *wait*–

Just now, just *now* we were in the square–

Just now she was in my arms–

She was *dying* in my arms–

"Where is she?" I spit into the dark, tasting blood, my voice croaking, my Noise rising like a sudden hurricane, high and red and furious. *"WHERE IS SHE?"*

"I will be the one doing the asking here, Todd."

That voice.

3

Somewhere in the dark.

Somewhere behind me, somewhere unseen.

Mayor Prentiss.

I blink again and the murk starts to turn into a vast room, the only light coming from a single window, a wide circle up high and far away, its glass not clear but coloured into shapes of New World and its two circling moons, the light from it slanting down onto me and nothing else.

"What have you done with her?" I say, loud, blinking against fresh blood trickling into my eyes. I try to reach up to clear it away but I find my hands are tied behind my back and panic rises in me and I struggle against the binds and my breathing speeds up and I shout again, *"WHERE IS SHE?"*

A fist comes from nowhere and punches me in the stomach.

I lean forward into the shock of it and realize I'm tied to a wooden chair, my feet bound to its legs, my shirt gone somewhere up on a dusty hillside and as I'm throwing up my empty stomach I notice there's carpet beneath me, repeating the same pattern of New World and its moons, over and over and over, stretching out for ever.

And I'm remembering we were in the square, in the square where I'd run, holding her, carrying her, telling her to stay alive, stay alive till we got safe, till we got to Haven so I could save her–

But there *weren't* no safety, no safety at all, there was just *him* and his men and they took her from me, they *took* her from my arms–

4

"You notice that he does not ask, *Where am I?*" says the Mayor's voice, moving out there, somewhere. "His first words are, *Where is she?*, and his Noise says the same. Interesting."

My head's throbbing along with my stomach and I'm waking up some more and I'm remembering I *fought* them, I fought them when they took her till the butt of a gun smashed against my temple and knocked me into blackness–

I swallow away the tightness in my throat, swallow away the panic and the fear–

Cuz this is the end, ain't it?

The end of it all.

The Mayor has me.

The Mayor has her.

"If you hurt her–" I say, the punch still aching in my belly. Mr Collins stands in front of me, half in shadow, Mr Collins who farmed corn and cauliflower and who tended the Mayor's horses and who stands over me now with a pistol in a holster, a rifle slung round his back and a fist rearing up to punch me again.

"She seemed quite hurt enough already, Todd," the Mayor says, stopping Mr Collins. "The poor thing."

My fists clench in their bindings. My Noise feels lumpy and half-battered but it still rises with the memory of Davy Prentiss's gun pointed at us, of her falling into my arms, of her bleeding and gasping–

And then I make it go even redder with the feel of my own fist landing on Davy Prentiss's face, of Davy Prentiss falling from his horse, his foot caught in the stirrup, dragged away like so much trash.

5

"Well," the Mayor says, "that explains the mysterious whereabouts of my *son*."

And if I didn't know better, I'd say he sounded almost *amused*.

But I notice the only way I can tell this is from the sound of his voice, a voice sharper and smarter than any old Prentisstown voice he might once have had, and that the nothing I heard coming from him when I ran into Haven is still a big nothing in whatever room this is and it's matched by a big nothing from Mr Collins.

They ain't got Noise.

Neither of 'em.

The only Noise here is mine, bellering like an injured calf.

I twist my neck to find the Mayor but it hurts too much to turn very far and all I can tell is that I'm sitting in the single beam of dusty, coloured sunlight in the middle of a room so big I can barely make out the walls in the far distance.

And then I do see a little table in the darkness, set back just far enough so I can't make out what's on it.

Just the shine of metal, glinting and promising things I don't wanna think about.

"He still thinks of me as Mayor," his voice says, sounding light and amused again.

"It's President Prentiss now, boy," grunts Mr Collins. "You'd do well to remember that."

"What have you done with her?" I say, trying to turn again, this way and that, wincing at the pain in my neck. "If you *touch* her, I'll–"

6

"You arrive in my town this very morning," interrupts the Mayor, "with nothing in your possession, not even the shirt on your back, just a girl in your arms who has suffered a terrible accident—"

My Noise surges. "It was no *accident*—"

"A very bad accident indeed," continues the Mayor, his voice giving the first hint of the impayshunce I heard when we met in the square. "So very bad that she is near death and here is the boy who we have spent so much of our time and energy trying to find, the boy who has caused us so much trouble, offering himself up to us *willingly*, offering to do anything we wish if we just *save the girl* and yet when we try to do just that—"

"Is she all right? Is she safe?"

The Mayor stops and Mr Collins steps forward and backhands me across the face. There's a long moment as the sting spreads across my cheek and I sit there, panting.

Then the Mayor steps into the circle of light, right in front of me.

He's still in his good clothes, crisp and clean as ever, as if there ain't a man underneath there at all, just a walking talking block of ice. Even Mr Collins has sweat marks and dirt and the smell you'd expect but not the Mayor, no.

The Mayor makes you look like yer nothing but a mess that needs cleaning up.

He faces me, leans down so he's looking into my eyes.

And then he gives me an asking, like he's only curious.

"What is her name, Todd?"

I blink, surprised. "What?"

"What is her name?" he repeats.

Surely he must know her name. Surely it must be in my Noise—

"You know her name," I say.

"I want you to tell me."

I look from him to Mr Collins, standing there with his arms crossed, his silence doing nothing to hide a look on his face that would happily pound me into the ground.

"One more time, Todd," says the Mayor lightly, "and I would very much like for you to answer. What is her name? This girl from across the worlds."

"If you know she's from across the worlds," I say, "then you must know her name."

And then the Mayor smiles, actually *smiles*.

And I feel more afraid than ever.

"That's not how this works, Todd. How this works is that I ask and you answer. Now. What is her name?"

"Where is she?"

"What's her name?"

"Tell me where she is and I'll tell you her name."

He sighs, as if I've let him down. He nods once to Mr Collins, who steps forward and punches me again in the stomach.

"This is a simple transaction, Todd," the Mayor says, as I gag onto the carpet. "All you have to do is tell me what I want to know and this ends. The choice is yours. Genuinely, I have no wish to harm you further."

I'm breathing heavy, bent forward, the ache in my gut making it difficult to get enough air in me. I can feel my weight pulling at the bonds on my wrists and I can feel the blood on my face, sticky and drying, and I look out bleary-eyed from my little prison of light in the middle of this room, this room with no exits–

This room where I'm gonna die–

This room–

This room where she ain't.

And something in me chooses.

If this is it, then something in me decides.

Decides not to say.

"You know her name," I say. "Kill me if you want but you know her name already."

And the Mayor just watches me.

The longest minute of my life passes with him watching me, reading me, seeing that I mean it.

And then he steps to the little wooden table.

I look to see but his back's hiding what he's doing. I hear him fiddling with things on top of it, a *thunk* of metal scraping against wood.

"*I'll do anything you want*," he says and I reckernize he's aping my own words back at me. "*Just save her and I'll do anything you want.*"

"I ain't afraid of you," I say, tho my Noise says otherwise, thinking of all the things that could be on that table. "I ain't afraid to die."

And I wonder if I mean it.

He turns to me, keeping his hands behind his back so I can't see what he's picked up. "Because you're a man, Todd? Because a man isn't afraid to die?"

"Yeah," I say. "Cuz I'm a man."

"If I'm correct, your birthday is not for another fourteen days."

"That's just a number. I'm breathing heavy, my stomach flip-flopping from talking like this. "It don't mean *nothing*. If I was on Old World, I'd be–"

"You ain't on Old World, *boy*," Mr Collins says.

"I don't believe that's what he means, Mr Collins," the Mayor says, still looking at me. "Is it, Todd?"

I look back and forth twixt the two of 'em. "I've killed," I say. "I've killed."

"Yes, I believe you've killed," says the Mayor. "I can see the shame of it all over you. But the asking is who? *Who* did you kill?" He steps into the darkness outside the circle of light, whatever he picked up from the table still hidden as he walks behind me. "Or should I say *what*?"

"I killed Aaron," I say, trying to follow him, failing.

"Did you, now?" His lack of Noise is an awful thing, especially when you can't see him. It's not like the silence of a girl, a girl's silence is still active, still a living thing that makes a shape in all the Noise that clatters round it.

(I think of her, I think of her silence, the ache of it)

(I don't think of her name)

But with the Mayor, however he's done it, however he's made it so he and Mr Collins don't got Noise, it's like it's nothing, like a dead thing, no more shape nor Noise nor life in the world than a stone or a wall, a fortress you ain't never gonna conquer. I'm guessing he's reading my Noise but how can you tell with a man who's made himself of stone?

I show him what he wants anyway. I put the church under the waterfall at the front of my Noise. I put up all the truthful fight with Aaron, all the struggle and the blood, I put me fighting him and beating him and knocking him to the ground, I put me taking out my knife.

I put me stabbing Aaron in the neck.

"There's truth there," says the Mayor. "But is it the whole truth?"

"It is," I say, raising my Noise loud and high to block out anything else he might hear. "It's the truth."

His voice is still amused. "I think you're lying to me, Todd."

"I ain't!" I practically shout. "I done what Aaron wanted! I murdered him! I became a man by yer own laws and you can have me in yer army and I'll do whatever you want, just tell me what you've done with her!"

I see Mr Collins notice a sign from behind me and he steps forward again, fist back and–

(I can't help it)

I jerk away from him so hard I drag the chair a few inches to the side–

(shut up)

And the punch never falls.

"Good," says the Mayor, sounding quietly pleased. "Good." He begins to move again in the darkness. "Let me explain a few things to you, Todd," he says. "You are in the main office of what was formerly the Cathedral of Haven and what yesterday became the Presidential Palace. I have brought you into my home in the hope of helping you. Helping you see that you are mistaken in this hopeless fight you put up against me, against us."

His voice moves behind Mr Collins–

His voice–

For a second it feels like he's not talking out loud–

Then it passes.

"My soldiers should arrive here tomorrow afternoon," he says, still moving. "You, Todd Hewitt, will first tell me what I ask of you and then you will be true to your word and you will assist me in our creation of a new society."

He steps into the light again, stopping in front of me, his hands still behind his back, whatever he picked up still hidden.

"But the process I want to begin here, Todd," he says, "is the one where you learn that I am not your enemy."

I'm so surprised I stop being afraid for a second.

Not my enemy?

I open my eyes wide.

Not my enemy?

"No, Todd," he says. "Not your enemy."

"Yer a murderer," I say, without thinking.

"I am a general," he says. "Nothing more, nothing less."

I stare at him. "You killed people on yer march here. You killed the people of Farbranch."

"Regrettable things happen in wartime, but that war is now over."

"I saw you shoot them," I say, hating how the words of a man without Noise sound so solid, so much like unmoveable stone.

"Me personally, Todd?"

I swallow away a sour taste. "No, but it was a war *you started*!"

"It was necessary," he says. "To save a sick and dying planet."

12

My breathing is getting faster, my mind getting cloudier, my head heavier than ever. But my Noise is redder, too. "You murdered Cillian."

"Deeply regrettable," he says. "He would have made a fine soldier."

"You killed my mother," I say, my voice catching (shut up), my Noise filling with rage and grief, my eyes screwing up with tears (shut up, shut up, shut up). "You killed all the women of Prentisstown."

"Do you believe everything you hear, Todd?"

There's a silence, a real one, as even my own Noise takes this in. "I have no desire to kill women," he adds. "I never did."

My mouth drops open. "Yes, you *did*–"

"Now is not the time for a history lesson."

"Yer a *liar*!"

"And you presume to know everything, do you?" His voice goes cold and he steps away from me and Mr Collins strikes me so hard on the side of the head I nearly fall over onto the floor.

"Yer a LIAR AND A MURDERER!" I shout, my ears still ringing from the punch.

Mr Collins hits me again the other way, hard as a block of wood.

"I am *not* your enemy, Todd," the Mayor says again. "Please stop making me do this to you."

My head is hurting so bad I don't say nothing. I *can't* say nothing. I can't say the word he wants. I can't say nothing else without getting beaten senseless.

This is the end. It's gotta be the end. They won't let me live. They won't let *her* live.

13

"I hope it *is* the end," the Mayor says, his voice actually making the sounds of truth. "I hope you'll tell me what I want to know so we can stop all this."

And then he says—

Then he says—

He says, "Please."

I look up, blinking thru the swelling coming up round my eyes.

His face has a look of concern on it, a look of almost *pleading*.

What the hell? What the ruddy hell?

And I hear the buzz of it inside my head again—

Different than just hearing someone's Noise—

PLEASE like it's said in my own voice—

PLEASE like it's coming from me—

Pressing on me—

On my insides—

Making me feel like I wanna say it—

PLEASE—

"The things you think you know, Todd," the Mayor says, his voice still twining around inside my own head. "Those things aren't true."

And then I remember—

I remember Ben—

I remember Ben saying the same thing to me—

Ben who I lost—

And my Noise hardens, right there.

Cutting him off.

The Mayor's face loses the look of pleading.

"All right," he says, frowning a little. "But remember that it is your choice." He stands up straight. "What is her name?"

"You know her name."

Mr Collins strikes me across the head, careening me sideways.

"What is her name?"

"You already know it–"

Boom, another blow, this time the other way.

"What is her name?"

"No."

Boom.

"Tell me her name."

"No!"

BOOM!

"What is her *name*, Todd?"

"EFF YOU!"

Except I don't say "eff" and Mr Collins hits me so hard my head whips back and the chair over-balances and I do topple sideways to the floor, taking the chair with me. I slam into the carpet, hands tied so I can't catch myself, my eyes filling up with little New Worlds till there ain't nothing else to see.

I breathe into the carpet.

The toes of the Mayor's boots approach my face.

"I am not your enemy, Todd Hewitt," he says one more time. "Just tell me her name and this will all stop."

I take in a breath and have to cough it away.

I take in another and say what I have to say.

"Yer a murderer."

15

"So be it," says the Mayor.

His feet move away and I feel Mr Collins pull my chair up from the floor, taking me up with it, my body groaning against its own weight, till I'm sat up again in the circle of coloured light. My eyes are so swollen now I can't hardly see Mr Collins at all even tho he's right in front of me.

I hear the Mayor at the small table again. I hear him moving things round on the top. I hear again the scrape of metal.

I hear him step up beside me.

And after all that promising, here it really, finally is.

My end.

I'm sorry, I think. *I'm so, so sorry.*

The Mayor puts a hand on my shoulder and I flinch away from it but he keeps it there, pressing down steadily. I can't see what he's holding, but he's bringing something towards me, towards my face, something hard and metal and filled with pain and ready to make me suffer and end my life and there's a hole inside me that I need to crawl into, away from all this, down deep and black, and I know this is the end, the end of all things, I can never escape from here and he'll kill me and kill her and there's no chance, no life, no hope, nothing.

I'm sorry.

And the Mayor lays a bandage across my face.

I gasp from the coolness of it and jerk away from his hands but he keeps pressing it gently into the lump on my forehead and onto the wounds on my face and chin, his body so close I can smell it, the cleanliness of it, the woody odour of his soap, the breath from his nose brushing over my cheek, his fingers touching my cuts almost tenderly, dressing the swelling round my eyes, the splits on my lip, and I can feel the bandages get to work almost instantly, feel the swelling going right down, the painkillers flooding into my system, and I think for a second how *good* the bandages are in Haven, how much like *her* bandages, and the relief comes so quick, so unexpected that my throat clenches and I have to swallow it away.

"I am not the man you think I am, Todd," the Mayor says quietly, almost right into my ear, putting another bandage on my neck. "I did not do the things you think I did. I asked my son to bring you back. I did not ask him to shoot anyone. I did not ask Aaron to kill you."

"Yer a liar," I say but my voice is weak and I'm shaking from the effort of keeping the weep out of it (shut up).

The Mayor puts more bandages across the bruises on my chest and stomach, so gentle I can barely stand it, so gentle it's almost like he cares how it feels.

"I *do* care, Todd," he says. "There will be time for you to learn the truth of that."

He moves behind me and puts another bandage around the bindings on my wrists, taking my hands and rubbing feeling back into them with his thumbs.

"There will be time," he says, "for you to come to trust me. For you, perhaps, to come to even *like* me. To even think of me, one day, as a kind of father to you, Todd."

It feels like my Noise is melting away with all the drugs, with all the pain disappearing, with me disappearing along with it, like he's killing me after all, but with the cure instead of the punishment.

"Please," I say. "Please."

But I don't know what I mean.

"The war is over, Todd," the Mayor says again. "We are making a new world. This planet finally and truly living up to its name. Believe me when I say, once you see it, you'll *want* to be part of it."

I breathe into the darkness.

"You could be a leader of men, Todd. You have proven yourself very special."

I keep breathing, trying to hold on to it but feeling myself slip away.

"How can I know?" I finally say, my voice a croak, a slur, a thing not quite real. "How can I know she's even still alive?"

"You can't," says the Mayor. "You only have my word."

And waits again.

"And if I do it," I say. "If I do what you say, you'll save her?"

"We will do whatever's necessary," he says.

Without pain, it feels almost like I don't have a body at all, almost like I'm a ghost, sitting in a chair, blinded and eternal.

Like I'm dead already.

Cuz how do you know yer alive if you don't hurt?

"We are the choices we make, Todd," the Mayor says. "Nothing more, nothing less. I'd like you to choose to tell me. I would like that very much indeed."

Under the bandages is just further darkness.

Just me, alone in the black.

Alone with his voice.

I don't know what to do.

I don't know anything.

(what do I do?)

But if there's a chance, if there's even a *chance*–

"Is it really such a sacrifice, Todd?" the Mayor says, listening to me think. "Here, at the end of the past? At the beginning of the future?"

No. No, I can't. He's a liar and a murderer, no matter what he says–

"I'm waiting, Todd."

But she might be alive, he might keep her alive–

"We are nearing your last opportunity, Todd."

I raise my head. The movement opens the bandages some and I squint up into the light, up towards the Mayor's face.

It's blank as ever.

It's the empty, lifeless wall.

I might as well be talking into a bottomless pit.

I might as well *be* the bottomless pit.

I look away. I look down.

"Viola," I say into the carpet. "Her name's Viola."

The Mayor lets out a long, pleased-sounding breath. "Good, Todd," he says. "I thank you."

He turns to Mr Collins.

"Lock him up."

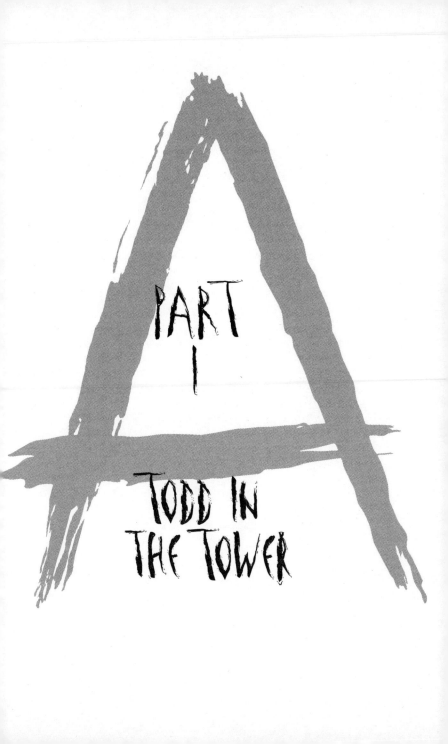

PART I

TODD IN THE TOWER

1

THE OLD MAYOR

[TODD]

MR COLLINS PUSHES ME up a narrow, windowless staircase, up and up and up, turning on sharp landings but always straight up. Just when I think my legs can't take no more, we reach a door. He opens it and shoves me hard and I go tumbling into the room and down onto a wooden floor, my arms so stiff I can't even catch myself and I groan and roll to one side.

And look down over a thirty-metre drop.

Mr Collins laughs as I scrabble back away from it. I'm on a ledge not more than five boards wide that runs round the walls of a square room. In the middle is just an enormous hole with some ropes dangling down thru the centre. I follow 'em up thru a tall shaft to the biggest set of bells I ever saw, two of 'em hanging from a single wooden beam, huge things, big as a room you could live in, archways cut into the sides of the tower so the bell-ringing can be heard.

I jump when Mr Collins slams the door, locking it with a *ker-thunk* sound that don't brook no thoughts of escape.

I get myself up and lean against the wall till I can breathe again.

I close my eyes.

I am Todd Hewitt, I think. *I am the son of Cillian Boyd and Ben Moore. My birthday is in fourteen days but I am a man.*

I am Todd Hewitt and I am a man.

(a man who told the Mayor her name)

"I'm sorry," I whisper. "I'm so sorry."

After a while, I open my eyes and look up and around. There are small rectangular openings at eye level all around this floor of the tower, three on each wall, fading light shining in thru the dust.

I go to the nearest opening. I'm in the bell tower of the cathedral, obviously, way up high, looking out the front, down onto the square where I first entered the town, only this morning but it already feels like a lifetime ago. Dusk is falling, so I musta been out cold for a bit before the Mayor woke me, time where he coulda done anything to her, time where he coulda–

(shut up, just shut up)

I look out over the square. It's still empty, still the quiet of a silent town, a town with no Noise, a town waiting for an army to come and conquer it.

A town that didn't even try to fight.

The Mayor just turned up and they handed it right over

to him. *Sometimes the rumour of an army is just as effective as the army itself*, he told me and wasn't he right?

All that time, running here as fast as we could, not thinking bout what Haven'd be like once we got here, not saying it out loud but hoping it'd be safe, hoping it'd be paradise.

I'm telling you there's hope, Ben said.

But he was wrong. It wasn't Haven at all.

It was New Prentisstown.

I frown, feeling my chest tighten and I look out west across the square, across the treetops that spread out into the farther silent houses and streets and on up to the waterfall, smashing down from the rim of the valley in the near distance, the zigzag road zipping up the hill beside it, the road where I fought Davy Prentiss Jr, the road where Viola—

I turn back into the room.

My eyes are adjusting to the fading light but there don't seem to be nothing here anyway but boards and a faint stink. The bell ropes dangle about two metres from any side. I look up to see where they're tied fast to the bells to make 'em chime. I squint down into the hole but it's too dark to see clearly what might be at the bottom. Probably just hard brick.

Two metres ain't that much at all, tho. You could jump it easy and grab onto a rope to climb yer way down.

But then—

"It's quite ingenious, really," says a voice from the far corner.

I jerk back, fists up, my Noise spiking. A man is standing up from where he was sitting, another Noiseless man.

Except—

25

"If you try to escape by climbing down the ropes left so temptingly available," he continues, "every person in town is going to know about it."

"Who are you?" I say, my stomach high and light but my fists clenching.

"Yes," he says. "I could tell you weren't from Haven." He steps away from the corner, letting light catch his face. I see a blackened eye and a cut lip that looks like it's only just scabbed over. No bandages spared for him, obviously. "Funny how quickly one forgets the *loudness* of it," he says, almost to himself.

He's a small man, shorter than me, wider, too, older than Ben tho not by much, but I can also see he's soft all over, soft even in his face. A softness I could beat if I had to.

"Yes," he says, "I imagine you could."

"Who are you?" I say again.

"Who am I?" repeats the man softly, then raises his voice like he's playing at something. "I am Con Ledger, my boy. Mayor of Haven." He smiles in a dazed way. "But not Mayor of New Prentisstown." He shakes his head a little as he looks at me. "We even gave the refugees the cure when they started pouring in."

And then I see that his smile ain't a smile, it's a *wince*.

"Good God, boy," he says. "How Noisy you are."

"I ain't a boy," I say, my fists still up.

"I completely fail to see how that's any sort of point."

I got ten million things I wanna say but my curiosity wins out first. "So there *is* a cure then? For the Noise?"

"Oh, yes," he says, his face twitching a bit at me, like he's tasting something bad. "Native plant with a natural neurochemical mixed with a few things we could synthesize and there you go. Quiet falls at last on New World."

"Not *all* of New World."

"No, well," he says, turning to look out the rectangle with his hands clasped behind his back. "It's very hard to make, isn't it? A long and slow process. We only got it right late last year and that was after twenty years of trying. We made enough for ourselves and were just on the point of starting to export it when…"

He trails off, looking firmly out onto the town below.

"When you surrendered," I say, my Noise rumbling, low and red. "Like cowards."

He turns back to me, the wincing smile gone, *way* gone. "And why should the opinion of a boy matter to me?"

"I *ain't* a boy," I say again and are my fists still clenched? Yes, they are.

"Clearly you are," he says, "for a *man* would know the necessary choices that have to be made when one is facing one's oblivion."

I narrow my eyes. "You ain't got nothing you can teach me bout oblivion."

He blinks a little, seeing the truth of it in my Noise as if it were bright flashes trying to blind him, and then his stance slumps. "Forgive me," he says. "This isn't me." He puts a hand up to his face and rubs it, smarting at the bruise around his eye. "Yesterday, I was the benevolent Mayor of a beautiful town." He seems to laugh at some private joke. "But that was yesterday."

"How many people in Haven?" I say, not quite ready to let it go.

He looks over at me. "Boy—"

"My name is Todd Hewitt," I say. "You can call me Mr Hewitt."

"He promised us a new beginning—"

"Even *I* know he's a liar. *How many people?*"

He sighs. "Including refugees, three thousand, three hundred."

"The army ain't a third that size," I say. "You coulda fought."

"Women and children," he says. "Farmers."

"Women and children fought in other towns. Women and children *died*."

He steps forward, his face getting stormy. "Yes, and now the women and children of this city will *not* die! Because *I* reached a peace!"

"A peace that blacked yer eye," I say. "A peace that split yer lip."

He looks at me for another second and then gives a sad snort. "The words of a sage," he says, "in the voice of a hick."

And he turns back to look out the opening.

Which is when I notice the low buzz.

Asking marks fill my Noise but before I can open my mouth, the Mayor, the *old* Mayor, says, "Yes, that's me you hear."

"You?" I say. "What about the cure?"

"Would you give your conquered enemy his favourite medicine?"

I lick my upper lip. "It comes back? The Noise?"

"Oh, yes." He turns to me again. "If you don't take your daily dose, it most definitely comes back." He returns to his corner and slowly sits himself down. "You'll notice there are no toilets," he says. "I apologize in advance for the unpleasantness."

I watch him sit, my Noise still rattling red and sore and full of askings.

"It *was* you, if I'm not mistaken?" he says. "This morning? The one who the town was cleared for, the one the new President greeted himself on horseback?"

I don't answer him. But my Noise does.

"So, who are you then, Todd Hewitt?" he says. "What makes you so special?"

Now *that*, I think, is a very good asking.

Night falls quick and full, Mayor Ledger saying less and less and fidgeting more and more till he finally can't stand it and starts to pace. All the while, his buzz gets louder till even if we wanted to talk, we'd have to shout to do it.

I stand at the front of the tower and watch the stars come out, night covering the valley below.

And I'm thinking and I'm trying not to think cuz when I do, my stomach turns and I feel sick, or my throat clenches and I feel sick, or my eyes wet and I feel sick.

Cuz she's out there somewhere.

(*please* be out there somewhere)

(*please* be okay)

(*please*)

"Do you always have to be so bloody *loud*?" Mayor Ledger snaps. I turn to him, ready to snap back, and he holds up his hands in apology. "I'm sorry. I'm not like this."

29

He starts fidgeting his fingers again. "It's difficult having one's cure taken away so abruptly."

I look back out over New Prentisstown as lights start coming on in people's houses. I ain't hardly seen no one out there the whole day, everyone staying indoors, probably under the Mayor's orders.

"They all going thru this out there, then?" I say.

"Oh, everyone will have their little stockpile at home," Mayor Ledger says. "They'll have to have it pried out of their hands, I imagine."

"I don't reckon that'll be a problem when the army gets here," I say.

The moons rise, crawling up the sky as if there was nothing to hurry about. They shine bright enough to light up New Prentisstown and I see how the river cuts thru town but that there ain't nothing much north of it except fields, empty in the moonlight, then a sharp rise of rocky cliffs that make up the north wall of the valley. To the north, you can also see a thin road coming outta the hills before cutting its way back into town, the other road that Viola and I didn't take after Farbranch, the other road the Mayor *did* take and got here first.

To the east, the river and the main road just carry on, going god knows where, round corners and farther hills, the town petering out as it goes. There's another road, not much paved, that heads south from the square and past more buildings and houses and into a wood and up a hill with a notch on the top.

And that's all there is of New Prentisstown.

Home to three thousand, three hundred people, all

hiding in their houses, so quiet they might be dead.

Not one of them lifting a hand to save theirselves from what's coming, hoping if they're meek enough, if they're *weak* enough, then the monster won't eat 'em.

This is where we spent all our time running to.

I see movement down on the square, a shadow flitting, but it's only a dog. **Home, home, home,** I can just about hear him think. **Home, home, home.**

Dogs don't got the problems of people.

Dogs can be happy any old time.

I take a minute to breathe away the tightness that comes over my chest, the water in my eyes.

Take a minute to stop thinking bout my own dog.

When I can look out again, I see someone not a dog at all.

He's got his head slumped forward and he's walking his horse slow across the town square, the hoofs clopping against the brick and, as he approaches, even tho Mayor Ledger's **buzz** has started to become such a nuisance I don't know how I'm ever gonna sleep, I can still hear it out there.

Noise.

Across the quiet of a waiting city, I can hear the man's Noise.

And he can hear mine.

Todd Hewitt? he thinks.

And I can hear the smile growing on his face, too.

Found something, Todd, he says, across the square, up the tower, seeking me out in the moonlight. **Found something of yers.**

31

I don't say nothing. I don't *think* nothing.

I just watch as he reaches behind him and holds something up towards me.

Even this far away, even by the light of the moons, I know what it is.

My ma's book.

Davy Prentiss has my ma's book.

2

THE FOOT UPON THE NECK

[TODD]

EARLY NEXT MORNING, a platform with a microphone on it gets built noisily and quickly near the base of the bell tower and, as the morning turns to afternoon, the men of New Prentisstown gather in front of it.

"Why?" I say, looking out over 'em.

"Why do you think?" Mayor Ledger says, sitting in a darkened corner, rubbing his temples, his Noise *buzz* sawing away, hot and metallic. "To meet the new man in charge."

The men don't say much, their faces pale and grim, tho who can know what they're thinking when you can't hear their Noise? But they look cleaner than the men in my town used to, shorter hair, shaved faces, better clothes. A good number of 'em are rounded and soft like Mayor Ledger.

Haven musta been a comfortable place, a place where men weren't fighting every day just to survive.

Maybe too much comfort was the problem.

33

Mayor Prentiss's men are on horseback at strategic spots across the square, ten or twelve of 'em, rifles ready, to make sure everyone behaves tho the threat of an army coming seems to have done most of the work. I see Mr Tate and Mr Morgan and Mr O'Hare, men I grew up with, men I used to see every day being farmers, men who were just men till suddenly they became something else.

I don't see Davy Prentiss nowhere and my Noise starts rumbling again at the thought of him.

He musta come back down the hillside from wherever his horse dragged him and found the rucksack. All it had in it any more was a bunch of ruined clothes and the book.

My ma's book.

My ma's words to me.

Written when I was born. Written till just before she died.

Before she was murdered.

My wondrous son who I swear will see this world come good.

Words read to me by Viola cuz I couldn't–

And now *Davy bloody Prentiss*–

"Can you please," Mayor Ledger says thru gritted teeth, "at least *try*–" He stops himself and looks at me apologetically. "I'm sorry," he says, for the millionth time since Mr Collins woke us up with breakfast.

Before I can say anything back I feel the hardest, sudden tug on my heart, so surprising I nearly gasp.

I look out again.

The women of New Prentisstown are coming.

They start to appear farther away, in groups down side streets away from the main body of men, kept there by the Mayor's men patrolling on horseback.

I feel their silence in a way I can't feel the men's. It's like a loss, like great groupings of sorrow against the sound of the world and I have to wipe my eyes again but I press myself closer to the opening, trying to see 'em, trying to see every single one of 'em.

Trying to see if she's there.

But she ain't.

She ain't.

They look like the men, most of 'em wearing trousers and shirts of different cuts, some of 'em wearing long skirts, but most looking clean and comfortable and well-fed. Their hair has more variety, pulled back or up or over or short or long and not nearly as many of 'em are blonde as they are in the Noise of the menfolk where I come from.

And I see that more of their arms are crossed, more of their faces looking doubtful.

More anger there than on the faces of the men.

"Did anyone fight you?" I ask Mayor Ledger while I keep on looking. "Did anyone not wanna give up?"

"This is a democracy, Todd," he sighs. "Do you know what that is?"

"No idea," I say, still looking, still not finding.

"It means the minority is listened to," he says, "but the majority rules."

I look at him. "All these people wanted to surrender?"

"The President made a *proposal*," he says, touching his

35

split lips, "to the elected Council, promising that the city would be unharmed if we agreed to this."

"And you believed him?"

His eyes flash at me. "You are either forgetting or do not know that we already fought a great war, a war to end *all* wars, at just about the time you would have been born. If any repeat of that can be avoided–"

"Then yer willing to hand yerselves over to a murderer."

He sighs again. "The majority of the Council, led by myself, decided this was the best way to save the most lives." He rests his head against the brick. "Not everything is black and white, Todd. In fact, almost nothing is."

"But what if–"

Ker-thunk. The lock on the door slides back and Mr Collins enters, pistol pointed.

He looks straight at Mayor Ledger. "Get up," he says.

I look back and forth twixt 'em both. "What's going on?" I say.

Mayor Ledger stands from his corner. "It seems the piper must be paid, Todd," he says, his voice trying to sound light but I hear his buzz rev up with fear. "This was a beautiful town," he says to me. "And I was a better man. Remember that, please."

"What are you talking about?" I say.

Mr Collins takes him by the arm and shoves him out the door.

"Hey!" I shout, coming after them. "Where are you taking him?"

Mr Collins raises a fist to punch me–

And I flinch away.

(shut *up*)

He laughs and locks the door behind him.

Ker-thunk.

And I'm left alone in the tower.

And as Mayor Ledger's *buzz* disappears down the stairs, that's when I hear it.

March march march, way in the distance.

I go to an opening.

They're here.

The conquering army, marching into Haven.

They flow down the zigzag road like a black river, dusty and dirty and coming like a dam's burst. They march four or five across and the first of them disappear into the far trees at the base of the hill as the last finally crest the top. The crowd watches them, the men turning back from the platform, the women looking out from the side streets.

The *march march march* grows louder, echoing down the city streets. Like a clock ticking its way down.

The crowd waits. I wait with them.

And then, thru the trees, at the turning of the road—

Here they are.

The army.

Mr Hammar at their front.

Mr Hammar who lived in the petrol stayshun back home, Mr Hammar who thought vile, violent things no boy should ever hear, Mr Hammar who shot the people of Farbranch in the back as they fled.

Mr Hammar leads the army.

I can hear him now calling out marching words to keep everyone in time together. *The foot*, he's yelling to the rhythm of the march.

The foot.

The foot.

The foot upon the neck.

They march into the square and turn down its side, cutting twixt the men and the women like an unstoppable force. Mr Hammar's close enough so I can see the smile, a smile I know full well, a smile that clubs, a smile that beats, a smile that dominates.

And as he gets closer, I grow more sure.

It's a smile without Noise.

Someone, one of those men on horseback maybe, has gone out to meet the army on the road. Someone carrying the cure with him. The army ain't making a sound except with its feet and with its chant.

The foot, the foot, the foot upon the neck.

They march round the side of the square to the platform. Mr Hammar stops at a corner, letting the men start to make up formayshuns behind the platform, lining up with their backs to me, facing the crowd now turned to watch them.

I start to reckernize the soldiers as they line up. Mr Wallace. Mr Smith the younger. Mr Phelps the store-keeper. Men from Prentisstown and many, many more men besides.

The army that grew as it came.

I see Ivan, the man from the barn at Farbranch, the man who secretly told me there were men in sympathy. He stands at the head of one of the formayshuns and everything that proves him right is standing behind him, arms at attenshun, rifles at the ready.

The last soldier marches into place with a final chant.

The foot upon the NECK!

And then there ain't nothing but silence, blowing over New Prentisstown like a wind.

Till I hear the doors of the cathedral open down below me.

And Mayor Prentiss steps out to address his new city.

"Right now," he says into the microphone, having saluted Mr Hammar and climbed his way up the platform steps, "you are afraid."

The men of the town look back up at him, saying nothing, making no sound of Noise nor buzzing.

The women stay in the side streets, also silent.

The army stands at attenshun, ready for anything.

I realize I'm holding my breath.

"Right now," he continues, "you think you are conquered. You think there is no hope. You think I come up here to read out your doom."

His back is to me but from speakers hidden in the four corners, his voice booms clear over the square, over the city, probably over the whole valley and beyond. Cuz who else is there to hear him talk? Who else is there on all of New World that ain't either gathered here or under the ground?

Mayor Prentiss is talking to the whole planet.

"And you're right," he says and I tell you I'm certain I

39

hear the smile. "You *are* conquered. You *are* defeated. And I read to you your doom."

He lets this sink in for a moment. My Noise rumbles and I see a few of the men look up to the top of the tower. I try to keep it quiet but who are these people? Who are these clean and comfortable and not-at-all-hungry people who just handed theirselves over?

"But it is not I who conquered you," the Mayor says. "It is not I who has beaten you or defeated you or enslaved you."

He pauses, looking out over the crowd. He's dressed all in white, white hat, white boots, and with the white cloths covering the platform and the afternoon sun shining on down, he's practically blinding.

"You are enslaved by your idleness," says the Mayor. "You are defeated by your complacency. You are *doomed*" – and here his voice rises suddenly, hitting *doomed* so hard half the crowd jumps – "by your good intentions!"

He's working himself up now, heavy breaths into the microphone.

"You have allowed yourselves to become so *weak*, so *feeble* in the face of the challenges of this world that in a single generation you have become a people who would surrender to *RUMOUR*!"

He starts to pace the stage, microphone in hand. Every frightened face in the crowd, every face in the army, turns to watch him move back and forth, back and forth.

I'm watching, too.

"You let an army *walk* into your town and instead of making them *take* it, you *offer it willingly*!"

He's still pacing, his voice still rising.

"And so you know what I did. I *took*. I took *you*. I took your freedom. I took your town. I took your future."

He laughs, like he can't believe his luck.

"I expected a war," he says.

Some of the crowd look at their feet, away from each other's eyes.

I wonder if they're ashamed.

I hope so.

"But instead of a war," the Mayor says, "I got a conversation. A conversation that began, *Please don't hurt us* and ended with *Please take anything you want*."

He stops in the middle of the platform.

"I expected a WAR!" he shouts again, thrusting his fist at them.

And they flinch.

If a crowd can flinch, they flinch.

More than a thousand men flinch under the fist of just one.

I don't see what the women do.

"And because you did not give me a war," the Mayor says, his voice light, "you will face the consequences."

I hear the doors to the cathedral open again and Mr Collins comes out pushing Mayor Ledger forward thru the ranks of the army, hands tied behind his back.

Mayor Prentiss watches him come, arms crossed. Murmurs finally start in the crowd of men, louder in the crowds of women, and the men on horseback do some waving of their rifles to stop it. The Mayor don't even look back at the sound, like it's beneath his notice. He just watches Mr Collins push Mayor Ledger up the stairs at the back of the platform.

Mayor Ledger stops at the top of the steps, looking out over the crowd. They stare back at him, some of them squinting at the shrillness of his Noise buzz, a buzz I realize is now starting to shout some real words, words of fear, *pictures* of fear, pictures of Mr Collins giving him the bruised eye and the split lip, pictures of him agreeing to surrender and being locked in the tower.

"Kneel," Mayor Prentiss says and tho he says it quietly, tho he says it away from the microphone, somehow I hear it clear as a bell chime in the middle of my head, and from the intake of breath in the crowd, I wonder if that's how they heard it, too.

And before it looks like he even knows what he's doing, Mayor Ledger is kneeling on the platform, looking surprised that he's down there.

The whole town watches him do it.

Mayor Prentiss waits a moment.

And then he steps over to him.

And takes out a knife.

It's a big, no-kidding, death of a thing, shining in the sun.

The Mayor holds it up high over his head.

He turns slowly, so everyone can see what's about to happen.

So that everyone can see the knife.

My gut falls and for a second I think–

But it ain't mine—

It ain't—

And then someone calls, "Murderer!" from across the square.

A single voice, carrying above the silence.

It came from the women.

My heart jumps for a second—

But of course it can't be her—

But at least there's someone. At least there's *someone*.

Mayor Prentiss walks calmly to the microphone. "Your victorious enemy addresses you," he says, almost politely, as if the person who shouted was simply not understanding. "Your leaders are to be executed as the inevitable result of your defeat."

He turns to look at Mayor Ledger, kneeling there on the platform. His face is trying to look calm but everyone can hear how badly he don't wanna die, how childlike his wishes are sounding, how loud his newly uncured Noise is spilling out all over the place.

"And now you will learn," Mayor Prentiss says, turning back to the crowd, "what kind of man your new President is. And what he will demand from you."

Silence, still silence, save for Mayor Ledger's mewling.

Mayor Prentiss walks over to him, knife glinting. Another murmur starts spreading thru the crowd as they finally get what they're about to see. Mayor Prentiss steps behind Mayor Ledger and holds up the knife again. He stands there, watching the crowd watch him, watching their faces as they look and listen to their former Mayor try and fail to contain his Noise.

He turns the knife to a stabbing angle, as if to say again, *behold–*

The murmuring of the crowd rises–

Mayor Prentiss raises his arm–

A voice, a female one, maybe the same one, cries out, "No!"

And then suddenly I realize I know exactly what's gonna happen.

In the chair, in the room with the circle of coloured glass, he brought me to defeat, he brought me to the edge of death, he made me *know* that it would come–

And then he put a bandage on me.

And *that's* when I did what he wanted.

The knife swishes thru the air and slices thru the binds on Mayor Ledger's hands.

There's a town-sized gasp, a *planet*-sized one.

Mayor Prentiss waits for a moment, then says once more, "Behold your future," quietly, not even into the microphone.

But there it is again, right inside yer mind.

He puts the knife away in a belt behind his back and returns to the microphone.

And starts to put bandages on the crowd.

"I am not the man you think I am," he says. "I am not a tyrant come to slaughter his enemies. I am not a madman come to destroy even that which would save himself. I am *not*—" he looks over at Mayor Ledger "—your executioner."

The crowds, men and women, are so quiet now the square might as well be empty.

"The war is *over*," the Mayor continues. "And a new peace will take its place."

He points to the sky. People look up, like he might be conjuring something up there to fall on them.

"You may have heard a rumour," he says. "That there are new settlers coming."

My stomach twists again.

"I tell you as your President," he says. "The rumour is true."

How does he know? How does he ruddy *know*?

The crowd starts to murmur at this news, men and women. The Mayor lets them, happily talking over them.

"We will be ready to greet them!" he says. "We will be a proud society ready to welcome them into a new Eden!" His voice is rising again. "We will show them that they have left Old World and entered PARADISE!"

Lots more murmuring now, talking everywhere.

"I am going to take your cure away from you," the Mayor says.

And boy, does the murmuring *stop*.

The Mayor lets it, lets the silence build up, and then he says, "For now."

The men look at one another and back to the Mayor.

"We are entering a new era," Mayor Prentiss says. "You will earn my trust by joining me in creating a new society. As that new society is built and as we meet our first challenges

be called men again. You will earn the right to have your cure returned to you and that will be the moment all men truly will be brothers."

He's not looking at the women. Neither are the men in the crowd. Women got no use for the reward of a cure, do they?

"It will be difficult," he continues. "I don't pretend otherwise. But it *will* be rewarding." He gestures towards the army. "My deputies have already begun to organize you. You will continue to follow their instructions but I assure you they will never be too onerous and you will soon see that I am not your conqueror. I am not your doom. I am not," he pauses again, "your enemy."

He turns his head across the crowd of men one last time.

"I am your saviour," he says.

And even without hearing their Noise, I watch the crowd wonder if there's a chance he's telling the truth, if maybe things'll be okay after all, if maybe, despite what they feared, they've been let off the hook.

You ain't, I think. *Not by a long shot.*

Even before the crowds have started to properly leave after the Mayor's finished, there's a *ker-thunk* at my door.

"Good evening, Todd," the Mayor says, stepping into the bell-ringing jail and looking around him, wrinkling his nose a little at the smell. "Did you like my speech?"

"How do you know there are settlers coming?" I say. "Have you been talking to her? Is she all right?"

He don't answer this but he don't hit me for it neither. He just smiles and says, "All in good time, Todd."

We hear Noise coming up the stairs outside the door. **Alive, I'm alive** it says **alive alive alive** and into the room comes Mayor Ledger, pushed by Mr Collins.

He pulls up his step when he sees Mayor Prentiss standing there.

"New bedding will arrive tomorrow," Mayor Prentiss says, still looking at me. "As will toilet privileges."

Mayor Ledger's moving his jaw but it takes a few tries before any words come out. "Mr President–"

Mayor Prentiss ignores him. "Your first job will also begin tomorrow, Todd."

"*Job*?" I say.

"Everyone has to work, Todd," he says. "Work is the path to freedom. I will be working. So will Mr Ledger."

"I will?" Mayor Ledger says.

"But we're in jail," I say.

He smiles again and there's more amusement in it and I wonder how I'm about to be stung.

"Get some sleep," he says, stepping to the door and looking me in the eye. "My son will collect you first thing in the morning."

}

THE NEW LIFE

[TODD]

BUT IT TURNS OUT IT ain't Davy that worries me when I get dragged into the cold of the next morning in front of the cathedral. It ain't even Davy I look at.

It's the horse.

Boy colt, it says, shifting from hoof to hoof, looking down at me, eyes wide in that horse craziness, like I need a good stomping.

"I don't know nothing bout horses," I say.

"She's from my private herd," Mayor Prentiss says atop his own horse, Morpeth. "Her name is Angharrad and she will treat you well, Todd."

Morpeth is looking at my horse and all he's thinking is **Submit, submit, submit**, making my horse even more nervous and that's a ton of nervous animal I'm sposed to ride.

"Whatsa matter?" Davy Prentiss sneers from the saddle of a third horse. "You scared?"

"Whatsa matter?" I say. "Daddy not give you the cure yet?"

His Noise immediately rises. "You little piece of–"

"My, my," says the Mayor. "Not ten words in and the fight's already begun."

"He started it," Davy says.

"And he would finish it, too, I wager," says the Mayor, looking at me, reading the red, jittery state of my Noise, filled with urgent red askings about Viola, with more askings I wanna take outta Davy Prentiss's hide. "Come, Todd," the Mayor says, reining his horse. "Ready to be a leader of men?"

"It's a simple division," he says as we trot thru the early morning, way faster than I'd like. "The men will move to the west end of the valley in front of the cathedral and the women to the east behind it."

We're riding east down the main street of New Prentisstown, the one that starts at the zigzag road by the falls, carries thru to the town square and around the cathedral and now out the back into the farther valley. Small squads of soldiers march up and down side roads and the men of New Prentisstown come past us the other way on foot, carrying rucksacks and other luggage.

"I don't see no women," Davy says.

"*Any* women," corrects the Mayor. "And no, Captain Morgan and Captain Tate supervised the transfer of the rest of the women last night."

"What are you gonna do with 'em?" I say, my knuckles gripping so hard on the saddle horn they're turning white.

treated with the care and dignity that befits their importance to the future of New World." He turns away. "But for
now, separate is best."

"You put the bitches in their place," Davy sneers.

"You will not speak that way in front of me, David," the
Mayor says, calmly but in a voice that ain't joking. "Women
will be respected at all times and given every comfort.
Though in a non-vulgar sense you are correct. We all have
places. New World made men forget theirs, and that means
men must be away from women until we all remember who
we are, who we were meant to be."

His voice brightens a little. "The people will welcome
this. I offer clarity where before there was only chaos."

"Is Viola with the women?" I ask. "Is she okay?"

He looks back at me again. "You made a promise, Todd
Hewitt," he says. "Need I remind you once more? *Just save
her and I'll do anything you want*, I believe were your exact
words."

I lick my lips nervously. "How do I know yer keeping yer
end of the bargain?"

"You don't," he says, his eyes on mine, like he's peering
right past every lie I could tell him. "I want your faith in me,
Todd, and faith with proof is no faith at all."

He turns back down the road and I'm left with Davy
snickering to my side so I just whisper "Whoa, girl," to my
horse. Her coat is dark brown with a white stripe down her
nose and a mane brushed so nice I'm trying not to grab onto
it less it make her mad. **Boy colt**, she thinks.

She, I think. She. Then I think an asking I ain't never

50

had a chance to ask before. Cuz the ewes I had back on the farm had Noise, too, and if women ain't got Noise–

"Because women are not animals," the Mayor says, reading me. "No matter what anyone claims I believe. They are merely naturally Noiseless."

He lowers his voice. "Which makes them different."

It's mostly shops that line this part of the road, dotted twixt all the trees, closed, re-opening who knows when, with houses stretching back from side streets both towards the river on the left and the hill of the valley on the right. Most of the buildings, if not all, are built a fair distance from one another, which I spose is how you'd plan a big town before you found a cure for the Noise.

We pass more soldiers marching in groups of five or ten, more men heading west with their belongings, still no women. I look at the faces of the men going by, most of them pointed to the road at their feet, none of them looking ready to fight.

"Whoa, girl," I whisper again cuz riding a horse is turning out to be powerfully uncomfortable on yer private bits.

"And there's Todd," Davy says, pulling up next to me. "Moaning already."

"Shut it, Davy," I say.

"You will address each other as Mr Prentiss Jr and Mr Hewitt," the Mayor calls back to us.

"*What*?" Davy says, his Noise rising. "He ain't a man yet! He's just–"

The Mayor silences him with a look. "A body was discovered in the river in the early hours of this morning," he

large knife sticking out of its neck, a body dead not more than two days."

He stares at me, looking into my Noise again. I put up the pictures he wants to see, making my imaginings seem like the real thing, cuz that's what Noise is, it's everything you think, not just the truth, and if you think hard enough that you did something, well, then, maybe you actually did.

Davy scoffs. "*You* killed Preacher Aaron? I don't believe it."

The Mayor don't say nothing, just gees Morpeth along a little faster. Davy sneers at me, then kicks his own horse to follow.

"Follow," Morpeth nickers.

"Follow," Davy's horse whinnies back.

Follow, thinks my own horse, taking off after them, bouncing me even worse.

As we go, I'm on the constant look out for her, even tho there's no chance of seeing her. Even if she's still alive, she'd still be too sick to walk, and if she weren't too sick to walk, she'd be locked up with the rest of the women.

But I keep looking–

(cuz maybe she escaped–)

(maybe she's looking for me–)

(maybe she's–)

And then I hear it.

I AM THE CIRCLE AND THE CIRCLE IS ME.

Clear as a bell, right inside my head, the voice of the Mayor, twining around my own voice, like it's speaking direktly into my Noise, so sudden and real I sit up and nearly fall off my horse. Davy looks surprised, his Noise wondering what I'm reacting to.

But the Mayor just rides on down the road, like nothing happened at all.

The town gets less shiny the farther east we get from the cathedral and soon we're riding on gravel. The buildings get plainer, too, long wooden houses set at distances from each other like bricks dropped into clearings of trees.

Houses that radiate the silence of women.

"Quite correct," the Mayor says. "We're entering the new Women's Quarter."

My heart starts to clench as we go past, the silence rising up like a grasping hand.

I try to sit up higher on my horse.

Cuz this is where she'd be, this is where she'd be healing.

Davy rides up next to me again, his pathetic, half-there moustache bending into an ugly smile. **I'll tell you where yer whore is**, his Noise says.

Mayor Prentiss spins round in his saddle.

And there's the weirdest flash of sound from him, like a shout but quiet and away from me, not in the world at all, like a million words all said together, so fast I swear I feel my hair brush back like in a wind.

But it's Davy who reacts–

His head jerks back like he's been hit, and he has to catch his horse's reins so he don't fall off, spinning the horse round, his eyes wide and dazed, his mouth open, some drool dripping out.

What the hell–?

"He doesn't know, Todd," the Mayor says. "Anything his Noise tells you about her is a lie."

I look at Davy, still dazed and blinking with pain, then back to the Mayor. "Does that mean she's safe?"

"It means he doesn't know. Do you, David?"

No, Pa, says Davy's Noise, still shaky.

Mayor Prentiss raises his eyebrows.

I see Davy clench his teeth. "No, Pa," he says out loud.

"I know my son is a liar," the Mayor says. "I know he is a bully and a brute and ignorant of the things I hold dear. But he is my son." He turns back down the road. "And I believe in redemption."

Davy's Noise is quiet as we follow on but there's a dark red seething in it.

New Prentisstown fades in the distance and the road becomes almost free of buildings. Farm fields start showing up red and green thru the trees and up the hills, with crops I reckernize and others I don't. The silence of the women starts to ease a little and the valley becomes a wilder place, flowers growing in the ditches and waxy squirrels chattering insults to each other and the sun shining clear and cool like nothing else was going on.

At a bend in the river, we curve round a hill and I see a

large metal tower poking out the top of it, stretching up into the sky.

"What's that?" I say.

"Wouldn't you like to know?" Davy says, tho it's obvious he don't know neither. The Mayor don't answer.

Just past the tower, the road bends again and follows a long stone wall emerging outta the trees. Down a little farther, the wall connects to a big arched gate with a huge set of wooden doors. It's the only opening in the long, long wall I see. The road beyond is dirt, like we've come to the end.

"New World's first and last monastery," the Mayor says, stopping at the gate. "Built as a refuge of quiet contemplation for our holiest of men. Built when there was still faith we could beat the Noise germ through self-denial and discipline." His voice goes hard. "Abandoned before it was even properly finished."

He turns to face us. I hear a strange spark of happiness rising in Davy's Noise. Mayor Prentiss gives him a warning look.

"You are wondering," he says to me, "why I appointed my son as your overseer."

I cast a look over to Davy, still smiling away.

"You need a firm hand, Todd," the Mayor says. "Your thoughts even now are of how you might escape at the first opportunity and try to find your precious Viola."

"Where is she?" I say, knowing I won't get no answer.

"And I have no doubt," the Mayor continues, "that David here will be quite a firm hand for you indeed."

Davy's face and Noise both smirk.

"And in return, David will learn what real courage looks

like." Davy's smirk vanishes. "He will learn what it's like to act with honour, what it's like to act like a real man. What it's like, in short, to act like you, Todd Hewitt." He gives his son a last glance and then turns Morpeth in the road. "I shall be exceedingly eager to hear how your first day together went."

Without another word, he sets off back to New Prentisstown. I wonder now why he came in the first place. Surely he's got more important things to do.

"Surely I do," the Mayor calls, not turning back. "But don't underestimate yourself, Todd."

He rides off. Davy and I wait till he's well outta hearing distance.

I'm the one who speaks first.

"Tell me what happened to Ben or I'll rip yer effing throat out."

"I'm yer boss, boyo," Davy says, smirking again, jumping off his horse and throwing his rucksack to the ground. "Best treat me with respect or pa ain't gonna–"

But I'm already off Angharrad and hitting him as hard as I can in the face, aiming right for that sad excuse for a moustache. He takes the punch but comes back fast with his own. I ignore the pain, he does, too, and we fall to the ground in a heap of fists and kicks and elbows and knees. He's still bigger than me but only just, only in a way that don't feel like much of a difference no more, but still enough so that after a bit he's got me on my back with his forearm pressed into my throat.

His lip's bleeding, so's his nose, the same as my own poor

face but that ain't concerning me now. Davy reaches behind him and pulls a pistol from a holster strapped to his back.

"Ain't no way yer pa's gonna let you shoot me," I say.

"Yeah," he says, "but I still got a gun and you don't."

"Ben beat you," I grunt, underneath his arm. "He stopped you on the road. We got away from you."

"He didn't stop me," Davy sneers. "I took him prisoner, didn't I? And I took him back to Pa and Pa let me torture him. Let me torture him right to *death*."

And Davy's Noise–

I–

I can't say what's in Davy's Noise (he's a liar, he's a *liar*) but it makes me strong enough to push him away. We fight more, Davy fending me off with the butt of the gun till finally, with an elbow to his throat, I knock him down.

"You remember *that*, boy," Davy says, coughing, gun still gripped. "When my pa says all those nice things about you. He's the one who had me torture yer Ben."

"Yer a liar," I say. "Ben beat you."

"Oh, yeah?" Davy says. "Where is he now then? Coming to rescue you?"

I step forward, my fists up, cuz of course he's right, ain't he? My Noise surges with the loss of Ben, like it's happening all over again right here.

Davy's laughing, scrambling back away from me till he's against the huge wooden door. "My pa can read you," he says, then his eyes widen into a taunt. "Read you like a *book*."

My Noise gets even louder. "You *give* me that book! Or I swear, I'll kill you!"

57

"You ain't gonna do nothing to me, Mr Hewitt," Davy says, rising, his back still against the door. "You wouldn't wanna put yer beloved bitch at risk now, would you?"

And there it is.

They know they got me.

Cuz I won't put her in no more danger.

My hands are ready to do more damage to Davy Prentiss, like they did before when he hurt her, when he *shot* her–

But they won't now–

Even tho they *could*–

Cuz he's weak.

And we both know it.

Davy's smile drops. "Think yer special, do you?" he spits. "Think Pa's got a treat for you?"

I clench my fists, unclench them.

But I keep my place.

"Pa knows you," Davy says. "Pa's *read* you."

"He don't know," I say. "You don't neither."

Davy sneers again. "That so?" His hand reaches for the cast iron handle of the door. "Come and meet yer new flock then, Todd Hewitt."

His weight opens the door behind him and he steps into the paddock and outta the way, giving me a clear view.

Of a hundred or more Spackle staring right back at me.

4

THE MAKING OF A NEW WORLD

[TODD]

MY FIRST THOUGHT is to turn and run. Run and run and run and never stop.

"I'd like to see *that*," Davy says, standing inside the gate, smiling like he just won a prize.

There's so many of 'em, so many long white faces looking back at me, their eyes too big, their mouths too small and toothy and high on their faces, their ears looking nothing like a man's.

But you can still see a man's face in there, can't you? Still see a face that feels and fears–

And suffers.

It's hard to tell which are male and which are female cuz they all got the same lichen and moss growing right on their skins for clothing but there seem to be whole Spackle *families* in there, larger spacks protecting their spack children and what must be spack husbands protecting spack wives, arms wrapped round each other, heads pressed

59

Silently.

"I *know*!" Davy says. "Can you believe they gave the cure to these *animals*?"

They look at Davy now and a weird clicking starts passing twixt 'em all with glances and nods moving along the crowd. Davy raises his pistol and steps further into the monastery grounds. "Thinking of trying something?" he spits. "Give me a reason! Go on! GIVE ME A REASON!"

The Spackle huddle closer together in their little groups, backing away from him where they can.

"Get in here, Todd," Davy says. "We got work to do."

I don't move.

"I said, get in here! They're animals. They ain't gonna do *nothing*."

I still don't move.

"He murdered one of y'all," Davy says to the Spackle.

"*Davy!*" I shout.

"Cut its head right off with a knife. Sawed and sawed—"

"Stop it!" I run at him to get him to shut his effing mouth. I don't know how he knows but he knows and he's gotta shut up right *effing now*.

The Spackle nearest the gate scoot way back at my approach, getting outta my way as fast as they can, looking at me with frightened faces, parents getting their children behind them. I push Davy hard but he just laughs and I realize I'm inside the monastery walls now.

And I see just how many Spackle there are.

* * *

The stone wall of the monastery surrounds a *huge* bit of land but only one little building, some kind of storehouse. The rest is divided up into smaller fields, separated by old wooden fences with low gates. Most of 'em are badly overgrown and you can see heavy grass and brambles stretching all the way to the back walls a good hundred metres away.

But mostly you can see Spackle.

Hundreds and hundreds of 'em spread out over the grounds.

Maybe even more than a thousand.

They're pushing themselves against the monastery wall, huddling behind the rotting fences, sitting in groups or standing in rows.

But all watching me, silent as the grave, as my Noise spills out all over the place.

"He's a liar!" I say. "It weren't like that! It weren't like that at all!"

But what was it like? What was it like that I can explain?

Cuz I *did* do it, didn't I?

Not how Davy said but nearly as bad and completely as big in my Noise, too big to cover with all their eyes looking back at me, too big to surround with lies and confuse the truth, too big to not think about as a crowd of Spackle faces just stare.

"It was an accident," I say, my voice trailing off, looking from face to weird face, not seeing no pictures of Spackle Noise, not understanding the clicking they make, so doubly not knowing what's happening. "I didn't mean it."

But not one of 'em says a thing back. They don't do nothing but stare.

There's a creak as the gate behind us opens up again. We turn to look.

It's Ivan from Farbranch, the one who joined the army rather than fight it.

And look how right he was. He's wearing an officer's uniform and he's got a group of soldiers with him.

"Mr Prentiss Jr," he says, nodding at Davy, who nods back. Ivan turns to me, a look in his eye I can't read and no Noise to be heard. "It's good to see you well, Mr Hewitt."

"You two *know* each other?" Davy says, sharp-like.

"We've had past acquaintance," Ivan says, still looking at me.

But I ain't saying a word to him.

I'm too busy putting up pictures in my Noise.

Pictures of Farbranch. Pictures of Hildy and Tam and Francia. Pictures of the massacre that happened there. The massacre that didn't include him.

A look of annoyance crosses his face. "You go where the power is," he says. "That's how you stay alive."

I put up a picture of his town burning, men and women and children burning with it.

He frowns harder. "These men will stay here as guards. Your orders are to set the Spackle a-clearing the fields and make sure they're fed and watered."

Davy rolls his eyes. "Well, we know *that*–"

But Ivan's already turning and heading out the gate, leaving behind ten men with rifles. They take up stayshuns standing on top of the monastery wall, already getting to work unrolling coils of barbed wire along its edge.

"Ten men with rifles and us against all these Spackle," I say, under my breath but all over my Noise.

"Ah, we'll be okay," Davy says. He raises his pistol at the Spackle nearest him, maybe a female, holding a Spackle baby. She turns the baby away so her body's protecting it. "They ain't got no fight in 'em anyway."

I see the face of the Spackle protecting her baby.

It's defeated, I think. They all are. And they know it.

I know how they feel.

"Hey, pigpiss, check it out," Davy says. He raises his arms in the air, getting all the Spackle eyes on him. "People of New Prentisstown!" he shouts, waving his arms about. "I read to you yer *doooooooom*!"

And he just laughs and laughs and laughs.

Davy decides to oversee the Spackle clearing the fields of scrub but that's only cuz that means I'm the one who'll have to shovel out the fodder from the storehouse for all of 'em to eat and then fill troughs for 'em to drink from.

But it's farm work. I'm used to it. All the chores Ben and Cillian set me to doing every day. All the chores I used to complain about.

I wipe my eyes and get on with it.

The Spackle keep their distance from me as best they can while I work. Which, I gotta say, is okay by me.

Cuz I find I can't really look 'em in the eyes.

I keep my head down and carry on shovelling.

Davy says his pa told him the Spackle worked as servants

Mayor's first orders was for everyone to keep 'em locked away in their homes till the army collected 'em last night while I slept.

"People had 'em living in their back *gardens*," Davy says, watching me shovel as the morning turns to afternoon, eating what's sposed to be lunch for both of us. "Can you believe that? Like they're effing members of the *family*."

"Maybe they were," I say.

"Well they ain't no more," Davy says, rising and taking out his pistol. He grins at me. "Back to work."

I empty most of the storehouse of fodder but it still don't look like nearly enough. Plus, three of the five water pumps ain't working and by sunset, I've only managed to fix one.

"Time to go," Davy says.

"I ain't done," I say.

"Fine," he says, walking towards the gate. "Stay here on yer own then."

I look back at the Spackle. Now that the work day's thru, they've pushed themselves as far away from the soldiers and the front gates as possible.

As far away from me and Davy as possible, too.

I look back and forth twixt them and Davy leaving. They ain't got enough food. They ain't got enough water. There ain't no place to go to the toilet and no shelter of any kind at all.

I hold out my empty hands towards 'em but that don't do no kind of explaining that'll make anything okay. They just stare at me as I drop my hands and follow Davy out the gate.

"So much for being a man of courage, eh, pigpiss?" Davy says, untying his horse, which he calls Deadfall but which only seems to answer to Acorn.

I ignore him cuz I'm thinking bout the Spackle. How I'll treat them well. I will. I'll see that they get enough water and food and I'll do everything I can to protect 'em.

I *will*.

I promise that to myself.

Cuz that's what she'd want.

"Oh, I'll tell you what she *really* wants," Davy sneers.

And we fight again.

New bedding's been put in the tower when I get back, a mattress and a sheet spread out on one side for me and another on the other side for Mayor Ledger, already sitting on his, Noise jangling, eating a bowl of stew.

The bad smell's gone, too.

"Yes," says Mayor Ledger. "And guess who had to clean it up?"

It turns out he's been put to work as a rubbish man.

"Honest labour," he says to me, shrugging, but there are other sounds in his greyish Noise that make me think he don't believe it's very honest at all. "Symbolic, I suppose. I go from the top of the heap to the bottom. It'd be poetic if it weren't so obvious."

There's stew for me by my bed, too, and I take it to the window to look out over the town.

Which is starting to *buzz*.

As the cure leaves the systems of the men of the town,

you begin to hear it. From inside the houses and buildings, from down the side streets and behind the trees.

Noise is returning to New Prentisstown.

It was hard for me to even walk thru *old* Prentisstown and that only ever had 146 men in it. New Prentisstown's gotta have ten times that many. And boys, too.

I don't know how I'm gonna be able to bear it.

"You'll get used to it," Mayor Ledger says, finishing his stew. "Remember, I lived here for twenty years before we found a cure."

I close my eyes but all I see is a herd of Spackle, looking back at me.

Judging me.

Mayor Ledger taps me on the shoulder and points at my bowl of stew. "Are you going to eat that?"

That night I dream–

About her–

The sun's shining behind her and I can't see her face and we're on a hillside and she's saying something but the roar of the falls behind us is too loud and I say "What?" and when I reach for her, I don't touch her but my hand comes back covered in blood–

"Viola!" I say, sitting up on my mattress in the dark, breathing heavy.

I look over to Mayor Ledger on his mattress, facing away from me, but his Noise ain't sleeping Noise, it's the grey-type Noise he has when he's awake.

"I know yer up," I say.

"You dream quite loud," he says, not looking back. "She someone important?"

"Never you mind."

"We just have to get through it, Todd," he says. "That's all any of us has to do now. Just stay alive and get through it."

I turn to the wall.

There ain't nothing I can do. Not while they got her.

Not while I don't know.

Not while they could still hurt her.

Stay alive and get thru it, I think.

And I think of her out there.

And I whisper it, whisper it to her, wherever she is. "Stay alive and get thru it."

Stay alive.

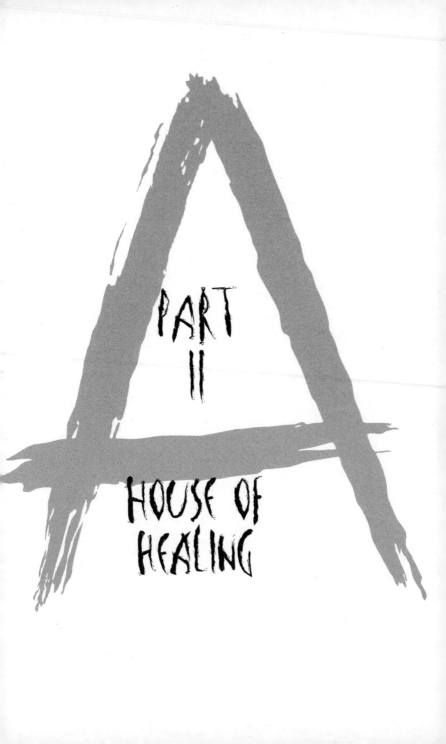

PART
II

HOUSE OF
HEALING

5

VIOLA WAKES

{VIOLA}

"CALM YOURSELF, MY GIRL."

A voice–

In the brightness–

I blink open my eyes. Everything is a pure white so bright it's almost a sound and there's a voice out there in it and my head is groggy and there's a pain in my side and it's too bright and I can't think–

Wait–

Wait–

He was carrying me down the hill–

Just *now* he was carrying me down the hill into Haven after–

"Todd?" I say, my voice a rasp, full of cotton and spit, but I run at it as hard as I can, forcing it out into the bright lights blinding my eyes. "*TODD?*"

"I said to calm yourself, now."

I don't recognize the voice, the voice of a woman–

"Who are you?" I ask, trying to sit up, pushing out my hands to feel what's around me, feeling the coolness of the air, the softness of–

A bed?

I feel panic begin to rise.

"*Where is he*?" I shout. "*TODD?*"

"I don't know any Todd, my girl," the voice says as shapes start to come together, as the brightness separates into lesser brightnesses, "but I do know you're in no shape to be demanding information."

"You were *shot*," says another voice, another woman, younger than the first, off to my right.

"Hush your mouth, Madeleine Poole," says the first woman.

"Yes, Mistress Coyle."

I keep on blinking and I start to see what's right in front of me. I'm in a narrow white bed in a narrow white room. I'm wearing a thin white gown, tied at the back. A woman both tall and plump stands in front of me, a white coat with a blue outstretched hand stitched into it draped over her shoulders, her mouth set in a line, her expression solid. Mistress Coyle. Behind her at the door holding a bowl of steaming water is a girl not much older than me.

"I'm Maddy," says the girl, sneaking a smile.

"Out," says Mistress Coyle, without even turning her head. Maddy catches my eye as she leaves, another smile sent my way.

"Where am I?" I ask Mistress Coyle, my breath still fast.

"Do you mean the room, my girl? Or the *town*?" She holds my eyes. "Or indeed the planet?"

"Please," I say and my eyes suddenly start to fill with water and I'm angry about that but I keep talking. "I was with a boy."

She sighs and looks away for a second, then she purses her lips and sits down in a chair next to the bed. Her face is stern, her hair pulled back in plaits so tight you could probably climb them, her body solid and big and not at all someone who you'd mess around.

"I'm sorry," she says, almost tenderly. Almost. "I don't know anything about a boy." She frowns. "I'm afraid I don't know anything about anything except that you were brought to this house of healing yesterday morning so close to death I wasn't at all sure we would be able to bring you back. Except that we were informed in no uncertain terms that *our* survival rather depended upon *yours*."

She waits to see how I take this.

I have no idea how I take this.

Where *is* he? What have they done with him?

I turn away from her to try and *think* but I'm wrapped so tight in bandages around my middle I can't properly sit up.

Mistress Coyle runs a couple of fingers across her brow. "And now that you're back," she says, "I'm not at all sure you're going to thank us for the world to which we've returned you."

She tells me of Mayor Prentiss arriving in Haven in front of the rumour of an army, a big one, big enough to crush the town without effort, big enough to set the whole world ablaze. She tells me of the surrender of someone called Mayor Ledger, of

73

how he shouted down the few people who wanted to fight, of how most people agreed to let him "hand over the town on a plate with a bow tied round it".

"And then the houses of healing," she says, real anger coming off her voice, "suddenly became prisons for the women inside."

"So you're a doctor, then?" I ask, but all I can feel is my chest pulling in on itself, sinking as if under an enormous weight, sinking because we failed, sinking because outrunning the army proved to be of no use at all.

Her mouth curls in a small smile, a secret one, like I just let something go. But it's not cruel and I'm finding myself less afraid of her, of what this room might mean, less afraid for myself, more afraid for *him*.

"No, my girl," she says, cocking her head. "As I'm sure you know, there are no women doctors on New World. I'm a healer."

"What's the difference?"

She runs her fingers across her brow again. "What's the difference indeed?" She drops her hands in her lap and looks at them. "Even though we're locked up," she says, "we still hear rumours, you see. Rumours of men and women being separated all over town, rumours of the army arriving perhaps this very day, rumours of slaughter coming over the hill to vanquish us all no matter how well we *surrendered*."

She's looking at me hard now. "And then there's you."

I look away from her. "I'm not anyone special."

"Are you not?" She looks unconvinced. "A girl whose arrival the whole town has to be cleared for? A girl whose life I am ordered to save on pain of my own? A girl," she leans forward to make sure I'm listening, "fresh from the great black beyond?"

I stop breathing for a second and hope she doesn't notice. "Where'd you get an idea like that?"

She grins again, not unkindly. "I'm a healer. The first thing I ever see is skin and so I know it well. Skin tells the story of a person, where they've been, what they've eaten, who they are. You've got some surface wear, my girl, but the rest of your skin is the softest and whitest I've seen in my twenty years of doing the good work. Too soft and white for a planet of farmers."

I'm still not looking at her.

"And then there are the rumours, of course, brought in by the refugees, of more settlers on the way. Thousands of them."

"Please," I say quietly, my eyes welling up again. I try to force them to stop.

"And no girl from New World would ever ask a woman if she was a doctor," she finishes.

I swallow. I put a hand to my mouth. Where is he? I don't care about any of this because *where is he?*

"I know you're frightened," Mistress Coyle says. "But we're suffering from an *excess* of fright here in this town and there's nothing I can do about that." She reaches out a rough hand to touch my arm. "But maybe you can do something to help *us.*"

I swallow but I don't say anything.

There's only one person I can trust.

And he's not here.

Mistress Coyle leans back in her chair. "We did save your life," she says. "A little knowledge could be a large comfort."

75

I breathe in deep, looking around the room, around at the sunlight streaming in from a window looking out onto trees and a river, *the* river, the one we followed into what was supposed to be safety. It seems impossible that anything bad could be happening anywhere on a day so bright, that there's any danger on the doorstep, that there's an army coming.

But there *is* an army coming.

There *is*.

And it won't be any friend to Mistress Coyle, no matter what's happened to–

I feel a little pain in my chest.

But I take a breath.

And I start to talk.

"My name," I say, "is Viola Eade."

"More settlers, huh?" Maddy says with a smile. I'm lying on my side as she unwraps the long bandage around my middle. The underside is covered in blood, my skin dusty and rust-coloured where it's dried. There's a little hole in my stomach, tied up with fine string.

"Why doesn't this hurt?" I say.

"Jeffers root on the bandages," Maddy says. "Natural opiate. You won't feel any pain but you won't be able to go to the toilet for a month either. Plus, you'll be sound asleep in about five minutes."

I touch the skin around the bullet wound, gently, gently. There's another on my back where the bullet went in. "Why aren't I dead?"

"Would you rather be dead?" She smiles again, which

changes to the smiliest frown I've ever seen. "I shouldn't joke. Mistress Coyle's always saying I lack the *proper serious-ness* to be a healer." She dips a cloth in a basin of hot water and starts washing the wounds. "You aren't dead because Mistress Coyle is the best healer in all of Haven, better than any of those so-called *doctors* they've got in this town. Even the bad guys know that. Why do you think they brought you here instead of a clinic?"

She's wearing the same long white coat as Mistress Coyle but she's also got on a short white cap with the blue out-stretched hand stitched on it, which she told me is something apprentices wear. She can't be more than a year or two older than me, whatever way they measure age on this planet, but her hands are sure, gentle and firm all around the wounds.

"So," she says, her voice deceptively light. "How bad *are* these bad guys?"

The door opens. A short girl in another apprentice cap leans in, young as Maddy but with dark brown skin and a storm cloud hanging over her head. "Mistress Coyle says you need to finish up right now."

Maddy doesn't look up from taping new bandages to my front. "Mistress Coyle knows I've only had time to get halfway done."

"We've been summoned," says the girl.

"You say that like we get *summoned* all the time, Corinne." The bandages are almost as good as the ones I had from my ship, the medicine on them already cooling my torso, already making my eyelids heavy. Maddy finishes on the front and turns to cut another set for my back. "I am in the middle of a healing."

"A man came by with a gun," Corinne says.

Maddy stops bandaging.

"Everyone's been called to the town square," Corinne continues. "Which includes you, Maddy Poole, healing or not." She crosses her arms hard. "I'll bet it's the army coming."

Maddy looks me in the eyes. I look away.

"We'll finally see what our end looks like," Corinne says.

Maddy rolls her eyes. "Always so cheerful, you," she says. "Tell Mistress Coyle I'll be out in two ticks."

Corinne gives her a sour look but leaves. Maddy finishes up the bandages on my back, by which time I can barely stay awake.

"You sleep now," Maddy says. "It'll be all right, you just watch. Why would they save you if they were going to..." She doesn't finish the thought, just scrunches her lips and then smiles. "I'm always *saying* Corinne's got enough proper seriousness in her for all of us put together."

Her smile is the last thing I see before I sleep.

"*TODD!*"

I jolt awake again, the nightmare dashing away, Todd slipping from me–

I hear a clunk and I see a book drop from Maddy's lap as she blinks herself awake in the chair by the bed. Night's fallen, and the room is dark, just a little lamp on where Maddy was meant to have been reading.

"Who's Todd?" she asks, yawning, already smiling through it. "Your *boyfriend?*" The look on my face makes her drop the tease immediately. "Someone important?"

I nod, still breathing heavily from the nightmare, my hair plastered to my forehead with sweat. "Someone important."

She pours me a glass of water from a pitcher on the bed-side table. "What happened?" I say, taking a drink. "You were summoned."

"Ah, yes, that," Maddy says, sitting back. "*That* was interesting."

She tells me about how everyone in the entire town – not Haven any more, New Prentisstown, a name that makes my stomach sink – gathered to watch the army march in and watch the new Mayor execute the old one.

"Except he didn't," Maddy says. "He spared him. Said he would spare all of us, too. That he was taking away the Noise cure, which the men weren't too happy about and good Lord it's been nice not to hear it yammering for the past six months, but that we should all know our place and remember who we were and that we would make a new home together in preparation for all the settlers that were coming."

She widens her eyes, waits for me to say something.

"I didn't understand half of that," I say. "There's a cure?"

She shakes her head but not to say no. "Boy, you really aren't from around here, are you?"

I set down the glass of water, leaning forward and lowering my voice to a whisper. "Maddy, is there a communications hub near here?"

She looks at me like I just asked her if she'd like to move with me to one of the moons. "So I can contact the ships," I say. "It might be a big, curved dish? Or a tower, maybe?"

She looks thoughtful. "There's an old metal tower up in the hills," she says, also whispering, "but I'm not even sure it is a communications tower. It's been abandoned for ages. Besides, you won't be able to get to it. There's a whole army out there, Vi."

"How big?"

"Big enough." We're both still whispering. "People are saying they're separating out the last of the women tonight."

"To do what?"

Maddy shrugs. "Corinne said a woman in the crowd told her they rounded up the Spackle, too."

I sit up, pressing against the bandages. "Spackle?"

"They're the native species here."

"I know who they are." I sit up even more, straining against the bandage. "Todd told me things, told me what happened before. Maddy, if the Mayor's separating out women and Spackle, then we're in danger. We're in the *worst kind* of danger."

I push back my sheets to get up but a sudden bolt of lightning rips through my stomach. I call out and fall back.

"Pulled a stitch," Maddy tuts, standing right up.

"Please." I grit my teeth against the pain. "We have to get out of here. We have to *run*."

"You're in no position to run anywhere," she says, reaching for my bandage.

Which is when the Mayor walks in the door.

SIDES OF THE STORY

{VIOLA}

MISTRESS COYLE LEADS HIM IN. Her face is sterner than ever, her forehead creased, her jaw set. Even having only met her once I can tell she's not happy.

He stands behind her. Tall, thin but broad-shouldered, all in white with a hat he hasn't taken off.

I've never properly seen him. I was bleeding, dying when he approached us in the town square.

But it's him.

It can only be him.

"Good evening, Viola," he says. "I've been wanting to meet you for a very long time."

Mistress Coyle sees me struggling with the sheet, sees Maddy reaching for me. "Is there a problem, Madeleine?"

"Nightmare," Maddy says, catching my eye. "I think she pulled a stitch."

"We'll ~~deal with that~~ later," Mistress Coyle says and the calm and serious way she says it gets Maddy's full attention. "Get her 400 units of Jeffers root in the meantime."

"400?" Maddy says, sounding surprised, but seeing the look on Mistress Coyle's face, all she says is, "Yes, Mistress." She gives my hand a last squeeze and leaves the room.

They both watch me for a long moment, then the Mayor says, "That'll be all, Mistress."

Mistress Coyle gives me a silent look as she leaves, maybe to reassure me, maybe to ask me something or *tell* me something, but I'm too frightened to figure it out before she backs out of the room, closing the door behind her.

And then I'm alone with him.

He lets the silence build until it's clear I'm meant to say something. I'm gripping the sheet to my chest with a fist, still feeling the lightning pain fire up my side if I move.

"You're Mayor Prentiss," I say. My voice shakes when I say it but I say it.

"*President* Prentiss," he says, "but you would know me as Mayor, of course."

"Where's Todd?" I look into his eyes. I do not blink. "What have you done with him?"

He smiles again. "Smart in your first sentence, courageous in your second. We may be friends yet."

"Is he hurt?" I swallow away the burn rising in my chest. "Is he alive?"

For a second, it looks like he's not going to tell me, not even going to acknowledge that I asked, but then he says,

82

"Todd is well. Todd is alive and well and asking about you every chance he gets."

I realize I've held my breath for his answer. "Is that true?"

"Of course it's true."

"I want to see him."

"And he wants to see you," says Mayor Prentiss. "But all things in their proper order."

He keeps his smile. It's almost friendly.

Here is the man we spent all those weeks running from, here he is, standing in my very own room, where I can barely move from the pain.

And he's *smiling*.

And it's almost friendly.

If he's hurt Todd, if he's laid a *finger* on him–

"Mayor Prentiss–"

"*President* Prentiss," he says again, then his voice brightens. "But you may call me David."

I don't say anything, just press down harder onto my bandage against the pain.

There's something about him. Something I can't quite place–

"That is," he says, "if I may call you Viola."

There's a knock on the door. Maddy opens it, a phial in her hand. "Jeffers," she says, keeping her eyes firmly on the floor. "For her pain."

"Yes, of course," the Mayor says, moving away from my bed, hands behind his back. "Proceed."

Maddy pours me a glass of water and watches me swallow four yellow gel caps, two more than I've taken before. She takes the glass from me and, with her back to the Mayor, gives me a firm look, a solid one, no smile but all kinds of bravery, and it makes me feel a little bit good, a little bit stronger.

"She'll grow tired very quickly," Maddy says to the Mayor, still not looking at him.

"I understand," the Mayor says. Maddy leaves, closing the door behind her. My stomach immediately starts to grow warm but it'll take a minute just yet to make the pain start to go or take away the quivering running all through me.

"So," the Mayor says. "May I?"

"May you what?"

"Call you Viola?"

"I can't stop you," I say. "If you want."

"Good," he says, not sitting, not moving, the smile still fixed. "When you are feeling better, Viola, I would very much like to have a talk with you."

"About what?"

"Why, your ships, of course," he says. "Coming closer by the moment."

I swallow. "What ships?"

"Oh, no, no, no." He shakes his head but still smiles. "You started out with intelligence and with courage. You are frightened but that has not stopped you from addressing me with calmness and clarity. All most admirable." He bends his head down. "But to that we must add honesty. We *must* start out honestly with each other, Viola, or how may we proceed at all?"

Proceed to where? I think.

"I have told you that Todd is alive and well," he says, "and what I tell you is true." He places a hand on the rail at the end of the bed. "And he will *stay* safe." He pauses. "And you will give me your honesty."

And I understand without having to be told that one depends on the other.

The warmth is starting to spread up from my stomach, making everything seem slower, softer. The lightning in my side is fading, but it's taking wakefulness along with it. Why *two* doses when that would put me to sleep so fast? So fast I won't even be able to talk to–

Oh.

Oh.

"I need to see him to believe you," I say.

"Soon," he says. "There is much to be done in New Prentisstown first. Much to be *un*done."

"Whether anyone wants it or not." My eyelids are getting heavy. I force them up. Only then do I realize I said it out loud.

He smiles again. "I find myself saying this with great frequency, Viola. The war is over. I am not your enemy."

I lift my groggy eyes to him in surprise.

I'm afraid of him. I am.

But–

"You were the enemy of the women of Prentisstown," I say. "You were the enemy of everyone in Farbranch."

He stiffens a little, though he tries not to let me see it. "A body was found in the river this morning," he says. "A body with a knife in its throat."

I try to keep my eyes from widening, even under the Jeffers. He's looking at me close now. "Perhaps the man's death was justified," he says. "Perhaps the man had *enemies*."

I see myself doing it–

I see myself plunging the knife–

I close my eyes.

"As for me," the Mayor says, "the war is over. My days of soldiering are at an end. Now come the days of leadership, of bringing people together."

By separating them, I think, but my breathing is slowing. The whiteness of the room is growing brighter but only in a soft way that makes me want to fall down into it and sleep and sleep and sleep. I press further into the pillow.

"I'll leave you now," he says. "We will meet again."

I begin to breathe through my mouth. Sleep is becoming impossible to avoid.

He sees me starting to drift off.

And he does the most surprising thing.

He steps forward and pulls the sheet straight across me, almost like he's tucking me in.

"Before I go," he says. "I have one request."

"What?" I say, fighting to keep awake.

"I'd like you to call me David."

"*What?*" I say, my voice heavy.

"I'd like you to say, *Good night, David*."

The Jeffers has so disconnected me that the words come out before I know I'm even saying them. "Good night, David."

Through the haze of the drug, I see him look a little surprised, even a little disappointed.

But he recovers quickly. "And to you, Viola." He nods at me and steps towards the door to leave.

And I realize what it is, what's so different about him.

"I can't hear you," I whisper from my bed.

He stops and turns. "I said, *And to–*"

"No," I say, my tongue barely able to move. "I mean I can't *hear* you. I can't hear you think."

He raises his eyebrows. "I should hope not."

And I think I'm asleep before he can even leave.

I don't wake for a long, long time, finally blinking again into the sunshine, wondering what was real and what was a dream.

(... my father, holding out his hand to help me up the ladder into the hatch, smiling, saying, "Welcome aboard, skipper...")

"You snore," says a voice.

Corinne is seated in the chair, her fingers flying a threaded needle through a piece of fabric so fast it's like it's not her doing it, like someone else's angry hands are using her lap.

"I do not," I say.

"Like a cow in oestrus."

I push back the covers. My bandages have been changed and the lightning pain is gone so the stitch must be repaired. "How long have I been asleep?"

"More than a day." She sounds disapproving. "The President's already sent men by twice to check on your condition."

I put a hand on my side, tentatively pushing on the wound. The pain is almost non-existent.

"Nothing to say to that then, my girl?" Corinne says, needle thrashing ferociously.

I furrow my forehead. "What's there to say? I'd never met him before."

"He was sure keen to know *you* though, wasn't he? Ow!" She breathes in a sharp hiss and sticks a fingertip in her mouth. "All the while he's got us trapped," she says around her finger. "All the while we can't even leave this building."

"I don't see how that's my fault."

"It isn't your fault, my girl," Mistress Coyle says, coming into the room. She looks sternly at Corinne. "And no one here thinks it is."

Corinne stands, bows slightly to Mistress Coyle and leaves without another word.

"How are you feeling?" Mistress Coyle asks.

"Groggy." I sit up more, finding it much easier to do so this time. I also notice my bladder is uncomfortably full. I tell Mistress Coyle.

"Well, then," she says, "let's see if you can stand on your own to help with that."

I take in a breath and turn to put my feet on the floor. My legs don't want to bend very fast but eventually they get there and eventually I can stand up and even walk to the door.

"Maddy *said* you were the best healer in town," I marvel.

"Maddy tells no lies."

She accompanies me down a long white hallway to a toilet. When I've finished and washed and opened the door again, Mistress Coyle is holding a heavier white gown for me to wear, longer and much nicer than the backwards robe I have on. I slip it over my head and we walk back up the hallway, a little wobbly, but walking all the same.

"The President has been asking after your health," she says, steadying me with her hand.

"Corinne told me." I look up at her out of the corner of my eye. "It's only because of the settler ships. I don't know him. I'm not on his side."

"Ah," Mistress Coyle says, getting me back through the door to my room and onto my bed. "You do recognize there are sides then?"

I lie back, my tongue pressed against the back of my teeth. "Did you give me two doses of Jeffers so I wouldn't have to speak to him for very long?" I say. "Or so I wouldn't be able to tell him very much?"

She gives a nod as if to say how clever I am. "Would it be the worst thing in the world if it was a little of both?"

"You could have asked."

"Wasn't time," she says, sitting down in the chair next to the bed. "We only know him by his history, my girl, and his history is bad, bad, bad. Whatever he might say about a new society, there is good reason to want to be better prepared if he starts a conversation."

"I don't know him," I say again. "I don't know anything."

"But, done rightly," she says, with a little smile, "you might *learn* things from a man who takes an interest."

I try to read her, read what she's trying to tell me, but of course women here don't have Noise either, do they?

"What are you saying?" I ask.

"I'm saying it's time for you to get something solid into your stomach." She stands, brushing invisible threads off her white coat. "I'll have Madeleine bring in some breakfast for you."

She walks to the door, taking hold of the handle but not turning it yet. "But know this," she says, without turning around. "If there *are* sides and our President is on one..." She glances back at me over her shoulder. "Then I am most definitely on the other."

I

MISTRESS COYLE

{VIOLA}

"THERE ARE SIX SHIPS," I say from my bed, for the third time in as many days, days where Todd is still out there somewhere, days where I don't know what's happening to him or to anyone else outside.

From the windows of my room, I see soldiers marching by all the time, but all they do is march. Everyone here at the house of healing half-expected them to come bursting through the doors at any moment, ready to do terrible things, ready to assert their victory.

But they haven't. They just march by. Other men bring us deliveries of food to the back doors, and the healers are left to their work.

We still can't leave, but the world outside doesn't seem to be ending. Which isn't what anyone expected, not least, it seems, Mistress Coyle, who's convinced it only means something worse is waiting to happen.

I can't help but think that she's probably right.

She frowns into her notes. "Just six?"

"Eight hundred sleeping settlers and three caretaker families in each," I say. I'm getting hungry, but I know by now there's no eating until she says the consultation is finished. "Mistress Coyle–"

"And you're sure there are eighty-one members of the caretaker families?"

"I should know," I say. "I was in school with their children."

She looks up. "I know this is tedious, Viola, but information is power. The information we give him. The information we learn *from* him."

I sigh impatiently. "I don't know anything *about* spying."

"It's not spying," she says, returning to her notes. "It's just finding things out." She writes something more in her pad. "Four thousand, eight hundred and eighty-one people," she says, almost to herself.

I know what she means. More people than the entire population of this planet. Enough to change everything.

But change it how?

"When he speaks with you again," she says, "you can't tell him about the ships. Keep him guessing. Keep him off the right number."

"While I'm also supposed to be finding out what I can," I say.

She closes her pad, consultation over. "Information is power," she repeats.

I sit up in the bed, pretty much sick to death of being a patient. "Can I ask you something?"

She stands and reaches for her cloak. "Certainly."

"Your face when he walked into your room," she says without hesitating. "You looked as if you'd just met your worst enemy."

She snaps the buttons of the cloak under her chin. I watch her carefully. "If I could just find Todd or get to that communications tower..."

"And be taken by the army?" She's not frowning but her eyes are bright. "Lose us our one advantage?" She opens the door. "No, my girl, the President will come a-calling and when he does, what you find out from him will help us."

I call out after her as she goes, "Who do you mean by *us*?"

But she's gone.

" ... and the last thing I really remember is him picking me up and carrying me down a long, long hill, and telling me that I wasn't going to die, that he'd save me."

"Wow," breathes Maddy softly, wisps of hair sneaking out from under her cap as we walk slowly up one hallway and down another to build my strength. "And he did save you."

"But he can't kill," I say, "not even to save himself. That's the thing about him, why they wanted him so bad. He isn't like them. He killed a Spackle once and you should have seen how he suffered for it. And now they've *got* him–"

I have to stop and blink a lot and look at the floor.

"I need to get *out* of here," I say, clenching my teeth. "I'm no spy. I need to find him and I need to get to that tower and *warn* them. Maybe they can send help. They have more scout ships that could reach here. They've got weapons..."

Maddy's face looks tense, like it always does when I talk this way. "We're not even allowed outside yet."

"You can't just accept what people tell you, Maddy. You can't just *do* that if they're wrong."

"And *you* can't fight an army on your own." She turns me gently back down the hallway, giving me a smile. "Not even the great and brave Viola Eade."

"I did it before," I say. "I did with *him*."

She lowers her voice. "Vi–"

"I lost my parents," I say and my voice is husky. "And there's no way I can get them back. And now I've lost him. And if there's a chance, if there's even a chance–"

"Mistress Coyle won't allow it," she says, but there's something in her voice that makes me look up.

"But?" I say.

Maddy says no more, just walks us over to the hall window that looks out onto the road. A troop of soldiers passes by in the bright sunlight, a cart full of dusty purple grain passing by the other way, the Noise we can hear from the town coming down the road like an army all on its own.

At first it was like no Noise I'd ever heard, this weird buzzing sound of metal grinding against metal. Then it got even louder than that, like a thousand men shouting at once, which I guess is pretty much what it is, too loud and messy to be able to pick out any individual person.

Too loud to pick out one boy.

"Maybe it's not as bad as we all think." Maddy's voice is slow, weighing every word as if she's testing them out for herself. "I mean, the town looks peaceful. *Loud,* but the men who deliver the food say the stores are about to re-open. I'll bet your Todd is out there working away at a job, safe and alive and waiting to see you."

I can't tell if she's saying this because she believes it or because she's trying to get *me* to believe it. I wipe my nose with my sleeve. "That could be true."

She looks at me for a long time, obviously thinking something but not saying it. Then she turns back to the glass.

"Just listen to them roar," she says.

There are three other healers here besides Mistress Coyle. Mistress Waggoner, a short round puff of a woman with wrinkles and a moustache, Mistress Nadari, who treats cancers and who I've only seen once closing a door behind her, and Mistress Lawson, who treats children in another house of healing but who was trapped here while having a consultation with Mistress Coyle when the surrender happened and who's been fretting ever since about the ill children she left behind.

There are more apprentices, too, a dozen besides Maddy and Corinne, who – because they work with Mistress Coyle – seem to be the top two apprentices out of the whole house, maybe even all of Haven. I rarely see the others except when they're trailing behind one of the healers, stethoscopes bouncing, white coats flapping behind them, off to find something to do.

Because the truth of it is, as the days go by and the town gets on with whatever it's doing beyond our doors, most of us patients are getting better and new ones aren't arriving. All the male patients were taken out of here the first night,

Maddy told me, whether they could travel or not, and no new women have been brought here even though invasion and surrender aren't bars to getting sick.

Mistress Coyle worries about this.

"Well, if she can't heal, then who is she?" Corinne says, snapping the elastic band around my arm a little too tight. "She used to run all of the houses of healing, not just this one. Everyone knew her, everyone respected her. For a while, she was even Chair of the Town Council."

I blink. "She used to be in charge?"

"Years ago. Quit moving around." She jabs the needle into my arm harder than she needs to. "She's always saying that being a leader is making the people you love hate you a little more each day." She catches my eye. "Which is something I believe, too."

"So what happened?" I ask. "Why isn't she still in charge?"

"She made a mistake," Corinne says primly. "People who didn't like her took advantage of it."

"What kind of mistake?"

Her permanent frown gets bigger. "She saved a life," she says and snaps loose the elastic band so hard it leaves a mark.

Another day passes, and another, and nothing changes. We're still not allowed out, our food still comes, and the Mayor still hasn't asked for me. His men check on my condition but the promised talk never happens. He's just leaving me here, so far.

Who knows why?

"And do you know what he's done?" Mistress Coyle says over dinner, my first one where I'm allowed out of bed and in the canteen. "The cathedral isn't just his base of operations. He's made it into his *home*."

There's a general clucking of disgust from the women around her. Mistress Waggoner even pushes her plate away. "He fancies himself *God* now," she says.

"He hasn't burned the town down, though," I say, wondering aloud from the other end of the table. Maddy and Corinne both look up from their plates with wide eyes. I carry on anyway. "We all thought he would, but he hasn't."

Mistresses Waggoner and Lawson give Mistress Coyle a meaningful look.

"You show your youth, Viola," Mistress Coyle says. "And you shouldn't challenge your superiors."

I blink, surprised. "That's not what I meant," I say. "I'm only saying it's not what we expected."

Mistress Coyle takes another bite while eyeing me. "He killed every woman in his town because he couldn't hear them, because he couldn't *know* them in the way that men could be known before the cure."

The other mistresses nod. I open my mouth to speak but she overrides me.

"What's also true, my girl," she says, "is that everything we've been through since landing on this planet – the surprise of the Noise, the chaos that followed – all of that remains unknown to your friends up there." She's watching me closely now. "Everything that happened to us is waiting to happen to them."

96

I don't reply, I just watch her.

"And who do you want in charge of that process?" she asks. "Him?"

She's done talking to me and returns to quieter conference with the mistresses. Corinne starts eating again, a smug grin on her face. Maddy's still staring at me wide-eyed, but all I can think of is the word left hanging in the air.

When she said *Him?*, did she also mean, *Or her?*

On our ninth day locked indoors, I'm no longer a patient. Mistress Coyle summons me to her office.

"Your clothes," she says, handing me a package over her desk. "You can put them on now, if you like. Make you feel like a real person again."

"Thank you," I say genuinely, heading behind the screen she's pointed out. I lift off the patient's robe and look for a second at my wound, almost healed both front and back.

"You really are the most amazing healer," I say.

"I do try," she says from her desk.

I unwrap the package and find all of my own clothes, freshly laundered, smelling so clean and crisp I feel a strange pull on my face and discover I'm smiling.

"You know, you're a brave girl, Viola," Mistress Coyle is saying, as I start to dress. "Despite not knowing when to keep quiet."

"Thank you," I say, a little annoyed.

"The crashing of your ship, the deaths of your parents, the amazing journey here. All faced with intelligence and resourcefulness."

"I had help," I say, sitting down to put on clean socks.

I notice Mistress Coyle's pad on a little side table, the one so full of notes from our little consultations. I look up but she's still on the other side of the screen. I reach over and flip open the cover.

"I sense big things in you, my girl," she says. "Leadership potential."

The notebook is upside down and I don't want to make a noise by moving it so I try to twist round to see what it says.

"I see a lot of myself in you."

On the first page, before her notes start, there's only a single letter, written in blue.

A.

Nothing else.

"We are the choices we make, Viola," Mistress Coyle is still talking. "And you can be so valuable to us. If you choose."

I lift up my head from the pad. "Us who?"

The door bursts open so loud and sudden I jump up and look around the screen. It's Maddy. "There was a messenger," she says, breathless. "Women can start leaving their houses."

"It's so loud out here," I say, wincing into the ROAR of all the New Prentisstown Noise twining together.

"You get used to it," Maddy says. We're sitting on a bench outside a store while Corinne and another apprentice named Thea buy supplies for the house of healing, stocking up for the expected flood of new patients.

I look around the streets. Stores are open, people pass by, mostly on foot but on fissionbikes and horses, too. If you don't look too closely, you'd almost think nothing was even wrong.

But then you see that the men who move down the road never talk to each other. And women are allowed out only in groups of four and only in daylight and only for an hour at a time. And the groups of four never interact. Even the men of Haven don't approach us.

And there are soldiers on every corner, rifles in hand.

A bell chimes as the door of the store opens. Corinne storms out, arms full of bags, face full of thunder, Thea struggling behind her. "The storekeeper says no one's heard from the Spackle since they were taken," Corinne says, practically dropping a bag in my lap.

"Corinne and her spacks," Thea says, rolling her eyes and handing me another bag.

"Don't call them that," Corinne says. "If *we* could never treat them right, what do you think *he's* going to be doing to them?"

"I'm sorry, Corinne," Maddy says before I can ask what Corinne means, "but don't you think it makes more sense to worry about us right now?" Her eyes are watching some soldiers who've noticed Corinne's raised voice. They aren't moving, haven't even shifted from the veranda of a feed store.

But they're looking.

"It was inhuman, what we did to them," Corinne says.

"Yes, but they *aren't* human," Thea says, under her breath, looking at the soldiers, too.

"Th— Reese!" A vein bulges out of Corinne's forehead. "How can you call yourself a healer and say—"

"Yes, yes, all right," Maddy says, trying to calm her down. "It was awful. I agree. You know we *all* agree, but what could we have done about it?"

"What are you talking about?" I say. "Did *what* to them?"

"The *cure*," Corinne says, saying it like a curse.

Maddy turns to me with a frustrated sigh. "They found out that the cure worked on the Spackle."

"By *testing* it on them," Corinne says.

"But it does more than that," Maddy says. "The Spackle don't *speak*, you see. They can click their mouths a little but it's hardly more than like when we snap our fingers."

"The Noise was the only way they communicated," Thea says.

"And it turned out we didn't really need them to talk to us to tell them what to do," Corinne says, her voice rising even more. "So who cares if they needed to talk to each *other*?"

I'm beginning to see. "And the cure..."

Thea nods. "It makes them docile."

"Better slaves," Corinne says bitterly.

My mouth drops open. "They were *slaves*?"

"Shhhh," Maddy shushes harshly, jerking her head toward the soldiers watching us, their lack of Noise among all the ROAR of the other men making them seem ominously blank.

"It's like we cut out their tongues," Corinne says, lowering her voice but still burning.

But Maddy is already getting us on our way, looking back over her shoulder at the soldiers.

Who watch us go.

100

* * *

We walk the short distance back to the house of healing in silence, entering the front door under the blue outstretched hand painted over the door frame. After Corinne and Thea go inside, Maddy takes my arm lightly to hold me back.

She looks at the ground for a minute, a dimple forming in the middle of her eyebrows. "The way those soldiers looked at us," she says.

"Yeah?"

She crosses her arms and shivers. "I don't know if I like this version of peace very much."

"I know," I say softly.

She waits a moment, then she looks at me square. "Could your people help us? Could they stop this?"

"I don't know," I say, "but finding out would be better than just sitting here, waiting for the worst to happen."

She looks around to see if we're being overheard. "Mistress Coyle is brilliant," she says, "but sometimes she can only hear her own opinion."

She waits, biting her upper lip.

"Maddy?"

"We'll watch out," she says.

"For what?"

"*If* the right moment arrives, and *only* if," she looks around again, "we'll see what we can do about contacting your ships."

8

THE NEWEST APPRENTICE

{VIOLA}

"BUT SLAVERY IS WRONG," I say, rolling up another bandage.

"The healers were always opposed to it." Mistress Coyle ticks off another box on her inventory. "Even after the Spackle War, we thought it inhuman."

"Then why didn't you stop it?"

"If you ever see a war," she says, not looking up from her clipboard, "you'll learn that war only destroys. No one escapes from a war. No one. Not even the survivors. You accept things that would appal you at any other time because life has temporarily lost all meaning."

"*War makes monsters of men,*" I say, quoting Ben from that night in the weird place where New World buried its dead.

"And women," Mistress Coyle says. She taps her fingers on boxes of syringes to count them.

"But the Spackle War was over a long time ago, wasn't it?"

"Thirteen years now."

"Thirteen years where you could have righted a wrong."

She finally looks at me. "Life is only that simple when you're young, my girl."

"But you were in charge," I say. "You could have done something."

"And who told you I was in charge?"

"Corinne said–"

"Ah, Corinne," she says, turning back to her clipboard, "doing her best to love me no matter what the facts."

I open up another bag of supplies. "But if you were head of this Council thing," I press on, "surely you could have done *something* about the Spackle."

"Sometimes, my girl," she says, giving me a displeased look, "you can lead people where they don't want to go, but most of the time you *can't*. The Spackle weren't going to be freed, not after we'd just beaten them in an awful and vicious war, not when we needed so much labour to rebuild. But they could be treated better, couldn't they? They could be fed properly and set to work humane hours and allowed to live together with their families. All victories *I* won for them, Viola."

Her writing on the clipboard is a lot more forceful than it was. I watch her for a second. "Corinne says you were thrown off the Council for saving a life."

She doesn't answer me, just sets down her clipboard and looks on one of the higher shelves. She reaches up and takes down an apprentice hat and a folded apprentice cloak. She turns and tosses them to me.

"Who are these for?" I say, catching them.

"You want to find out about being a leader?" she says. "Then let's put you on the path."

I look at her face.

I look down at the cloak and the cap.

From then on, I barely have time to eat.

The day after women were allowed to move again, there were eighteen new patients, all female, who'd been suffering all kinds of things – appendicitis, heart problems, lapsed cancer treatments, broken bones – all trapped in houses where they'd been stuck after being separated from husbands and sons. The next day, there were eleven more. Mistress Lawson went back to the children's house of healing the second she was able, but Mistresses Coyle, Waggoner and Nadari were suddenly rushing from room to room, shouting orders and saving lives. I don't think anyone's been to sleep since.

There's certainly no time for me and Maddy to look for our moment, no time to even notice that the Mayor still hasn't come to see me. Instead, I run around a lot, getting in the way, helping out where I can, and squeezing apprentice lessons in.

I turn out not to be a natural healer.

"I don't think I'm ever going to get this," I say, failing yet again to tell the blood pressure of a sweet old patient called Mrs Fox.

"It sure feels that way," Corinne says, glancing up at the clock.

"Patience, pretty girl," Mrs Fox says, her face wrinkling up in a smile. "A thing worth learning is worth learning well."

"You're right there, Mrs Fox," Corinne says, looking back at me. "Try it again."

I pump up the armband to inflate it, listen through the stethoscope for the right kind of *whoosh, whoosh* in Mrs Fox's blood and match that up to the little dial. "Sixty over twenty?" I guess weakly.

"Well, let's find out," Corinne says. "Have you died this morning, Mrs Fox?"

"Oh, dearie me, no," Mrs Fox says.

"Probably not sixty over twenty then," Corinne says.

"I've only been doing this for three days," I say.

"I've been doing it for six years," Corinne says, "since I was *way* younger than you, my girl. And here you are, can't even work a blood pressure sleeve, yet suddenly an apprentice just like me. Funny how life works, huh?"

"You're doing fine, sweetheart," Mrs Fox says to me.

"No, she isn't, Mrs Fox," Corinne says. "I'm sorry to contradict you, but some of us regard healing as a sacred duty."

"I regard it as a sacred duty," I say, almost as a reflex.

This is a mistake.

"Healing is more than a *job*, my girl," Corinne says, making *my girl* sound like the worst insult. "There is nothing more important in this life than the preservation of it. We're God's hands on this world. We are the opposite of your friend the tyrant."

"He's not my–"

"To allow someone, *anyone*, to suffer is the greatest sin there is."

"Corinne–"

"You don't understand anything," she says, her voice low

and fierce. "Quit pretending that you do."

Mrs Fox has shrunk down nearly as far as I have.

Corinne glances at her and back at me, then she straightens her cap and tugs the lapels on her cloak, stretching out her neck from right to left. She closes her eyes and lets out a long, long breath.

Without looking at me, she says, "Try it again."

"The difference between a clinic and a house of healing?" Mistress Coyle asks, ticking off boxes on a sheet.

"The main difference is that clinics are run by male doctors, houses of healing by female healers," I recite, as I count out the day's pills into separate little cups for each patient.

"And why is that?"

"So that a patient, male or female, can have a choice between knowing the thoughts of their doctor or not."

She raises an eyebrow. "And the real reason?"

"Politics," I say, returning her word.

"Correct." She finishes the paperwork and hands it to me. "Take these and the medicines to Madeleine, please."

She leaves and I finish filling up the tray of medicines. When I come out with it in my hands, I see Mistress Coyle down at the end of the hallway, passing by Mistress Nadari.

And I swear I see her slip Mistress Nadari a note, without either of them pausing.

We can still only go out for an hour at a time, still only in groups of four, but that's enough to see how New Prentisstown is putting itself together. As my first week as an apprentice comes to an end, we hear tell that some women are even being sent out into fields to work in women-only groups.

We hear tell that the Spackle are being kept somewhere on the edge of town, all together as one group, awaiting "processing", whatever that might mean.

We hear tell the old Mayor is working as a dustman.

We hear nothing about a boy.

"I missed his birthday," I tell Maddy, as I practise tying bandages around a rubber leg so ridiculously realistic everyone calls it Ruby. "It was four days ago. I lost track of how long I was asleep and–"

I can't say any more, just pull the bandage tight–

And think of when he put a bandage on me–

And when I put bandages on him.

"I'm sure he's fine, Vi," Maddy says.

"No, you're not."

"No," she says, looking back out the window to the road, "but against all odds the city's not at war. Against all odds, we're still alive and still working. So, against all odds, Todd could be alive and well."

I pull tighter on the bandage. "Do you know anything about a blue A?"

She turns to me. "A what?"

I shrug. "Something I saw in Mistress Coyle's notebook."

"No idea." She looks back out the window.

"What are you looking for?"

"I'm counting soldiers," she says. She looks back again at me and Ruby. "It's a good bandage." Her smile makes it almost seem true.

I head down the main hallway, Ruby kicking from one hand. I have to practise injecting shots into her thigh. I already feel sorry for the poor woman whose thigh gets my first real jab.

I come round a corner as the hallway reaches the centre of the building, where it turns ninety degrees down the other wing, and I nearly collide with a group of mistresses, who stop when they see me.

Mistress Coyle and four, five, *six* other healers behind her. I recognize Mistress Nadari and Mistress Waggoner, and there's Mistress Lawson, too, but I've never seen the other three before and didn't even see them come into the house of healing.

"Have you no work, my girl?" Mistress Coyle says, some edge in her voice.

"Ruby," I stammer, holding out the leg.

"Is this her?" asks one of the healers I don't recognize.

Mistress Coyle doesn't introduce me.

She just says, "Yes, this is the girl."

I have to wait all day to see Maddy again, but before I can ask her about it, she says, "I've figured it out."

"Did one of them have a scar on her upper lip?" Maddy whispers in the dark. It's well past midnight, well past lights out, well past when she should be in her own room.

"I think so," I whisper back. "They left really quickly."

We watch another pair of soldiers march down the road. By Maddy's reckoning, we've got three minutes.

"That would have been Mistress Barker," she says. "Which means the others were probably Mistress Braithwaite and Mistress Forth." She looks back out the window. "This is crazy, you know. If she catches us, we'll get it good."

"I hardly think she's going to fire you under the circumstances."

Her face goes thoughtful. "Did you hear what the mistresses were saying?"

"No, they shut up the second they saw me."

"But you were *the girl*?"

"Yeah," I say. "And Mistress Coyle avoided me the rest of today."

"Mistress Barker..." Maddy says, still thinking. "But how could that accomplish anything?"

"How could what accomplish what?"

"Those three were on the Council with Mistress Coyle. Mistress Barker still *is*. Or was, before all this. But why would they be–" She stops and leans closer to the window. "That's the last foursome."

I look out and see four soldiers marching up the road.

If the pattern Maddy's spotted is right, the time is now.

If the pattern's right.

"You ready?" I whisper.

"Of *course* I'm not ready," Maddy says, with a terrified smile. "But I'm going."

I see how she's flexing her hands to keep them from shaking. "We're just going to look," I say. "That's all. Out and back again before you know it."

Maddy still looks terrified but nods her head. "I've never done anything like this before in my whole life."

"Don't worry," I say, lifting the sash on my window all the way up. "I'm an expert."

The ROAR of the town, even when it's sleeping, covers our footsteps pretty well as we sneak across the dark lawn. The only light is from the two moons, shining down on us, half-circles in the sky.

We make it to the ditch at the side of the road, crouching in the bushes.

"What now?" Maddy whispers.

"You said two minutes, then another pair."

Maddy nods in the shadows. "Then another break of seven minutes."

In that break, Maddy and I will start moving down the road, sticking to the trees, staying under cover, and see if we can get to the communications tower, if that's even what it *is*.

See what's there when we do.

"You all right?" I whisper.

"Yeah," she whispers back. "Scared but excited, too."

I know what she means. Out here, crouching in a ditch under the cover of night, it's crazy, it's dangerous, but I finally feel like I'm *doing* something, finally feel like I'm taking charge of my own life for the first time since being stuck in that bed.

Finally feel like I'm doing something for Todd.

We hear the crunch of gravel on the road and crouch a

little lower as the expected pair of soldiers march past us and away.

"Here we go," I say.

We stand up as much as we dare and move quickly down the ditch, away from the town.

"Do you still have family on the ships?" Maddy whispers. "Someone besides your mother and father?"

I wince a little at the sound she's making but I know she's only talking to cover her nerves. "No, but I know everyone else. Bradley Tench, he's lead caretaker on the *Beta*, and Simone Watkin on the *Gamma* is really smart."

The ditch bends with the road and there's a crossroads coming up that we'll have to negotiate.

Maddy starts up again. "So Simone's the one you'd–"

"Shh," I say because I think I heard something.

Maddy comes close enough to press against me. Her whole body is shaking and her breath is coming in short little puffs. She has to come this time because she knows where the tower is, but I can't ask her to do it again. When I come back, I'll come on my own.

Because if anything goes wrong–

"I think we're okay," I say.

We step slowly out from the ditch to cross the crossroads, looking all around us, stepping lightly in the gravel.

"Going somewhere?" says a voice.

Maddy takes in a sharp breath behind me. There's a soldier

leaning against a tree, his legs crossed like he couldn't be more relaxed.

Even in the moonlight I can see the rifle hanging lazily from his hand.

"Little late to be out, innit?"

"We got lost," I sputter. "We were separated from–"

"Yeah," he interrupts. "I'll bet."

He strikes a match against the zip of his uniform jacket. In the flare of light, I see SERGEANT HAMMAR written across his pocket. He uses the match to light a cigarette in his mouth.

Cigarettes were banned by the Mayor.

But I guess if you're an officer.

An officer without Noise who can hide in the dark.

He takes a step forward and we see his face. He's got a smile on over the cigarette, an ugly one, the ugliest I've ever seen.

"You?" he says, recognition in his voice as he gets nearer.

As he raises his rifle.

"Yer the girl," he says, looking at me.

"Viola?" Maddy whispers, a step behind me and to my right.

"Mayor Prentiss knows me," I say. "You won't harm me."

He inhales on the cigarette, flashing the ember, making a streak against my vision. "*President* Prentiss knows you."

Then he looks at Maddy, pointing at her with the rifle.

"I don't reckon he knows you, tho."

And before I can say anything–

Without giving any kind of warning–

As if it was as natural to him as taking his next breath–

Sergeant Hammar pulls the trigger.

9

WAR IS OVER

[TODD]

"YOUR TURN TO DO THE BOG," Davy says, throwing me the canister of lime.

We never see the Spackle use the corner where they've dug a bog to do their business but every morning it's a little bit bigger and stinks a little bit more and it needs lime powdered over it to cut down on the smell and the danger of infeckshun.

I hope it works better on infeckshun than it does on smell.

"Why ain't it never *yer* turn?" I say.

"Cuz Pa may think yer the *better man*, pigpiss," Davy says, "but he still put me in charge."

And he grins at me.

I start walking to the bog.

The days passed and they kept passing, till there was two full weeks of 'em gone and more.

I stayed alive and got thru.

(did she?)

(*did* she?)

Davy and I ride to the monastery every morning and he "oversees" the Spackle tearing down fences and pulling up brambles and I spend the day shovelling out not enough fodder and trying and failing to fix the last two water pumps and taking every turn to do the bog.

The Spackle've stayed silent, still not doing nothing that could save themselves, fifteen hundred of 'em when we finally got 'em counted, crammed into an area where I wouldn't herd two hundred sheep. More guards came, standing along the top of the stone wall, rifles pointed twixt rows of barbed wire, but the Spackle don't do nothing that even comes close to threatening.

They've stayed alive. They've got thru it.

And so has New Prentisstown.

Every day, Mayor Ledger tells me what he sees out on his rubbish rounds. Men and women are still separated and there are more taxes, more rules about dress, a list of books to be surrendered and burned, and compulsory church attendance, tho not in the cathedral, of course.

But it's also started to act like a real town again. The stores are back open, carts and fissionbikes and even a fissioncar or two are back on the roads. Men've gone back to work. Repairmen returned to repairing, bakers returned to baking, farmers returned to farming, loggers returned to logging, some of 'em even signing up to join the army itself, tho you can tell who the new soldiers are cuz they ain't been given the cure yet.

"You know," Mayor Ledger said one night and I could see it in his Noise before he said it, see the thought forming, the thought I hadn't thought myself, the thought I hadn't *let* myself think. "It's not nearly as bad as I thought," he said. "I expected slaughter. I expected my own death, certainly, and perhaps the burning of the entire town. The surrender was a fool's chance at best, but maybe he's not lying."

He got up and looked out over New Prentisstown. "Maybe," he said, "the war really is over."

"Oi!" I hear Davy call as I'm halfway to the bog. I turn round. A Spackle has come up to him.

It's holding its long white arms up and out in what may be a peaceful way and then it starts clicking, pointing to where a group of Spackle have finished tearing down a fence. It's clicking and clicking, pointing to one of the empty water troughs, but there ain't no way of understanding it, not if you can't hear its Noise.

Davy steps closer to it, his eyes wide, his head nodding in sympathy, his smile dangerous. "Yeah, yeah, yer thirsty from the hard work," he says. "Course you are, course you are, thank you for bringing that to my attenshun, thank you very much. And in reply, let me just say this."

He smashes the butt of his pistol into the Spackle's face. You can hear the crack of bone and the Spackle falls to the ground clutching at his jaw, long legs twisting in the air.

There's a wave of clicking around us and Davy lifts his pistol again, bullet end facing the crowd. Rifles cock on the fence-top, too, soldiers pointing their weapons. The Spackle clink back, the broken-jawed one still writhing and writhing in the grass.

"Know what, pigpiss?" Davy says.

"What?" I say, my eyes still on the Spackle on the ground, my Noise shaky as a leaf about to fall.

He turns to me, pistol still out. "It's *good* to be in charge."

Every minute I've expected life to blow apart.

But every minute, it don't.

And every day I've looked for her.

I've looked for her from the openings outta the top of the bell tower but all I ever see is the army marching and men working. Never a face I reckernize, never a silence I can feel as hers.

I've looked for her when Davy and I ride back and forth to the monastery, seeking her out in the windows of the Women's Quarter, but I never see her looking back.

I've even half-looked for her in the crowds of Spackle, wondering if she's hiding behind one, ready to pop out and yell at Davy for beating on 'em and then saying to me, like everything's okay, "Hey, I'm here, it's me."

But she ain't there.

She ain't there.

I've asked Mayor Prentiss bout her every time I've seen him and he's said I need to trust him, said he's not my enemy, said if I put my faith in him that everything will be all right.

But I've looked.

And she ain't there.

"Hey, girl," I whisper to Angharrad as I saddle her up at the end of our day. I've got way better at riding her, better at talking to her, better at reading her moods. I'm less nervous about being on her back and she's less nervous about being underneath me. This morning after I gave her an apple to eat, she clipped her teeth thru my hair once, like I was just another horse.

Boy colt, she says, as I climb on her back and me and Davy set off back into town.

"Angharrad," I say, leaning forward twixt her ears, cuz this is what horses like, it seems, constant reminders that everyone's there, constant reminders that they're still in the herd.

Above anything else, a horse hates to be alone.

Boy colt, Angharrad says again.

"Angharrad," I say.

"Jesus, pigpiss," Davy moans, "why don't you marry the effing–" He stops. "Well, goddam," he says, his voice suddenly a whisper, "would you look at this?"

I look up.

There are women coming out of a store.

Four of 'em, together in a group. We knew they were being let out but it's always daylight hours, always while me and Davy are at the monastery, so we always return to a city of men, like the women are just phantoms and rumour.

It's been ages since I even seen one more than just thru a window or from up top of the tower.

They're wearing longer sleeves and longer skirts than I saw before and they each got their hair tied behind their heads the same way. They look nervously at the soldiers that line the streets, at me and Davy, too, all of us watching 'em come down the store's front steps.

And there's still the silence, still the pull at my chest and I have to wipe my eyes when I'm sure Davy ain't looking.

Cuz none of 'em is her.

"They're late," Davy says, his voice so quiet I guess he ain't seen a woman for weeks neither. "They're all sposed to be in way before sundown."

Our heads turn as we watch 'em pass by, parcels held close, and they carry on down the road back to the Women's Quarter and my chest tightens and my throat clenches.

Cuz *none* of 'em is *her*.

And I realize–

I realize all over again how much–

And my Noise goes all muddy.

Mayor Prentiss has used her to control me.

Duh.

Any effing idiot would know it. If I don't do what they say, they kill her. If I try to escape, they kill her. If I do anything t Davy, they kill her.

If she ain't dead already.

My Noise gets blacker.

No.

No, I think.

Cuz she might not be.

She mighta been out here, on this very street, in another group of four.

Stay alive, I think. *Please please please stay alive.*
(please be alive)

I stand at an opening as me and Mayor Ledger eat our dinners, looking for her again, trying to close my ears against the **ROAR**.

Cuz Mayor Ledger was right. There's so many men that once the cure left their systems, you stopped being able to hear individual Noise. It'd be like trying to hear one drop of water in the middle of a river. Their Noise became a single loud wall, all mushed together so much it don't say nothing but

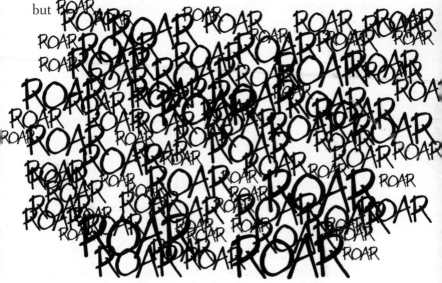

But it's actually something you can sorta get used to. In a way, Mayor Ledger's words and thoughts and feelings bubbling round his own personal grey Noise are more distracting.

"Quite correct," he says, patting his stomach. "A man is capable of thought. A crowd is not."

"An army is," I say.

"Only if it has a general for a brain."

He looks out the opening next to mine as he says it. Mayor Prentiss is riding across the square, Mr Hammar, Mr Tate, Mr Morgan and Mr O'Hare riding behind him, listening to the orders he's giving.

"The inner circle," Mayor Ledger says.

And for a second, I wonder if his Noise sounds jealous.

We watch the Mayor dismount, hand his reins to Mr Tate and disappear into the cathedral.

Not two minutes later, *ker-thunk*, Mr Collins opens our door.

"The President wants you," he says to me.

"One moment, Todd," the Mayor says, opening up one of the crates and looking inside.

We're in the cellar of the cathedral, Mr Collins having pushed me down the stairs at the back of the main lobby. I stand there waiting, wondering how much of my dinner Mayor Ledger will eat before I can get back.

I watch Mayor Prentiss look thru another crate.

"*President* Prentiss," he says, without looking up. "Do try to remember that." He stands up straight. "Used to be wine stored down here. Far more than was ever needed for communion."

I don't say nothing. He looks at me, curious. "You aren't going to ask, are you?"

120

"Bout what?" I say.

"The cure, Todd," he says, thumping one of the crates with his fist. "My men have retrieved every last trace of it from every home in New Prentisstown and here it all is."

He reaches in and takes out a phial of the cure pills. He pops the lid off and takes out a small white pill twixt his finger and thumb. "Do you never wonder why I haven't given the cure to you or David?"

I shift from foot to foot. "Punishment?"

He shakes his head. "Does Mr Ledger still fidget?"

I shrug. "Sometimes. A little."

"They made the cure," the Mayor says. "And then they made themselves *need* it." He indicates row after row of crates and boxes. "And if I have *all* of what they need..."

He puts the pill back in the phial and turns more fully to me, smiling wider.

"You wanted something?" I mumble.

"You really don't know, do you?" he asks.

"Know what?"

He pauses again, and then he says, "Happy birthday, Todd."

I open my mouth. Then I open it wider.

"It was four days ago," he says. "I'm surprised you didn't mention it."

I don't believe it. I completely forgot.

"No celebrations," the Mayor says, "because of course we both know you are *already* a man, now, aren't you?"

And again I raise the pictures of Aaron.

"You have been very impressive these past two weeks," he says, ignoring them. "I know it's been a great struggle for

121

you not knowing what to believe about Viola, not knowing exactly how you should behave to keep her safe." I can feel his voice buzzing in my head, searching around. "But you have worked hard nonetheless. You have even been a good influence on David."

I can't help but think of the ways I'd like to beat Davy Prentiss into a bloody pulp but Mayor Prentiss just says, "As a reward, I bring you two belated birthday presents."

My Noise rises. "Can I see her?"

He smiles like he expected it. "You may not," he says, "but I will promise you this. On the day that you can bring yourself to trust me, Todd, truly bring yourself to understand that I mean good for this town and good for you, then on that day, you will see that I am indeed trustworthy."

I can hear myself breathing. It's the closest he's come to saying she's all right.

"No, your first birthday present is one you've earned," he says. "You'll have a new job starting tomorrow. Still with our Spackle friends, but added responsibility and an important part of our new process." He looks me hard in the eye again. "It's a job that could take you far, Todd Hewitt."

"All the way up to be a leader of men?" I say, my voice a bit more sarcastic than he'd probably like.

"Indeed," he says.

"And the second present?" I say, still hoping it might be her.

"My second present to you, Todd, surrounded by all this cure." He gestures at the crates again. "Is not to give you any at all."

I screw up my mouth. "Huh?"

But he's already walking towards me as if we're thru talking.

And as he passes me—

I AM THE CIRCLE AND THE CIRCLE IS ME.

Rings thru my head, just the once, coming right from the centre of me, of who I am.

I jump from the surprise of it.

"Why can I hear it if yer taking the cure?" I say.

But he just gives me a sly smile and disappears up the staircase, leaving me there.

Happy late birthday to me.

I am Todd Hewitt, I think, as I lie in bed, staring up into the dark. *I am Todd Hewitt and four days ago I was a man.*

Sure don't feel no different, tho.

All that reaching for it, all that importance on the date, and I'm still the same ol' stupid effing Todd Hewitt, powerless to do anything, powerless to save myself much less her.

Todd effing Hewitt.

And lying here in the dark, Mayor Ledger snoring away over on his mattress, I hear a faint *pop* outside, somewhere in the distance, some stupid soldier firing off his gun at who knows what (or who knows who) and that's when I think it.

That's when I think getting thru it ain't enough.

Staying alive ain't enough if yer barely living.

They'll play me as long as I let 'em.

And she coulda been out there.

She coulda been out there *today*.

I'm gonna find her—

her–

And when I do–

And then I notice Mayor Ledger ain't snoring no more.

I raise my voice into the dark. "You got something to say?"

But then he's snoring again and his Noise is grey and muzzy and I wonder if I imagined it.

10

IN GOD'S HOUSE

{ VIOLA }

"I CAN'T TELL YOU HOW SORRY I AM."

I don't take the cup of root coffee he offers.

"Please, Viola," he says, holding it out towards me.

I take it. My hands are still shaking.

They haven't stopped since last night.

Since I watched her fall.

First to her knees, then onto her side down to the gravel, her eyes still open.

Open, but already unseeing.

I watched her fall.

"Sergeant Hammar will be punished." The Mayor takes a seat across from me. "He was by no means and under no circumstances following my orders."

"He killed her," I say, hardly any sound to my voice. Sergeant Hammar dragged me back to the house of healing, pounding on the door with the butt of his rifle, waking everyone up, sending them out after Maddy's body.

I couldn't speak, I could barely even cry.

They wouldn't look at me, the mistresses, the other apprentices. Even Mistress Coyle refused to meet my eye.

What did you think you were doing? Where did you think you were taking her?

And then Mayor Prentiss summoned me here this morning to his cathedral, to his home, to God's house.

And then they *really* wouldn't look at me.

"I'm sorry, Viola," he says. "Some of the men of Prentisstown, *old* Prentisstown, still bear grudges against women over what happened all those years ago."

He sees my look of horror. "The story you think you know," he says, "is not the story that's true."

I'm still gaping at him. He sighs. "The Spackle War was in Prentisstown, too, Viola, and it was a terrible thing, but women and men fought side by side to save ourselves." He puts his fingertips together in a triangle, his voice still calm, still gentle. "But there was division in our little outpost even as we were victorious. Division between men and women."

"I'll say there was."

"They made their own army, Viola. They splintered off, not trusting men whose thoughts they could read. We tried to reason with them, but eventually, they wanted war. And I'm afraid they got it."

He sits up, looking at me sadly. "An army of women is still an army with guns, still an army that can defeat you."

I can hear myself breathing. "You killed every single one."

"I did not," he says. "Many of them died in battle, but when they saw the war was lost, they spread the word that we were their murderers and then they killed themselves so

126

that the remaining men would be doomed either way."

"I don't believe you," I say, remembering that Ben told us a different version. "That's not how it happened."

"I was there, Viola. I remember it all far more clearly than I want to." He catches my eye. "I am also the one most keen that history doesn't repeat itself. Do you understand me?"

I think I do understand him and my stomach sinks and I can't help it – I start to cry, thinking of how they brought Maddy's body back, how Mistress Coyle insisted I be the one to help her prepare the body for burial, how she wanted me to see up close the cost of trying to find the tower.

"Mistress Coyle," I say, fighting to control myself. "Mistress Coyle wanted me to ask if we can bury her this afternoon."

"I've already sent word that she can," the Mayor says. "Everything Mistress Coyle requires is being delivered to her as we speak."

I set the coffee down on a little table next to my chair. We're in a huge room, bigger than any place indoors I've ever seen except for the launch hangars of my ship. Too large for just a pair of comfortable chairs and a wooden table. The only light shines down through a round window of coloured glass showing this world and its two moons.

Everything else is in shadow.

"How are you finding her?" the Mayor asks. "Mistress Coyle."

The weight on my shoulders, the weight of Maddy being gone, the weight of Todd still out there, sits so heavily I'd forgotten for a minute he was even there. "What do you mean?"

He shrugs a little. "How is she to work with? How is she as a teacher?"

Lowallow "She's the best healer in Haven."

"And now the best healer in New Prentisstown," he corrects. "People tell me she used to be quite powerful around here. A force to be reckoned with."

I bite my lip and look back at the carpet. "She couldn't save Maddy."

"Well, let's forgive her for that, shall we?" His voice is low, soft, almost kind. "Nobody's perfect."

He sets down his cup. "I'm sorry about your friend," he says again. "And I'm sorry it has taken this long for us to speak again. There has been much work to do. I look to *stop* the suffering on this planet, which is why your friend's death grieves me so. That's been my whole mission. The war is over, Viola, it truly is. Now is the time for healing."

I don't say anything to that.

"But your mistress doesn't see it that way, does she?" he asks. "She sees me as the enemy."

In the early hours of this morning, as we dressed Maddy in her white burial cloths, she said, *If he wants a war, he's got a war. We haven't even* started *fighting.*

But then when I was summoned here, she said to tell him no such thing, to ask only about the funeral.

And to find out what I could.

"You see me as the enemy, too," he says, "and I truly wish that weren't the case. I am so disappointed that this terrible incident has made you even more suspicious of me."

I feel Maddy rising again in my chest. I feel Todd rising, too. I have to breathe through my mouth for a minute.

"I know how appealing it seems that there should be sides, that you should be on *her* side," he says. "I don't blame

128

you. I haven't even asked you about your ships because I know you would lie to me. I know she would have asked you to. If I were in Mistress Coyle's position, I would do exactly the same thing. Push you to help me. Use an asset that's fallen into my lap."

"She's not using me," I say quietly.

You can be so valuable to us, I remember, *if you choose.*

He leans forward. "Can I tell you something, Viola?"

"What?" I ask.

He cocks his head. "I really do wish you would call me David."

I look back down to the carpet. "What is it, David?"

"Thank you, Viola," he says. "It really does mean something to me." He waits until I look up again. "I've met the Council that ran Haven as was. I've met the former Mayor of Haven. I've met the former police chief and the chief medical officer and the head of education. I've met everyone of any importance in this town. Some of them now work for me. Some of them don't fit into the new administration and that's fine, there's plenty of work to be done rebuilding this city, making it ready for *your* people, Viola, making it the proper paradise that they need and want and expect."

He's still looking right into my eyes. I notice how dark blue his own are, like water running over a slate.

"And of all the people I've met in New Prentisstown, your Mistress Coyle is the only one who truly knows what leading is like. Leadership isn't grown, Viola. It's *taken*, and she may be the only person on this entire planet besides myself who has enough strength, enough *will* to take it."

I keep looking at his eyes and a thought comes.

and eyes give away nothing either.

But I do begin to wonder–

Right there, just at the back of my thinking–

Is he *afraid* of her?

"Why do you think I had you taken to her for your gun-shot wound?" he asks.

"She's the best healer. You said it yourself."

"Yes, but she's far from the only one. Bandages and medicine do most of the work. Mistress Coyle just applies them especially skilfully."

My hand goes unconsciously to my front scar. "It's not just that."

"It is not, you're correct." He leans even farther forward. "I want her on my side, Viola. I *need* her on my side if I'm going to make this new society any kind of success. If we worked together, Mistress Coyle and I," he leans back, "well, what a world we could make."

"You locked her up."

"But I wasn't going to *keep* her locked up. The borders between men and women had become blurred, and the reintroduction of those borders is a slow and painful process. The formation of mutual trust takes time, but the important thing to remember is, as I've said, the war is *over*, Viola. It truly is. I want no more fighting, no more bloodshed."

For something to do, I pick up the cooling cup of coffee. I put it to my lips but I don't drink it.

"Is Todd okay?" I ask, not looking at him.

"Happy and healthy and working in the sun," the Mayor says.

"Can I see him?"

He's silent, as if he's considering it. "Will you do something for me?" he asks.

"What?" Another idea begins to form in my head. "You want me to spy on her for you."

"No," he says. "Not *spying*, not at all. I just want your help in convincing her that I'm not the tyrant she thinks, that history isn't as she knows it, that if we work together, we can make this place into the home we *both* wanted when our people left Old World all those many years ago. I am not her enemy. And I am not yours."

He seems so sincere. He really does.

"I'm asking for your help," he says.

"You're in complete control," I say. "You don't need my help."

"I do," he says insistently. "You've grown closer to her than I ever possibly could."

Have I? I think.

This is the girl, I remember.

"I also know that she drugged you that first night so you would fall asleep before you told me anything."

I sip my cold coffee. "Wouldn't you have done the same?"

He smiles. "So you agree we're not that different, her and I?"

"How can I trust you?"

"How can you trust her if she drugged you?"

"She saved my life."

"After I delivered you to her."

"She's not keeping me locked up in the house of healing."

"You came here unchaperoned, didn't you? The restrictions are being lessened this very day."

"And who are all those other healers she's been meeting with?" He folds his fingers back into a tent. "What are they up to, do you suppose?"

I look down into the coffee cup and swallow, wondering how he knows.

"And what do they have planned for *you*?" he asks.

I still don't look at him.

He stands. "Come with me, please."

He leads me out of the huge room and across the short lobby at the front of the cathedral. The doors are wide open onto the town square. The army is doing marching exercises out there and the *pound pound pound* of their feet pours in and the ROAR of the men who no longer have the cure floods in right behind it.

I wince a little.

"Look there," says the Mayor.

Past the army, in the centre of the square, some men are assembling a small platform of plain wood, a bent pole up on the top.

"What's that?"

"It's where Sergeant Hammar is going to be hanged tomorrow afternoon for his terrible, terrible crime."

The memory of Maddy, of her lifeless eyes, rises in my chest again. I have to press my hand to my mouth to hold it back.

"I spared the old Mayor of this town," he says, "but I will not spare one of my most loyal and long-standing sergeants."

132

He looks at me. "Do you honestly think I would go to such lengths just to please one girl who has information I could use? Do you honestly think I would go to that much trouble when, as you say, I'm in complete control?"

"Why are you doing it then?" I ask.

"Because he broke the law. Because this is a civilized world and acts of barbarity will not be tolerated. Because the *war* is *over*." He turns to me. "I would very much like you to convince Mistress Coyle of that." He steps closer. "Will you do that? Will you at least tell her the things I'm doing to remedy this tragic situation?"

I look down at my feet. My mind is whirling, spinning like a meteor.

The things he says could be true.

But Maddy is dead.

And it's my fault.

And Todd's still gone.

What do I do?

(what do I do?)

"Will you, Viola?"

At least, I think, *it's information to give to Mistress Coyle.*

I swallow. "I'll try?"

He smiles again. "Wonderful." He touches me gently on the arm. "Run along back now. They'll be needing you for the funeral service."

I nod and step out onto the front steps and away from him, moving into the square a little bit, the ROAR of it all beating down on me as hard as the sun. I stop and try to catch the breath that seems to have run away from me.

"Viola." He's still watching me, watching me from the

with me here tomorrow night?"

He grins, seeing how I try to hide how much I don't want to come.

"Todd will be there, of course," he says.

I open my eyes wide. Another wave rises from my chest, bringing the tears again and surprising me so much I hiccup. "Really?"

"Really," he says.

"You mean it?"

"I mean it," he says.

And then he opens his arms to me for an embrace.

11

SAVED YER LIFE

[TODD]

"WE GOTTA NUMBER 'EM," Davy says, getting out a heavy canvas bag that's been left in the monastery storeroom and dropping it loudly to the grass. "That's our new job."

It's the morning after the Mayor wished me a late happy birthday, the morning after I vowed I'd find her.

But ain't nothing's changed.

"Number 'em?" I ask, looking out at the Spackle, still staring back at us in the silence that don't make no sense. Surely the cure shoulda worn off by now? "Why?"

"Don't you *never* listen to Pa?" Davy says, getting out some of the tools. "Everyone's gotta know their place. Besides, we gotta keep track of the animals somehow."

"They ain't animals, Davy," I say, not too heated cuz we've had this fight before a coupla times. "They're just aliens."

"Whatever, pigpiss," he says and pulls out a pair of bolt cutters from the bag, setting them on the grass. He reaches

ful of metal bands, strapped together with a longer one. I take them from him.

Then I reckernize what I'm holding.

"We're not," I say.

"Oh, yes, we are." He holds up another tool, which I also reckernize.

It's how we marked sheep back in Prentisstown. You take the tool Davy's holding and you wrap a metal band around a sheep's leg. The tool bolts the ends together tight, too tight, so tight it cuts into the skin, so tight it starts an infeckshun. But the metal's coated with a medicine to fight it so what happens is that the infeckted skin starts to heal around the band, grow *into* it, replacing that bit of skin with the metal band itself.

I look up again at the Spackle, looking back at us.

Cuz the catch is, it don't heal if you take it off. The sheep'll bleed to death if you do. You put on a band and it's yers till it dies. There ain't no going back from it.

"Then all you gotta do is think of 'em as sheep," Davy says, standing up with the bolting tool and looking out over the Spackle. "Line up!"

"We'll do one field at a time," he shouts, gesturing at the Spackle with the bolting tool in one hand and the pistol in the other. The soldiers on the stone walls keep their rifles pointed into the herd. "Once you get yer number, you stay in that field and you don't leave it, unnerstand?"

And they seem to unnerstand.

136

That's the thing.

They unnerstand way more than a sheep would.

I look at the packet of metal bands I'm holding. "Davy, this is—"

"Just get a move on, pigpiss," he says impayshuntly. "We're meant to get thru two hundred today."

I swallow. The first Spackle in line is watching the metal bands as well. I think it's female cuz sometimes you can tell by the colour of the lichen they've got growing for their clothes. She's shorter than usual, too, for a Spackle. My height or less.

And I'm thinking, if I don't do it, if I'm not the one who does this, then they'll just get someone else who won't care if it hurts. Better they have me who'll treat 'em right. Better than just Davy on his own.

Right?

(right?)

"Just wrap the effing band round its arm or we'll be here all effing morning," Davy says.

I gesture for her to hold out her arm. She does, staring at my eyes, not blinking. I swallow again. I unwrap the packet of bands and peel off the one marked 0001. She's still staring, still not blinking.

I take hold of her outstretched hand.

The flesh is warm, warmer than I expected, they look so white and cold.

I wrap the band round her wrist.

I can feel her pulse beating under my fingertips.

She still looks into my eyes.

"I'm sorry," I whisper.

bolting tool, gives it a twist so sharp and hard the Spackle lets out a pained hiss, and then he slams the bolting tool together, locking the metal strip into her wrist, making her 0001 for ever and ever.

She bleeds from under the band. 0001 bleeds red.

(which I already knew)

Holding her wrist with her other hand, she moves away from us, still staring, still unblinking, silent as a curse.

None of 'em fight. They just line up and stare and stare and stare. Once in a while they make their clicking sounds to one another but no Noise, no struggles, no resistance.

Which makes Davy angrier and angrier.

"Damn things," he says, holding the twist for a second before he bolts it off just to see how long he can make 'em hiss. And a second or two longer than that.

"How d'you like *that*, huh?" he yells at a Spackle as it walks away, holding its wrist, staring back at us.

0038 is next in line. It's a tall one, probably male, skinny as anything and getting skinnier cuz even a fool can see that the fodder we put out every morning ain't enough for fifteen hundred Spackle.

"Put the band round its neck," Davy says.

"What?" I say, my eyes widening. "*No!*"

"Put it round its effing neck!"

"I'm not–"

He lunges forward suddenly, clonking me on the head with the bolting tool and ripping the metal bands outta my hand. I fall to one knee, clutching at my skull and the pain keeps me from looking up for a few seconds.

And when I do, it's too late.

Davy's got the Spackle kneeling in front of him, the 0038 band twisted tight around its neck, and is using the bolting tool to twist it tighter. The soldiers on the top of the wall are laughing and the Spackle's gasping for air, clawing at the band with its fingers, blood coming from round its neck.

"Stop it!" I shout, struggling to get to my feet.

But Davy slams the bolting tool shut and the Spackle tumbles over into the grass, making loud gagging sounds, its head starting to turn a cruel-looking pink. Davy stands above it, not moving, just watching it choke to death.

I see the bolt cutters Davy set on the grass and I stumble to 'em, grabbing 'em and rushing back over to 0038. Davy tries to stop me but I swing the bolt cutters at him and he jumps back and I kneel beside 0038 and try to get to the metal band but Davy's twisted it so tight and the Spackle's thrashing so much from suffocating that I finally have to force him down with one fist.

I cut the band free. It flies off in a mess of blood and skin. The Spackle takes in a rake of air so loud it hurts yer ears and I lean back away from him, bolt cutters still in my hand.

And as I watch the Spackle struggle to breathe again and possibly fail and as Davy hovers behind me, bolting tool in his hand, I realize how much *clicking* I'm hearing running thru the Spackle and it's now, of all times, of all moments, of all reasons—

It's *right now* they decide to attack.

The first punch glances lightly off the crown of my head. They're thin and they're light so there's not much weight behind the punch.

But there are fifteen hundred of 'em.

And they come in a wave, so thick it's like being plunged under water–

More fists, more punching, scratches across my face and the back of my neck and I'm knocked farther to the ground and the weight of 'em presses down on me, grabbing at my arms and legs, grabbing at my clothes and hair, and I'm calling out and yelling and one of 'em's taken the bolt cutters from my hand and swings it hard into my elbow and the pain of it is more than I can actually stand–

And my only thought, my only stupid thought is–

Why are they attacking *me*? I tried to *save* 0038.

(but they know, they know–)

(they know I'm a killer–)

Davy cries out as I hear the first gunshots from the top of the stone walls. More punches and more scratches but more gunshots, too, and the Spackle start to scatter which is something I can hear more than see cuz of the pain radiating up from my elbow.

And there's still one on top of me, scratching at me from behind as I lie face-down on the grass and I manage to turn myself over and tho the guns are still firing and the smell of cordite is filling the air and Spackle are running and running, this one stays on me, scratching and slapping away.

And the same second I realize it's 0001, the first one in line, the first one I touched, there's a bang and she spins and falls to the grass beside me. Dead.

Davy's standing over me with his pistol, smoke still coming from its barrel. His nose and lip are bleeding, he's got as many scratches as I do, and he's leaning heavily to one side.

But he's smiling.

"Saved yer life, didn't I?"

The firing of rifles carries on. The Spackle keep running but there's nowhere to go. They fall and they fall and they fall.

I look down at my elbow. "I think my arm's broke."

"I think my *leg's* broke," Davy says, "but you go back to Pa. Tell him what's happened. Tell him I *saved yer life*."

Davy's not looking at me, still raising his pistol, firing it, keeping his weight all weird on his legs.

"Davy–"

"Go!" he says and there's a grim kinda joy coming from him. "I got me a job to finish here." He fires the gun again. Another Spackle falls. They're falling all over the place.

I take a step towards the gate. And another.

And then I'm running.

My arm throbs with every step but Angharrad says **boy colt** when I get to her and snuffles my face with a wet nose. She kneels down so I can flop forward onto her saddle. When she takes off down the road, she waits till I'm upright before she hits the fastest gallop I ever seen from her. I'm

141

under me, and I'm trying not to throw up from the pain.

I look up now and then to see women watch me ride past from their windows, quiet and distant. I see men watch the horse run by, looking at my face all bloody and injured.

And I wonder who they think they're seeing.

Are they seeing one of them?

Or are they seeing their enemy?

Who do they think I am?

I close my eyes but I nearly lose my balance so I open them again.

Angharrad takes me down the road on the side of the cathedral, her shoes striking sparks on the cobbles as she turns the corner to go round to the entrance. The army's in the square doing marching exercises. Most of them still ain't got Noise but the pounding of their feet is loud enough to bend the air.

I wince at it all and look up to where we're going, to the front door of the cathedral–

And my Noise gives such a shock, Angharrad stops up short, scrabbling on the cobbles, flanks foaming from getting me here so fast.

I barely notice–

My heart has stopped beating–

I've stopped breathing–

Cuz there she is.

In front of my eyes, walking up the steps of the cathedral–
  There she *is*.

And my heart jump-starts again and my Noise is ready to scream her name and my pain is disappearing–
  Cuz she's alive–
  She's *alive*–
  But then I'm seeing more–
  I'm seeing her walking up the steps–
  Towards Mayor Prentiss–

Into his open arms–

And he's *embracing* her–

And she's *letting* him–

And all I can think–
  All I can say–
  Is–

"Viola?"

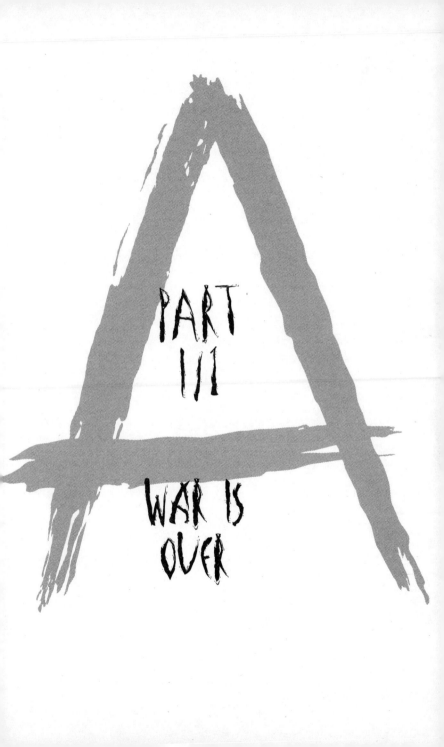

PART
III

WAR IS
OVER

12

BETRAYAL

MAYOR PRENTISS STANDS THERE.

The leader of this town, this world.

Arms wide.

As if this is the price.

Do I pay it?

It's just one hug, I think.

(isn't it?)

One hug to see Todd.

I step forward–

(just one hug)

– and he puts his arms around me.

I try not to go rigid at his touch.

"I never told you," he says into my ear. "We found your ship in the swamp as we marched here. We found your parents."

I let out a little gasp of tears and try to swallow them back.

how lonely you must be, and nothing would please me more
than if, one day, maybe, you could consider me as your–"

There's a sudden sound above the ROAR–

One bit of Noise flying higher than the rest, clear as an
arrow–

An arrow fired directly at me–

Viola! it screams, knocking the words right out of the
Mayor's mouth–

I step back from his embrace, his arms falling away–

I turn–

And there, in the afternoon sunshine, in the square, on
the back of a horse not ten metres away–

There he is.

It's him.

It's *him*.

"TODD!" I yell and I'm already running.

He's standing where he slid off the horse, holding his arm
at a bad angle, and I hear **Viola!** roaring through his Noise
but I can also hear the pain in his arm and confusion lacing
through everything but my own mind is racing too fast and
my heart is pounding too loud for me to hear any of it clearly.

"TODD!" I yell again and I reach him and his Noise opens
even farther and wraps around me like a blanket and I'm

grabbing him to me, grabbing him to me like I'll never let him go and he calls out in pain but his other arm is grabbing me back, it's grabbing me back, it's grabbing me back–

"I thought you were dead," he's saying, his breath on my neck. "I thought you were dead."

"Todd," I say and I'm crying and the only thing I can say is his name. "*Todd*."

He gasps sharply again and the pain flashes so loud in his Noise I'm almost blinded by it. "Your arm," I say, pulling back.

"Broken," he pants, "broken by–"

"Todd?" the Mayor says, right behind us, staring hard into him. "You're back early."

"My arm," Todd says. "The Spackle–"

"The *Spackle*?" I say.

"That looks bad, Todd," the Mayor says, talking over us. "We need to get you healed right away."

"He can come to Mistress Coyle!"

"Viola," the Mayor says and I hear Todd think **"Viola"?**, wondering all over how the Mayor speaks to me like this. "Your house of healing is too far for Todd to walk with an injury this bad."

"I'll come with you!" I say. "I'm training as an apprentice!"

"Yer what?" Todd says. His pain is wailing like a siren but he's still looking back and forth between me and the Mayor. "What's going on? How do you know–"

"I'll explain everything," the Mayor says, taking Todd's free arm, "after we get you healed." He turns to me. "The invitation is still on for tomorrow. You have a funeral to get to just now."

"Funeral?" Todd says. "What funeral?"

149

Todd away.

"Wait–" I say.

"Viola!" Todd shouts, jerking away from the Mayor's grasp but the movement shakes his broken arm and he falls to one knee with the pain of it, pain so sharp, so loud and clear in his Noise that soldiers from the army stop to hear it. I jump forward to help but the Mayor holds out a hand to stop me.

"Go," he says and it's not a voice that's asking for discussion. "I'll help Todd. You go to your funeral and mourn your friend. You'll see Todd tomorrow night, good as new."

Viola? Todd's Noise says again, choking back a weep from pain so heavy now I don't think he can speak.

"Tomorrow, Todd," I say loudly, trying to get through his Noise. "I'll see you tomorrow."

Viola! he calls again but the Mayor is already leading him away.

"You promised!" I call after them. "Remember that you promised!"

The Mayor gives me a smile. "Remember you promised, too."

Did I? I think.

And then I'm watching them go, so fast it's like it didn't even happen.

But Todd–

Todd is alive.

I have to bend down close to the ground for a minute and just let it be true.

* * *

"And with burdened hearts, we commit you to the earth."

"Here." Mistress Coyle takes my hand after the priest-ess finishes speaking and puts some loose dirt into it. "We sprinkle it over the coffin."

I stare at the dirt in my hand. "Why?"

"So that she's been buried by the efforts of all of us." She directs me to a place with her in the line of healers gathering by the graveside. We pass by the hole one by one, each of us throwing our handful of dry soil onto the wooden box where Maddy now rests. Everyone stands as far away from me as they can.

No one but Mistress Coyle will even speak to me.

They blame me.

I blame me, too.

There are more than fifty women here, healers, appren-tices, patients. Soldiers are spread out in a circle around us, more than you'd think necessary for a funeral. Men, including Maddy's father, are kept separate on the other side of the grave. Maddy's father's weeping Noise is the saddest thing I think I've ever heard.

And in the middle of everything, I can only feel even more guilty because what I'm mostly thinking about is Todd.

Now that I'm away from it, I can see the confusion in his Noise more clearly, see how it must have looked to find me in the arms of the Mayor, how friendly we must have seemed together.

Even though I can explain it all, I still feel ashamed.

And then he was gone.

I throw my dirt on Maddy's coffin, then Mistress Coyle takes me by the arm. "We need to talk."

"He wants to *work* with me?" Mistress Coyle says, over a cup of tea in my small bedroom.

"He says he admires you."

Her eyebrows raise. "Does he now?"

"I know," I say. "I know how it sounds, but maybe if you *heard* him–"

"Oh, I think I've heard enough from our President to last me a good while."

I lean back on my bed. "But he could have, I don't know, *forced* me to tell him about the ships. And he's not forcing me to do anything." I look away. "He's even letting me see my friend tomorrow."

"Your Todd?"

I nod. Her expression is solid as stone.

"And I suppose that makes you grateful to him, does it?"

"No," I say, rubbing my face with my hands. "I saw what his army did as they marched. I saw it with my own two eyes."

There's a long silence.

"But?" Mistress Coyle finally says.

I don't look at her. "But he's hanging the man who shot Maddy. He's executing him tomorrow."

She makes a dismissive sound with her lips. "What's one more killing to a man like him? What's one more life to take? Typical that he should think that solves the problem."

"He seemed genuinely sorry."

She looks at me sideways. "I'm sure he did. I'm sure that's exactly how he *seemed*." She lowers her voice. "He's the

President of Lies, my girl. He will lie so well you'll believe it's the truth. The Devil tells the best stories. Didn't your mama teach you that?"

"He doesn't think he's the Devil," I say. "He thinks he's just a soldier who won a war."

She looks at me carefully. "Appeasement," she says. "That's what it's called. Appeasement. It's a slippery slope."

"What does it mean?"

"It means you want to work with the enemy. It means you'd rather join him than beat him, and it's a sure-fire way to stay beaten."

"I don't want *that*!" I yell. "I just want this all to *stop*! I want this to be a home for all the people on their way, the home that we were all looking forward to. I want there to be peace and happiness." My voice starts to thicken. "I don't want anyone else to die."

She sets down her teacup, puts her hands on her knees and looks hard at me. "Are you sure that's what you want?" she says. "Or is it your boy you'll do anything for?"

And I wonder for a minute if she can read my mind.

(because, yes, I want to see Todd–)

(I want to *explain* to him–)

"Clearly your loyalty doesn't lie with *us*," Mistress Coyle says. "After your little stunt with Maddy, there are those of us who aren't so sure you're not more of a danger than an asset."

Asset, I think.

She sighs, long and hard. "For the record," she says, "I don't blame you for Maddy's death. She was old enough to make her own decisions and if she chose to help you, well,

153

then." She runs her fingers across her forehead. "I see so much of myself in you, Viola. Even when I'd rather not." She stands to leave. "So please know, I don't blame you. Whatever happens."

"What do you mean, *whatever happens?*"

But she doesn't say anything more.

That night, they have something called a wake, where everyone at the house of healing drinks lots of weak beer and sings songs that Maddy liked and tells stories about her. There are tears, including my own, and they're not happy tears but they're not as sad as they could be.

And I'm going to see Todd again tomorrow.

And that's as close as I can feel to all right about anything just now.

I wander around the house of healing, around the other healers and apprentices and patients talking to one another. None of them will talk to me. I see Corinne sitting by herself in a chair by the window, looking especially stormy. She's refused to speak to anyone since Maddy's death, even declining to say something over the grave. You'd have to have been sitting right next to her to see how many tear tracks were on her cheeks.

It must be the beer working in me, but she looks so upset I go over and sit down next to her.

"I'm sorry–" I start to say but she stands up before I can even finish and walks away, leaving me there.

Mistress Coyle comes over, two glasses of beer in her hands. She hands one to me. We both watch Corinne as she leaves the room. "Don't be too bothered about her," Mistress Coyle says, sitting down.

"She's always hated me."

"She hasn't. She's just had a hard time of it, that's all."

"How hard?"

"It's her place to tell you, not mine. Drink up."

I take a drink. It's sweet and wheaty-tasting, the bubbles sharp against the roof of my mouth but not in a bad way. We sit and drink for a minute or two.

"Have you ever seen an ocean, Viola?" Mistress Coyle asks.

I cough away a little of the beer. "An ocean?"

"There's oceans on New World," she says, "big as anything."

"I was born on the settler ship," I say, "but I saw them from orbit as we flew in on the scout."

"Ah, well, then you've never stood on a beach as the waves came crashing in, the water stretching out from you until it's beyond sight, moving and blue and alive and so much bigger than even the black beyond seems because the ocean hides what it contains." She shakes her head in a happy way. "If you ever want to see how small you are in the plan of God, just stand at the edge of an ocean."

"I've only ever been to a river."

She puffs out her bottom lip, regarding me. "This river goes to the ocean, you know. It's not even all that far. Two days on horseback at most. A long morning in a fissioncar, though the road's not that great."

"There's a road?"

"Not much left of it any more."

"Is there something there?"

"I used to be my home," she says, shifting in her chair. "When we first landed, going on twenty-three years ago now. Meant to be a fishing settlement, boats and everything. In a hundred years' time, it might have even been a port."

"What happened?"

"What happened all over this planet, all our grand plans just sort of falling by the wayside in the first couple of years in the face of difficulty. It was harder to start a new civilization than we thought. You have to crawl before you can walk." She takes a sip of her beer. "And then sometimes you go back to crawling." She smiles to herself. "Probably for the best, though. Turns out New World's oceans aren't really for fishing."

"Why not?"

"Oh, the fish are the size of your boat and they swim up alongside and look you in the eye and tell you how they're going to eat you." She laughs a little. "And then they eat you."

I laugh a little, too. And then I remember all that's happened.

She looks at me again, catching my eye. "It's beautiful, though, the ocean. Like nothing you've ever seen."

"You miss it." I drink the last of my beer.

"To see the ocean once is to learn how to miss it," she says, taking my glass. "Let me get you another."

That night, I dream.

I dream of oceans and of fish that will eat me. I dream of armies that swim by and of Mistress Coyle leading them. I dream of Maddy taking my hand and holding me up from the water.

I dream of thunder making a single loud *BOOM!* that almost breaks the sky in two.

Maddy smiles when I jump at the sound of it. "I'm going to see him," I tell her.

She glances over my shoulder and says, "There he is."

I turn to look.

I wake but the sun's all wrong. I sit up, my head feeling like it's a boulder, and I have to close my eyes to make everything stop spinning.

"Is this what a hangover feels like?" I say out loud.

"There was no alcohol in that beer," Corinne says.

I snap my eyes open, which is a mistake as black spots form everywhere in my vision. "What are you doing here?"

"Waiting for you to wake up so the President's men can take you."

"What?" I say, as she stands. "What's going on?"

"She drugged you. Jeffers in your beer, plus bandy root to disguise the taste. She left you this." She holds out a small piece of paper. "You're to destroy it after you read it."

I take the paper. It's a note from Mistress Coyle.

Forgive me, my girl, it says, *but the President is wrong. The war is not over. Keep to the side of right, keep gathering information, keep leading him astray. You'll be contacted.*

"They blew up a storefront and left in the confusion," Corinne says.

"They did *what*?" My voice starts to rise. "Corinne, *what's going on*?"

But she's not even looking at me. "I told them they were

157

abandoning their sacred trust, that *nothing* was more important than saving lives."

"Who else is here?"

"Just you and me," she says. "And the soldiers waiting
outside to take you to your President." She looks down at
her shoes and for the first time I notice the anger, the *rage*
burning off her. "I expect I'll be interrogated by someone less
handsome."

"Corinne–"

"You'll have to start calling me Mistress Wyatt now," she
says, turning towards the door. "That is, in the unlikely event
that both of us get back here alive."

"They're gone?" I say, still not believing it.

Corinne just glares at me, waiting for me to rise.

They're gone.

She left me here alone with Corinne.

She *left* me here.

To go off and start a war.

13

SPLINTERS

[TODD]

"FISSION FUEL, SIR, soaked into clay powder to make a paste–"

"I know how to make a bush bomb, Corporal Parker," says the Mayor, surveying the damage from his saddle. "What I do not know is how a group of unarmed women managed to *plant* one in full view of soldiers under your command."

We see Corporal Parker swallow, actually see it move in his throat. He's not a man from old Prentisstown, so he musta been picked up along the way. *You go where the power is,* Ivan said. But what about when the power wants answers you ain't got? "It may not have been just women, sir," Parker says. "People are talking about something called–"

"Look at this, pigpiss," Davy says to me. He's ridden Deadfall/Acorn over to a tree trunk, near where we've stopped across the road from the blown-out storefront.

I chirrup to Angharrad, using my one good hand to tap

159

the rain. She picks her feet lightly over the bits of wood and plaster and glass and foodstuffs that are scattered everywhere, like the store finally let go of a sneeze it was holding in. We get over to Davy, who's pointing at a bunch of light-coloured splinters sticking straight outta the tree trunk.

"Explozhun so big it rammed 'em straight into the tree," he says. "Those bitches."

"It was late at night," I say, readjusting my arm in the sling. "They didn't hurt no one."

"Bitches," Davy repeats, shaking his head.

"You'll turn in your supply of cure, Corporal," we hear the Mayor say, loud enough so Corporal Parker's men hear the punishment, too. "All of you will. Privacy is a privilege for those who've earned it."

The Mayor ignores Corporal Parker's mumbled, "Yes, sir," and turns to have a short, quiet word with Mr O'Hare and Mr Morgan, who then ride off in different direkshuns. The Mayor comes over to us next, not saying nothing, face frowning like a slap. Morpeth stares viciously at our mounts, too. **Submit**, says his Noise. **Submit. Submit**. Deadfall and Angharrad both lower their heads and step back.

All horses are a little bit crazy.

"Want me to go hunting for 'em, Pa?" Davy says. "The bitches who did this?"

"Mind your language," the Mayor says. "You both have work to be getting on with."

Davy gives me a sideways glance and holds out his left leg. The whole bottom half is covered in a cast. "Pa?" he

160

says. "If you ain't noticed, I can barely walk and pigpiss here's in a sling and–"

He don't even finish the sentence before there's that *whoosh* of sound, flying from the Mayor faster than thought, like a bullet made of Noise. Davy flinches back in his saddle, yanking the reins so hard Deadfall rears up, nearly dumping Davy to the ground. Davy recovers, breathing heavy, eyes unfocused.

What the hell *is* that?

"Does this look like a day you can take off?" the Mayor says, indicating all the wreckage of the store stretched around us, the husk of the building still smoking in some parts.

Blown up.

(I've been hiding it in my Noise, doing my best to keep it down–)

(but it's there, hidden away, bubbling below the surface–)

(the thought of a bridge that blew up once–)

I look back to see the Mayor staring at me so hard I'm blurting it out before I can barely think. "It wasn't her," I say. "I'm sure it wasn't."

He keeps on staring. "I never thought it might be, Todd."

Fixing my arm didn't take very long yesterday once he'd dragged me cross the square to a clinic where men in white coats set it and gave me two injeckshuns of bone-mending that hurt more than the break but by then he was already gone, promising I'd see Viola the next night (tonight, tonight) and already outta reach of a million and calling her all friendly-like by her first name and how she's working as a doctor or something and how she had to leave to go to a funeral and–

(and how my heart just exploded from my chest when I saw her–)

(and how it hurt all over again when she left–)

And then off she went somehow to a life of her own already being lived out there somewhere without me in it and then there was just me and my arm going back to the cathedral with the painkillers making me so sleepy I barely had time to fall on my mattress before blinking right out.

I didn't wake when Mayor Ledger came back in with his grey day-of-rubbish-collecting Noise complaints. I didn't wake when dinner came and Mayor Ledger ate both servings. I didn't wake when we were locked inside for the night *ker-thunk*.

But I surely did wake when a *BOOM!* shook the entire city.

And even as I sat up in the darkness and felt the queasy of the painkillers in my stomach, even without knowing what the *BOOM* was or where it had come from or what it meant, even then I knew things had changed again, that the world had suddenly become different one more time.

And sure enough, out we came with the Mayor and his men at first light, injuries or no, straight to the bombsite. I look at him on Morpeth. The morning sun's shining behind him, casting his shadow over everything.

"Will I still see her tonight?" I ask.

There's a long, quiet moment where he just stares.

"Mr President?" calls Corporal Parker, as his men take away a long plank of wood that was blown against another tree.

Something's been drawn onto the trunk underneath.

Even with not knowing how to–

Well, even with not knowing much, I can tell what it is.

A single letter, smeared on the trunk in blue.

A, it says. Just the letter **A**.

"I can't believe he's making us effing go back there one day after we fought off the attack," Davy grumbles as we make our way down the long road to the monastery.

I can't believe it neither, frankly. Davy can barely walk and even with the bone-mending doing its work on my arm, it'll be a coupla days before everything's back to normal. I can start to bend it already but I sure as hell can't fight off a Spackle army with it.

"Did you tell him I saved yer life?" Davy asks, looking both angry and shy.

"Didn't *you* tell him?" I say.

Davy's mouth flattens, pulling his sad little moustache fluff even thinner. "He don't believe me when I tell him stuff like that."

I sigh. "I told him. He saw it in my Noise anyway."

We ride in silence for a bit before Davy finally says, "Did he say anything?"

I hesitate. "He said, *Good for him*."

"That all?"

"He said it was good for me, too."

"That's it."

"I see." He don't say no more, just jigs Deadfall along a bit faster.

Even tho it was only one building that got blown up in the night, the whole city looks different as we ride. The patrols of soldiers are suddenly larger and there's more of 'em, marching up and down the roads and side streets so fast it's like they're running. There are soldiers on rooftops now, too, here and there, holding rifles, watching watching watching.

The only non-soldier men out are hustling as fast as they can from place to place, staying outta the way, not looking up.

I ain't seen no women this morning. Not one.

(not her)

(what was she *doing* with him?)

(is she lying to him?)

(is he believing her?)

(did she have something to do with the explozhun?)

"Did *who* have something to do with it?" Davy asks.

"Shut up."

"Make me," he says. But his heart ain't in it.

We ride past a group of soldiers escorting a beat-up look-ing man with his wrists bound. I press my slinged arm closer to my chest and we keep on riding. The morning sun's high in the sky by the time we pass the hill with the metal tower and come round the final bend to the monastery.

Ain't no putting off getting there any longer.

"What happened after I left?" I say.

"We beat 'em," Davy says, huffing a little with the rising pain in his leg, pain I can see in his Noise. "We beat 'em back good and proper."

Something lands on Angharrad's mane. I brush it away and something else lands on my arm. I look up.

"What the hell?" Davy says.

It's snowing.

I only ever seen snow once in my whole life, back when I was too young to really know how I'd hardly never see it again.

Flakes of white fall thru the trees and onto the road, catching on our clothes and hair. It's a silent fall and it's weird how it makes everything else seem quiet, too, like it's trying to tell you a secret, a terrible, terrible secret.

But the sun is blazing.

And this ain't snow.

"Ash," Davy spits when a flake lands near his mouth. "They're burning the bodies."

They're burning the bodies. The men are still on the tops of the stone walls with their rifles, making the Spackle that lived pile up the bodies of the ones that died. The burning pile is huge, taller than the tallest living Spackle, and more bodies are being brought to it by Spackle with their heads down and their mouths shut.

lands askew and tumbles down the side, rolling over other bodies, thru the flames, till it reaches the mud below and comes to a stop facing straight up, holes in its chest, blood dried on its wounds–

(a dead-eyed Spackle, face up in a campsite–)

(a Spackle with a knife in its chest–)

I breathe a heavy breath and I look away.

Apart from some of the clicking, the living Spackle still ain't got no Noise. No sounds of mourning nor anger nor nothing at all bout the mess they're having to clean up.

It's like someone cut out their tongues.

Ivan's there waiting for us, rifle in the crook of his arm. He's quieter this morning and his face ain't happy.

"You're to be a-carrying on with the numbers," he says, kicking over the bag with the numbering bands and tools. "Though there's less to do now."

"How many'd we get?" Davy says, smiling.

Ivan shrugs, annoyed. "Three hundred, three-fifty, can't say for sure."

I feel another greasy twist in my stomach at that but Davy's grin gets even higher. "That's hot stuff, right there."

"I'm to give you this," Ivan says, holding out the rifle to me.

"Yer *arming* him?" Davy says, his Noise rising right up.

"President's orders," Ivan snaps. He's still holding out the rifle. "You're to give it to the night watch when you leave. It's only for your protection while you're in here." He looks at me, frowning. "The President says to tell you he knows you'll do the right thing."

166

I'm just staring at the rifle.

"I don't effing believe this," Davy says, under his breath and shaking his head.

I know how to use a rifle. Ben and Cillian taught me how to use one so I didn't blow my own head off, how to hunt safely with it, how to use it only when necessary.

The right thing.

I look up. Most of the Spackle are back and away in the far fields, as far as they can get from the entrance. The rest are dragging broken and torn bodies to the fire that's burning in the middle of the next field over.

But the ones that can see me are watching me.

And they're watching me watch the rifle.

And they ain't thinking nothing I can hear.

So who knows what they're planning?

I take the rifle.

It don't mean nothing. I won't use it. I just take it.

Ivan turns and walks back to the gate to leave and as he goes, I notice it.

A low *buzz*, just barely beyond hearing, but there. And growing.

No wonder he looked so pissed off.

The Mayor took away *his* cure, too.

We spend the rest of the morning shovelling out the fodder, refilling the troughs and putting lime on the bogs, me one-handed, Davy one-legged, but taking more time than even that would allow for cuz brag tho he may I don't think Davy wants to get back to the numbering just yet either. We may

~~both have guns now but~~ touching an enemy that almost killed you, well, that takes a bit of leading up to.

Morning turns to early afternoon. For the first time, instead of taking both our lunches for himself, Davy throws a sandwich at me, hitting me in the chest with it.

So we eat and watch the Spackle watching us, watch the pile of bodies burn, watch the eleven hundred and fifty Spackle left over from the attack that went wrong, wrong, wrong. They're gathered round the edges of the fields we opened up and along the wall of the monastery, as far from us and from the burning pile as they can be.

"The bodies should go in a swamp," I say, eating my sandwich with one tired arm. "That's what Spackle bodies are for. You put 'em in water and then–"

"Fire's good enough for 'em," Davy says, leaning against the bag of numbering tools.

"Yeah, but–"

"There's no buts here, pigpiss." He frowns. "And what're you moaning for their sakes anyway? All yer blessed kindness didn't stop 'em from trying to rip yer arm off, now did it?"

He's right but I don't say nothing to that, just keep on watching them, feeling the rifle at my back.

I could take it. I could shoot Davy. I could run from here.

"You'd be dead before you got to the gate," Davy mumbles, looking at his sandwich. "And so would yer precious girl."

I don't say nothing to that neither, just finish my lunch. Every pile of food is out, every trough has been refilled, every bog has been limed up. There ain't nothing left to do except the thing we gotta do.

Davy sits up from where he was leaning against the bag. "Where were we?" he says, opening it up.

"0038," I say, keeping my gaze on the Spackle.

He sees from the metal bands that I'm right. "How'd you remember that?" he says, amazed.

"I just do."

They're looking back at us now, all of 'em. Their faces are hollowed-out, bruised, blank. They know what we're doing. They know what's coming. They know what's in the bag. They know there ain't nothing they can do about it except die if they resist us.

Cuz I got a rifle on my back to make that happen.

(what's the right thing?)

"Davy," I start to say but it's all that comes out cuz–

BOOM!

– in the distance, almost not a sound at all, more like the faraway thunder of a storm you know is gonna get here quick and do its best to knock yer house down.

We turn, as if we could see over the walls, as if the smoke's already rising over the treetops outside the gates.

We can't and it ain't yet.

"Those bitches," Davy whispers.

But I'm thinking–

(is it her?)

(is it her?)

(what is she *doing*?)

14

THE SECOND BOMB

{VIOLA}

THE SOLDIERS WAIT until midday to take me and Corinne. They practically have to tear her away from treating the remaining patients and they march us down the road, eight soldiers to guard two small girls. They won't even look at us, the one next to me so young he's barely older than Todd, so young he's got a large angry spot on his neck that for some stupid reason I can't keep my eyes off.

Then I hear Corinne gasp. They've marched us past the storefront where the bomb went off, the front of the building collapsed on itself, soldiers guarding what's left of it. Our escort slows to take a look.

And that's when it happens.

BOOM!

A sound so big it makes the air as solid as a fist, as a wave of bricks, as if the world's dropped out beneath you and you're falling sideways and up and down all at once, like the weightlessness of the black beyond.

There's a blankness where I can't remember anything and then I open my eyes to find myself lying on the ground with smoke twirling around me in spinning, floating ribbons and bits of fire drifting down from the sky here and there and for a minute it seems almost peaceful, almost beautiful, and then I realize I can't hear anything except a high-pitched whine that's drowning out all the sounds the people around me are making as they stagger to their feet or open their mouths in what must be shouting and I sit up slowly, the world still gone in whining silence and there's the soldier with the spot on his neck, there he is on the ground next to me, covered in wooden splinters, and he must have shielded me from the blast because I'm mostly okay but he's not moving.

He's not moving.

And sound begins to return and I start to hear the screaming.

"This is exactly the kind of history I did *not* want to repeat," the Mayor says, staring up thoughtfully into the shaft of light coming down from the coloured-glass window.

"I didn't know anything about a bomb," I say for a second time, my hands still shaking and my ears ringing so loud it's hard to hear what he's saying. "Neither one."

"I believe you," he says. "You were very nearly killed yourself."

"A soldier blocked most of it for me," I stutter out,

171

splinters that were stuck in nearly every part of him–

"She drugged you again, didn't she?" he asks, staring back up into the coloured window, as if the answers might be there. "She drugged you and abandoned you."

This hits me like a punch.

She did abandon me.

And set off a bomb that killed a young soldier.

"Yes," I finally say. "She left. They all did."

"Not all." He walks behind me, becoming just a voice in the room, talking loud and clear enough so I can hear. "There are five houses of healing in this city. One remains fully staffed, three others are partially depleted of their healers and apprentices. It's only yours where there's been complete desertion."

"Corinne stayed," I whisper and then I'm suddenly pleading. "She tended the soldiers who were hurt in the second bomb. She didn't hesitate. She went right to the worst injured and tied tourniquets and cleared airways and–"

"Duly noted," he interrupts, even though it's true, even though she called me over to help her and we did the best we could until other stupid soldiers who couldn't or *wouldn't* see what we were doing grabbed us and dragged us away. Corinne struggled against them but they hit her in the face and she stopped.

"Please don't hurt her," I say again. "She has nothing to do with this. She stayed behind out of choice. She tried to help those–"

"I'm not going to *hurt* her!" he shouts suddenly. "Enough of this *cowering*! There will be no harm to women as long as I am President! Why is that so difficult for you to understand?"

I think of the soldiers hitting Corinne. I think of Maddy falling to the ground.

"Please don't hurt her," I whisper again.

He sighs and lowers his voice. "We just need answers from her, that's all. The same answers I'll be needing from you."

"I don't know where they went," I say. "She didn't tell me. She didn't mention anything."

And I stop myself and he notices. Because she did mention something, didn't she?

She told me a story about–

"Something you'd like to share, Viola?" the Mayor asks, coming around to face me, looking suddenly interested.

"Nothing," I say quickly. "Nothing, just..."

"Just what?" His eyes are keen on me, flitting over my face, trying to read me, even though I have no Noise, and I realize briefly how much he must *hate* that.

"Just that she spent her first years on New World in the hills," I lie, swallowing. "Out west of town past the waterfall. I thought it was just idle talk."

He's still staring deep into me and there's a long silence while he looks and looks before starting his walk again.

"The most important issue," he says, "is whether the second bomb was a mistake, part of the first bomb that went off later by accident?" He comes round again to read my face. "Or was it on purpose? Was it set to go off later deliberately so that my men would be surrounding a crime scene, so that there would be maximum loss of life?"

"No," I say, shaking my head. "She wouldn't. She's a healer. She wouldn't kill–"

173

"A general would do anything to win a war," he says. "That's why it's war."

"No," I keep saying. "No, I don't believe–"

"I know you don't believe it." He steps away from me again, turning his back. "That's why you were left behind."

He goes to the small table next to his chair and picks up a piece of paper. He holds it up so I can see it.

There's a blue *A* written across it.

"Does this mean anything to you, Viola?"

I try to keep any look off my face.

"I've never seen that before." I swallow again, cursing myself as I do. "What is it?"

He looks at me long and hard again, then he puts the paper back down on the table. "She will contact you." He watches my face. I try to give him nothing. "Yes," he says, as if to himself. "She will, and when she does, pass along one message in particular, please."

"I don't–"

"Tell her that we can stop this bloodshed at once, that we can end all this before it even begins, before more people die and peace is for ever put aside. Tell her that, Viola."

He's staring so hard at me, I say, "Okay."

He's not blinking, his eyes black holes I can't turn away from. "But also tell her that if she wants war, she can have her war."

"Please–" I start to say.

"That'll be all," he says, gesturing me to my feet and towards the door. "Go back to your house of healing. Treat what patients you can."

"But–"

He opens the door for me. "There'll be no hanging this afternoon," he says. "Some civic functions will have to be curtailed in light of recent terrorist activities."

"*Terrorist–?*"

"And I'm afraid I'll be far too busy sweeping up the mess your mistress has made to host the dinner I promised you tonight."

I open my mouth but nothing comes out.

He closes the door on me.

My head spins as I stagger back down the main road. Todd is out here somewhere and all I can think of is how I can't see him and won't be able to tell him anything about what's happened or explain myself or anything.

And it's her fault.

It is. I hate to say it but it's her fault. All of this. Even if it was for reasons she thought were right, it's all her fault. Her fault that I won't see Todd tonight. Her fault that war is coming. Her fault–

I come upon the wreckage again.

There are four bodies lying in the road, covered in white sheets that don't quite conceal the pools of blood beneath them. Nearest to me but behind a cordon of soldiers guarding the site is the sheet covering the soldier who accidentally saved me.

I didn't even know his name.

And then all of a sudden he was dead.

If she'd just waited, if she'd just seen what the Mayor wanted her to do–

But the bodies here in the road–

But Maddy dying–

But the boy soldier who saved me–

But Corinne being hit to stop her from helping–

(oh, Todd, where are you?)

(what do I do? what's the right thing?)

"Move along there," a soldier barks at me, making me jump.

I hurry along the road and before I even realize it, I'm running.

I return to the nearly empty house of healing out of breath and slam the front door behind me. There were yet more soldiers on the road, more patrols, men on rooftops with rifles who watched me run very closely, one of them even whistling rudely as I went by.

There'll be no getting to the communications tower now, not any more.

Another thing she screwed up.

As I catch my breath, it sinks in that I'm the only thing even resembling a healer here now. Many of the patients were well enough to follow Mistress Coyle out to wherever she's gone and, who knows, might have even been the ones to plant the bombs, but there's still at least two dozen in beds here, with more coming in every day.

And I'm just about the worst healer New Prentisstown has ever seen.

"Oh, help," I whisper to myself.

"Where'd everybody go?" Mrs Fox asks as soon as I open the door to her room. "There's been no food, no medicine—"

"I'm sorry," I say, bustling up her bedpan. "I'll get you food as soon as I can."

"Good heavens, dear!" she says as I turn, her eyes widening. I look at the back of my white coat where her eyes have gone. There's a dirty smear of the young soldier's blood all the way down to the hem.

"Are you all right?" Mrs Fox asks.

I look at the blood, and all I can say is, "I'll get your food."

The next hours pass in a blur. The help staff are all gone, too, and I do my best to cook for the remaining patients, serving them and asking at the same time which medicines they take and when and how much and though they're all wondering what's going on, they see how I must look and try to be as helpful as they can.

It's well past nightfall when I come round a corner with a tray full of dirty dinner dishes and there's Corinne, just inside the entrance, pressing on the wall with one hand to hold herself up.

I throw the tray on the floor and run to her. She holds up her other hand to stop me before I reach her. She winces as I get close.

And I see the swelling around her eyes.

And the swelling in her lower lip.

And the way she's holding her body up too straight, like it hurts, like it really hurts.

"Oh, Corinne," I say.

"Just," she says, taking a breath, "just help me to my room."

I take her hand to help her along and feel something hidden in her palm, pressed into mine. She holds up a finger to her lips to shush the wonderings about to come from my open mouth.

"A girl," she whispers. "Hidden in the bushes by the road." She shakes her head angrily. "No more than a girl."

I don't look at it until I've got Corinne to her room and left again to get bandages for her face and compresses for her ribs. I wait until I'm alone in the supply room and open my palm.

It's a note, folded, with *V* written on the outside. Inside, it's only a few lines, saying almost nothing at all.

My girl, it says. *Now is the time you must choose.*

And then there's a single asking.

Can we count on you?

I look up.

I swallow.

Can we count on you?

I fold the note into my pocket and I take up the bandages and compresses and I go to help Corinne.

Who was beaten by the Mayor's men.

But who wouldn't have been beaten if she hadn't had to speak for Mistress Coyle.

But who was beaten even though the Mayor said she wouldn't be hurt.

Can we count on you?

And it wasn't signed with a name.

It just said, The Answer.

And Answer was spelled with a bright blue *A*.

15

LOCKED IN

BOOM!

– and the sky tears open behind us and a rush of wind comes up the road and Angharrad rears back in terror and I tumble off her to the ground and there's dust and screaming and a throbbing in my ears as I lay there and wait to see if I'm dead or not.

Another bomb. The third this week since the first two. Not two hundred metres away from us this time.

"Bitches," I hear Davy spit, getting to his own feet and looking back down the road.

My ears are ringing and my body's shaking as I get to my feet. The bombs've come at different times of day and night, at different spots in the city. Once it was an aqueduct that fed water to the western part of town, once it was the two main bridges to the farmlands north of the river. Today, it's–

"That's that caff," Davy says, trying to stop Deadfall/ Acorn from bolting. "Where the soldiers eat."

179

He gets Deadfall ~~...~~ and climbs back up on the saddle. "Come on!" he barks. "We'll go see if they need help."

I put my hands on Angharrad who's still frightened, still saying **bɘy cɘlt bɘy cɘlt** over and over again. I say her name a buncha times and finally get back up on her.

"Don't you go getting no funny ideas," Davy says. He takes out his pistol and points it at me. "You ain't sposed to leave my sight."

Cuz that's also how life's gone since the bombs started.

Davy with a gun on me, every waking minute of every waking day.

So I can't never go looking for her.

"The women certainly aren't helping their own cause any," says Mayor Ledger, mouth filled with chook.

I don't say nothing, just eat my own dinner and field off the asking marks coming from his Noise. The caff was bombed at a time when it was closed, like everything else this Answer thing bombs, but just cuz it's sposed to be empty don't mean it always is. Davy and I found two dead soldiers when we got there and one other dead guy who probably mopped the floors or something. Three more soldiers have died in the other bombs.

It's all really pissing off Mayor Prentiss.

I don't hardly see him no more, not since the day of my arm break, not since the day I sorta got to see Viola again. Mayor Ledger says he's arresting people and stuffing 'em in prisons west of town but not getting the knowledge he wants out of 'em. Mr Morgan, Mr O'Hare and Mr Tate are leading parts of the army off into the hills west of town looking for the camps of the bomb-planters, who are all these women who disappeared the night of the first bombs.

But the army ain't finding nothing and the Mayor just gets madder and madder, making more and more curfews, taking away more and more cure from his soldiers.

New Prentisstown gets louder by the day.

"The Mayor's denying the Answer even exists," I say.

"Well, the *President* can say anything he likes." Mayor Ledger pokes at his dinner with a fork. "But people talk." He takes another bite. "Oh, yes, they do."

In addishun to the mattresses wedged in on the tower ledges, they've put in a basin with fresh water every morning and a little chemical toilet back in the darkest corner. We're also getting better food, brought to us by Mr Collins, who then locks us back inside.

Ker-thunk.

That's where I am, locked up here every minute I'm not with Davy. The Mayor obviously don't want me out looking for Viola, despite what he says about *trust*.

"We don't know it's just women," I say, trying to keep her outta my Noise. "We don't know for sure."

"A group calling themselves the Answer played a role in the Spackle War, Todd. Covert bombing, night-time operations, that sort of thing."

"And?"

"And it was all women. No Noise to be heard by the enemy, you see." He shakes his head. "But they got out of hand at the end, became a law unto themselves. After the

181

peace, they even attacked ~~our~~ ~~~~~~ ~~~~~~ we were finally forced to execute some of them. A nasty business."

"But if you executed them, how can it be them?"

"Because an idea lives on after the death of the person." He burps quietly. "I don't know what they think they're going to accomplish, though. It's only a matter of time before the President finds them."

"Men have gone missing, too," I say, cuz it's true but what I'm thinking is–

(did she go with 'em?)

I lick my lips. "These healing houses where women work," I say, "are they marked somehow? Some way to tell what they are?"

He takes a sip of his water, watching me over his cup. "Why do you want to know a thing like that?"

I rustle my Noise a little to hide anything that might give me away. "No reason," I say. "Never mind." I set my dinner on the little table they've given us, our agreed sign that he can eat the rest of mine. "I'm gonna sleep."

I lay back on my bed and face the wall. The last of the setting sun's coming thru the openings in the tower. There ain't no glass in the openings and winter's coming. I don't know how we're gonna get thru the cold. I put my arm under my pillow and pull my legs up to me, trying not to think too loud. I can hear Mayor Ledger eating the rest of my dinner.

But then a picture comes floating from his Noise, floating right over to me, a picture of an outstretched hand, painted in blue.

I turn to look at him. I've seen the hand on at least two different buildings on the way to the monastery.

"There are five of them," he says, his voice low. "I can tell you where they are. If you want."

I look into his Noise. He looks into mine. We're both covering something, hiding something beneath all the other strands of our thoughts. All these days locked together and we're still wondering if we can trust each other.

"Tell me," I say.

"1017," I read out to Davy as he spins the bolting tool around, latching the band to a Spackle who instantly becomes 1017.

"That's enough for today," Davy says, tossing the bolting tool in the bag.

"We've still got–"

"I said that's enough." He limps back over to our bottle of water and takes a swig. His leg should be healed by now. My *arm* is, but he still limps.

"We were sposed to be done with this in a week," I say. "We're going on *two* now."

"I don't see no one hurrying us along." He spits out some water. "Do you?"

"No, but–"

"And no further instruckshuns and no new jobs..." He trails off, takes another swig of water and spits some more. He glares to my left. "What're you looking at?"

1017 is still standing there, holding the band with one hand and staring at us. I think it's a male and I think it's young, not quite an adult. It clicks at us once and then once again and even tho it ain't got Noise the click sure sounds like something rude.

Davy thinks so, too. "Oh yeah?" He ~~reached for the rifle~~ slung on his back, his Noise firing it again and again at fleeing Spackle.

1017 stands his ground. He looks me in the eye and clicks again.

Yeah, definitely rude.

He backs off, walking away but still staring at us, one hand rubbing his metal band. I turn to Davy, who's got his rifle up and pointed at 1017 as he goes.

"Don't," I say.

"Why not?" Davy says. "Who's gonna stop us?"

I don't got the answer, cuz it seems there's nobody.

The bombs have come every third or fourth day. No one knows where they'll be or how they're planted, but *BOOM! BOOM! BOOM!* The evening of the sixth bomb, a small fission reactor this time, Mayor Ledger comes in with a blackened eye and a swollen nose.

"What happened?" I ask.

"Soldiers," he spits. He takes up his dinner plate, stew again, and winces as he takes the first bite.

"What did you do?"

His Noise rises a little and he turns an angry eye on me. "I didn't *do* anything."

"You know what I mean."

He grumbles some, eats some more stew, then says, "Some of them got the brilliant idea that *I* was the Answer. *Me*."

"You?" I say, maybe a bit too surprised.

He stands, setting down his stew, mostly uneaten, so I know he must be *really* sore. "They can't find the women responsible and the soldiers are looking for someone to blame." He stares outta one of the openings, watching night fall across the town that was once his home. "And did our President do anything to stop my beating?" he says, almost to himself. "No, he did not."

I keep eating, trying to keep my Noise quiet of things I don't wanna think.

"People are talking," Mayor Ledger says, keeping his voice low, "about a new healer, a young one no one's ever seen before, going in and out of this very cathedral a while back, now working at the house of healing Mistress Coyle used to run."

Viola, I think, loud and clear before I can cover it.

Mayor Ledger turns to me. "That's one you won't have seen. It's off the main road and down a little hill towards the river about halfway to the monastery. There are two barns together on the road where you need to turn." He looks out the opening again. "You can't miss it."

"I can't get away from Davy," I say.

"I'm sure I don't know what you're talking about," Mayor Ledger says, lying back down on his bed. "I'm merely telling you idle facts about our fair city."

My breathing gets heavier, my mind and Noise racing thru possibilities about how I can get there, how I can get away from Davy to find the house of healing.

(to find her)

It isn't till later that I think to ask, "Who's Mistress Coyle?"

Even tho it's dark, I can feel Mayor Ledger's Noise get a little redder. "Ah, well," he says, into the night. "She'd be your Answer, wouldn't she?"

"That's the last of 'em," I say, watching Spackle 1182 slink away, rubbing her wrist.

"About effing time," Davy says, flopping down onto the grass. There's a crispness to the air but the sun is out and the sky is mostly clear.

"What are we sposed to do now?" I say.

"No effing idea."

I stand there and watch the Spackle. If you didn't know no better, you really wouldn't think they were much smarter than sheep.

"They *ain't*," Davy says, closing his eyes to the sun.

"Shut up," I say.

But I mean, *look* at 'em, tho.

They just sit on the grass, still no Noise, not saying nothing, half of 'em staring at us, half of 'em staring at each other, clicking now and then but hardly ever moving, not doing nothing with their hands or their time. All these white faces, looking drained of life, just sitting by the walls, waiting and waiting for *something*, whatever that something's gonna be.

"And the time for that something is now, Todd," booms a voice behind us. Davy scrambles to his feet as the Mayor comes in thru the main opening, his horse tied up outside.

But he looks at me, only me. "Ready for your new job?"

*   *   *

"Ain't barely talked to me for weeks," Davy's fuming as we ride home. Things didn't go so well twixt him and his pa. "Just *keep watch on Todd* this and *hurry up with the Spackle* that." His hands're gripped tightly round the reins. "Do I even get a *thank you*? Do I even get a *nice job, David*?"

"We were sposed to band the Spackle in a week," I say, repeating what the Mayor told him. "It took us more'n twice that."

He turns to me, his Noise really rising red. "We got *attacked*! How's that sposed to be *my* fault?"

"I ain't saying it was," I say back but my Noise is remembering the band around 0038's neck.

"So you blame me, *too*, do you?" He's stopped his horse and is glaring at me, leaning forward in the saddle, ready to jump off.

I open my mouth to answer but then I glance down the road behind him.

There's two barns by a turning in the road, a turning that heads down to the river.

I look back to Davy quickly.

He's got an evil smile. "What's down there?"

"Nothing."

"Yer girl, ain't it?" he sneers.

"Eff you, Davy."

"No, pigpiss," he says, sliding off his saddle to the ground, his Noise rising even redder. "Eff *you*."

There ain't nothing for it but to fight.

"Soldiers?" Mayor Ledger asks, seeing my bruises and blood as I come into the tower for dinner.

"Never you mind," I growl. It was me and Davy's worst fight in ages. I'm so sore I can barely reach my bed.

"You going to eat that?" Mayor Ledger asks.

A certain word in my Noise lets him know that no, I ain't gonna eat that. He picks it up and starts chomping away without even a thank you.

"You trying to eat yer way to freedom?" I say.

"Says a boy who's always had food provided for him."

"I ain't a boy."

"The supplies we brought when we landed only lasted a year," he says, twixt mouthfuls, "by which time our hunting and farming wasn't quite up to where it should have been." He takes another bite. "Lean times make you appreciate a hot meal, Todd."

"What is it about men that makes them need to turn everything into a lesson?" I cover my face with my arm, then take it away cuz of how much my blackening eye hurts.

Night falls again. The air is even cooler and I leave most of my clothes on as I get under the blanket. Mayor Ledger starts to snore, dreaming about walking in a house with endless rooms and not being able to find the exit.

This is the safest time I got to think about her.

Cuz is she really out there?

And is she part of this Answer thing?

And other things, too.

Like what would she say if she saw me?

If she saw what I did every day?

And with *who*?

I swallow the cool night air and blink away the wet in my eyes.

(are you still with me, Viola?)

(are you?)

An hour later and I'm still not asleep. Something's nagging at me and I'm turning in my sheets, trying to clear my Noise of whatever it is, trying to calm down enough so I can be ready for the new job the Mayor's got planned for us tomorrow, one which don't sound all that bad, if I'm honest.

But it's like I'm missing something, something obvious, right in front of my face.

Something–

I sit up, listening to the snoring Noise of Mayor Ledger, the sleeping roar of New Prentisstown outside, the night birds chirping, even the river rushing by in the distance.

There was no *ker-thunk* sound after Mr Collins let me in.

I think back.

Definitely not.

I look thru the darkness towards the door.

He forgot to lock it.

Right now, right this second.

It's unlocked.

16

WHO YOU ARE

{VIOLA}

"I HEAR NOISE OUTSIDE," Mrs Fox says as I refill her water jug for the night.

"It'd only be remarkable if you *didn't*, Mrs Fox."

"Just by the window–"

"Soldiers smoking their cigarettes."

"No, I'm sure it was–"

"I'm really very busy, Mrs Fox, if you don't mind."

I replace her pillows and empty her bedpan. She doesn't speak again until I'm almost ready to go.

"Things aren't like they used to be," she says quietly.

"You can say that again."

"Haven used to be better," she says. "Not perfect. But better than this."

And she just looks out of her window.

I'm dying with tiredness at the end of my rounds but I sit

down on my bed and take out the note that hasn't left my pocket. I read it for the hundredth, thousandth time.

My girl,

Now is the time you must choose.

Can we count on you?

The Answer

Not even a name, not even *her* name.

Almost three weeks I've had this note. Three weeks and nothing, so maybe that's how much they think they can count on me. Not another note, not another sign, just stuck here in this house with Corinne – or Mistress Wyatt, as I have to call her now – and the patients. Women who've fallen sick in the normal course of things, yes, but also women who've returned from "interviews" with the Mayor's men about the Answer, women with bruises and cuts, women with broken ribs, broken fingers, broken arms. Women with burns.

And those are the lucky ones, the ones who aren't in prison.

And every third or fourth day, *BOOM! BOOM! BOOM!*

And more are arrested and more are sent here.

And there's no word from Mistress Coyle.

And no word from the Mayor.

No word about why I'm being left alone. You'd think I'd be the one who'd be taken in first, the one who'd have interview after interview, the one who'd be sitting rotting in a prison cell.

"But nothing," I whisper. "Nothing at all."

And no word from Todd.

I close my eyes. I'm too tired to feel anything. Every day, I look for ways to get to the communications tower but there are soldiers everywhere now, way too many to find a pattern, and it only gets worse with each new bomb.

"I've got to do *something*," I say out loud. "I have to or I'll go crazy." I laugh. "I'll go crazy and start talking to myself."

I laugh some more, a lot more than how funny it actually is.

And there's a knock at my window.

I sit up, my heart pumping.

"Mistress Coyle?" I say.

Is this it? Is it now?

Is this where I have to choose?

Can they count on me?

(but is that *Noise* I can hear...?)

I get to my knees on the bed and pull the curtains back just far enough to look through a slit outside, expecting that frown, those fingers going over her forehead–

But it's not her.

It's not her at all.

"Todd!"

And I'm throwing back the sash and lifting up the glass and he's leaning in and his Noise is saying my name and I'm putting my arms around him and dragging him inside, actually *lifting* him off the ground and pulling him through my window and he's climbing up and we fall onto my bed and I'm on my back and he's lying on top of me and my face is close to his and I remember how we were like this after we'd jumped under the waterfall with Aaron right behind us and I looked right into his eyes.

And I knew we'd be safe.

"*Todd.*"

In the light of my room, I see his eye is blacked and there's blood on his nose and I'm saying, "What happened? Are you hurt? I can–"

But he just says, "It's you."

I don't know how much time passes with us just lying there, just feeling that the other is really there, really true, really *alive*, feeling the safety of him, his weight against mine, the roughness of his fingers touching my face, his warmth and his smell and the dustiness of his clothes, and we barely speak and his Noise is roiling with feeling, with complicated things, with memories of me being shot, of how he felt when he thought I was dying, of how I feel now at his fingertips, but at the front of it all, he's just saying, Viola, Viola, Viola.

And it's Todd.

Bloody hell, it's *Todd.*

And everything's all right.

And then there are footsteps in the hall.

Footsteps that stop right outside my room.

We both look towards the door. A shadow is cast underneath it, two legs of someone standing just on the other side.

I wait for the knock.

I wait for the order to get him out of here.

I wait for the fight I'll put up.

But then the feet walk away.

"Who was that?" Todd asks.

"Mistress Wyatt," I say, and I can hear the surprise in my own voice.

"And then the bombs started going off," I finish, "and he only called for me twice, early on, to ask me if I knew anything and I didn't, I truly didn't, and then that was it. Nothing. That's all I know about him, I swear."

"He ain't barely spoken to me since the bombs neither," Todd says, looking down at his feet. "I was worried it was you setting 'em off."

I see the bridge blowing up in his Noise. I see me being the one to do it. "No," I say, thinking of the note in my pocket. "It wasn't me."

Todd swallows, then he says simply, clearly, "Should we run?"

"Yes," I say, betraying Corinne so fast I feel a red blush of shame already coming over me, but yes, we should run, we should run and run.

"Where, tho?" he asks. "Where is there to go?"

I open my mouth to answer–

But I hesitate.

"Where are the Answer hiding?" he asks. "Can we go there?"

And I notice some tension in his Noise, disapproval and reluctance.

The bombs. He doesn't like the bombs either.

I see a picture of some dead soldiers in the wreckage of a cafe.

But there's more, too, isn't there?

I hesitate again.

I'm wondering, just for the briefest moment, just as if it's a fly I'm brushing away, I'm wondering–

I'm wondering if I can tell him.

"I don't know," I say. "I really don't. They didn't tell me in case I couldn't be trusted."

Todd looks up at me.

And for a second, I see the doubt on his face, too.

"You don't trust me," I say, before I think to stop.

"You don't trust me neither," he says. "Yer wondering if I'm working for the Mayor right now. And yer wondering what took me so long to find you." He looks down sadly at the floor again. "I can still read you," he says. "Nearly as well as my own self."

I look at him, into his Noise. "*You* wonder if I'm part of the Answer. You think it's something I'd do."

He doesn't look at me, but he nods. "I was just trying to stay alive, looking for ways to find you, hoping you hadn't left me behind."

"Never," I say. "Not ever."

He looks back up at me. "I'd never leave you neither."

"You promise?"

"Cross my heart, hope to die," he says, grinning shyly.

"I promise, too," I say and I smile at him. "I ain't never leaving you, Todd Hewitt, not never again."

He smiles harder when I say *ain't* but it fades and then I see him gathering his Noise to tell me something, something difficult, something he's ashamed of, but before he does, I want him to *know*, I want him to know for *sure*.

"_____ they're at the ocean," I say. "Mistress Coyle told me a story about it before she left. I think she was trying to tell me that's where they were going."

He looks back up at me.

"Now tell me I don't trust you, Todd Hewitt."

And then I see my mistake.

"What?" he says, seeing the look on my face.

"It's in your Noise," I say, standing up. "Todd, it's all *over* your Noise. *Ocean*, over and over and over again."

"It ain't on purpose," he says but his eyes are widening and I see the door of his cell left unlocked and I see a man in the cell with him telling him where I am and I see asking marks rising–

"I'm so *stupid*," Todd says, standing, too. "Such an effing *idiot!* We need to go. Now!"

"Todd–"

"How far away is the ocean?"

"Two days' ride–"

"Four days' walk then." He's pacing now. His Noise says Ocean again, clear as a bomb itself. He sees me looking at him, sees me seeing it. "I'm not spying on you," he says. "I'm *not*, but he musta left the door open so I'd–" He pulls his hair in frustration. "I'll hide it. I hid the truth about Aaron and I can hide this."

My stomach flutters, remembering what the Mayor said to me about Aaron.

"But we have to go," Todd's saying. "Do you have any food we can take?"

"I can get some," I say.

"*Hurry.*"

As I turn to leave, I hear my name in his Noise. Viola, it says, and it's covered in worry, worry that we've been set up, worry that I think he was sent here on purpose, worry that I think he's lying, and all I can do is just look at him and think his name.

Todd.

And hope he knows what I mean.

I burst into the canteen and run to the cabinets. I leave most of the lights off, trying to keep quiet as I grab meal-packs and loaves of bread.

"That fast, huh?" Corinne says.

She's sitting at a table far back in the darkness, cup of coffee in front of her. "Your friend shows up and you just leave." She stands and walks over to me.

"I have to," I say. "I'm sorry."

"You're sorry?" she says, eyebrows raised. "And what happens here, then? What happens to all the patients who need you?"

"I'm a *terrible* healer, Corinne, all I do is wash and feed them-"

"So that I can have time to do the very little healing that I'm capable of."

"Corinne-"

Her eyes flash. "*Mistress Wyatt.*"

I sigh. "Mistress Wyatt," I say and then I think and say it at the same time. "Come with us!"

"Can't you see where this is all headed? Women in prison, women with injuries. Can't you see this isn't going to get any better?"

"Not with bombs going off every day, it isn't."

"It's the President who's the enemy," I say.

She crosses her arms. "You think you can have just one enemy?"

"Corinne–"

"A healer doesn't take life," she says. "A healer *never* takes life. Our first oath is to do no harm."

"The bombs are set for empty targets."

"Which aren't always empty, are they?" She shakes her head, her face looking suddenly sad, sadder than I've ever seen it. "I know who I am, Viola. In my *soul*, I know it. I heal the sick, I heal the wounded, that's who I am."

"If we stay here, they'll eventually come for us."

"If we leave, patients will die." She doesn't even sound angry any more, which is scarier than before.

"And if you're taken in?" I say, my voice getting challenging. "Who'll heal them then?"

"I was hoping you would."

I just breathe for a second. "It's not that simple."

"It is to me."

"Corinne, if I can get away, if I can contact my people–"

"Then what? They're still five months away, you said. Five months is a long time."

I turn back to the cabinets, continue filling the sack with food. "I have to try," I say. "I have to do *something*." I turn back to her, bag full. "That's who *I* am." I think of Todd, waiting for me, and my heart races faster. "That's who I've become, anyway."

She regards me quietly and then she quotes something Mistress Coyle once said to me. "We are the choices we make."

It takes me a second to realize she's just said goodbye.

"What took so long?" Todd says, anxiously looking out of the window.

"Nothing," I say. "I'll tell you later."

"You got the food?"

I hold up the bag.

"And I'm guessing we just follow the river again?" he says.

"I guess so."

He takes a second to look at me awkwardly, trying not to smile. "Here we go again."

And I feel this funny rush and I know that however much danger we're in, the rush is *happiness* and he feels it, too, and we clasp hands hard for just a second and then he stands on the bed, puts a leg on the sill and jumps through.

I pass the bag of food to him and climb out, my shoes thudding on the hard mud. "Todd," I whisper.

"Yeah?"

"Someone told me there's a communications tower some-where outside of town," I say. "It's probably surrounded by soldiers but I was thinking if we could find it–"

"Big metal tower?" he interrupts. "Higher than the trees?"

I blink. "Probably," I say and my eyes open wide. "You know where it is?"

...noods. I pass it every day."

"*Really?*"

"Yes, really," he says and I see it in his Noise, I see the road–

"And I think finally that's enough," says a voice from the darkness.

A voice we both recognize.

The Mayor steps out of the blackness, a row of soldiers behind him.

"Good evening to you both," he says.

And I hear a flash of Noise from the Mayor.

And Todd collapses.

17

HARD LABOUR

[TODD]

IT'S A SOUND but it's not a sound and it's louder than anything possible and it would burst yer eardrums if you were hearing it with yer ears rather than the inside of yer head and everything goes white and it's not just like I'm blind but deaf and dumb and frozen, too, and the pain of it comes from right deep down within so there's no part of yerself you can grab to protect it, just a stinging, burning slap right into the middle of who you are.

This is what Davy felt, every time he got hit with the Mayor's Noise.

And it's words–

All it is is *words*–

But it's *every* word, crammed into yer head all at once, and the whole world is shouting at you that YER NOTHING YER NOTHING YER NOTHING and it rips away every word of yer own, like pulling yer hair out at the roots and taking skin with it–

A flash of words and I'm nothing–

201

I'm nothing–

YER NOTHING–

And I fall to the ground and the Mayor can do whatever he wants with me.

I don't wanna talk about what happens next.

The Mayor leaves some soldiers behind to guard the house of healing and the others drag me back to the cathedral and he don't say nothing as we go, not a word as I beg him not to hurt her, as I promise and scream and cry (shut up) that I'll do anything he wants as long as he don't hurt her.

(shut up, shut up)

When we get back, he ties me to the chair again.

And lets Mr Collins go to town.

And–

And I don't wanna talk about it.

Cuz I cry and I throw up and I beg and I call out her name and I beg some more and it all shames me so much I can't even say it.

And all thru it, the Mayor says nothing. He just walks round me, over and over again, listening to me yell, listening to me plead.

Listening to my Noise beneath it all.

And I tell myself that I'm doing all this yelling, all this begging, to hide in my Noise what she told me, to keep her safe, to keep him from knowing. I tell myself I have to cry and beg as loud as I can so he won't hear.

(shut up)

That's what I tell myself.

And I don't wanna say no more about it.

(just effing shut the hell up)

By the time I get back in the tower, it's nearly morning and Mayor Ledger's waiting up for me and even tho I'm in no fitness to do anything, I'm wondering if maybe he played a part in all this somehow but his instant concern for me, his horror at the shape I'm in, it all sounds true in his Noise, so true that I just lay slowly down on the mattress and don't know what to think.

"They barely even came in," he says, standing behind me. "Collins just opened the door, took a look, then locked me in again. It's like they knew."

"Yeah," I say into my pillow. "It sure is like they knew."

"I had nothing to do with it, Todd," he says, reading me. "I swear to you. I'd never help that man."

"Just leave me be," I say.

And he does.

I don't sleep.

I burn.

I burn with the stupidity of how easy they trapped me, how easy it was to use her against me. I burn with the shame of crying at the beating (shut *up*). I burn with the ache of being taken from her again, the ache of her promise to me, the ache of not knowing what's going to happen to her now.

I don't care nothing bout what they do to me.

Eventually, the sun rises and I find out my punishment.

"Put yer back into it, pigpiss."

"Shut it, Davy."

Our new job is putting the Spackle to work in groups, digging up foundayshuns for new buildings in the monastery grounds, new buildings that'll house the Spackle for the coming winter.

My punishment is, I'm working right down there with 'em.

My punishment is, Davy's in complete charge.

My punishment is, he's got a new whip.

"C'mon," he says, slashing it against my shoulders. "Work!"

I spin round, every bit of me sore and aching. "You hit me with that again, I'll tear yer effing throat out."

He smiles, all teeth, his Noise a joyous shout of triumph. "Like to see you try, *Mr Hewitt*."

And he just *laughs*.

I turn back to my shovel. The Spackle in my group are all staring at me. I ain't had no sleep and my fingers are cold in the sharp, morning sun and I can't help myself and I shout at 'em. "Get back to work!"

They make a few clicking sounds one to another and start digging at the ground again with their hands.

All except one, who looks at me a minute longer.

I stare him out, seething, my Noise riled and raging right at him. He just takes it silently, his breath steaming from his mouth, his eyes daring me to do something. He holds up his wrist, like he's identifying himself, as if I don't know which one he is, then he returns to working the cold earth as slowly as he can.

1017 is the only one who ain't afraid of us.

I take my shovel and stab it hard into the ground.

"Enjoying yerself?" Davy calls.

I put something in my Noise, rude as I can think of.

"Oh, my mother's long dead," he says. "Just like yers." Then he laughs. "I wonder if she talked as much in real life as she wrote in her little book."

I straighten up, my Noise rising red. "Davy–"

"Cuz boy, don't she go on for *pages*."

"One of these days, Davy," I say, my Noise so fierce I can almost see it bending the air like a heat shimmer. "One of these days, I'm gonna–"

"You're going to what, dear boy?" the Mayor says, riding thru the entrance on Morpeth. "I can hear you two arguing from out on the road." He turns his gaze to Davy. "And arguing is not working."

"Oh, I got 'em working, Pa," Davy says, nodding out to the fields.

And it's true. Me and the Spackle are all separated into teams of ten or twenty, spread out among the whole enclosed bit of the monastery, removing stones from the low internal walls and pulling up the sod in the fields. Others are piling the dug-up dirt in other fields and my group here near the front have already dug parts of the trenches for the foundayshuns of the first building. I've got a shovel. The Spackle have to use their hands.

"Not bad," the Mayor says. "Not bad at all."

Davy's Noise is so pleased it's embarrassing. Nobody looks at him.

"And you, Todd?" The Mayor turns to me. "How is your morning progressing?"

"Please don't hurt her," I say.

"For the last time, Todd," the Mayor says, "I'm not going to hurt her. I'm just going to *talk* with her. In fact, I'm on my way to speak with her right now."

My heart jumps and my Noise raises.

"Oh, he don't like *that*, Pa," Davy says.

"Hush," the Mayor says. "Todd, is there anything you'd like to tell me that might make my visit with her go more quickly, more pleasantly for everyone?"

I swallow.

And the Mayor's just *staring* at me, staring into my Noise, and words form in my brain, PLEASE DON'T HURT HER said in my voice and his voice all twisted together, pressing down on the things I think, the things I know and it's different from the Noise slap, this voice pokes around where I don't want him, trying to open locked doors and turn over stones and shine lights where they shouldn't never be shone and all the while saying PLEASE DON'T HURT HER and I can feel myself starting to *want* to tell (*ocean*), starting to *want* to unlock those doors (*the ocean*), starting to *want* to do just exactly what he says, cuz he's right, he's right about everything and who am I to resist–

"She don't know nothing," I say, my voice wobbly, almost gasping.

He arches an eyebrow. "You seem distressed, Todd." He angles Morpeth to approach. **Submit**, Morpeth says. Davy watches the Mayor's attenshuns on me and even from here I can hear him getting jealous. "Whenever my passions need calming, Todd, there's something I like to do."

He looks into my eyes.

I AM THE CIRCLE AND THE CIRCLE IS ME.

Hatched right in the middle of my brain, like a worm in an apple.

"Reminds me who I am," the Mayor says. "Reminds me of how I can control myself."

"What does?" Davy says and I realize he's not hearing it.

I AM THE CIRCLE AND THE CIRCLE IS ME.

Again, right on the inside of me.

"What does it mean?" I almost gasp cuz it's sitting so heavy in my brain I'm finding it hard to speak.

And then we hear it.

A whining in the air, a buzzing that ain't Noise, a buzz more like a fat purple bee coming in to sting you.

"What the–?" Davy says.

And then we're all turning, looking at the far end of the monastery, looking up over the heads of the soldiers along the top of the wall.

Buzzzz–

It's in the sky, a shape making an arc, high and sharp, coming up thru some trees behind the monastery, trailing smoke behind it, but the buzzing is getting louder and the smoke is starting to thicken into black.

And then the Mayor pulls Viola's binos out of his shirt pocket to get a closer look.

I stare at them, my Noise churning, slopping out with asking marks that he ignores.

Davy musta brought them back down the hill, too.

I clench my fists.

"Whatever it is," Davy says, "it's coming this way."

I look back round. The thing has reached the high point of its arc and is heading back down to earth.

Down towards the monastery where we're all standing.

Buzzzz–

"I'd get out of the way if I were you," the Mayor says. "That's a bomb."

Davy runs so fast back to the gate he drops the whip. The soldiers on the wall start jumping off to the outside. The Mayor readies his horse but he don't move yet, waiting to see where the bomb's gonna land.

"Tracer," he's saying, his voice full of interest. "Antiquated, practically useless. We used them in the Spackle War."

The *buzzzzzzz* is getting louder. The bomb's still falling, but picking up speed.

"Mayor Prentiss?"

"President," he corrects but he's still looking thru the binos almost like he's hypnotized. "The sound and the smoke," he says. "Far too obvious for covert use."

"Mayor Prentiss!" My Noise is getting higher with nerves.

"The city's all been bush bombs, so why–"

"RUN!" I yell.

Morpeth starts and the Mayor looks at me.

But I ain't talking to him.

"RUN!" I'm yelling and waving my hands and the shovel at the Spackle nearest me, the Spackle in my field.

The field the bomb is heading right for.

Buzzzzz–

They don't understand. Most of 'em are just watching the bomb coming right for them. "RUN!" I keep shouting and I'm sending explozhuns out in my Noise, showing 'em what'll happen when that bomb lands, imagining blood and guts and the **BOOM** that's on its way. "*RUN*, GODDAMMIT!"

It finally gets thru and some start to scatter, maybe just to get away from me screaming and waving my shovel, but they run and I chase them further up the field. I look back. The Mayor's moved to the entrance of the monastery, ready to ride further if necessary.

But he's watching me.

"RUN!" I keep yelling, getting the Spackle to move up and away, fleeing from the centre of this field. The last few hop over the nearest internal wall and I hop over with 'em, gasping for breath and turning round again to watch it land–

And I see 1017, still there in the middle of the field, just staring up at the sky.

At the bomb that's gonna kill him where he stands.

I'm jumping back over the internal wall before I even know it–

My feet pounding over the grass–

Leaping over the trenches we've dug–

Running so hard there ain't nothing in my Noise–

Just the *BUZZ* of the bomb–

Getting louder and lower–

And 1017 raising up his hand to shield his eyes from the sun–

...y ain't he running?
And *pound pound* go my feet–
And I'm chanting "*Damn you, damn you*" –
BUZZZZZZZZZZZZZZZZZZZZ–
And 1017 don't see me coming–

I slam into him hard enough to lift him off his feet, feeling
the air punched from his lungs as we fly across the grass, as
we hit the ground rolling, as we go end over end across the
dirt and into a shallow trench, as one titanic–

BOOM

eats the entire planet in a single bite of sound

blasting away every thought and bit of Noise

picking up yer brain and shattering it into pieces

and every bit of air is sucked up and blown past us
and dirt and grass hits us in hard, heavy clods
and smoke fills our lungs

And then there's silence.

Loud silence.

*   *   *

"Are you hurt?" I hear the Mayor shout, as if he's miles and miles away and deep under water.

I sit back up in the trench, see the huge smoking crater in the middle of the field, smoke already thinning cuz there's nothing to burn, row upon row of Spackle watching huddled from the far fields.

I'm breathing but I can't hear it.

I turn back to 1017, still mostly under me in the trench, scrabbling to get up, and I'm opening my mouth to ask him if he's all right even tho there's no way for him to answer–

And he hits me in a hard slap that leaves a rake of scratches across my face.

"Hey!" I shout, tho I can barely hear myself–

He's twisting out from under me and I reach out a hand to hold him there–

And he bites it hard with his rows of little sharp teeth–

And I pull it back, already bleeding–

And I'm ready to punch him, ready to *pound* him–

And he's out from under me, running away across the crater, back towards the other Spackle–

"Hey!" I shout again, my Noise rising into red.

He's just running and staring back and the rows of Spackle are all looking back at me, too, their stupid silent faces with less expresshun than the dumbest sheep I ever had back on the farm and my hand is bleeding and my ears are ringing and my face is stinging from the scratches and I saved his stupid life and this is the thanks I get?

Animals, I think. *Stupid, worthless, effing animals.*

* * *

"Todd?" says the Mayor again, riding over to me. "Are you hurt?"

I turn my face up towards him, not even sure if I'm calm enough to answer, but when I open my mouth–

The ground heaves.

My hearing's still gone so I feel it more than hear it, feel the rumble thru the dirt, feel the air pulse with three hard vibrayshuns, one right after the other, and I see the Mayor turn his head suddenly back towards town, see Davy and all the Spackle do the same.

More bombs.

In the distance, towards the city, the biggest bombs that've ever exploded in the history of this world.

18

TO LIVE IS TO FIGHT

{VIOLA}

I'M SO STUPIDLY UNDONE after the Mayor and his soldiers take Todd away Corinne finally has to give me something for it, though I feel the prick of the needle in my arm as little as I feel her hand on my back, not moving, not caressing, not doing anything to make it feel better, just holding me there, keeping me to earth.

I'm sorry to say, I'm not grateful.

When I wake in my bed, it's only just dawn, the sun so low it's not quite over the horizon yet, everything else in morning shadow.

Corinne is in the chair next to me.

"As much as it would do you good to sleep longer," she says, "I'm afraid you can't."

I lean forward in the bed until I'm almost bent in half. There's a weight in my chest so heavy, it's like I'm being pulled into the ground. "I know," I whisper. "I know."

I don't even know why he collapsed. He was dazed,

unconscious, foam coming from his mouth, and then the soldiers lifted him to his feet and dragged him away.

"They'll come for me," I say, having to swallow away the tightness in my throat. "After they're done with Todd."

"Yes, I expect they will," Corinne says simply, looking at her hands, at the cream-coloured calluses raised on her fingertips, at the ash-coloured skin that flakes off the top of her hands because of so much time under hot water.

The morning is cold, surprisingly, harshly so. Even with my window closed, I can feel a shiver coming. I wrap my arms around my middle.

He's gone.

He's gone.

And I don't know what'll happen now.

"I grew up in a settlement called the Kentish Gate," Corinne suddenly says, keeping her eyes off mine, "on the edge of a great forest."

I look up. "Corinne?"

"My father died in the Spackle War," she presses on, "but my mother was a survivor. From the time I could stand, I worked with her in our orchards, picking apples and crested pine and roisin fruit."

I stare at her, wondering why now, why this story now?

"My reward for all that hard work," she continues, "was a camping trip every year after final harvest, just me and my mother, as deep in the forest as we dared to go." She looks out into the dark dawn. "There's so much life here, Viola. So much, in every corner of every forest and stream and river and mountain. This planet just *hums* with it."

She runs a fingertip over her calluses. "The last time we

went, I was eight. We walked south for three whole days, a present for how grown-up I was getting. God only knows how many miles away we were, but we were alone, just me and her and that was all that mattered."

She lets a long pause go by. I don't break it.

"She was bitten by a Banded Red, on her heel, as she cooled her feet in a stream." She's rubbing her hands again. "It's fatal, red snake venom, but slow."

"Oh, Corinne," I say, under my breath.

She stands suddenly, as if my sympathy is almost rude. She walks over to my window. "It took her seventeen hours to die," she says, still not looking at me. "And they were awful and painful and when she went blind, she grabbed onto me and begged me to save her, begged me over and over to save her life."

I remain silent.

"What we know now, what the healers have discovered, is that I *could* have saved her life just by boiling up some Xanthus root." She crosses her arms. "Which was all around us. In abundance."

The ROAR of New Prentisstown is only just starting to rise with the sun. Light shoots in from the far horizon, but we stay silent for a moment longer.

"I'm sorry, Corinne," I finally say. "But why–?"

"Everyone here is someone's daughter," she says quietly. "Every soldier out there is someone's son. The only crime, the *only* crime is to take a life. There is nothing else."

"And that's why you don't fight," I say.

She turns to me sharply. "To live *is* to fight," she snaps. "To preserve life is to fight *everything* that man stands for."

215

an angry huff of air. "And now her, too, with all the bombs. I fight them every time I bandage the blackened eye of a woman, every time I remove shrapnel from a bomb victim."

Her voice has raised but she lowers it again. "That's my war," she says. "That's the war I'm fighting."

She walks back to her chair and picks up a bundle of cloth sat next to it. "And to that end," she says, "I need you to put these on."

She doesn't give me time to argue or even ask about her plan. She takes my apprentice robes and my own few much-washed clothes and has me put on poorer rags, a long-sleeved blouse, a long skirt, and a headscarf that completely covers my hair.

"Corinne," I say, tying up the scarf.

"Shut up and hurry."

When I'm dressed, she takes me down to the end of the long hallway leading out to the riverside by the house of healing. There's a heavy canvas bag of medicines and bandages loaded up by the door. She hands it to me and says, "Wait for the sound. You'll know it when you hear it."

"Corinne–"

"Your chances aren't very good, you have to know that." She's looking me in the eye now. "But if you get to wherever they're hiding, you put these supplies to use as a *healer*, do you hear me? You've got it in you whether you know it or not."

My breathing is heavy, nervous, but I look at her and I say, "Yes, Mistress."

"*Mistress* is right," she says and looks out of the window in the door. We can see a single bored soldier at the corner of the building, picking his nose. Corinne turns to me. "Now. Strike me, please."

I blink. "What?"

"Strike me," she says again. "I'll need a bloody nose or a split lip at least."

"Corinne—"

"Quickly or the streets will grow too crowded with soldiers."

"I'm not going to *hit* you!"

She grabs me by the arm, so fiercely I flinch back. "If the President comes for you, do you honestly think you'll return? He's tried to get the truth from you by asking and then by trapping your friend. Do you honestly think the patience of a man like that lasts forever?"

"Corinne—"

"He will eventually hurt you," she says. "If you refuse to help him, he will kill you."

"But I don't *know*—"

"He doesn't *care* what you don't know!" she hisses through her teeth. "If I can prevent the taking of a life, I will do so, even one as irritating as yours."

"You're hurting me," I say quietly, as her fingers dig into my arm.

"Good," she says. "Get angry enough to strike me."

"But why—"

"Just do it!" she shouts.

I take in a breath, then another, then I hit her across the face as hard as I can.

* * *

I wait, crouched by the window in the door, watching the soldier. Corinne's footsteps fade down the corridor as she runs to the reception room. I wait some more. The soldier is one of the many now who have had the cure taken from them and in the relative quiet of the morning I can hear what he thinks. Thoughts of boredom, thoughts of the village he lived in before the army invaded, thoughts of the army he was forced to join.

Thoughts of a girl he knew who died.

And then I hear the faint shout of Corinne coming from the front. She'll be screaming that the Answer snuck in during the night, beat her senseless and kidnapped me under their very noses but that she saw us all flee in the opposite direction I'm going to be running.

It's a poor story, there's no way it's going to work, how could anyone sneak in with guards everywhere?

But I know what she's counting on. A legend that's been rising, a legend about the Answer.

How can the bombs be planted with no one seeing?

With no one being caught?

If the Answer can do that, could they sneak past armed guards?

Are they invisible?

I hear thoughts just like this as soon as I see the soldier's head snap up when he hears the ruckus. It grows louder in his Noise as he runs around the corner and out of view.

And as fast as that, it's time.

I hoist the bag of medicines up onto my shoulder.

I open the door.

I run.

I run towards a line of trees and down to the river. There's a path along the riverbank but I stick to the trees beside it and as the bag bashes my shoulders and back with heavy corners, I can't help but think of me and Todd running down this same river, this same riverbank, running from the army, running and running and running.

I have to get to the ocean.

As much as I want to save Todd, my only chance is to find her first.

And then I'll come back for him.

I will.

I ain't never leaving you, Todd Hewitt.

My heart aches as I remember saying it.

As I break my promise.

(you hold on, Todd)

(you stay alive)

I run.

I make my way downriver, avoiding patrols, cutting across back gardens, running behind back fences, staying as far clear of houses and housing blocks as I can.

The valley is narrowing again. The hills approach the road and the houses begin to thin out. Once, I hear marching and I have to dive deep into the undergrowth as soldiers pass, holding my breath, crouching as low to the ground as

man. I wait until there's only bird call (**Where's my safety?**) and the now-distant **ROAR** of the town, wait for a breath or two more, then I raise my head and look down the road.

The river bends in the distance and the road is lost from view behind further rolling hills and forests. Across the road here, this far from town, there are mostly farms and farmhouses, working their way up sloping hillsides, back towards more forest. Directly across, there's a small drive leading to a farmhouse with a little stand of trees in the front garden. The farming fields spread out to the right, but above and beyond the farmhouse, thicker forest begins again. If I can get up the drive, that'll be the safest place for me. If I have to, I'll hide until nightfall and make my way in the dark.

I look up and down the road again and once more. I listen out for marching, for stray Noise, for the rattle of a cart.

I take in a breath.

And I bolt across the road.

I keep my eyes on the farmhouse, the bag banging into my back, my arms pumping the air, my lungs gasping as I run faster and faster and faster–

Up the drive–

Nearly to the trees–

Nearly there–

And a farmer steps out from behind them.

I skid to a stop, sliding in the dirt and nearly falling. He jumps back, obviously surprised to see me appearing suddenly in front of him.

We stare at each other.

His Noise is quiet, disciplined, almost gentlemanly, which is why I didn't hear it from a distance. He's holding a basket under one arm and a red pear in his free hand.

He looks me up and down, sees the bag on my back, sees me alone out on the road in a break of the law, sees from the heaviness of my breath that I've obviously been running.

And it comes in his Noise, fast and clear as morning.

The Answer, he thinks.

"No," I say. "I'm not–"

But he holds a finger up to his lips.

He cocks his head in the direction of the road.

And I hear the distant sound of soldiers marching down it.

"That way," the farmer whispers. He points up a narrow path, a small entrance to the woods above that would be easy to miss if you didn't know it was there. "Quickly now."

I look at him again, trying to see a trap, trying to *tell* but there's no time. There's no time.

"Thank you," I say and I take off running.

The path leads almost immediately into thicker woods, all uphill. It's narrow and I have to push back vines and branches to make my way. The trees swallow me and I can only go forward and forward, hoping that I'm not being led into a trap. I get to the top of the hill only to find a small slope down and then another hill to climb. I run up that, too. I'm still heading east but I can't see enough over anything to tell where the road is or the river or which way I'm–

I nearly stumble out into a clearing.

221

where there's a soldier not ten metres from me.

His back is to me (thank god, thank god) and it's not until my heart has leapt out of my chest and I've caught myself and fallen back into the bushes that I see what he's guarding.

There it is.

In the middle of a clearing cresting the hill, stretching up on three metal legs almost fifty metres into the sky. The trees around it have been felled, and across the clearing underneath it I can see a small building and a road that leads back down the other side of the hill to the river.

I've found the communications tower.

It's here.

And there aren't that many soldiers around it. I count five, no, six.

Just six. With big gaps.

My heart rises.

And rises.

I've found it.

And a *BOOM!* echoes in the distance beyond the tower.

I flinch, along with the soldiers. Another bomb. Another statement from the Answer. Another–

The soldiers are leaving.

They're running, running towards the sound of the explosion, running away from me and down the other side of the hill, towards where I can already see a white pillar of smoke rising.

The tower stands in front of me.
All of a sudden, it's completely unguarded.

I don't even wait to think how stupid I'm being–
    I'm just running–
    Running towards the tower–
    If this is my chance to save us then–
    I don't know–
    I'm just running–
    Across the open ground–
    Towards the tower–
    Towards the building underneath–
    I can save us–
    Somehow I can save all of us–

And out of the corner of my eye, I see someone else break
cover from the trees to my left–
    Someone running straight towards me–
    Someone–
    Someone saying my name–

"Viola!" I hear. "Get back!"
    "Viola, *NO!*" Mistress Coyle is screaming at me.

I don't stop–
    Neither does she–

"GET BACK!" she's yelling–

And she's crossing the clearing in front of me–

Running and running and running–

And then I realize–

Like a blow to the stomach–

The reason why she's yelling–

No–

Even as I'm skidding to a stop–

No, I think–

No, you can't–

And Mistress Coyle reaches me–

You CAN'T–

And pushes us both to the ground–

NO!

And the legs of the tower explode in three blinding flashes of light.

PART IV

NIGHT FALLING

19

WHAT YOU DON'T KNOW

{VIOLA}

"GET OFF ME!"

She slaps her hand over my mouth, holding it there, holding *me* there with the weight of her body as clouds of dust billow around us from the rubble of the communications tower. "*Quit shouting*," she hisses.

I bite her hand.

She makes a pained face, fierce and angry, but she doesn't let go, just takes the bite and doesn't move.

"You can scream and shout all you want later, my girl," she says, "but in two seconds, this place is going to be swarming with soldiers and do you honestly think they're going to believe you just *happened by*?"

She waits to see my reaction. I glare at her but finally nod. She takes away her hand.

"Don't you call me *my girl*," I say, keeping my voice low but just as fierce as hers. "Don't you call me that ever again."

I follow her down a steep slope, heading back towards the road, sliding on fallen leaves and gathered dew but always down and down. I hop over logs and roots, the canvas bag like a stone around my shoulders.

I have no choice but to go with her.

I'd be captured and god knows what else if I went back to town.

And she took my other choice away.

She reaches a stand of bushes at the bottom of a steepening in the slope. She ducks fast under them and beckons for me to follow. I slide down next to her, my breath almost gone, and she says, "Whatever you do, don't scream."

Before I can even open my mouth, she's jumped out through the bushes. They close up behind her and I have to fight my way through leaves and branches to follow. I'm still pushing them back when I practically tumble out the other side.

Onto the road.

Where two soldiers stand by a man with a cart, all of them looking straight at me and Mistress Coyle.

The soldiers look more astonished than angry, but they have no Noise, so there's no way to know.

But they're carrying rifles.

And they're raising them at us.

"And who the hell is *this*?" one barks, a middle-aged man with a shaved head and a scar down his jaw line.

"Don't shoot!" Mistress Coyle says, hands out and up.

"We heard the explosion," says the other soldier, a younger one, not much older than me, with blond, shoulder-length hair.

Then the older soldier says something else, something unexpected.

"You're *late*."

"That's enough, Magnus," Mistress Coyle says, lowering her hands and stepping forward to the cart. "And put your rifles down, she's with me."

"What?" I say, still frozen to my spot.

"The tracer malfunctioned completely," the younger soldier says to her. "We're not even sure where it came down."

"I told you they were too old," Magnus says.

"It did its job," Mistress Coyle says, bustling around the cart, "wherever it landed."

"Hey!" I say. "What's going on?"

And then I hear, "Hildy?"

Mistress Coyle stops in her tracks, the two soldiers do, too, and stare at the man driving the cart.

"Iss you, ain it?" he says. "Hildy hoo's also called Viola."

My mind's been racing so fast, so completely focused on the soldiers, that I barely took in the man driving the cart, the nearly expressionless face, the clothes, the hat, the voice, the Noise flat and calm as the far horizon.

The man that once drove me and Todd across a sea of things.

"*Wilf*," I gasp.

Now everyone looks at *me*, Mistress Coyle's eyebrows so high it's like they're trying to crawl into her hair.

"Hey," Wilf says, in greeting.

"Hey," I say back, too stunned to say any more.

He touches two fingers to the brim of his hat. "Ah'm glad to see yoo mayde it."

Mistress Coyle's mouth is moving but no sound comes out for a second or two. "There'll be time for that later," she finally says. "We have to go *now*."

"Will there be room for two?" the younger soldier asks.

"There'll have to be." She ducks down under the cart and removes a panel from the underside. She motions to me. "Get in."

"In where?" I bend down and see a compartment hidden like a trick of the eye in the width of the cart, narrow and thin as a cot above the rear axle.

"Pack won't fit," Wilf says, pointing at the bag on my back. "Ah'll take it."

I slip it off and hand it to him. "Thank you, Wilf."

"*Now*, Viola," Mistress Coyle says.

I give Wilf a last nod, duck under the cart and crawl in, forcing my way across the compartment until my head's nearly touching the far side. Mistress Coyle doesn't wait and forces herself in after me. The younger soldier was right. There isn't enough room. She's pressed right up against me, face to face, her knees digging into my thighs, our noses less than a centimetre apart. She's barely drawn her feet inside when the panel is replaced, plunging us into almost complete darkness.

"Where are we–" I start to say but she shushes me harshly.

And outside I hear soldiers marching fast up the road, led by the clopping of horse's hooves.

*   *   *

"Report!" one of them shouts as they stop by the cart.

His voice–

It's up high and I hear the horse whinnying beneath it–

But his voice–

"Heard the explosion, sir," the older of our soldiers replies. "This man says he saw women heading past him down the river road about an hour ago."

We hear the real soldier spit. "Bitches."

I recognize his voice–

It's Sergeant Hammar.

"Whose unit you two in?" he says.

"First, sir," says our younger soldier, after the briefest of pauses. "Captain O'Hare."

"*That* pansy?" Sergeant Hammar spits. "You wanna do some *real* soldiering, transfer to the Fourth. I'll show you what's what."

"Yes, sir," says our older soldier, sounding more nervous than I'd want him to.

I can hear the Noise of the soldiers in Sergeant Hammar's unit. They're thinking of the cart. They're thinking of the explosions. They're thinking about shooting women.

But there's no Noise coming from Sergeant Hammar.

"Arrest this man," Sergeant Hammar finally says, meaning Wilf.

"We were just doing that, sir."

"Bitches," Sergeant Hammar says again, and we hear him spur his horse (**Yield**, it thinks) and he and his men march off at speed.

231

I let out the breath I didn't realize I was holding. "He wasn't even *punished*," I whisper, more to myself than to Mistress Coyle.

"Later," she whispers back.

I hear Wilf snap the reins and we rock as the cart plods slowly forward.

So the Mayor was a liar. All along.

Of course he was, you *idiot*.

And Maddy's killer walks free to kill again, his cure still in place.

And I'm bumping and juddering against the woman who destroyed the only hope of contacting the ships that might save us.

And Todd is out there. Somewhere. Being left behind.

I've never felt so lonely in my life.

The compartment is hellishly small. We share too much of each other's air, elbows and shoulders bruising away as we ride along, the heat soaking our clothes.

We don't speak.

Time passes. And then more. And more after that. I fall into a kind of doze, the close warmth sucking the life right out of me. The rocking of the cart eventually flattens all my worries and I close my eyes against it.

I'm awakened by the older soldier knocking on the wood and I think we're going to finally get out, but he just says, "We're at the rough bit. Hold on."

"To what?" I say, but I don't say any more as the cart feels like it drops off a cliff.

Mistress Coyle's forehead smacks into my nose and I smell blood almost at once. I hear her gasp and choke as my stray hand is shoved into her neck and still the cart tumbles and bumps and I wait for the moment where we topple end over end.

And then Mistress Coyle is working both arms around me, pulling me close to her and bracing us in the compartment with one hand and one foot pressed against the opposite side. I resist her, resist the implied comfort, but there's wisdom in it as almost immediately we stop knocking each other about, even though the cart lurches and stutters.

And so it's in Mistress Coyle's arms that the last bit of my journey is taken. And it's in Mistress Coyle's arms that I enter the camp of the Answer.

Finally the cart stops and the panel is removed almost immediately.

"We're here," says the younger soldier, the blond one. "Everyone okay?"

"Why wouldn't we be?" Mistress Coyle says sourly. She lets go of me and scoots her way out of the compartment, extending a hand to help me out, too. I ignore it, getting myself out and looking at my surroundings.

We've come down a steep rocky path that's barely fit for a cart and into what looks like a gash of rocks in the middle of a forest. Trees press in on every side, a row of them on the level ground in front of us.

The ocean must be beyond them. Either I dozed off for longer than I thought or she lied and it's closer than she said.

which wouldn't surprise me.

The blond soldier whistles when he sees our faces, and I can feel caked blood under my nose. "I can get you something for that," he says.

"She's a healer," Mistress Coyle says. "She can do it herself."

"I'm Lee," he says to me, a grin on his face.

For a brief second, I'm completely aware of how terrible I must look with my bloody nose and this ridiculous outfit.

"I'm Viola," I say to the ground.

"'Ere's yer bag," Wilf says, suddenly next to me, holding out the canvas sack of medicines and bandages. I look at him for a second and then I pretty much throw myself at him in a hug, pulling him tight to me, feeling the big, safe bulk of him. "Ah'm glad to see yoo, Hildy," he says.

"You, too, Wilf," I say, my voice thick. I let him go and take the bag.

"Corinne pack that?" Mistress Coyle asks.

I fish out a bandage and start cleaning the blood from my nose. "What do you care?"

"You can accuse me of many things," she says, "but not caring isn't one of them, my girl."

"I told you," I say, catching her eye, "never call me that again."

Mistress Coyle licks her teeth. She makes a quick glance to Lee and to the other soldier, Magnus, and they leave, quickly, disappearing into the trees ahead of us. "You, too, Wilf."

Wilf looks at me. "Yoo gone be all right?"

"I think so, Wilf," I say, swallowing, "but don't you go far."

234

He nods, touching the brim of his hat again and walking after the soldiers. We watch him go.

"All right." Mistress Coyle turns to me, crossing her arms. "Let's hear it."

I look at her, at her face full of defiance, and I feel my breath quicken, the anger rising up again so fast, so easily, it feels like I might crack in two. "How *dare you*–"

But she's interrupting, *already*. "Whoever contacts your ships first has the advantage. If he's first, he tells them all about the nasty little terrorist organization he's got on his hands and can they please use their guidance equipment to track us down and blow us off the face of New World."

"Yes but if we–"

"If we got to them first, yes, of course, we could have told them all about our local tyrant, but that was never going to happen."

"We could have tried–"

"Did you know what you were doing when you ran towards that tower?"

I clench my fists. "*No*, but at least I could have–"

"Could have what?" Her eyes challenge me. "Sent out a message to the very coordinates the President's been searching for? Don't you think he was counting on you *try-ing*? Just why exactly do you think you haven't been arrested yet?"

I dig my nails into my palms, forcing myself not to hear what she's saying.

"We were running out of time," she says. "And if *we* can't

235

_____ it to contact help, then at the very least we prevent him from doing the same."

"And when they land? What's your brilliant plan then?"

"Well," she says, uncrossing her arms and taking a step towards me, "if we haven't overthrown him, then there's a race to get to them first, isn't there? At least this way, it's a fair fight."

I shake my head. "You had no right."

"It's a war."

"That you started."

"*He* started it, my girl."

"And you escalated it."

"Hard decisions have to be made."

"And who put you in charge of making them?"

"Who put *him* in charge of locking away half the population of this planet?"

"You're blowing people up!"

"Accidents," she says. "Deeply regrettable."

Now it's my turn to take a step towards her. "That sounds exactly like something *he* would say."

Her shoulders rise and if she had Noise, it would be taking the top of my head off. "Have you *seen* the women's prisons, my girl? What you don't know could fill a *crater*–"

"Mistress Coyle!" A voice calls from the trees. Lee steps back into the rocky gash. "There's a report just come in."

"What is it?" Mistress Coyle says.

He looks from her to me. I look at the ground again.

"Three divisions of soldiers marching down the river road," he says, "full out for the ocean."

* * *

I look up sharply. "They're coming *here*?"

Both Mistress Coyle and Lee look at me.

"No," Lee says. "They're going to the ocean."

I blink back and forth between them. "But aren't we–?"

"Of course not," Mistress Coyle says, her voice flat, mocking. "Whatever made you think we were? And whatever, I wonder, makes the *President* think we are?"

I feel an angry chill, despite the sun, and I notice I'm shaking inside these big stupid puffy sleeves.

She was *testing* me.

As if I would tell the Mayor where–

"How *dare* you–" I start to say again.

But the anger suddenly fades as it comes flooding back.

"Todd," I whisper.

Ocean all over his Noise.

How he promised to hide it.

And how I know he'd keep that promise–

If he could.

(oh, Todd, did he–?)

(are you–?)

Oh, *no*.

"I have to go back," I say. "I have to *save* him–"

She's already shaking her head. "There's nothing we can do for him right now–"

"He'll kill him."

She looks at me, not without pity. "He's probably dead already, my girl."

I feel my throat closing up but I fight it. "You don't know that."

"If he's not dead, then he must have told the President

army. She cocks her head. "Which would you rather be true?"

"No," I say, shaking my head. "No–"

"I'm sorry, my girl." Her voice is a little calmer than before, a little softer, but still strong. "I truly am, but there are thousands of lives at stake. And like it or not, you've picked a side." She looks over to where Lee stands. "So why don't you let me show you your army?"

20

RUBBLE

"BITCHES," Mr Hammar says from atop his horse.

"Your analysis was not asked for, Sergeant," says the Mayor, riding Morpeth thru the smoke and the twisted metal.

"They've left the mark, tho," Mr Hammar says, pointing at the trunk of a large tree at the edge of the clearing.

The blue **A** of the Answer is smeared across it.

"Your concern for my eyesight does you credit," says the Mayor, sharply enough that even Mr Hammar shuts up.

We rode up here straight from the monastery, meeting Mr Hammar's squadron coming up the hill, looking ready for battle. When we got to the top, we found Ivan and the soldiers who were meant to be guarding the tower. Ivan got promoted here, I guess, after all the Spackle were rounded up, but now he's looking like he wishes he never *heard* of a tower.

Cuz it ain't here no more. It's just a heap of smoking metal, mostly in a long line where it fell, like a drunk man

239

forward onto the ground and deciding to just stay there and sleep.

(and I do my damnedest not to think about her asking me how to get here)

(saying we should go here first)

(oh, Viola, you didn't–)

"If they got enough to blow up something this big…" Davy says to my right, looking across the field. He don't finish his sentence cuz it's the same thing we're all thinking, the thing that's in everyone's Noise.

Everyone that's *got* Noise, that is, cuz Mr Hammar seems to be one of the lucky ones. "Hey, boy," he sneers at me. "You a man yet?"

"Don't you have somewhere you need to be heading, Sergeant?" the Mayor asks, not looking at him.

"With haste, sir," Mr Hammar says again, giving me an evil wink, then spurring his horse and shouting for his men to follow. They speed down the hill in the fastest march I've seen, leaving us with Ivan and his soldiers, all of their Noise regretting to a man how they ran towards the monastery after hearing the tracer bomb hit.

It's obvious, tho, when you look back. A smaller bomb in one place to get people running away from where you want to plant yer bigger bomb.

But what the hell were they doing bombing the monastery?

Why attack the Spackle?

Why attack *me*?

"Private Farrow," the Mayor says to Ivan.

"It's *Corporal* Farrow, actually–" Ivan says.

The Mayor turns his head slowly and Ivan stops talking as he comes to understand. "Private Farrow," the Mayor says again. "You will salvage what metal and scrap you can and then report to your commanding officer to relinquish your supply of cure–"

He stops. We can all hear Ivan's Noise clear as day. The Mayor looks round. Every soldier in the squadron has Noise. Every one of 'em's already been punished for one thing or another.

"You will submit yourselves to your commanding officer for appropriate punishment."

Ivan don't reply but his Noise rumbles.

"Is something unclear, Private?" the Mayor says, his voice dangerously bright. He looks into Ivan's eyes, holding his gaze. "You will submit yourselves to your commanding officer for appropriate punishment," he says again, but there's something in his voice, some weird vibrayshun.

I look at Ivan. His eyes are going foggy, unfocused, his mouth a little slack. "I will submit to my commanding officer for appropriate punishment," he says.

"Good," the Mayor says, looking back at the wreckage.

Ivan slumps a little when the eye contact is broken, blinking as if he's just woken up, forehead furrowing.

"But, sir," he says to the Mayor's back.

The Mayor turns round again, looking *very* surprised at still being spoken to.

Ivan presses on. "We were coming to your aid when–"

The Mayor's eyes flash. "When the Answer watched you do exactly what it wanted you to do and then blew up *my tower*."

Without changing his expresshun, the Mayor pulls out a pistol from his holster and shoots Ivan in the leg.

Ivan tumbles over, wailing. The Mayor looks at the other soldiers.

"Anyone else care to contribute before you get to work?"

As the rest of the soldiers ignore Ivan's screams and start clearing up the wreckage, the Mayor moves Morpeth right in front of that **A**, loud and clear like the announcement it is. "The Answer," he says, in a low voice like he's talking to himself. "The Answer."

"Let *us* go after 'em, Pa," Davy says.

"Hmm?" The Mayor turns his head slowly, like he forgot we were there.

"We can fight," Davy says. "We proved that. And instead you got us babysitting animals that are already beat."

The Mayor considers us for a minute, tho I don't know how or when Davy turned him and me into an *us*. "If you think they're already beaten, David," he finally says, "then you know very little about the Spackle."

Davy's Noise ruffles a little. "I think I've learnt a thing or two by now."

And as much as I hate to, I have to agree with him.

"Yes," says the Mayor. "I suppose you have. Both of you." He looks me in the eye and I can't help thinking of me saving 1017 from the bomb, risking my own life to get him outta the way.

And him biting and scratching me by way of thanks.

"Then how about a new project?" the Mayor says, steering Morpeth over to us. "One where you can put all your expertise to work."

Davy's Noise ain't sure of this. There's pride but doubt, too.

All I got in mine is dread.

"Are you ready to lead, Todd?" the Mayor asks lightly.

"*I'm* ready, Pa," Davy says.

The Mayor still looks only at me. He knows I'm thinking about her but he's ignoring all my askings.

"The Answer," he says, turning back to the *A*. "If that's who they want to be, then let them." He looks back at us. "But if there's an Answer, then someone must first…"

He lets his voice fade and he gets a faraway smile on his face, like he's laughing at his own private joke.

Davy unfolds the big white scroll onto the grass, not caring that it's getting wet in the cold morning dew. There's words written across the top and diagrams and squares and things drawn in below it.

"Measurements mostly," Davy reads. "Too effing many. I mean, *look* at that."

He holds the scroll up to me, trying to get me to agree.

And, well–

Yeah, okay, I–

Whatever.

"Too effing many," I say, feeling sweat come up under my arms.

...the day after the tower fell and we're back at the monastery, back to putting teams of Spackle to work. My escape seems to be forgotten, like it was part of another life and now we've all got new things to think about. The Mayor won't talk to me about Viola and I'm back working for Davy, who ain't too happy.

So it's like old times.

"There's fighting to be done and he's got us building an effing *palace*," Davy frowns, looking over the plans.

It ain't a palace but he's got a point. Before it was just gonna be rough shacks to shelter the Spackle for the winter but this looks like a whole new building for men, taking up most of the inside of the monastery.

It's even got a name written across the top.

A name my eye stumbles over, trying to–

Davy turns to me, his eyes widening. I make my Noise as Noisy as possible.

"We should get started," I say, standing up.

But Davy's still looking at me. "What do you think about what it says right here?" he asks, putting his finger on a block of words. "Ain't that something amazing what it says?"

"Yeah," I shrug. "I guess."

His eyes get even wider with delight. "It's a list of materials, pigpiss!" His voice is practically celebrating. "You can't read, can you?"

"Shut up," I say, looking away.

"You can't even *read*!" Davy's smiling up into the cold sun and around at all the Spackle watching us. "What kinda idiot gets thru life–"

"I said, *shut up*!"

244

Davy's mouth drops open as he realizes.

And I know what he's gonna say before he says it.

"Yer ma's book," he says. "She wrote it for you and you can't even–"

And what can I do but hit him across his stupid lughole of a mouth?

I'm getting taller and bigger and he comes off worst in the fight but he don't seem to mind all that much. Even when we get back to work, he's still giggling and making a big show outta reading the plans.

"Mighty complicated, these instruckshuns," he says, a big smile across his bloody lips.

"Just effing get on with it!"

"Fine, fine," he says. "First step is what we were already doing. Tearing down all the internal walls." He looks up. "I could write it down for you."

My Noise rages red at him but Noise is useless as a weapon.

Unless yer the Mayor.

I didn't think life could turn more to crap but it always does, don't it? Bombs and towers falling and having to work with Davy and the Mayor paying me special attenshun and–

(and I don't know where she is)

(and I don't know what the Mayor's gonna do to her)

(and did she plant the bombs?)

(did she?)

I turn back round to the work site.

1150 pairs of Spackle eyes are watching us, watching *me*, like they're just effing farm animals looking up from their grazing cuz they heard a loud noise.

Stupid effing *sheep*.

"GET TO WORK!" I shout.

"You look like hell," Mayor Ledger says, as I fall onto my bed.

"Stuff it," I say.

"Working you hard, is he?" He brings me over the dinner that's already waiting for us. It don't even look like he ate too much of mine before I got here.

"Ain't he working *you* hard?" I say, digging in to the food.

"I think he's forgotten about me, truth to tell." He sits back on his own bed. "I haven't spoken to him in I don't know how long."

I look up at him. His Noise is grey, like he's hiding something, tho that ain't unusual.

"I've just been doing my rubbish duties," he says, watching me eat. "Listening to people talk."

"And what're they saying?" I ask, cuz it seems like he wants to talk.

"Well," he says. His Noise shifts uncomfortably.

"Well what?"

And then I see the reason his Noise is so flat is cuz there's something he don't wanna tell me but feels like he has to, so here it comes.

"That house of healing," he says. "That one in particular."

"What about it?" I say, trying not to make it sound important, failing.

"It's closed down," he says. "Empty."

I stop eating. "What do you mean, empty?"

"I mean *empty*," he says gently, cuz he knows it's bad news. "There's no one there, not even the patients. Everyone's gone."

"Gone?" I whisper.

Gone.

I stand up tho there ain't nowhere to go, my stupid plate of dinner still in my hand.

"Gone where? What's he done with her?"

"He hasn't done anything," Mayor Ledger says. "Your friend ran. That's what I heard. Ran off with the women just before the tower fell." He rubs his chin. "Everyone else was arrested and taken to the prisons. But your friend … got away."

He says *got away* like that's not what he means, like what he means is she was planning to get away all along.

"You can't know that," I say. "You can't know that's true about her."

He shrugs. "Maybe not," he says. "But I heard it from one of the soldiers who was guarding the house of healing."

"No," I say, but I don't know what I mean. "No."

"How well did you really know her?" Mayor Ledger says.

"You shut up."

I'm breathing hard, my chest rising and falling.

It's good that she ran, ain't it?

Ain't it?

She was in danger and now—

(but)

(but did she blow up the tower?)

(why didn't she tell me she was going to?)

(did she lie to me?)

And I shouldn't think it, I shouldn't think it, but here it comes—

She promised.

And she left.

She left *me*.

(Viola?)

(did you leave me?)

21

THE MINE

{VIOLA}

I OPEN MY EYES to the sound of wings flapping outside the door, something I already know in the few days I've been here means that the bats have returned to the caves after their night's hunting, that the sun is about to rise, that it's almost time to get myself out of bed.

Some women start to stir, stretching in their cots. Others are still dead to the world, still snoring, still farting, still drifting on in the empty nothing of sleep.

I spend a second wishing I was still there, too.

The sleeping quarters is basically just a long shack, swept earth floor, wood walls, wood door, barely any windows and only an iron stove in the centre for not enough heat. The rest is just a row of cots stretched from one end to the other, full of sleeping women.

As the newest arrival, I'm at one end.

And I'm watching the occupant of the bed at the other end. She sits up straight, body fully under her command, like

249

she ~~actually~~ sleeps, just puts herself on pause until she can start work again.

Mistress Coyle turns in her cot, sets her feet on the floor, and looks over the other sleepers straight at me.

Checking on me first.

To see, no doubt, if I've run off sometime in the night to find Todd.

I don't believe he's dead. And I don't believe he told the Mayor on us, either.

There must be another answer.

I look back at Mistress Coyle, unmoving.

Not gone, I think. *Not yet.*

But mainly because I don't even know where we are.

We're not by the ocean. Not even close, as far as I can tell, though that's not saying much because secrecy is the watchword of the camp. No one gives information out unless it's absolutely necessary. That's in case anyone gets captured on a bombing raid or, now that the Answer has started running out of things like flour and medicine, raids for supplies as well.

Mistress Coyle guards information as her most valuable resource.

All I know is that the camp is at an old mine, started up – like so many other things seem to have been on this planet – with great optimism after the first landings but abandoned after just a few years. There are a number of shacks around the openings to a couple of deep caves. The shacks, some new, some from the mining days, serve as sleeping quarters and meeting rooms and dining halls and so on.

The caves – the ones where there aren't bats, anyway – are the food and supply stores, always worryingly low, always guarded fiercely by Mistress Lawson, still fretting over the children she left behind and taking out her fretting on anyone who requests another blanket for the cold.

Deeper in the caves are the mines, originally sunk to find coal or salt and then when none were found, diamonds and then gold, which weren't found either, as if they'd do anyone any good in this place anyway. The mines are now where the weapons and explosives are hidden. I don't know how they got here or where they came from, but if the camp is found, they'll be detonated, probably wiping us all off the map.

But for now it's a camp that's near a natural well and hidden by the forest around it. The only entrance is through the trees at the bottom of the path Mistress Coyle and I bumped our way down, and it's so steep and hard you'd hear intruders come from a long way away.

"And they'll come," Mistress Coyle said to me on my first day. "We'll just have to make sure we're ready to meet them."

"Why haven't they come already?" I asked. "People must know there's a mine here."

All she did was wink at me and touch the side of her nose.

"What's *that* supposed to mean?" I asked.

But that was all I got, because information is her most valuable resource, isn't it?

At breakfast, I get my usual snubbing by Thea and the other apprentices I recognize, none of whom will say a word to me,

... blaming me for Maddy's death, blaming me for somehow

being a traitor, blaming me for this whole sodding war, for all I know.

Not that I care.

Because I don't.

I leave them to the dining hall, and I take my plate of grey porridge out in the cold morning to some rocks near the mouth of one of the caves. As I eat, I watch the camp start to wake itself, start to put itself together for the things that terrorists spend their days doing.

The biggest surprise is how few people there are. Maybe a hundred. That's all. That's the big Answer causing all the fuss in New Prentisstown by blowing things up. One hundred people. Mistresses and apprentices, former patients and others, too, disappearing in the night and returning in the morning, or keeping the camp running for those that come and go, tending to the few horses the Answer has and the oxes that pull the carts and the hens we get our eggs from and a million other things that need doing.

But only a hundred people. Not enough to have a whisper of a prayer if the Mayor's *real* army comes marching down towards us.

"All right, Hildy?"

"Hi, Wilf," I say, as he comes up to me, a plate of porridge in his hands, too. I scoot over so he can sit near me. He doesn't say anything, just eats his porridge and lets me eat mine.

"Wilf?" we both hear. Jane, Wilf's wife, is coming for us, two steaming mugs in her hands. She picks her way over the rocks towards us, stumbling once, spilling some coffee and

252

causing Wilf to rise halfway up, but she recovers. "Here ya go!" she practically shouts, thrusting the mugs at us.

"Thank you," I say, taking mine.

She shoves her hands under her armpits against the cold and smiles, eyes wide and searching around, like she eats with them. "Awful cold to be eating outside," she says, like an overly friendly demand that we explain ourselves.

"Yup," Wilf says, going back to his porridge.

"It's not too bad," I say, also going back to eating.

"Didja hear they got a grain store last night?" she says, lowering her voice to a whisper but somehow making it louder at the same time. "We can have *bread* again!"

"Yup," Wilf says again.

"D'you like bread?" she asks me.

"I do."

"Ya gotta have bread," she says, to the ground, to the sky, to the rocks. "Ya gotta have bread."

And then she's back off to the dining hall, not another word, though Wilf doesn't seem to much mind or even notice. But I know, I *definitely* know that Wilf's clear and even Noise, his lack of words, his seeming blankness doesn't describe all of him, not even close.

Wilf and Jane were refugees, fleeing into Haven as the army swept behind them, passing us on the road as Todd slept off his fever in Carbonel Downs. Jane fell ill on the trip and, after asking directions, Wilf took her straight to Mistress Forth's house of healing, where Jane was still recovering when the army invaded. Wilf, whose Noise is as free of deception as anyone's on this planet, was assumed by the soldiers to be an idiot and so allowed to visit his wife when no other man was.

When the women ran, Wilf helped. When I asked him why, all he did was shrug and say, "They were gone take Jane." He hid the less able women on his cart as they fled, built a hidey-hole in it so others could return for missions, and for weeks on end has risked his life taking them to and fro because the soldiers have always assumed a man so transparent couldn't be hiding anything.

All of which has been a surprise to the leaders of the Answer.

But none of which is a surprise to me.

He saved me and Todd once when he didn't have to. He saved Todd again when there was even more danger. He was even ready the first night I was here to turn right back around to help me find him, but Sergeant Hammar knows Wilf's face now, knows that he should have been arrested, so any trip back is pretty much a death sentence.

I take a last spoonful of my porridge and sigh heavily as I pop it into my mouth. I could be sighing at the cold, sighing at the boring porridge, sighing at the lack of anything to do in camp.

But, somehow, Wilf knows. Somehow, Wilf always knows.

"Ah'm shur he's okay, Hildy," he says, finishing up his own porridge. "He survives, does our Todd."

I look up into the cold morning sun and I swallow again, though there's no porridge left in my throat.

"Keep yerself strong," Wilf stays, standing. "Strong for what's comin."

I blink. "What's coming?" I ask as he walks on towards the dining hall, drinking his mug of coffee.

He just keeps on going.

I finish my coffee, rubbing my arms to gather some heat, thinking I'll ask her again today, no, I'll *tell* her I'm coming on the next mission, that I need to find–

"You're sitting out here all by yourself?"

I look up. Lee, the blond soldier, is standing there, smiling all toothy.

I immediately feel my face go hot.

"No, no," I say, standing straight up, turning away from him and picking up the plate.

"You don't have to leave–" he's saying.

"No, I'm finished–"

"Viola–"

"All yours–"

"That's not what I meant–"

But I'm already stomping back to the dining hall, cursing myself for the redness of my face.

Lee isn't the only man. Well, he's hardly a *man*, but like Wilf, he and Magnus can no longer pretend to be soldiers and go to the city, now that their faces are known.

But there are others who can. Because that's the biggest secret of all about the Answer.

At least a third of the people here are men, men who pretend to be soldiers to shuttle women in and out of the

men who help Mistress Coyle with the planning and targets, men with expertise on handling explosives, men who believe in the cause and want to fight against the Mayor and all he stands for.

Men who've lost wives and daughters and mothers and who are fighting to save them or fighting to avenge their memories.

Mostly it's memories.

I suppose it's useful if everyone thinks it's only women; it allows men to come and go, even if the Mayor surely knows what's what, which is probably why he's denying the cure to so much of his own army, why the Answer's own supply of cure is becoming more burden than blessing.

I cast a glance quickly back to Lee behind me and forward again.

I'm not sure of his reason for being here.

I haven't been able–

I haven't had the *chance* to ask him yet.

I'm not paying attention as I reach the dining room door and don't really notice when it opens before I can take the handle.

I look up into Mistress Coyle's face.

I don't even greet her.

"Take me with you on the next raid," I say.

Her expression doesn't change. "You know why you can't."

"Todd would join us," I say. "In a *second*."

"Others aren't so sure about that, my girl." I open my mouth to reply but she interrupts. "If he's even still alive.

Which matters not, because we can't afford to have you captured. You're the most valuable prize of all. The girl who can help the President when the ships land."

"I–"

She holds up her hand. "I won't have this fight with you again. There is too much important work to do."

The camp feels silent now. The people behind her have stopped moving as we stare at one another, no one willing to ask her to get out of the way, not even Mistresses Forth and Nadari, who wait there patiently. Like Thea, they've barely spoken to me since my arrival, all these acolytes of Mistress Coyle, all these people who wouldn't dare to dream of speaking to her the way I'm speaking to her now.

They treat me as if I'm a little dangerous.

I'm slightly surprised to find I kind of like it.

I look into her eyes, into the unyieldingness of them. "I won't forgive you," I say quietly, as if I'm only talking to her. "I won't. Not now, not ever."

"I don't want your forgiveness," she says, equally quietly. "But one day, you *will* understand."

And then her eyes glint and she pulls her mouth into a smile. "You know," she says, raising her voice. "I think it's time you had some employment."

22

1017

[TODD]

"CAN'T YOU EFFING THINGS move any faster?"

The four or five Spackle nearest to me flinch away, tho I ain't even spoken that loud.

"Get a *move* on!"

And as ever, no thoughts, no Noise, no nothing.

They can only be getting the cure in the fodder I still have to shovel out. But why? Why when no one else is? It makes them a sea of silent clicking and white backs bent into the cold and white mouths sending out puffs of steam and white arms pulling up handfuls of dirt and when yer looking out across the monastery grounds, all those white bodies working, well, they could be a herd of sheep, couldn't they?

Even tho if you look close you can see family groups and husbands and wives and fathers and sons. You can see older ones lifting smaller amounts more slowly. You can see younger ones helping 'em, trying to keep us from seeing that the older ones can't work too hard. You can see a baby strapped to its mother's chest with an old piece of cloth. You can see an especially tall one directing others along a faster work chain. You can see a small female packing mud around the infected number band of a larger female. You can see 'em working together, keeping their heads down, trying not to be the one who gets seen by me or Davy or the guards behind the barbed wire.

You can see all that if you look close.

But it's easier if you don't.

We can't give 'em shovels, of course. They could use 'em against us as weapons and the soldiers on the walls get twitchy if a Spackle even stretches its arms up too high. So there they all are, bending to the ground, digging, moving rocks, silent as clouds, suffering and not doing nothing about it.

I got a weapon, tho. They gave me the rifle back.

Cuz where am I gonna go?

Now that she's gone.

"Hurry it *up*!" I shout at the Spackle, my Noise rising red at the thought of her.

I catch Davy looking over at me, a surprised grin on his face. I turn away and cross the field to another group. I'm halfway there when I hear a louder click.

I look round till I find the source.

But it's only ever the same one.

1017, staring at me again, with that look that ain't forgiveness. He moves his eyes to my hands.

It's only then I realize I've got them both clenched hard around my rifle.

I can't even remember taking it off my shoulder.

* * *

Even with all this Spackle labour, it's still gonna take a coupla months to even come close to finishing this building, whatever it is, and by that time it'll be mid-winter and the Spackle won't have the shelter they were sposed to be building for themselves and I know they live outside more than men do but I don't think even they can live unsheltered in the winter frost and I ain't heard of nowhere else they're gonna be going yet.

Still, we had all the internal walls torn down in seven days, two ahead of schedule, and no Spackle even died, tho we did have a few with broken arms. Those Spackle were taken away by soldiers.

We ain't seen 'em since.

By the end of the second week after the tower bomb, we've nearly dug all the trenches and blocks for the foundayshuns to be poured, something Davy and I are sposed to supervize even tho it's gonna be the Spackle who know how to do it.

"Pa says they were the labour that rebuilt the city after the Spackle War," Davy says. "Tho you wouldn't know it from this bunch."

He spits out a shell from the seeds he's eating. Food's getting a bit scarce what with the Answer adding supply raids to the ongoing bombs but Davy always manages to scrounge up something. We're sitting on a pile of rocks, looking out over the one big field, now dug up with square holes and ditches and so full of rock piles there's barely any room for the Spackle to crowd into.

But they do, cramming onto the edges and huddling together in the cold. And they don't say nothing about it.

Davy spits out another shell. "You ever gonna talk again?"

"I talk," I say.

"No, you scream at yer workforce and you grunt at me. That ain't talking." He's spits out another shell, high and long, hitting the nearest Spackle in the head. It just brushes it away and keeps on digging out the last of a trench.

"She left ya," Davy says. "Get over it."

My Noise rises. "*Shut up*."

"I don't mean it in a bad way."

I turn to look at him, eyes wide.

"*What?*" he says. "I'm just saying, you know? She left, don't mean she's dead or nothing." Spit. "From what I remember, that filly can take plenty care of herself."

There's a memory in his Noise of being electrocuted on the river road. It should make me smile, but it don't, cuz she's standing right there in his Noise, standing right there and taking him down.

Standing right there and not standing right here.

(where'd she go?)

(where'd she effing *go*?)

Mayor Ledger told me just after the tower bombs that the army had gone straight for the ocean cuz they'd got a tip-off that that's where the Answer were hiding–

(was it me? did he hear it in me? I burn at the thought–)

But when Mr Hammar and his men got there, they didn't find nothing but long-abandoned buildings and half-sunken boats.

Cuz the informayshun turned out to be false.

And I burn at that, too.

(did she lie to me?)

(did she do it on purpose?)

"Jesus, pigpiss." Davy spits again. "It's not like any of the *rest* of us got girlfriends. They're all in ruddy *jail* or setting off bombs every week or walking around in groups so big you can't even talk to 'em."

"She ain't my girlfriend," I say.

"Not the point," he says. "All it means is that yer just as alone as the rest of us, so get over it."

There's a sudden, ugly strength of feeling in his Noise, which he wipes away in an instant when he sees me watching him. "What're you looking at?"

"Nothing," I say.

"Damn right." He stands, takes his rifle and stomps back into the field.

Somehow 1017 keeps ending up in my part of the work. I'm mainly in the back part of the fields, finishing up digging the trenches. Davy's near the front, getting Spackle to snap together the pre-formed guide walls we'll be using once the concrete gets poured. 1017's sposed to be doing that, but every time I look up, there he is, nearest me again no matter how many times I send him back.

He's working, sure, digging up his handfuls of dirt or piling up the sod in even rows, but always looking for me, always trying to catch my eye.

Clicking at me.

I walk towards him, my hand up on the stock of my rifle, grey clouds starting to move in overhead. "I sent you over to Davy," I bark. "What're you doing here?"

Davy, hearing his name, calls from far across the field. "What?"

I call back, "Why do you keep letting this one back over here?"

"What the hell are you talking about?" Davy yells. "They all look the same!"

"It's 1017!"

Davy gives an exaggerated shrug. "*So?*"

I hear a click, a rude and sarcastic one, from behind me.

I turn and I swear 1017 is *smiling* at me.

"You little piece of–" I start to say, reaching my rifle round my front.

Which is when I see a flash of Noise.

Coming from 1017.

Quick as anything but clear, too, me standing in front of him, reaching for my rifle, nothing more than what he's seeing with his eyes–

Except a flash as he grabs the rifle from me–

And then it's gone.

I've still got the rifle in my hands, 1017 still knee-deep in the ditch.

No Noise at all.

I look him up and down. He's skinnier than he used to be, but they *all* are, they never get quite enough fodder of a day, and I'm wondering if 1017's been skipping meals altogether.

So he don't take no cure.

"What're you playing at?" I ask him.

But he's back at work, arms and hands digging for more dirt, ribs showing thru the side of his white, white skin.

And he don't say nothing.

"Why do we keep giving 'em the cure if yer pa's taking it away from everyone else?"

Me and Davy are lunching the next day. The clouds are heavy in the sky and it'll probably start raining soon, the first rain in a good long while, and it'll be cold rain, too, but we've got orders to keep working no matter what so we're spending the day watching the Spackle pour out the first concrete from the mixer.

Ivan brought it in this morning, healed but limping, his Noise raging. I wonder where he thinks the power is *now*.

"Well, it keeps 'em from plotting, don't it?" Davy says. "Keeps 'em from passing along ideas to each other."

"But they can do that with the clicking." I think for a second. "Can't they?"

Davy just gives a *who cares, pigpiss* shrug. "Got any of that sandwich left?"

I hand him my sandwich, keeping an eye out over the Spackle. "Shouldn't we know what they're thinking?" I say. "Wouldn't that be a good thing to know?"

I look out over the field for 1017 who, sure enough, is looking back at me.

Plick. The first drop of rain hits me on the eyelash.

"Aw, crap," Davy says, looking up.

* * *

It don't let up for three days. The site gets muckier and muckier but the Mayor still wants us to keep on somehow so those three days are spent slipping and sliding thru mud and putting up huge tarpaulins on frames to cover big parts of the field.

Davy's got the inside work, bossing Spackle around to keep the tarpaulin frames in place. I spend most of my time out in the rain, trying to keep the edges of the tarpaulin pinned to the ground with heavy stones.

It's ruddy *stupid* work.

"Hurry up!" I shout to the Spackle helping me get one of the last edges pinned to the ground. My fingers are freezing cuz no one's given us gloves and there ain't been no Mayor round to ask. "Ow!" I put a bloodied knuckle up to my lips, having scraped my hand for the millionth time.

The Spackle keep at it with the rocks, seeming oblivious to the rain, which is good cuz there ain't room under the tarpaulins for all of 'em to shelter.

"Hey," I say, raising my voice. "Watch the edge! Watch that—"

A gust of wind rips away the whole sheet of tarpaulin we just pinned down. One of the Spackle keeps hold of it as it flies up, taking him with it and tumbling him hard down to the ground. I leap over him as I chase after the tarpaulin, twisting and rolling away across the muddy field and up a little slope, and I've just about got a hand on it—

And I slip badly, skidding right down the other side of the slope on my rump—

And I realize where I've run, where I've slipped—

I'm heading right down into the bog.

I grab at the mud to stop myself but there's nothing to hold on to and I drop right in with a *splat*.

"Gah!" I shout and try to stand. I'm up to my thighs in lime-covered Spackle shit, splattered all up my front and back, the stink of it making me retch–

And I see another flash of Noise.

Of me standing in the bog.

Of a Spackle standing right over me.

I look up.

There's a wall of Spackle staring.

And right in front of 'em all.

1017.

Above me.

With a huge stone in his hands.

He don't say nothing, just stands there with the stone, more'n big enough to do a lot of harm if thrown right.

"Yeah?" I say up to him. "That's what you want, ain't it?"

He just stares back.

I don't see the Noise again.

I reach up for my rifle, slowly.

"What's it gonna be?" I ask and he can see in my Noise just how ready I am, how ready I am to fight him.

How ready I am to–

I've got the rifle stock in my hand now.

But he's just staring at me.

And then he tosses the rock down on the ground and turns back towards the tarpaulin. I watch him go, five steps, then ten, and my body relaxes a bit.

It's when I'm pulling myself outta the bog that I hear it.

The click.

His rude click.

And I lose it.

I'm running towards him and I'm yelling but I don't know what I'm saying and Davy's turning round in shock as I reach the shelter of the tarpaulin just after 1017 and I'm running in with the rifle up above my head like I'm some stupid madman and 1017's turning to me but I don't give him a chance to do nothing and I knock him hard in the face with the butt of the rifle and he falls back on the ground and I lift the rifle again and bring it down and he raises his hands to protect himself and I hit him again and again and again—

In the hands—

And the face—

And in those skinny ribs—

And my Noise is raging—

And I hit—

And I hit—

And I hit—

And I'm screaming—

I'm screaming out—

"WHY DID YOU LEAVE?"

"WHY DID YOU LEAVE ME?"

And I hear the cold, crisp *snick* of his arm breaking.

*   *   *

It fills the air, louder than the rain or the wind, turning my stomach upside down, making a thick lump in my throat.

I stop, mid-swing.

Davy's staring at me, his mouth open.

All the Spackle are edging back, terrified.

And from the ground, 1017 is looking back up at me, red blood pouring from his weird nose and the corner of his too-high eyes but there's no sound coming from him, no Noise, no thoughts, no clicks, no nothing–

(and we're in the campsite and there's a dead Spackle on the ground and Viola's looking so scared and she's backing away from me and there's blood everywhere and I've done it again I've done it again and why did you go oh jesus dammit Viola why did you *leave*–)

And 1017 just looks at me.

And I swear to God, it's a look of triumph.

23

SOMETHING'S COMING

{VIOLA}

"WATER PUMP'S workin agin, Hildy."

"Thank you, Wilf." I hand him a tray of bread, the heat still coming off it. "Could you take these to Jane, please? She's setting the tables for breakfast."

He takes the tray, a flat little tune coming from his Noise. As he leaves the kitchen shack, I hear him call out, "Wife!"

"Why does he call you Hildy?" Lee says, appearing at the back door with a basket of flour he just pounded. He's wearing a sleeveless shirt and the skin up to his elbows is dusty white.

I look at his bare arms for a second and look away quickly.

Mistress Coyle put us to work together since he can't go back to New Prentisstown any more either.

No, I will certainly *not* forgive her.

"Hildy was the name of someone who helped us," I say. "Someone worth being called after."

269

And by us, you mean–"

"Me and Todd, yes." I take the basket of flour from him and thump it down heavily on the table.

There's a silence, as there always seems to be when Todd's name comes up.

"No one's seen him, Viola," Lee says gently. "But they mostly go in at night so that doesn't–"

"She wouldn't tell me even if she did." I start separating the flour into bowls. "She thinks he's dead."

Lee shifts from foot to foot out. "But you say different."

I look at him. He smiles and I can't help but smile back. "And you believe me, do you?"

He shrugs. "Wilf believes you. And you'd be surprised how far the word of Wilf goes around here."

"No." I look out the window to where Wilf disappeared. "No, actually I wouldn't."

That day passes like the others and still we cook. That's our new employment, Lee and me, cooking. All of it, for the entire camp. We've learned how to make bread from a starting point of *wheat*, not even flour. We've learned how to skin squirrels, de-shell turtles and gut fish. We've learned how much base you need for soup to feed a hundred. We've learned how to peel potatoes and pears faster than possibly anyone on this whole stupid planet.

Mistress Coyle swears this is how wars are won.

"This isn't really why I signed up," Lee says, pulling another handful of feathers off the sixteenth forest fowl of the afternoon.

"At least signing up was your idea," I say, fingers cramping on my own fowl. The feathers hover in the air like a swarm of sticky flies, catching everywhere they touch. I've got little green puffs under my fingernails, in the crooks of my elbows, glopped in the corner of my eyes.

I know this because Lee's got them all over his face, too, all through his long golden hair and in the matching golden hair on his forearms.

I feel my face flush again and pull out a furious rip of feathers.

A day turned into two, turned into three, turned into a week, turned into the week after and the week after that, cooking with Lee, washing up with Lee, sitting out three days of solid rain stuck in this shack with Lee.

And still. And *still*.

Something's coming, something's being prepared for, no one's telling me anything.

And I'm still stuck *here*.

Lee tosses a plucked fowl onto the table and picks up another one. "We're going to make this species extinct if we're not careful."

"It's the only thing Magnus can shoot," I say. "Everything else is too fast."

"A whole animal lost," Lee says, "because the Answer lacked for an optician."

I laugh, too loud. I roll my eyes at myself.

I finish my own fowl and pick up a new one. "I'm doing three of these for every two of yours," I say. "*And* I did more loaves this morning *and*–"

"You burnt half of them."

"...because *you* stoked the oven too hot!"

"I'm not made for cooking," he says, smiling. "I'm made for soldiering."

I gasp. "And you think *I'm* made for cooking–"

But he's laughing and keeps laughing even when I throw a handful of wet feathers at him, smacking him straight on the eye. "Ow," he says, wiping it away. "You got some aim, Viola. We really need to get a gun in your hands."

I turn my face quickly back down to the millionth fowl in my lap.

"Or maybe not," he says, more quietly.

"Have you–?" I stop.

"Have I what?"

I lick my lips, which is a mistake because then I have to spit out a mouthful of feathery puffs, so when I do finally say it, it comes out more exasperated than I meant. "Have you ever shot someone?"

"No." He sits up straighter. "Have you?"

I shake my head and see him relax, which makes me immediately say, "But I've *been* shot."

He sits back up. "No way!"

I say it before I mean to, before I even know it's coming, and then I'm saying it and I realize I've never said it, not out loud, not to myself, not ever, not since it happened, and yet here it is, tumbling out in a room full of floating feathers.

"And I've stabbed someone." I stop plucking. "To death."

My body feels suddenly twice as heavy in the silence that follows.

When I start to cry, Lee just hands me a kitchen towel and lets me, not crowding me or saying anything stupid or even asking about it, though he must be dying of curiosity. He just lets me cry.

Which is exactly right.

"Yes, but we're gaining sympathy," Lee says near the end of dinner with Wilf and Jane. I'm putting off finishing because as soon as I do, we have go back to the kitchens to start preparing the yeasts to cook *tomorrow's* bread. You wouldn't believe how much bloody bread a hundred people can eat.

I take half of my last bite. "I'm just saying there aren't very many of you."

"Of *us*," Lee says, looking at me seriously. "And we've got spies working throughout the city and people join us when they can. Things are only getting worse there. They're rationing *food* now and no one's getting the cure any more. They're going to have to start turning against him."

"And so many in prisons," Jane adds. "Hundreds of women, all locked up, all chained together underground, starving and dying by the dozen."

"Wife!" Wilf snaps.

"Ah'm only sayin what Ah heard!"

"Yoo din't hear nothin of the sort."

Jane looks sullen. "Don't mean it's not true."

"There are a lot of people who'd support us in prison, though," Lee says. "And so that might turn out—"

He stops.

"What?" I ask, looking up. "Turn out what?"

He doesn't answer me, just looks over to another table where Mistress Coyle is sitting with Mistresses Braithwaite, waggoner and Barker, and Thea, too, like they always do, discussing things, whispering in low voices, devising secret orders for other people to carry out.

"Nothing," Lee says, seeing Mistress Coyle stand and come towards us.

"I'm going to need the cart hitched up for tonight, Wilf, please," she says, approaching our table.

"Yes, Mistress," he says, getting to his feet.

"Eat a little longer," she says, stopping him. "This isn't forced labour."

"Ah'm happy to do it," Wilf says, brushing off his trousers and leaving us.

"Who are you blowing up tonight?" I ask.

Mistress Coyle pulls her lips tight. "I think that's enough for now, Viola."

"I want to come," I say. "If you're going back into the city tonight, I want to come with you."

"Patience, my girl," she says. "You'll have your day."

"Which day?" I ask as she walks off. "*When?*"

"Patience," she says again.

But she says it impatiently.

It gets dark earlier and earlier every day. I sit outside on a pile of rocks as night falls, watching tonight's mission-takers head on out to the carts, their bags packed with secret things. Some of the men have Noise now, taking reduced amounts of cure from our own dwindling supply stashed in the cave. They take enough to blend in with the city but not enough to give anything away. It's a tricky balance, and it's getting more and more dangerous for our men to be on city streets, but still they go.

And as the people of New Prentisstown sleep tonight, they'll be stolen from and bombed, all in the name of what's right.

"Hey," Lee says, hardly more than a shadow in the twilight as he sits down next to me.

"Hey," I say back.

"You okay?"

"Why wouldn't I be?"

"Yeah." He picks up a stone and tosses it into the night. "Why wouldn't you be?"

Stars start to appear in the sky. My ships are up there somewhere. People who might've been able to help us, no, who *would* have helped us if I could've contacted them. Simone Watkin and Bradley Tench, good people, *smart* people who would have stopped all this stupidity and the explosions and–

I feel my throat clench again.

"You really killed someone," Lee says, tossing another stone.

"Yeah," I say, pulling my knees up to my chest.

Lee waits a moment. "With Todd?"

"*For* Todd," I say. "To save him. To save *us*."

Now that the sun's gone, the real cold moves in swiftly. I hold my knees tighter.

"She's afraid of you, you know," he says. "Mistress Coyle. She thinks you're powerful."

I look over at him, trying to see him in the dark. "That's stupid."

I heard her say it to Mistress Braithwaite. Said you could lead whole armies if you put your mind to it."

I shake my head but of course he can't see. "She doesn't even know me."

"Yeah, but she's smart."

"And everyone here follows her like little lambs."

"Everyone but you." He bumps me with his shoulder in a friendly way. "Maybe that's what she's talking about."

We start to hear the low rumble from the caves that means the bats are readying themselves.

"Why are *you* here?" I ask. "Why do you follow her?"

I've asked before but he's always changed the subject.

But maybe tonight's different. It sure *feels* different.

"My father died in the Spackle War," he says.

"Lots of fathers did," I say and I think of Corinne, wondering where she is, wondering if–

"I don't really remember him," Lee's saying. "It was just me and my mother and my older sister growing up, really. And my sister–" he laughs. "You'd like her. All mouth and fire and we had some fights you wouldn't believe."

He laughs again but more quietly. "When the army came, Siobhan wanted to fight but Mum didn't. I wanted to fight, too, but Siobhan and Mum really went at it, Siobhan ready to take up arms and Mum practically having to bar the door to keep her from running out into the streets when the army came marching in."

The rumbling is getting louder and the bats' Noise starts to echo through the cave opening. **Fly, fly**, they say. **Away, away**.

"And then it was out of our hands, wasn't it?" he says.

"The army was here and that night they took all the women away to the houses east of town. Mum said to cooperate, you know, 'just for now, just to see where it goes, maybe he's not all that bad.' That sort of thing."

I don't respond and I'm glad it's dark so he can't see my face.

"But Siobhan wasn't going to go without a fight, was she? She shouted and screamed at the soldiers and refused to go along and Mum's just begging for her to stop, to not make them angry, but Siobhan–" He stops and makes a clicking sound with his tongue. "Siobhan punched the first soldier who tried to move her by force."

He takes a deep breath. "And then it was uproar. I tried to fight and the next thing I know I'm on the ground with my ears ringing and a soldier's knee in my back and Mum is screaming but there's nothing from Siobhan and I black out and when I wake up, I'm alone in my house."

Fly, fly, we hear, just inside the cave mouth. *Away, away, away.*

"I looked for them when the restrictions eased," he says, "but I never found them. I looked in every cabin and dormitory and at every house of healing. And finally, at the last one, Mistress Coyle answered."

He pauses and looks up. "Here they come."

The bats swarm out of the caves, like the world's been tipped on its side and they're being poured out over the top of us, a flood of greater darkness against the night sky. The sheer *whoosh* of them makes it impossible to talk for a minute so we just sit and watch them.

Each is at least two metres across, with furred wings and

277

short stubby ~~~~~ green glowing dot of phosphorus on each outstretched wingtip which they use somehow to confuse and stun the moths and bugs they eat. The dots glow in the night, making a blanket of temporary fluttering stars above us. We sit, surrounded by the slapping of wings, the cheeping of their Noise, the **fly fly away away away**.

And in five minutes they're gone, out into the surrounding forest, not to return until just before dawn.

"Something's coming," Lee says in the quiet that follows. "You know that. I can't say what but I'm going along because there's one more place to look for them."

"Then I'll go, too," I say.

"She won't let you." He turns to me. "But I promise you, I'll look for Todd. With the same eyes I look for Siobhan and my mother, I'll look for him."

A bell chimes out over the camp, signalling all raiding teams are off into town and all remaining people in camp are to go to bed. Lee and I sit in the dark for a while longer, his shoulder brushed up against mine, and mine brushed up against his.

24

PRISON WALLS

[TODD]

"NOT BAD," says the Mayor from atop Morpeth, "for an unskilled workforce."

"There'd be more," Davy says, "but it rained and then everything was just *mud*."

"No, no," the Mayor says, casting his eyes around the field. "You've done admirably, both of you, managing so much in just a month."

We all take a minute to look at what we've managed admirably. We've got all the concrete foundayshuns poured for a single long building. Every guide wall is up, some have even started to be filled in by the stones we took from the monastery's internal walls, and the tarpaulin makes a kind of roof. It already looks like a building.

He's right, we have done admirably.

Us and 1150 Spackle.

"Yes," says the Mayor. "Very pleasing."

Davy's Noise is taking on a pinkish glow that's

"So what is it?" I ask.

The Mayor looks my way. "What's what?"

"This." I gesture at the building. "What's it sposed to be?"

"You finish building it, Todd, and I promise to invite you to the grand opening."

"It's not for the Spackle, tho, is it?"

The Mayor frowns slightly. "No, Todd, it's not."

I rub the back of my neck with my hand and I can hear some clanking in Davy's Noise, clanks that are gonna get louder if he thinks I'm messing up his moment of praise. "It's just," I say, "there's been frost the past three nights and it's only getting colder."

The Mayor turns Morpeth to face me. **BOY COLT**, he thinks. **BOY COLT STEPS BACK**.

I step back without even thinking.

The Mayor's eyebrows raise. "Are you wanting heaters for your workforce?"

"Well," I look at the ground and at the building and at the Spackle who are doing their best to stay at the far end, as much away from the three of us as is possible to do when there are so many crowded into such a limited space. "Snow might come," I say. "I don't know that they'll survive."

"Oh, they're tougher than you think, Todd." The Mayor's voice is low and full of something I can't put my finger on. "A lot tougher."

I look down again. "Yeah," I say. "Okay."

"I'll have Private Farrow bring in some small fission heaters if that will make you feel better."

280

I blink. "Really?"

"*Really?*" Davy says.

"They've done good work," the Mayor says, "under your direction, and you've shown real dedication these past weeks, Todd. Real *leadership*."

He smiles, almost warmly.

"I know you're the kind of soul who hates to see others suffer." He keeps hold of my eye, almost daring me to break it. "Your tenderness does you credit."

"*Tenderness*," Davy snickers.

"I'm proud of you." The Mayor gathers up his reins. "*Both* of you. And you will be rewarded for your efforts."

Davy's Noise beams again as the Mayor rides outta the monastery gates. "Didja hear that?" he says, waggling his eyebrows. "Rewards, my tender pigpiss."

"Shut up, Davy." I'm already walking down the guide wall and towards the back of the building where there's the last of the clear ground and so that's where all the Spackle are having to crowd themselves. They get outta my way as I move thru them. "Heaters're coming," I say, putting it in my Noise, too. "Things'll be better."

But they just keep doing all they can not to touch me.

"I *said* things'll be better!"

Stupid ungrateful—

I stop. I take in a breath. I keep walking.

I get to the back of the building where we've leaned a few unused guide walls against the building frame, forming a nook. "You can come out now," I say.

and 1017 emerges, his arm in a sling made up from one of my few shirts. He's skinnier than ever, some redness still creeping up his arm from the break but it seems to be finally fading. "I managed to scrounge some painkillers," I say, taking 'em outta my pocket.

He snatches 'em from my hand with a slap, scratching my palm.

"Watch it," I say, thru clenched teeth. "You wanna be taken away to whatever they do with lame Spackle?"

There's a burst of Noise from him, one I've grown to expect, and it's the usual thing, him standing over me with a rifle, him hitting me and hitting me, me pleading for him to stop, him breaking *my* arm.

"Yeah," I say. "Whatever."

"Playing with yer pet?" Davy's come round, too, leaning against the building with his arms crossed. "You know, when horses break their legs, they shoot 'em."

"He ain't a horse."

"Nah," Davy says. "He's a sheep."

I puff out my lips. "Thanks for not telling yer pa."

Davy shrugs. "Whatever, pigpiss, as long as it don't screw up our reward."

1017 makes his rude clicking at both of us, but mostly at me.

"He don't seem too grateful, tho," Davy says.

"Yeah, well, I saved him twice now." I look at 1017, look right into eyes that never leave mine. "I ain't doing it again."

"You say that," Davy says, "but everyone knows you will." He nods at 1017. "Even him." Davy's eyes widen in a mock.

"It's cuz yer *tender*."

"Shut up."

But he's already laughing and leaving and 1017 just stares at me and stares at me.

And I stare back.

I saved him.

(I saved him for her)

(if she was here, she could see, see how I saved him)

(if she was here)

(but she ain't)

I clench my fists and then force myself to unclench them.

New Prentisstown has changed in the past month, I see it every day as we ride home.

Part of it's winter coming. The leaves on the trees have turned purple and red and dropped to the ground, leaving the tall winter skeletons behind them. The evergreens have kept their needles but dropped their cones and the reachers have pulled their branches tight into their trunks, leaving naked poles to sit out the cold. All of it plus the constant darker skies makes it look like the town's going hungry.

Which it is. The army invaded at the end of harvest, so there were food stocks, but there's no one left in the outer settlements to bring in food to trade and the Answer are keeping up their bombs and food raids. One night a whole storehouse of wheat was taken, so completely and successfully it's obvious now there's people in the town and the army who've been helping 'em.

The curfew got lowered two weeks ago and again last week till no one's allowed out after dark at all except for a few patrols. The square in front of the cathedral has become a place for bonfires, of books, of the wordly belongings of people found to have helped the Answer, of a bunch of healer uniforms from when the Mayor closed the last house of healing. And practically no one takes the cure no more, except some of the Mayor's closest men, Mr Morgan, Mr O'Hare, Mr Tate, Mr Hammar, men from old Prentisstown who've been with him for years. Loyalty, I guess.

Me and Davy ain't never been given it in the first place so there weren't never a chance for him to take it away.

"Maybe that's our reward," Davy says as we ride. "Maybe he'll get some outta the cellar and we'll finally see what it's like."

Our *reward*, I think. *We*.

I run my hand along Angharrad's flank, feeling the chill in her skin. "Almost home, girl," I whisper twixt her ears. "Nice warm barn."

Warm, she thinks. **Boy colt**.

"Angharrad," I say back.

Horses ain't pets and they're half-crazy all the time but I've been learning if you treat 'em right, they get to know you.

Boy colt, she thinks again and it's like I'm part of her herd.

"Maybe the reward is women!" Davy says suddenly. "Yeah! Maybe he's gonna give us some women and finally make a real man outta you."

"Shut up," I say, but it don't turn into a fight. Come to think of it, we ain't had a fight in a good long while.

We're just used to each other, I guess.

We don't hardly see women no more neither. When the communicayshuns tower fell, they were all confined to their houses again, except when teams of 'em are working the fields, readying for next year's planting, under guard from armed soldiers. The visits from husbands and sons and fathers are now once a week at most.

We hear stories about soldiers and women, stories about soldiers getting into dormitories at night, stories about awful things going on that no one gets punished for.

And that don't even count the women in the prisons, prisons I've only seen from the cathedral tower, a group of converted buildings in the far west of town down near the foot of the waterfalls. Who knows what goes on inside? They're way far away, outta sight of everyone 'cept for those that guard 'em.

Kinda like the Spackle.

"Jesus, Todd," Davy says, "the racket you make by *thinking* all the time."

Which is exactly the kinda thing I've learned to ignore from Davy. Except this time, he called me *Todd*.

We leave our horses in the barn near the cathedral. Davy walks me back to the cathedral, tho I don't really need a guard no more.

Cuz where would I go?

I go in the front door and I hear, "Todd?"

"Yes, sir?" I say.

"Always so polite," he smiles, walking towards me, boots clicking on the marble. "You seem better lately, calmer." He stops a metre away. "Have you been using the tool?"

Huh?

"What tool?" I ask.

He sighs a little. And then–

I AM THE CIRCLE AND THE CIRCLE IS ME.

I put a hand up to the side of my head. "How do you do that?"

"Noise can be used, Todd," he says. "If you're disciplined enough. And the first step is using the tool."

"I am the Circle and the Circle is me?"

"It's a way of centring yourself," he nods, "a way of aligning your Noise, of reining it in, *controlling* it, and a man who can control his Noise is a man with an advantage."

I remember him chanting away back in his house in old Prentisstown, how sharp and scary his Noise sounded compared to other men's, how much it felt like–

Like a weapon.

"What's the Circle?" I ask.

"Your destiny, Todd Hewitt. A circle is a closed system. There's no way of getting out, so it's easier if you don't fight it."

I AM THE CIRCLE AND THE CIRCLE IS ME.

But this time, my voice is in there, too.

"There's so much I look forward to teaching you," he says and leaves without saying good night.

*   *   *

I pace the walls of the bell tower, looking out towards the falls in the west, the hill with the notch on it in the south, and to the east, the hills that lead towards the monastery, tho you can't see it from here. All you can see is New Prentisstown, indoors and huddled together as a cold night settles in.

She's out there somewhere.

A month and she ain't come.

A month and–

(shut up)

(just effing shut up your effing whiny *mouth*)

I start pacing again.

We've got glass in the openings now and a heater to protect us from the autumn nights. More blankets, too, and a light and approved books for Mayor Ledger to read.

"Still a prison, though, isn't it?" he says behind me, mouth full. "You'd think he'd have at least found a better place for *you* by now."

"I sure wish everyone would stop thinking it's okay to read me all the damn time," I say, without turning around.

"He probably wants you out of the town," he says, finishing up his meal, which is just over half what we used to get. "Wants you away from all the rumours."

"What rumours?" I say, tho I'm barely interested.

"Oh, rumours of the great mind-control powers of our Mayor. Rumours of weapons made from Noise. Rumours he can fly, I don't doubt."

I don't look back at him and I keep my Noise quiet.

I am the Circle, I think.

And then I stop.

It's after midnight when the first one goes off.

Boom!

I jump a little on my mattress but that's all.

"Where do you think that was?" Mayor Ledger asks, also not rising from his bed.

"Sounded near east," I say, looking up into the dark of the tower bells. "Maybe a food store?"

We wait for the second. There's always a second now. As the soldiers rush to the first, the Answer take the chance for a second–

Boom!

"There it is," Mayor Ledger says, sitting up in bed and looking out of an opening. I get up, too.

"Damn," he says.

"What?" I say, moving next to him.

"I think that was the water plant down by the river."

"What does that mean?"

"It means we'll have to boil every stupid cup of–"

BOOM!

There's a huge flash that causes me and Mayor Ledger to flinch back from the window. The glass shakes in its frames.

And every light in New Prentisstown goes off.

"The power station," Mayor Ledger says, unbelieving. "But that's guarded every hour of the day. How could they possibly get to *that*?"

"I don't know," I say, my stomach sinking. "But there's gonna be hell to pay."

Mayor Ledger runs a tired hand over his face as we hear sirens and soldiers shouting down in the city below. He's shaking his head. "I don't know *what* they think they're accomp–"

BOOM!
BOOM!
BOOM!
BOOM!
BOOM!

Five huge explosions, one right after the other, shaking the tower so much that me and Mayor Ledger are thrown to the floor and a bunch of our windows shatter, busting inwards, covering us in shards and powdery glass.

We see the sky light up.

The sky to the west.

A cloud of fire and smoke shooting so high above the prisons it's like a giant's flinging it there.

Mayor Ledger is breathing heavy beside me.

"They've done it," he says, gasping. "They've really done it."

They've really done it, I think.

They've started their war.

And I can't help it–

I can't help but think it–

Is she coming for me?

25

THE NIGHT IT HAPPENS

{ VIOLA }

"I NEED YOUR HELP," Mistress Lawson says, standing in the doorway of the kitchen.

I hold up my hands, covered in flour. "I'm kind of in the middle of–"

"Mistress Coyle specifically asked me to fetch you."

I frown. I don't like the word *fetch*. "Then who's going to finish these loaves for tomorrow? Lee's out getting firewood–"

"Mistress Coyle said you had experience in medical supplies," Mistress Lawson interrupts. "We've brought a lot more in and the girl I have now is hopeless at sorting them out."

I sigh. It's better than cooking, at least.

I follow her out into the dusk, into the mouth of a cave and through a series of passages until we get to the large cavern where we keep our most valuable supplies.

"This might take a while," Mistress Lawson says.

We spend most of the evening and into the night counting just how many medicines, bandages, compresses, bed linens, ethers, tourniquets, diagnostic bands, blood pressure straps, stethoscopes, gowns, water purification tablets, splints, cotton swabs, clamps, Jeffers root pills, adhesives, and everything else we have, sorting them out into smaller piles and spreading them across the supply cavern, right up the lip of the main tunnel.

I wipe cold sweat from my forehead. "Shouldn't we be stacking these up already?"

"Not just yet," Mistress Lawson says. She looks around at the neat piles of everything we've done. She rubs her hands together, a worried frown creasing her face. "I hope it's enough."

"Enough for what?" I follow her with my eyes as she goes from pile to pile. "Enough for *what*, Mistress Lawson?"

She looks up at me, biting her lip. "How much of your healing do you remember?"

I stare at her for a second, suspicions rising and rising, then I take off running out of the cavern. "Wait!" she calls after me, but I'm already out into the central tunnel, running out of the main mouth of the cave and shooting into the camp.

Which is deserted.

"Don't be angry," Mistress Lawson says after I've searched every cabin.

I stand there, stupidly, hands on my hips, staring around at the empty camp. Having found a distraction for me, Mistress Coyle left, along with all the other mistresses except for Mistress Lawson. Thea and the apprentices are gone, too.

And everyone else. Every cart, horse and ox.

Wilf's gone, too, though Jane is here, the only other one who stayed behind.

Tonight's the night.

Tonight's the night it happens.

"You know why she couldn't take you," Mistress Lawson says.

"She doesn't trust me," I say. "None of you do."

"That's neither here nor there right now," she says, her voice taking on that stern mistress tone I've grown to hate. "What matters is that when they come back, we're going to need all the healing hands we can get."

I'm about to argue but I see how much she's still wringing her hands, how worried her face looks, how much is going on beneath the surface.

And then she says, "If any of them make it back at all."

There's nothing left to do but wait. Jane makes us coffee, and we sit in the increasing cold, watching the path out of the woods, watching to see who returns down it.

"Frost," Jane says, digging her toe across the small breath of ice frozen on a stone near her foot.

"We should have done it earlier," Mistress Lawson says into her cup, face over the rising steam. "We should have done it before the weather turned."

"Done *what*?" I ask.

"Rescue," Jane says simply. "Wilf tole me when he was leavin."

"Rescue of who?" I say, though of course it can only be–

We hear rocks fall on the path. We're already on our feet when Magnus comes barrelling over the hill. "Hurry!" he's shouting. "Come on!"

Mistress Lawson grabs some of the most urgent of the medical supplies and starts running after him up the path. Jane and I do the same.

We're halfway up when they start to come out of the forest.

On the backs of carts, across the shoulders of others, on stretchers, on horseback, with more people pouring down the path behind them and more cresting the hill behind *them*.

All the ones who needed rescuing.

The prisoners locked away by the Mayor and his army.

And the *state* of them–

"Oh, m'Gawd," Jane says, quietly, next to me, both of us stopped, stunned.

Oh, my God.

The next hours are a blur, as we rush to bring the wounded into camp, though some of them are hurt so bad we have to treat them where they are. I'm ordered from one healer to another and another, racing from wound to wound, running back for more supplies, going so fast it's only after a while that I start to realize that most of the wounds being treated aren't from fighting.

"They've been beaten," I say.

"And starved," Mistress Lawson says angrily, setting up a fluid injection into the arm of a woman we've carried into the cave. "And tortured."

The woman is just one of a growing number that threatens

293

never to stop. Most of them too shocked to speak, staring at you in the most horrible silence or keening at you without words, burn scars on their arms and faces, old wounds left untreated, the sunken eyes of women who haven't eaten for days and days and days.

"He did this," I say to myself. "He did this."

"Hold it together, my girl," Mistress Lawson says. We rush back outside, arms full of bandages that don't begin to cover what's needed. Mistress Braithwaite waves me over with a frantic hand. She tears the bandages from me, furiously wrapping up the leg of a woman screaming beneath her. "Jeffers root!" Mistress Braithwaite snaps.

"I didn't bring any," I say.

"Then bloody well get some!"

I go back to the cave, twisting around healers and apprentices and fake soldiers crouched over patients everywhere, up the hillsides, on backs of carts, everywhere. It's not just women injured either. I see male prisoners, also starved, also beaten. I see people from the camp wounded in the fighting, including Wilf with a burn bandage up the side of his face, though he's still helping carry patients on stretchers into the camp.

I run into the cave, grab more bandages and Jeffers root, and run back to the gully for the dozenth time. I cross the open ground and look up the path, where a few more people are still arriving.

I stop a second and check the new faces before running back to Mistress Braithwaite.

Mistress Coyle hasn't returned yet.

Neither has Lee.

*   *   *

"He was right in the thick of it," Mistress Nadari says, as I help her get a freshly-drugged woman to her feet. "Like he was looking for someone."

"His mother and sister," I say, taking the woman's weight against me.

"We didn't get everyone," Mistress Nadari says. "There was a whole other building where the bomb didn't go off–"

"Siobhan!" we hear someone shout in the distance.

I turn, my heart racing a lot faster and bigger than I expect, a smile breaking my cheeks. "He's found them!"

But you can see right away it's not true.

"Siobhan?" Lee is coming down the path from the forest, the arm and shoulder of his uniform blackened, his face covered in soot, his eyes looking everywhere, this way and that through all the people in the gully as he walks through them. "Mum?"

"Go," Mistress Nadari says to me. "See if he's hurt."

I let the woman lean onto Mistress Nadari and I run towards Lee, ignoring the other mistresses calling my name.

"Lee!" I call.

"Viola?" he says, seeing me. "Are they here? Do you know if they're here?"

"Are you hurt?" I reach him, taking the blackened sleeve and looking at his hands. "You're burned."

"There were fires," he says, and I look into his eyes. He's looking at me but he's not seeing me, he's seeing what he saw at the prisons, he's seeing the fires and what was behind them, he's seeing the prisoners they found, maybe he's seeing guards he had to kill.

He's not seeing his sister or his mother.

"Are they *here*?" he pleads. "Tell me they're here."

Lee stares at me, his mouth open, his breath heavy and raspy, like he's breathed in a lot of smoke. "It was..." he says. "Oh, God, Viola, it was..." He looks up and past me, over my shoulder. "I've got to find them. They've got to be here."

He steps past me and down the gully. "Siobhan? *Mum*?"

I can't help it and I call after him. "Lee? Did you see Todd?"

But he keeps on walking, stumbling away.

"Viola!" I hear and at first I think it's just another mistress calling for my help.

But then a voice beside me says, "Mistress Coyle!"

I turn and look up. At the top of the path is Mistress Coyle, on horseback, clopping down the rocks of the path as fast as she can make the horse go. She's got someone in the saddle behind her, someone tied to her to keep them from falling off. I feel a jolt of hope. Maybe it's Siobhan. Or Lee's mum.

(or him, maybe it's him, maybe–)

"Help us, Viola!" Mistress Coyle shouts, working the reins.

And as I start to run up the hill towards them, the horse turns to find its footing and I see who it is, unconscious and leaning badly.

Corinne.

"No," I keep saying, under my breath, hardly realizing it. "No, no, no, no, no," as we get her down onto a flat of rock and as Mistress Lawson runs towards us with armfuls of bandages and medicines. "No, no, no," as I take her head in my hands to cradle it from the hard rock and Mistress Coyle tears off Corinne's sleeve to prepare for injections. "No," as Mistress

Lawson reaches us and gasps as she sees who it is.

"You found her," Mistress Lawson says.

Mistress Coyle nods. "I found her."

I feel Corinne's skull under my hands, feel how the skin burns with fever. I see how sharp her cheeks look, how the bruising that discolours her eyes is against skin sagging and limp. And the collarbones that jut up from above the neckline of her torn and dirty mistress cloak. And the circles of burns against her neck. And the cuts on her forearms. And the tearing at her fingernails.

"Oh, Corinne," I whisper and wet from my eyes drops onto her forehead. "Oh, no."

"Stay with us, my girl," Mistress Coyle says, and I don't know whether she's talking to me or Corinne.

"Thea?" Mistress Lawson asks, not looking up.

Mistress Coyle shakes her head.

"Thea's dead?" I ask.

"And Mistress Waggoner," Mistress Coyle says, and I notice the smoke on her face, the red angry burns on her forehead. "And others." Her mouth draws thin. "But we got some of *them*, too."

"Come on, my girl," Mistress Lawson says to Corinne, still unconscious. "You were always the stubborn one. We need that now."

"Hold this," Mistress Coyle says, handing me a bag of fluid connected to a tube injected into Corinne's arm. I take it in one hand, keeping Corinne's head in my lap.

"Here it is," Mistress Lawson says, peeling away a strap of crusted cloth on Corinne's side. A terrible smell hits all of us at the same time.

It's worse than ~~I~~ ~~...~~ ~~...ing it stinks.~~ It's worse because of what it means.

"Gangrene," Mistress Coyle says pointlessly, because we can all see that it's way past infection. The smell means the tissue's dead. It means it's started to eat her alive. Something I wish I didn't remember that Corinne taught me herself.

"They didn't even give her basic bloody treatment," grunts Mistress Lawson, getting to her feet and running back towards the cave to get the heaviest medicines we've got.

"Come on, my difficult girl," Mistress Coyle says quietly, stroking Corinne's forehead.

"You stayed until you found her," I say. "That's why you were last."

"She'd never yield, this one," Mistress Coyle says, her voice rough and not just because of smoke. "No matter what they did to her."

We look down at Corinne's face, her eyes still closed, her mouth dropped open, her breath faltering.

Mistress Coyle's right. Corinne would never yield, would never give names or information, would take the punishment to keep other daughters, other mothers, from feeling it themselves.

"The infection," I say, my throat swelling. "The smell, it means–"

Mistress Coyle just bites her lips hard and shakes her head.

"Oh, Corinne," I say. "Oh, no."

And right there, right there in my hands, in my lap, her face turned up to mine–

She dies.

*　*　*

There's only silence when it happens. It isn't loud or struggled against or violent or anything at all. She just falls quiet, a
certain type of quiet you know is endless as soon as you hear
it, a quiet that muffles everything around it, turning off the
volume of the world.

The only thing I *can* hear, in fact, is my own breathing,
wet and heavy and like I'll never feel lightness again. And in
the silence of my breath I look down the hillside, I see the rest
of the wounded around us, their mouths open to cry out in
pain, their eyes blank with horrors still being seen even after
rescue. I see Mistress Lawson, running towards us with medicine, too late, too late. I see Lee, coming back up the path,
calling out for his mother and sister, not willing to believe yet
that in all this mess, they're still not here.

I think of the Mayor in his cathedral, making promises,
telling lies.

(I think of Todd in the Mayor's hands)

I look down at Corinne in my lap, Corinne who never liked
me, not ever, but who gave her life for mine anyway.

We are the choices we make.

When I look up at Mistress Coyle, the wet in my eyes
makes everything shine with pointed lights, makes the first
peek of the rising sun a smear across the sky.

But I can see her clearly enough.

My teeth are clenched, my voice thick as mud.

"I'm ready," I say. "I'll do anything you want."

26

THE ANSWER

"OH, GOD," Mayor Ledger keeps saying under his breath. "Oh, God."

"What're *you* so upset about?" I finally snap at him.

The door ain't unlocked at its usual time. Morning's come and gone with no sign of anyone remembering that we're here. Outside the city burns and ROARs but a sour part of me can't help thinking he's moaning cuz they're late with our breakfast.

"The surrender was supposed to bring *peace*," he says. "And that bloody woman has ruined *everything*."

I look at him strangely. "It's not like it's paradise here or nothing. There's curfews and prisons and–

But he's shaking his head. "Before she started her little *campaign,* the President was relaxing the laws. He was easing the restrictions. Things were going to be okay."

I stand and look out the windows to the west, where smoke still rises and fires still rage and the Noise of men don't show no sign of stopping.

"You've got to be *practical*," Mayor Ledger says, "even in the face of tyrants."

"Is that what you are then?" I say. "Practical?"

He narrows his eyes. "I don't know what you're getting at, *boy*."

I don't really know what I'm getting at neither but I'm frightened and I'm hungry and we're stuck in this stupid tower while the world falls to bits around us and we can *watch* it but we can't do nothing to *change* it and I don't know what Viola's part in all this is or *where* she is and I don't know where the future's heading and I don't know how any good can possibly come outta any of this but what I *do* know is that Mayor Ledger telling me how *practical* he's been is kinda pissing me off.

Oh, yeah, and one more thing.

"Don't you call me boy."

He takes a step towards me. "A man would understand that things are more complicated than just right or wrong."

"A man trying to save his own skin surely would." And my Noise is saying *Try it, come on, try it*.

Mayor Ledger clenches his fists. "What you don't know, Todd," he says, nostrils flaring. "What you don't know."

"*What* don't I know?" I say but then the door goes *ker-thunk*, making us both jump.

Davy comes busting in, rifles in hand. "Come on," he says, shoving one at me. "Pa wants us."

I go without another word, leaving Mayor Ledger shouting "Hey!" behind us as Davy locks the door.

* * *

"Fifty-six soldiers killed," Davy says as we trundle down the stairs on the inside of the tower. "We killed a dozen of 'em and captured a dozen more but they got away with almost two hundred prisoners."

"*Two hundred?*" I say, stopping for a second. "How many people were in prison?"

"Come on, pigpiss, Pa's waiting."

I run to catch up. We cross the lobby of the cathedral and head out the front door. "Those bitches," Davy's saying, shaking his head. "You wouldn't believe the things they're capable of. They blew up a bunkhouse. A *bunkhouse*! Where men were *sleeping!*"

We exit the cathedral to chaos in the square. Smoke is still blowing in from the west, making everything hazy. Soldiers, both by themselves and in squads, run this way and that, some of them pushing people before them, beating them with their rifles. Others are standing guard around groups of terrified-looking women and separate smaller groups of terrified-looking men.

"But we showed them, tho," Davy says, grimacing.

"You were there?"

"No." He looks down at his rifle. "But I will be next time."

"David!" we hear. "Todd!" The Mayor's riding towards us from across the square, moving so heavy and fast Morpeth's shoes are striking sparks from the bricks.

"Something's happened at the monastery," he's shouting. "Get there. *Now!*"

* * *

The chaos is city-wide. We see soldiers everywhere as we ride, herding townspeople before them, forcing them into bucket-lines to help put out the smaller fires from the first three bombs of last night, the ones that *did* take out the power stayshun, the water plant and a food store, all still burning cuz New Prentisstown's fire hoses are busy trying to put out the prisons.

"They won't know what hit 'em," Davy says as we ride, fast.

"Who won't?"

"The Answer and any man who helps them."

"There ain't gonna be no one *left*."

"There'll be us," Davy says, looking at me. "That'll be a start."

The road gets quieter as we get away from the city, till you can almost believe things are still normal, unless you look back and see the columns of smoke rising in the air. There ain't no one on the roads down this far and it starts to get so quiet it's like the world's ended.

We ride past the hill where the tower rubble lies but don't see no soldiers going up the path towards it. We turn the last corner and come round to the monastery.

And pull back hard on our reins.

"Holy shit," Davy says.

The whole front wall of the monastery has been blown open. There ain't any guards on the walls, just a gaping hole in the masonry where the gate used to be.

"Those bitches," Davy says. "They set them *free*."

(is this what she did?)

"Now we're gonna have to bloody fight them, *too*," Davy whines.

But I'm hopping off Angharrad, my stomach all funny and light. *Free*, I think. *They're free*.

(is this why she joined them?)

I feel so–

So *relieved*.

I pick up the pace as I near the opening, my hands gripping my rifle but I have a feeling I ain't gonna need it.

(ah, Viola, I knew I could count–)

Then I reach the opening and stop.

Everything stops.

My stomach falls right thru my feet.

"They all gone?" Davy says, coming up beside me.

Then he sees what I see.

"What the–?" Davy says.

The Spackle ain't all gone.

They're still here.

Every single one.

All 1150 of them.

Dead.

"I don't unnerstand this at all," Davy says, looking round.

"Shut up," I whisper.

The guide walls have all been knocked down till it's just a field again and bodies are piled everywhere, thrown on top of each another and tumbled across the grass, too, like someone tossed 'em away, males and females and children and babies, tossed away like they were trash.

Something's burning somewhere and white smoke twists thru the field, circling the piles, pushing at them with smoky fingers, finding nothing alive.

And the quiet.

No clicking, no shuffling, no *breathing*.

"I gotta tell Pa," Davy says, already turning back. "I gotta tell Pa."

And he's off back out the front, hopping on Deadfall and riding back up the road.

I don't follow.

My feet will only go forward, thru them all, my rifle dragging behind me.

The piles of bodies are higher than my head. I have to look up to see the dead faces flung back, the eyes still open, grassflies already picking at the bullet wounds in their heads. Looks like all of 'em were shot, most of 'em in the middle of their high foreheads, but some of the bodies look slashed, too, cut across the throat or the chest and I start to see ripped-off limbs and heads twisted all the way round and—

I drop my rifle to the grass. I barely even notice.

I keep walking, not blinking, mouth open, not believing what I'm seeing, not taking in the scale of it—

Cuz I have to step over bodies with arms flung out, arms with bands round 'em that *I* put there, twisted mouths that I fed, broken backs that I—

That I—

Oh, God.

I tried not to but I couldn't help it–

(no, I could–)

I think of all the times I cursed 'em–

All the times I imagined 'em as sheep–

(a knife in my hand, plunging down–)

But I didn't want *this*–

Never, I–

And I come round the biggest pile of bodies, stacked near the east wall–

And I see it.

And I fall to my knees in the frozen grass.

Written on the wall, tall as a man–

The *A*.

The *A* of the Answer.

Written in blue.

I lean my head forward slowly till it's touching the ground, the cold sinking into my skull.

(no)

(no, it can't be her)

(it *can't* be)

My breath comes up around me as steam, melting a little spot of mud. I don't move.

(have they done this to you?)

(have they changed you?)

(Viola?)

(*Viola?*)

The blackness starts to overwhelm me, starts to fall over me like a blanket, like water rising above my head, no Viola no, it can't be you, it can't be you (can it?) no no no it can't–

No–

No–

And I sit up–

And I lean back–

And I strike myself in the face.

I punch myself hard.

Again.

And again.

Not feeling nothing as I hit.

As my lips crack open.

As my eyes swell.

No–

God no–

Please–

And I reach back to punch myself again–

But I switch off–

I feel it go cold inside me–

Deep down inside–

(where are you to save me?)

I switch off.

I go numb.

I look at the Spackle, dead, everywhere dead.

And Viola gone–

Gone in ways that I can't even say–

(you did *this*?)

And inside I just *die*.

And a body tumbles from the pile, knocking right into me.

I scoot back fast, rolling over other bodies, scrambling to my feet, wiping my hands on my trousers, wiping the dead away.

And then another body falls.

I look up at the pile.

1017 is working his way out.

He sees me and freezes, his head and arms sticking out from the rest of the bodies, bones showing thru his skin, thin as the dead.

Course he survived. *Course* he did. If any of 'em is spiteful enough to find a way to live, it's him.

I run to the pile and I start pulling on his shoulders to get him out, to get him out from under the dead, all the dead.

We fall back as he pops free, tumbling to the ground, rolling apart and then staring at each other across the ground.

Our breaths are heavy, clouds of steam huffing into the air.

He don't look injured, tho the sling's gone from his arm. He's just staring, eyes probably open as wide as mine.

"Yer alive," I say stupidly. "Yer alive."

He just stares back, no Noise this time, no clicking, nothing. Just the silence of us in the morning, the smoke sneaking thru the air like a vine.

"How?" I say. "How did–?"

But there ain't no answer from him, just staring and staring.

"Did you–?" I say, then I have to clear my throat. "Did you see a girl?"

And then I hear, *Thump budda-thump–*

Hoofbeats down the road. Davy musta caught his pa coming the other way.

I look hard at 1017.

"Run," I say. "You gotta get outta here."

Thump budda-thump–

"Please," I whisper. "Please, I'm so sorry, I'm *so* sorry, but please, just run, just run, just get outta here–"

I stop cuz he's getting to his feet. He's still eyeing me, not blinking, his face almost dead of expresshun.

Thump budda-THUMP–

He takes one step away, then two, then faster, heading for the blown open gate.

And then he stops and looks back.

Looks back at me.

A clear flash of Noise coming right at me.

Of me, alone.

Of 1017 with a gun.

Of him pulling the trigger.

Of me dying at his feet.

Then he turns and runs out the gate and into the woods beyond.

"I know how hard this must be for you, Todd," says the Mayor, looking at the blown out gate. We've come outside. No one wanted to see the bodies any more.

"But *why*?" I say, trying to keep the tightness outta my voice. "Why would they do it?"

The Mayor looks at the blood on my face from where I hit myself but he don't say nothing about it. "They thought we would have used them as soldiers, I expect."

"But to kill them *all*?" I look up at him on his horse. "The Answer never killed no one before except by accident."

"Fifty-six soldiers," Davy says.

"Seventy-five," the Mayor corrects. "And three hundred escaped prisoners."

"They tried to bomb us here before, remember?" Davy adds. "The bitches."

"The Answer have stepped up their campaign," the Mayor says, looking mainly at me. "And we will respond in kind."

"Damn right, we will," Davy says, cocking his rifle for no reason.

"I'm sorry about Viola," the Mayor says to me. "I'm as disappointed as you are that she's a part of this."

"We don't know that," I whisper.

(is she?)

(are you?)

"Regardless," the Mayor says. "The time for your boyhood is well and truly past. I need leaders now. I need *you* to be a leader. Are you ready to lead, Todd Hewitt?"

"*I'm* ready," Davy says, his Noise feeling like it's being left out.

"I already know I can count on you, son."

And there's the pink Noise again.

"It's Todd I need to hear from." He comes a bit closer to me. "You're no longer my prisoner, Todd Hewitt. We're beyond that now. But I need to know if you'll join *me*–" he nods his head towards the opening in the wall "– or them. There is no other choice."

I look into the monastery, at all those bodies, all those shocked and dead faces, all that pointless end.

"Will you help me, Todd?"

"Help you how?" I say to the ground.

But he just asks it again. "Will you help me?"

I think of 1017, alone now, alone in the entire world.

His friends, his family for all I know, piled like rubbish, left for the flies.

I can't stop seeing it, even when I close my eyes.

I can't stop seeing that bright blue *A*.

Oh don't deceive me, I think.

Oh never leave me.

(but she's gone)

(she's gone)

And I'm dead.

Inside, I'm dead dead dead.

There ain't nothing left.

"I will," I say. "I'll help."

"Excellent," the Mayor says, with feeling. "I knew you'd be special, Todd. I've known it all along."

Davy's Noise squeaks at this but the Mayor ignores it.

He turns M̶o̶r̶p̶e̶t̶h̶ ̶t̶o̶ ̶f̶a̶c̶e̶ ̶t̶h̶e̶ killing grounds of the monastery.

"As to how you'll help me," he says. "Well, we have met the Answer, have we not?" He turns back to look at us, his eyes glinting. "It is time for them to meet the Ask."

PART V

THE OFFICE OF THE ASK

27

THE WAY WE LIVE NOW

[TODD]

"DON'T LET THIS period of quiet fool you," says the Mayor, standing atop the platform, voice booming thru the square from speakers set at every corner, extra loud to be heard above the **ROAR**. The people of New Prentisstown stare up at him in the cold morning, the men gathered in front of the platform, surrounded by the army, with the women back on the side streets.

Here we all are again.

Davy and I are behind the platform on our horses, directly behind the Mayor.

Kinda like an honour guard.

Wearing our new uniforms.

I think, *I am the Circle and the Circle is me*.

Cuz when I think it, I don't gotta think about nothing else at all.

"Even now our enemies move against us. Even now they plot our destruction. Even now we have reason to believe an

The Mayor takes a long sweeping look across the crowd. It's easy to forget how many people are still here, still working, still trying to eat, still getting on with their daily lives. They're tired-looking, hungry, many of 'em dirty, but still staring, still listening.

"The Answer could strike in any place, at any time, against any*one*," he says, tho the Answer ain't done no such thing, not for almost a month now. The prison break was the last we heard from 'em before they disappeared into the wild, the soldiers who woulda chased 'em killed while sleeping in their bunkers.

But that just means they're out there, gloating on their victory and planning the next.

"Three hundred escaped prisoners," the Mayor says. "Almost two hundred soldiers and civilians dead."

"Up they go again," Davy mutters under his breath, talking about the numbers. "Next time he gives this speech, the whole *city'll* be dead." He looks to me to see if I'll laugh. I don't. I don't even look at him. "Yeah, whatever," he says, turning back.

"And not to mention the genocide," says the Mayor.

The crowd murmurs at this and the **ROAR** gets a bit louder and redder.

"The very same Spackle who served in your homes so peacefully for the past decade, the ones we had all grown to admire for their pluck under duress, the ones we had come to regard as our partners on New World."

He pauses again. "All dead, all gone."

The crowd **ROAR**s some more. The deaths of the Spackle

really did affect the people, even more than the deaths of the soldiers or the townspeople caught up in the attack. Men even started joining the army again. Then the Mayor let some of the women who remained in prison out, some of 'em even back with their families and not even in dormitories. He upped everyone's food rashuns, too.

And he started holding these rallies. Explaining things.

"The Answer says it fights for freedom. But are these the people in whom you put your faith for salvation? The ones who would kill an entire *unarmed* population?"

I feel a choke rising and I make my Noise empty space, make it a wasteland, thinking nothing, *feeling* nothing, except–

I am the Circle and the Circle is me.

"I know these past weeks have been difficult. The food and water shortages, the necessary curfews, the power cuts, especially during the cold nights. I applaud your forti- tude. The only way we're going to get thru this is by pulling together against those who would destroy us."

And people have pulled together, ain't they? They obey the curfew and take their assigned amounts of water and food without fuss and stay inside when they're sposed to and turn off their lights after a certain hour and generally keep getting on with things even as it gets colder. You ride thru the town, you even see stores open, big lines of people outside 'em, waiting to get what they need.

Their eyes looking at the ground, waiting it out.

At night, Mayor Ledger tells me the townsfolk still grumble against Mayor Prentiss, but now there's even louder grumbles against the Answer, for blowing up the water plant,

317

for blowing up the ~~power system~~, and specially for killing all the Spackle.

Better the devil you know, Mayor Ledger says.

We're still up in that tower, me and Mayor Ledger, for some reason best known to Mayor Prentiss, but I got a key now and I lock him in when I ain't there. He don't like it but what's he gonna do?

Better the devil you know.

I wonder why the only choice is twixt two devils, tho.

"I also want to express my thanks," says the Mayor to the people, "for your continued help in coming forward with information. It is only eternal vigilance that will lead us into the light. Let your neighbour know he is watched. Only then are we truly safe."

"How long is this gonna go *on*?" Davy says, accidentally spurring Deadfall/Acorn, who has to be reined back when he steps forward. "I'm effing freezing over here."

Angharrad moves from foot to foot below me. **Go?** her Noise asks, her breath heavy and white in the cold. "Almost," I say, rubbing my hand against her flank.

"Effective tonight," says the Mayor, "curfew is pushed back by two hours and visiting times for wives and mothers is extended by thirty minutes."

There's some nodding in the crowd of men, some relieved crying from the crowd of women.

They're grateful, I think. *Grateful* to the Mayor.

Ain't that something.

"Finally," says the Mayor. "It is my pleasure to announce that building work has been completed on a new Ministry, one that will keep us safe from the threat of the Answer, a building where no secret may be kept, where anyone who tries to undermine our way of life will be re-educated into understanding our ideals, where our future will be secured against those who would steal it from us."

The Mayor pauses, to give his words maximum impact.

"Today we launch the Office of the Ask."

Davy catches my eye and taps the sharp, silver *A* sewn on the shoulders of our new uniforms, the *A* that the Mayor picked special cuz it's got all kinda associashuns, don't it?

Me and Davy are now Officers of the Ask.

I don't share his excitement.

But that's cuz I don't feel nothing much at all no more.

I am the Circle and the Circle is me.

"Good speech, Pa," Davy says. "Long."

"It wasn't for you, David," the Mayor says, not looking at him.

The three of us are riding down the road to the monastery.

Tho it ain't the monastery no more.

"Everything *is* ready, I trust?" the Mayor says, barely turning his head. "I'd hate to be made a liar of."

"It ain't gonna get less ready if you keep asking," Davy mumbles.

The Mayor turns to him, a deep frown on his face, but I speak before anyone gets slapped with Noise.

"It's as ready as it can be," I say, my voice flat. "The walls and roof are up but the inside–"

"No need to sound so morose, Todd," the Mayor says.

319

that's all that's important. They can look at the outside and they can tremble."

He's got his back to us now, riding on ahead, but I can *feel* him smile at *they can tremble*.

"Are we gonna have a part in it?" Davy asks, Noise still stormy. "Or are you just gonna find a way for us to be babysitters again?"

The Mayor turns Morpeth in the road, blocking our way. "Do you ever hear Todd complain this much?" he asks.

"No," Davy says, sullen. "But he's just, you know, *Todd*."

The Mayor raises his eyebrows. "And?"

"And I'm yer *son*."

The Mayor walks Morpeth towards us, making Angharrad step back. **Submit**, Morpeth says. **Lead**, Angharrad says in answer, lowering her head. I stroke her mane, untangling a bit with my fingers, trying to calm her down.

"Let me tell you something interesting, David," the Mayor says, looking hard at him. "The officers, the army, the townspeople, they see the two of you riding together, in your new uniforms, with all your new authority, and they know that *one* of you is my son." He's almost side on to Davy now, pushing him back down the road. "And as they watch you ride by, as they watch you go about your business, do you know? They often guess wrong. They often guess wrong as to which one of you is my own flesh and blood."

The Mayor looks over to me. "They see Todd with his devotion to duty, with his modest brow and his serious face, with his calm exterior and mature handling of his Noise, and they never even consider that his loud, sloppy, *insolent* friend is the one who's actually my son."

Davy's looking at the ground, his teeth clenched, his Noise boiling. "He don't even *look* like you."

"I know," says the Mayor, turning Morpeth back down the road. "I just thought it was interesting. How often it happens."

We keep on riding, Davy in a silent, red storm of Noise, lagging behind. I keep Angharrad in the middle with the Mayor clopping on ahead.

"Good girl," I murmur to her.

BQy cๆlt, she says back, and then she thinks **Tๆdd**.

"Yeah, girl," I whisper twixt her ears. "I'm here."

I've taken to hanging round her stables at the end of the day, taken to unsaddling her myself and brushing her mane and bringing her apples to eat. The only thing she needs from me is assurance that I'm there, proof I haven't left the herd, and as long as that's true, she's happy and she calls me **Tๆdd** and I don't have to explain myself to her and I don't have to ask her nothing and she don't need nothing from me.

Except that I don't leave her.

Except that I don't never *leave*.

My Noise starts getting cloudy and I think it again, *I am the Circle and the Circle is me.*

The Mayor looks back at me. And he smiles.

* * *

Even the _____ _____, we ain't in the army, the Mayor was particular about that. We don't got ranks except Officer but the uniform and the **A** on its sleeve is enough to keep people outta our way as we ride towards the monastery.

Our job till now has been guarding the men and women who're still in prison, tho it's mostly women. After the prisons were busted into and burnt down, the prisoners left over were moved to a former house of healing down by the river.

Guess which one?

For the past month, Davy and I've been escorting work crews of prisoners back and forth from the house of healing to the monastery to finish the work the Spackle started, women and men working faster than Spackle, I guess. The Mayor didn't ask us to supervise the building this time, something I'm grateful for.

When everyone's in for the night back at the house of healing, Davy and I ain't got much to do except ride our horses round the building, doing what we can so as not to hear the screams coming from inside.

Some of the ones still in prison, see, are from the Answer, the ones the Mayor caught the night of the prison break. We don't never see them, they don't get sent out with the work parties, they just get Asked all day long till they answer with something. So far, all the Mayor's got from 'em is the locayshun of a camp around a mine, which was deserted by the time the soldiers got there. Anything else useful is slow in coming.

There are others in there, too, found guilty of helping the Answer or whatever, but the ones who said they saw the Answer kill the Spackle and saw women writing the **A** on the wall, those prisoners are the ones who've been set free and sent back to their families. Even tho there ain't really no way they coulda been there to see it.

The others, well, the others keep being Asked till they answer.

Davy talks loud to cover the sounds we hear while the Asking's going on inside, trying to pretend it don't bother him when any fool could see it does.

I just keep myself in myself, closing my eyes, waiting for the screaming to stop.

I have an easier time than Davy.

Cuz like I say, I don't feel nothing much, not no more.

I am the Circle and the Circle is me.

But today, everything's sposed to change. Today, the new building is ready, or ready enough, and Davy and I are gonna guard it instead of the house of healing, while sposedly learning the business of Asking.

Fine. It don't matter.

Nothing matters.

"The Office of the Ask," the Mayor says as we round the final corner.

The front wall of the monastery has been rebuilt and you can see the new building sticking over the top, a big stone block that looks like it'd happily knock yer brains out if you stood too close. And on the newly built gate, there's a great, shiny silver **A** to match the ones on our uniforms.

There are guards in army uniforms on either side of the door. One of them is Ivan, still a Private, still sour-faced as anything, tries to catch my eye as I ride up, his Noise clanging loud with things he don't want the Mayor to hear, I reckon.

I ignore him. So does the Mayor.

"Now we find out when the real war begins," the Mayor says.

The gate opens and out walks the man in charge of all the Asking, the man charged with finding out where the Answer are hiding and how best to track them down.

Our newly promoted boss.

"Mr President," he says.

"Captain Hammar," says the Mayor.

28

SOLDIER

{VIOLA}

"QUIET," Mistress Coyle says, a finger to her lips.

The wind has died and you can hear our footsteps snapping the twigs on the ground at the foot of the trees. We stop, ears open for the sounds of soldiers marching.

Nothing.

More nothing.

Mistress Coyle nods and continues moving down the hill and through the trees. I follow her. It's just the two of us.

Me and her and the bomb strapped to my back.

The rescue saved 132 prisoners. 29 of them died either on the way to or back in the camp. Corinne was number 30. There are others unrescued, like poor old Mrs Fox, whose fates I'm probably never going to know. But Mistress Coyle estimates we killed at least twenty of their soldiers. Miraculously, only six members of the Answer on the original raid were killed,

captured and there was no possibility they wouldn't be tortured for information about where the Answer was hiding.

So we moved. In a hurry.

Even before many of the injured could walk for themselves, we loaded up supplies and weapons, anything and everything we could carry on carts, horses, the backs of the able-bodied, and we fled into the woods, keeping moving all through the night, the next day, and the night after that until we came to a lake at the base of a rock cliff, where at least we might have water and some shelter.

"It'll do," Mistress Coyle said.

We pitched camp along the shore.

And then we began our preparations for war.

She makes a movement with the palm of her hand and I instantly duck below some shrubs. We've reached a narrow drive up from the main road and I can hear a troop of soldiers Noisily moving away from us in the distance.

Our own supply of cure is getting lower by the day, and Mistress Coyle has set up a rationing system, but since the raid, it's too dangerous for any man, with or without Noise, to go into town anyway, which means they can no longer ferry us in hidden compartments to easy targets. We have to take a cart to a certain point outside of town and walk the rest of the way.

Escaping will be more difficult, so we'll just have to be more careful.

"Okay," Mistress Coyle whispers.

I stand. The moons are our only light.

We cross the road, keeping low.

After we moved to the lake, after the rescue of all those people, after the death of Corinne–

After I joined the Answer–

I began to learn things.

"Basic training," Mistress Coyle called it. Led by Mistress Braithwaite and done not only for me but for every patient who improved enough to join in, which was most of them, more than you'd think, we were taught how to load a rifle and fire it, basics of infiltration, night-time manoeuvres, tracking, hand communications, code words.

How to wire and set a bomb.

"How do you know how to do this?" I asked one night at dinner, my body weary and aching from the running and diving and carrying we'd done all throughout the day. "You're healers. How do you know how–"

"To run an army?" Mistress Coyle said. "You forget about the Spackle War."

"We were our own division," Mistress Forth said, down the table, snuffling up some broth.

The mistresses talked to me, now that they could see how hard I was training.

"We weren't very popular," giggled Mistress Lawson, across from her.

"We didn't like how some of the generals were waging the war," Mistress Coyle said to me. "We thought an underground approach would be more effective."

"And si— ——— ——n't have Noise," said Mistress Nadari, down the table, "we could sneak into places, couldn't we?"

"The men in charge didn't think we were the answer to their problem, though," Mistress Lawson said, still giggling.

"Hence the name," Mistress Coyle said.

"And when the new government was formed and the city rebuilt, well," Mistress Forth said, "it wouldn't have been sensible not to keep important materials available should the need ever arise."

"The explosives in the mine," I said, realizing. "You hid them there years ago."

"And what a good decision it turned out to be," Mistress Lawson said. "Nicola Coyle always was a woman of fore-sight."

I blinked at the name Nicola, as if it was hardly possible that Mistress Coyle had a first name.

"Yes, well," said Mistress Coyle. "Men are creatures of war. It's only prudent to remember that."

Our target is deserted, as we expect it to be. It's small, but symbolic, a well above a tract of farmland east of the city. The well and the apparatus above it only bring water for the field below, not any huge system or set of buildings. But if the city goes on allowing the Mayor to imprison, torture and kill, then the city won't eat.

It's also a good way away from the city centre, so no chance of me seeing Todd.

Which I won't argue about. For now.

We've come up the cut-off road, keeping to the ditch

beside it, holding our breaths as we move past the sleeping farmhouse, a light still on in the upper floor but it's so late it can only be for security.

Mistress Coyle makes another hand signal and I move past her, ducking under a wire carriage of laundry, hung outside to dry. I trip on a child's toy scooter but manage to keep my balance.

The bomb's supposed to be safe, supposed to be impervious to any kind of jostling or shaking.

But.

I let out a breath and keep on towards the well.

Even in the weeks when we hid, when we didn't approach the city at all, the weeks where we laid low and kept quiet, training and preparing, even then a few escapees from the city found us.

"They're saying *what*?" Mistress Coyle said.

"That you killed all the Spackle," the woman said, pressing the poultice against her bleeding nose.

"Wait," I said. "*All* the Spackle are dead?"

The woman nodded.

"And they're saying we did it," Mistress Coyle repeated.

"Why would they say that?" I asked.

Mistress Coyle stood and looked out across the lake. "Turn the city against us. Make us look like the bad guys."

"That's exactly what he's saying," the woman said. I found her on a training run through the woods. She'd tripped down a rocky embankment, managing to break only her nose. "There's rallies every other day," she said. "People are listening."

I looked up at her. "You didn't do it, did you? You didn't kill them?"

Her face could've lit a match. "Exactly what sort of people do you think we are, my girl?"

I kept her gaze. "Well, I don't know, do I? You blew up a bunker. You killed soldiers."

But she just shook her head, though I didn't know if that was an answer.

"You're sure you weren't followed?" she asked the woman.

"I was wandering in the woods for three days," she said. "I didn't even find you." She pointed at me. "*She* found *me*."

"Yes," Mistress Coyle said, eyeing me. "Viola's useful that way."

There's a problem at the well.

"It's too close to the house," I whisper.

"It's not," Mistress Coyle whispers back, going behind me and unzipping my pack.

"Are you sure?" I say. "The bombs you blew up the tower with were—"

"There are bombs and there are bombs." She makes a few adjustments to the contents of my pack, then turns me around to face her. "Are you ready?"

I look over to the house, where anyone could be sleeping inside, women, innocent men, children. I won't kill anyone, not unless I have to. If I'm doing this for Todd and Corinne, well, then. "Are you sure?" I ask.

"Either you trust me, Viola, or you do not." She tilts her head. "Which will it be?"

The breeze has picked up again and it blows a bit of the sleeping Noise of New Prentisstown down the road. One indefinable, snuffling, snoring ROAR, almost quiet, if such a thing could be.

Todd somewhere in it all.

(not dead, no matter what she says)

"Let's get this done," I say, taking off the pack.

The rescue wasn't a rescue for Lee. His sister and his mother weren't among the prisoners saved or the prisoners who died. It's possible they were in the one prison the Answer didn't manage to break.

But.

"Even if they're dead," he said, one night as we sat on the shore of the lake, throwing in stones, aching again after yet another long day's training. "I just want to know."

I shook my head. "If you don't know, then there's still a chance."

"Knowing or not knowing doesn't keep them alive." He sat down, close to me again. "I think they're dead. I *feel* like they're dead."

"Lee–"

"I'm going to kill him." His voice was that of a man making a promise, not a threat. "If I get close enough, I swear to you."

The moons rose over us, making two more of themselves in the surface of the lake. I threw in another stone, watching it skip across the moons' reflections. The camp gave a low bustle in the ~~tree~~ ~~behind us~~ and up the bank. You could hear Noise here and there, including a growing buzz from Lee, not lucky enough to qualify for Mistress Coyle's ration.

"It's not what you think it's going to be like," I said quietly.

"Killing someone?"

I nodded. "Even if it's someone who deserves it, someone who will kill you if you don't kill them, even then it's not what you think."

There was more silence, until he finally said. "I know."

I looked over at him. "You killed a soldier."

He didn't answer, which was its own answer.

"Lee?" I said. "Why didn't you tell–?"

"Because it's not what you think it's going to be like, is it?" he said. "Even if it's someone who deserves it."

He threw another stone into the lake. We weren't resting our shoulders on each other. We were a space apart.

"I'm still going to kill him," he said.

I peel off the backing paper and press the bomb into the side of the well, sticking it there with a glue made from tree sap. I take two wires out of my pack and twist the ends on two more wires already sticking out of the bomb, hooking two together and leaving one end dangling.

The bomb is now armed.

I take a small green number pad from the front pocket of my pack and twist the end of the dangling wire around a point at the end of the pad. I press a red button on the pad and then a grey one. The green numbers light up.

The bomb is now ready for timing.

I click a silver button until the digits count up to 30:00. I press the red button again, flip over the green pad, slide one metal flap into another, then press the grey button one more time. The green numbers immediately change to 29:59, 29:58, 29:57.

The bomb is now live.

"Nicely done," Mistress Coyle whispers. "Time to go."

And then after almost a month of hiding in the forest, waiting for the prisoners to recuperate, waiting for the rest of us to train, waiting for a real army to have life breathed into it, there came a night when that waiting was over.

"Get up, my girl," Mistress Coyle said, kneeling at the foot of my cot.

I blinked myself awake. It was still pitch black. Mistress Coyle's voice was low so as not to wake the others in the long tent.

"Why?" I whispered back.

"You said you'd do anything."

I got up and went out into the cold, hopping to get my boots on while Mistress Coyle readied a pack for me to wear.

"We're going into town, aren't we?" I said, tying my laces.

"She's a genius, this one," Mistress Coyle muttered into the pack.

"Why tonight? Why now?"

She looked up at me. "Because we need to remind them that we're still here."

* * *

against my back. We cross the yard and sidle up to the house, stopping to listen for anyone stirring.

No one does.

I'm ready to go but Mistress Coyle is leaning back from the outer wall of the house, looking at the white expanse of it.

"This should do fine," she says.

"For what?" I look around us, spooked now that there's a timer running.

"Have you forgotten who we are?" She reaches into a pocket of her long healer's skirt, still worn even though trousers are so much more practical. She pulls out something and tosses it to me. I catch it without even thinking.

"Why don't you do the honours?" she says.

I look in my hand. It's a crumbling piece of blue charcoal, pulled from our wood fires, the remains of the reacher trees we burn to keep warm. It smears dusty blue across my hand, across my skin.

I look at it for a moment longer.

"Tick tock," says Mistress Coyle.

I swallow. Then I raise the charcoal and make three quick slashes against the white wall of the house.

A, looking back at me, by my hand.

I find myself breathing heavily.

When I look round, Mistress Coyle's already off down the ditches of the drive. I hurry after her, keeping my head low.

Twenty-eight minutes later, just as we reach our cart, deep in the woods, we hear the *Boom*.

"Congratulations, soldier," Mistress Coyle says, as we set off back to camp. "You have just fired the first shot of the final battle."

29

THE BUSINESS OF ASKING

[TODD]

THE WOMAN IS STRAPPED against a metal frame, her arms out behind her and up, each tied at the wrist to a bar of the frame.

It looks like she's diving into a lake.

Except for the watery blood on her face.

"She's gonna get it now," Davy says.

But his voice is oddly quiet.

"One more time, my female friend," Mr Hammar says, walking behind her. "Who set the bomb?"

The first bomb since the prison break went off last night, taking out a well and pump on a farm.

It's begun.

"I don't know," says the woman, her voice strangled and coughing. "I haven't even left Haven since–"

"Haven't left *where*?" Mr Hammar says. He grabs a handle on the frame and tips the whole thing forward, plunging the woman face first into a tub of water, holding her there

335

I look down at my feet.

"Raise your head, please, Todd," the Mayor says, standing behind us. "How else will you learn?"

I raise my head.

We're on the other side of a two-way mirror, in a small room looking in on the Arena of the Ask, which is just a room with high concrete walls and similar mirrored rooms off of each side. Davy and I sit next to each other on a short bench.

Watching.

Mr Hammar pulls up the frame. The woman rises outta the water, gasping for air, straining against where her arms are tied.

"*Where* do you live?" Mr Hammar's got his smile on, that nasty thing that hardly ever leaves his face.

"New Prentisstown," the woman gasps. "New Prentisstown."

"Correct," says Mr Hammar, then watches as the woman coughs so hard she throws up down her front. He takes a towel from a side table and gently wipes the woman's face, cleaning as much of the vomit off her as he can.

The woman's still gasping but her eyes don't leave Mr Hammar as he cleans her.

She looks even more frightened than before.

"Why's he doing that?" Davy says.

"Doing what?" the Mayor says.

Davy shrugs. "Being, I don't know, *kind.*"

I don't say nothing. I keep my Noise clear of the Mayor putting bandages on me.

All those months ago.

I hear the Mayor shift his stance, rustling himself to cover up my Noise so Davy don't hear it. "We're not inhuman, David. We don't do this for our own joy."

I look out at Mr Hammar, look at his smile.

"Yes, Todd," the Mayor says, "Captain Hammar does show a certain *glee* that is perhaps unseemly, but you have to admit, he does get results."

"Are you recovered?" Mr Hammar asks the woman. We can hear his voice over a microphone system, pumped into the room. It separates it oddly from his mouth, making it seem like we're watching a vid rather than a real thing.

"I'm sorry to have to keep Asking you," Mr Hammar says. "This can end as quick as you want."

"Please," says the woman in a whisper. "Please, I don't know anything."

And she starts to weep.

"Christ," Davy says, under his breath.

"The enemy will try many tricks to win our sympathy," says the Mayor.

Davy turns to him. "So this is a trick?"

"Almost certainly."

I keep watching the woman. It don't look like a trick.

I am the Circle and the Circle is me, I think.

"Just so," says the Mayor.

"Yer in control here," says Mr Hammar, starting round the woman again. Her head turns to try and follow him but there ain't much movement from where she's strapped to the frame. He hovers just outside of her vision. To keep her off balance, I'm guessing.

Me and Davy do, tho.

"Only muffled sounds, Todd," the Mayor says, reading my asking. "Do you see the metal rods coming out of the frame by the sides of her head?"

He points. Davy and I see them.

"They play a whining buzz into her ears at all times," the Mayor says. "Muffles any Noise she might hear from the observation rooms. Keeps her focused on the Officer of the Ask."

"Wouldn't want 'em hearing what we already know," Davy says.

"Yes," the Mayor says, sounding a little surprised. "Yes, that's it exactly, David."

Davy smiles and his Noise glows a bit.

"We saw the **A** written in blue on the side of the farmhouse," Mr Hammar says, still hovering behind the woman. "The bomb was the same as all the others planted by your organizayshun—"

"It's not *my* organization!" says the woman but Mr Hammar continues like she didn't even speak.

"And we know you've worked in that field for the past month."

"So have other women!" she yells, sounding more and more desperate. "Milla Price, Cassia MacRae, Martha Sutpen—"

"So they were in on it, too?"

"No! No, just that—"

"Cuz Mrs Price and Mrs Sutpen have already been Asked."

The woman stops, her face suddenly even more frightened.

Davy chuckles next to me. "Got you," he whispers.

But I can hear a weird sense of relief in him.

I wonder if the Mayor hears it, too.

"What did–" the woman says, stopping and then having to go on. "What did they say?"

"They said you tried to get 'em to help," Mr Hammar says calmly. "Said you tried to enlist 'em as terrorists and when they refused, you said you'd carry on alone."

The woman goes pale, her mouth falling open, her eyes wide in disbelief.

"That's not true, is it?" I say, my voice level. *I am the Circle and the Circle is me.* "He's trying to make her confess by pretending he don't need her to."

"Excellent, Todd," says the Mayor. "You may end up having a flair for this."

Davy looks first at me, then at his pa, then at me again, askings left unsaid.

"We already know yer responsible," Mr Hammar says. "We already have enough to stick you in prison for the rest of yer life." He stops in front of her. "I stand before you as yer friend," he says. "I stand before you as the one who can save you from a fate worse than prison."

The woman swallows and looks like she's going to vomit again.

"But I don't *know* anything," she says weakly. "I just don't *know*."

Mr Hammar sighs. "Well, that's a real disappointment, I must say."

her into the water.

And holds her there–

And holds her there–

He looks up to the mirror where he knows we're watching–

He smiles at us–

And still holds her there–

The water churns with the limited thrashing she can do–

I am the Circle and the Circle is me, I think, closing my eyes–

"Open them, Todd," the Mayor says–

I do–

And still Mr Hammar holds her there–

The thrashing gets worse–

So hard the binds on her wrists start to bleed–

"Jesus," Davy says, under his breath–

"He's gonna kill her," I say, voice still low–

It's only a vid–

It's only a vid–

(except it ain't–)

(feeling nothing–)

(cuz I'm dead–)

(I'm dead–)

The Mayor leans past me and presses a button on the wall. "I should think that's enough, Captain," he says, his voice carrying into the Arena of the Ask.

Mr Hammar raises the frame outta the water. But he does it slowly.

The woman hangs from it, chin down on her chest, water pouring from her mouth and nose.

"He killed her," Davy says.

"No," says the Mayor.

"Tell me," Mr Hammar says to the woman, "and this will all stop."

There's a long silence, longer still.

And then a croaking sound from the woman.

"What was that?" Mr Hammar says.

"I did it," croaks the woman.

"*No way!*" says Davy.

"What did you do?" Mr Hammar asks.

"I set the bomb," the woman says, her head still down.

"And you tried to get yer worksisters to join you in a terrorist organizayshun."

"Yes," the woman whispers. "Anything."

"Ha!" Davy says, and again there's relief, relief that he tries to cover. "She confessed! She did it!"

"No, she didn't," I say, still looking at her, still not moving on the bench.

"*What?*" Davy says to me.

"She's making it up," I say, still looking thru the mirror. "So he'll stop drowning her." I move my head just slightly to show I'm talking to the Mayor. "Ain't she?"

The Mayor waits before answering. Even without Noise, I can tell he's impressed. Ever since I started with *the Circle*, things have taken on the worst kinda clarity.

Maybe that's the point.

"Almost certainly she's making it up," he finally says. "But now we've got her confession, we can use it against her."

and his pa. "You mean, yer gonna ... Ask her some more?"

"All women are part of the Answer," the Mayor says, "if only in sympathy. We need to know what she thinks. We need to know what she *knows*."

Davy looks back at the woman, still panting against the frame.

"I don't get it," he says.

"When they send her back to prison," I say, "all the other women will know what happened to her."

"Quite," says the Mayor, putting a hand briefly on my shoulder. Almost like affecshun. When I don't move, he takes it away. "They'll know what's in store for them if they don't answer. And that way, we'll find out what we need to know from whoever knows it. The bomb last night was a resumption of aggressions, the start of something larger. We need to know what their next move is going to be."

Davy's still looking at the woman. "What about her?"

"She'll be punished for the crime she confessed to, of course," the Mayor says, carrying on talking when Davy tries to interrupt with the obvious. "And who knows? Maybe she really *does* know something." He looks back up thru the mirror. "There's only one way to find out."

"I want to thank you for yer help today," Mr Hammar says, putting his hand under the woman's chin to lift it. "You've been very brave and can be proud of the fight you put up." He smiles at her but she won't meet his eye. "You've shown more spirit than many a man I've seen under Asking."

He steps away from her, going to a little side table and removing a cloth that's lying on top. Underneath are several shiny bits of metal. Mr Hammar picks one up.

"And now for the second part of our interview," he says, approaching the woman.

Who starts to scream.

"That was," Davy says, pacing around as we wait outside but it's all he can get out. "That was." He turns to me. "Holy crap, Todd."

I don't say nothing, just take the apple I been saving outta my pocket. "Apple," I whisper to Angharrad, my head close to hers. **Apple**, she says back, clipping at it with her teeth, lips back. **Todd**, she says, munching it and then she makes an asking of it, **Todd?**

"Nothing to do with you, girl," I whisper, rubbing her nose.

We're down from the gate where Ivan's still guarding, still trying to catch my eye. I can hear him calling quietly to me in his Noise.

I still ignore him.

"That was effing intense," Davy says, trying to read my Noise, trying to see what I might think about it all, but I'm keeping it as flat as I can.

Feeling nothing.

Taking nothing in.

"Yer a cool customer these days," Davy says, voice scornful, ignoring Deadfall, who's wanting an apple, too. "You didn't even flinch when he–"

"Gentlemen," the Mayor says, coming outta the gate, a long, heavy sack in one hand.

343

"Pa," Davy says in greeting.

"Is she dead?" I say, looking into Angharrad's eyes.

"She's no use to us dead, Todd," the Mayor says.

"She sure *looked* dead," Davy says.

"Only when she lost consciousness," the Mayor says. "Now, I've got a new job for the two of you."

There's a beat as we take in the words, *a new job*.

I close my eyes. *I am the Circle and the Circle is me.*

"Would you quit effing *saying* that?" Davy shouts at me.

But we can all hear the horror in his own Noise, the anxiety that's rising, the fear of his pa, of the *new job*, fear he won't be able to–

"You won't be leading the Askings, if that's what you're afraid of," says the Mayor.

"I ain't afraid," Davy says, too loud. "Who's saying I'm afraid?"

The Mayor drops the bag at our feet.

I reckernize its shape.

Feeling nothing, taking nothing in.

Davy's looking down at the bag, too. Even *he's* shocked.

"Just the prisoners," says the Mayor. "So we can fight against enemy infiltration on the inside."

"You want us to–?" Davy looks up at his pa. "On *people*?"

"Not people," says the Mayor. "Enemies of the state."

I'm still looking at the bag.

The bag that we all know carries a bolting tool and a supply of numbered bands.

10

THE BAND

{VIOLA}

I'VE JUST SET THE TIMER running and turned to Mistress Braithwaite to tell her we can leave when a woman comes tumbling out of the bushes behind us.

"Help me," she says, so gently it's almost as if she doesn't know we're there and is just asking the universe to help her somehow.

Then she collapses.

"What *is* this thing?" I say, taking another bandage from the too-small first aid kit we keep hidden in the cart, trying to tend her wound as we rock back and forth. There's a metal band encircling the middle of her forearm, so tight it seems like the skin around it is trying to grow *into* it. It's also so red with infection I can almost feel the heat coming off it.

"It's for branding livestock," Mistress Braithwaite says, angrily snapping the reins on the oxes, bumping us along

bastard."

"Help me," the woman whispers.

"I'm helping you," I say. Her head is in my lap to cushion it from the bumps in the road. I wrap a bandage around the metal band but not before I see a number etched into the side.

1391.

"What's your name?" I ask.

But her eyes are half-closed and all she says is, "Help me."

"And we're sure she's not a spy?" Mistress Coyle says, arms crossed.

"Good *God*," I snap. "Is there a stone where your heart should be?"

Her brow darkens. "We have to consider all manner of tricks–"

"The infection is so bad we're not going to be able to save her arm," Mistress Braithwaite says. "If she's a spy, she's in no position to return with information."

Mistress Coyle sighs. "Where was she?"

"Near that new Office of the Ask we've been hearing about," Mistress Braithwaite says, frowning even harder.

"We planted a device on a small storehouse nearby," I say. "It was as close as we could get."

"*Branding* strips, Nicola," Mistress Braithwaite says, anger puffing out of her like the steam of her breath.

Mistress Coyle rubs her fingers along her forehead. "I know."

"Can't we just cut it off?" I ask. "Heal the wound?"

Mistress Braithwaite shakes her head. "Chemicals make it so the banded skin never heals, that's the point. You can never remove it unless you want to bleed to death. They're permanent. *Forever.*"

"Oh, my God."

"I need to talk to her," Mistress Coyle says.

"Nadari's treating her," Mistress Braithwaite says. "She might be lucid before the surgery."

"Let's go then," Mistress Coyle says and they head off towards the healing tent. I move to follow, but Mistress Coyle stops me with a look. "Not you, my girl."

"Why not?"

But off they keep walking, leaving me standing in the cold.

"Y'all right, Hildy?" Wilf asks as I wander among the oxes. He's brushing them down where they strained against the harnesses. **Wilf**, they say.

That's pretty much all they ever say.

"Rough night," I say. "We rescued a woman who'd been branded with some kind of metal band."

Wilf looks thoughtful for a minute. He points to a metal band around the right front leg of each ox. "Like these 'ere?"

I nod.

"On a person?" He whistles in amazement.

"Things are turning, Wilf," I say. "Turning for the worse."

"Ah know," he says. "We'll make a move soon and that'll be it, one way or t'other."

I look up at him. "Do you kn— ... what she's plan ning?"

He shakes his head and runs his hand around the metal band on one of the oxes. **Wilf**, says the ox.

"Viola!" I hear, called across the camp.

Wilf and I both see Mistress Coyle treading through the darkened camp towards us. "She's gone wake everyone up," Wilf says.

"She's a little delirious," Mistress Nadari says as I kneel down by the cot of the rescued woman. "You've got a minute, tops."

"Tell her what you told us, my girl," Mistress Coyle says to the woman. "Just once more and we'll let you sleep."

"My arm?" says the woman, her eyes cloudy. "It don't hurt no more."

"Just tell her what you said, my love," Mistress Coyle says, her voice as warm as it ever gets. "And everything'll be all right."

The woman's eyes focus briefly on mine and widen slightly. "You," she says. "The girl who was there."

"Viola," I say, touching her non-banded arm.

"We haven't got much time, Jess." Mistress Coyle's voice gets a little sterner, even as she says what must be the woman's name. "Tell her."

"Tell me what?" I say, getting a little annoyed. It's cruel to keep her awake like this and I'm about to say as much when Mistress Coyle says, "Tell her who did this to you."

Jess's eyes grow frightened. "Oh," she says. "Oh, oh."

348

"Just this one thing and we'll leave you be," Mistress Coyle says.

"Mistress Coyle–" I start to say, getting angry.

"*Boys*," the woman says. "Boys. Not even men."

I take in a breath.

"Which boys?" Mistress Coyle asks. "What were their names?"

"Davy," says the woman, her eyes not seeing the inside of the tent any more. "Davy was the older one."

Mistress Coyle catches my eye. "And the other?"

"The quiet one," the woman says. "Didn't say nothing. Just did his job and didn't say nothing."

"What was his name?" Mistress Coyle insists.

"I need to go," I say, standing up, not wanting to hear. Mistress Coyle grabs my hand and holds me there firmly.

"What was his name?" she says again.

The woman is breathing harshly now, almost panting.

"That's enough," Mistress Nadari says. "I didn't want this in the first–"

"One second more," Mistress Coyle says.

"Nicola–" Mistress Nadari warns.

"Todd," says the woman on the cot, the woman I saved, the woman with the infected arm she's going to lose, the woman I now wish was at the bottom of the ocean I've never seen. "The other one called him Todd."

"Get away from me," I say, as Mistress Coyle follows me out of the tent.

"He's alive," she's saying, "but he's one of them."

how loud I'm being.

Mistress Coyle races forward and grabs my arm. "You've lost him, my girl," she says. "If you ever really had him in the first place."

I slap her face so fast and hard she doesn't have time to defend herself. It's like smacking a tree trunk. The solid weight of her staggers back and my arm rings with pain.

"You don't know what you're talking about," I say, my voice blazing.

"How *dare* you," she says, her hand to her face.

"You haven't even *seen* me fight yet," I say, standing my ground. "*I* knocked down a bridge to stop an army. *I* put a knife through the neck of a crazy murderer. *I* saved the lives of others while you just ran around at night blowing them up."

"You ignorant child–"

I step towards her.

She doesn't step back.

But she stops her sentence.

"I hate you," I say slowly. "Everything you do makes the Mayor respond with something *worse*."

"I did *not* start this war–"

"But you *love* it!" I take another step towards her. "You love everything about it. The bombs, the fighting, the rescues."

Her face is so angry I can even see it in the moonlight.

But I'm not afraid of her.

And I think she can tell.

"You want to see it as simple good and evil, my girl," she says. "The world doesn't work that way. Never has, never will, and don't forget," she gives me a smile that could curdle milk, "you're fighting the war *with* me."

I lean in close to her face. "He needs to be overthrown, so I'm helping you do it. But when it's done?" I'm so close I can feel her breath. "Are we going to have to overthrow you next?"

She doesn't say anything.

But she doesn't back down either.

I turn on my heels and I walk away from her.

"He's gone, Viola!" Mistress Coyle shouts after me.

But I just keep walking.

"I need to go back to the city."

"Now?" Wilf says, looking up at the sky. "Be dawn soon. T'ain't safe."

"It's *never* safe," I say, "but I have no choice."

He blinks at me. Then he starts gathering ropes and bindings to get the cart ready again.

"No," I say, "you'll have to show me how to do it. I can't ask you to risk your life."

"Yer goin for Todd?"

I nod.

"Then Ah'll take yoo."

"Wilf–"

"Still early," he says, backing the oxes into position. "Ah'll at least get yoo close."

He doesn't say another word as he re-harnesses the oxes to his cart. They ask him **Wilf? Wilf?** in surprise at being used so quickly again after thinking their night of work was finished.

her Wilf into danger.

But all I say is, "Thank you."

"I'm coming, too." I turn around. Lee is there, rubbing sleep out of his eyes but dressed and ready.

"What are you doing up?" I ask. "And no, you're not."

"Yes, I am," he says, "and who can sleep with all that shouting?"

"It's too dangerous," I say. "They'll hear your Noise–"

He keeps his mouth shut and says to me, Then they can just hear it.

"Lee–"

"You're going to look for him, aren't you?"

I sigh in frustration, beginning to wonder if I should abandon the idea altogether before I put anyone else in danger.

"You're going to the Office of the Ask," Lee says, lowering his voice.

I nod.

And then I understand.

Siobhan and his mum might be there.

I nod again, and this time he knows I've agreed.

No one tries to stop us, though half the camp must know we're going. Mistress Coyle must have her reasons.

We don't talk much as we go. I just listen to Lee's Noise and its thoughts of his family, of the Mayor, of what he'll do if he ever gets his hands on him.

Thoughts of me.

"You'd better say something," Lee says. "Listening that close is rude."

"So I've heard," I say.

But my mouth is dry and I find I don't have much to say.

The sun rises before we get to the city. Wilf pushes the oxes as fast as they'll go, but even so, it's going to be a dangerous trip back, with the city awake, with Noisy men on our cart. We're taking a terrible risk.

But on Wilf drives.

I've explained what I want to see, and he says he knows a place. He stops the cart deep in some woods and directs us up a bluff.

"Keep yer heads down now," he says. "Don't be seen."

"We won't," I say. "But if we're not back in an hour, don't wait for us."

Wilf just looks at me. We all know how likely him leaving us is.

Lee and I make our way up the bluff, keeping down in the cover of the trees, until we reach the top and see why Wilf chose the place. It's a hill near where the tower fell, one where we've got a clear view of the road coming down towards the Office of the Ask, which we've heard is some kind of prison or torture chamber or something like that.

I don't even want to know.

We lie on our stomachs, side by side, looking out from some bushes.

"Keep your ears open," Lee whispers.

As if we need to. As soon as the sun rises, New Prentisstown

his Noise so much. How could it not be possible to drown in it?

"Because drowning is the right word," Lee says when I ask. "If you disappeared into it, you'd suffocate."

"I can't imagine what it's like growing up inside it all," I say.

"No," he says. "No, you can't."

But he doesn't say it in a mean way.

I squint down the road as the sun brightens. "I wish I had some binos."

Lee reaches into a pocket and pulls out a pair.

I give him a look. "You were just waiting for me to ask so you could look all impressive."

"I don't know what you're talking about," he says, smiling, putting the binos to his eyes.

"C'mon." I push him with my shoulder. "Give them to me."

He stretches away to keep them out of my grabbing range. I start to giggle, so does he. I grab onto him and try to hold him down while I snatch at the binos but he's bigger than me and keeps twisting them away.

"I'm not afraid to hurt you," I say.

"I don't doubt that," he laughs, turning the binos back to the road.

His Noise spikes, loud enough to make me afraid someone'll hear us.

"What do you see?" I say, not giggling any more.

He hands the binos to me, pointing. "There," he says. "Coming down the road."

But I'm already seeing them in the binos.

354

Two people on horseback. Two people in shiny new uniforms, riding their horses. One of them talking, gesturing with his hands.

Laughing. Smiling.

The other keeping his eyes on his horse, but riding along to work.

Riding along to his job at the Office of the Ask.

In a uniform with a shiny *A* on the shoulder.

Todd.

My Todd.

Riding next to Davy Prentiss.

Riding to work with the man who shot me.

31

NUMBERS AND LETTERS

[TODD]

THE DAYS KEEP PASSING. They keep getting worse.

"*All* of 'em?" Davy asks, his Noise ringing with badly hidden alarm. "Every single one?"

"This is a vote of confidence, David," the Mayor says, standing with us at the door of the stables while our horses are made ready for the day's work. "You and Todd did such an excellent job with permanently identifying the female prisoners, who else would I want to be in charge of expanding the programme?"

I don't say nothing, not even acknowledging Davy's looks at me. His Noise is confused with the pink of his pa's praise.

But then there's also his thoughts about banding all the women.

Every single one.

Cuz banding the ones in the Office of the Ask was even worse than we thought.

"They keep leaving," the Mayor says. "In the dead of night, they slip away and cast their lot with the terrorists."

Davy's watching Deadfall get saddled in a small paddock, his Noise clanking with the faces of the women who get banded, the cries of pain they make.

The words they speak to us.

"And if they keep getting out," the Mayor says, "they obviously keep getting in, too."

He means the bombs. One every night for the past two weeks nearly, so many they must be increasing for a reason, they must be leading up to something bigger, and no women have been caught planting 'em except once when a bomb blew up while the woman was still putting it in place. They didn't find much left of her except bits of clothing and flesh.

I close my eyes when I think of it.

Feeling nothing, taking nothing in.

(was it her?)

Feeling *nothing*.

"You want us to number *all* the women," Davy says again quietly, looking away from his pa.

"I've said it before," the Mayor sighs. "*Every* woman is part of the Answer, if only because she is a woman and therefore sympathetic to other women."

The groomsmen bring Angharrad into a nearby paddock. She sticks her head over the rail to bump me with her nose. **Todd**, she says.

"They'll resist," I say, stroking her head. "The men won't like it neither."

"Ah, yes," says the Mayor. "You missed yesterday's rally, didn't you?"

357

yesterday and didn't hear nothing bout no rally.

"I spoke to the men of New Prentisstown," the Mayor says. "Man to man. I explained to them the threat the Answer poses us and how this is the next prudent step forward to ensure safety for all." He rubs a hand down Angharrad's neck. I try and hide how prickly my Noise gets at the sight. "I encountered no resistance."

"There weren't no women at this rally," I say, "were there?"

He turns to me. "I wouldn't want to encourage the enemy among us, now would I?

"But there's effing *thousands* of 'em!" Davy says. "Banding 'em all will take forever."

"There will be other teams working, David," the Mayor says calmly, making sure he's got his son's full attenshun. "But I'm sure the two of you will outwork any of them."

Davy's Noise perks up a bit at this. "You bet we will, Pa," he says.

He looks at me, tho.

And there's worry there.

I stroke Angharrad's nose again. The groomsmen bring out Morpeth, freshly brushed and shiny with oil. **Submit**, he says.

"If you're worried," the Mayor says, taking Morpeth's reins. "Ask yourselves this." He hoists himself up in the saddle in one smooth movement, like he's made of liquid. He looks down at us.

"Why would any innocent woman object to being identified?"

358

*　*　*

"You won't get away with this," the woman says, her voice almost steady.

Mr Hammar cocks his rifle behind us and aims it at her head.

"You blind?" Davy says to the woman, voice a little too squeaky. "I'm getting away with it *right now*."

Mr Hammar laughs.

Davy twists the bolting tool with a hard turn. The band snaps into the woman's skin halfway up her forearm. She calls out, grabbing the band and falling forward, catching herself on the floor with her unbanded arm. She stops there a minute, panting.

Her hair is pulled back into a severe knot, blondy and brown mixed together, like the wire filaments in the back of a vid player. There's a small patch on the back where the hair is grey, all growing together, a river across a dusty land.

I stare at the grey patch, letting my eyes blur a little.

I am the Circle and the Circle is me.

"Get up," Davy says to the woman. "So the healers can treat you." He looks back at the line of women staring at us down the hall to the front of the dormitory, waiting their turn.

"The boy said get up," Mr Hammar says, waving his rifle.

"We don't need you here," Davy snaps, his voice tight. "We're doing just fine without no babysitter."

"I ain't babysitting," Mr Hammar smiles. "I'm protecting."

The woman stands, her eyes on me.

don't have to be.

I am the Circle and the Circle is me.

"Where's your heart?" she asks. "Where is your heart if you can do these things?" And then she turns to where the healers, who we've already banded, wait to give her treatment.

I watch her go.

I don't know her name.

Her number, tho, is 1484.

"1485!" Davy calls out.

The next woman in line steps forward.

We spend the day riding from one women's dormitory to another, getting thru almost three hundred bands, much faster than we ever did the Spackle. We start for home when the sun begins to set, as New Prentisstown turns its thoughts to curfew.

We ain't saying much.

"What a day, eh, pigpiss?" Davy says, after a while.

I don't say nothing but he don't want an answer.

"They'll be all right," he says. "They got the healers to take away the pain and stuff."

Clop, clop, along we go.

I hear what he's thinking.

Dusk is falling. I can't see his face.

Maybe that's why he ain't covering it up.

"When they cry, tho," he says.

I keep quiet.

"Ain't you got nothing to say?" Davy's voice gets a little harder. "All silent now, like you don't wanna talk no more, like I ain't worth talking to."

His Noise starts to crackle.

"Not like I got anyone *else* to talk to, pigpiss. Not like I got any *choice* in the situashun. Not like no matter what I effing *do* can I get moved up for it, given the good work, the *fighting* work. All that stupid Spackle babysitting crap. Then we turn right around and do the same thing to the women. And for what? For *what*?"

His voice gets low.

"So they can cry at us," he says. "So they can look at us like we ain't even human."

"We ain't," I say, surprised to find I said it out loud.

"Yeah, that's the new you, ain't it?" he says, sneering. "All Mister No-Feeling I-Am-The-Circle Tough Guy. You'd put a bullet thru yer own *ma*'s head if Pa told you to."

I don't say nothing but I grind my teeth together.

Davy's quiet for a minute, too. Then he says, "Sorry."

Then he says, "Sorry, Todd," using my name.

Then he says, "What the hell am *I* saying sorry for? Yer the stupid can't-read pigpiss all getting on my pa's good side. Who cares about you?"

I still don't say nothing and *clop, clop*, along we go.

"Forward," Angharrad neighs to Deadfall, who nickers back, "Forward."

Forward, I hear in her Noise and then **boy colt, Todd**.

"Angharrad," I whisper twixt her ears.

"Todd?" Davy says.

I hear him breathe out thru his nose. "Nothing." Then he changes his mind. "How d'you *do* it?"

"Do what?"

I see him shrug in the dusk. "Be so calm bout it all. Be so, I don't know, *unfeeling*. I mean…" He drifts off and says, almost too quietly to hear, one more time, "when they cry."

I don't say nothing cuz how can I help him? How can he not know about *The Circle* unless his pa don't want him to?

"I *do* know," he says, "but I tried that crap and it don't work for me and he won't–"

He stops abruptly, like he's said too much.

"Ah, screw it," he says.

We keep riding, letting the **ROAR** of New Prentisstown enfold us as we enter the main part of town, the horses calling their orders to each other, reminding theirselves of who they are.

"Yer the only friend I got, pigpiss," Davy finally says. "Ain't that the biggest tragedy you ever heard?"

"Tiring day?" Mayor Ledger says to me when I come into our cell. His voice is oddly light and he keeps his eyes on me.

"What do you care?" I sling my bag on the floor and flop down on the bed without taking my uniform off.

"I suppose it must be exhausting torturing women all day."

I blink in surprise. "I don't torture 'em," I growl. "You shut yer mouth about that."

"No, of *course* you don't torture them. What was I

thinking? You just strap a corrosive metal band into their skin that can never be removed without them bleeding to death. How could that possibly be construed as *torture*?"

"Hey!" I sit up. "We do it fast and without fuss. There are lots of ways to make it worse and we don't do that. If it's gotta be done, then it's best that it's done by *us*."

He crosses his arms, his voice still light. "That excuse going to help you sleep tonight?"

My Noise roars up. "Oh, yeah?" I snap. "Was that you the Mayor didn't hear shouting at the rally yesterday? Was that you who weren't making that brave stand against him?"

His face goes stormy and I hear a flash of grey resentment in his Noise. "And get shot?" he says. "Or dragged away to be Asked? How would that help anything?"

"And that's what yer doing?" I say. "*Helping*?"

He don't say nothing to that, just turns to look out one of the windows, out over the few lights that come on only in essenshul places, out over the **ROAR** of a town wondering when the Answer are gonna make their big move and from where and how bad it'll be and who's gonna save 'em.

My Noise is raised and red. I close my eyes and take in a deep, deep breath.

I am the Circle and the Circle is me.

Feeling nothing, taking nothing in.

"They were getting used to him again," Mayor Ledger says out the window. "They were uniting behind him because what're a few curfews against being blown up? But this is a tactical mistake."

I open my eyes at *tactical* cuz it seems a weird word to choose.

they're going to be next." He looks down at his own fore-arm, rubbing a spot where a band might go. "Politically, he's made a mistake."

I squint at him. "What do you care if he's made a mis-take?" I ask. "Whose side are you on?"

He turns to me as if I've insulted him, which I guess I have. "The *town's*," he steams. "Whose side are *you* on, Todd Hewitt?"

There's a knock on the door.

"Saved by the dinner bell," Mayor Ledger says.

"The dinner bell don't knock," I say, getting to my feet. I unlock the door with my key *ker-thunk* and open it.

It's Davy.

He don't say nothing at first, just looks nervous, eyes here and there. I figure there's a problem at the dormitories so I sigh and move back to my bed to get my few things. I ain't even had time to get my boots off.

"It'll take a minute," I say to him. "Angharrad'll still be eating. She won't like being saddled up again so soon."

He still ain't said nothing so I turn to look at him. He's still nervous, not meeting my eye. "*What*?" I say.

He chews on his upper lip and all I can see in his Noise is embarrassment and asking marks and anger at Mayor Ledger being there and more asking marks and there behind it all, a weird strong feeling, almost guilty, almost *clear*–

Then he covers it up fast and the anger and embarrass-ment come foremost.

"Effing pigpiss," he says to himself. He pulls angrily at a strap on his shoulder and I see he's carrying a bag. "Effing…" he says again but don't finish the thought. He unsnaps the flap on it and takes something out.

"*Here,*" he practically shouts, thrusting it at me.

My ma's book.

He's giving me back my ma's book.

"Just take it!"

I reach out slowly, taking it twixt my fingers and pulling it away from him like it was a fragile thing. The leather of the cover is still soft, the gash still cut thru the front where Aaron stabbed me and it was stopped by the book. I run my hand over it.

I look up at Davy but he won't meet my eye.

"Whatever," he says and turns again, stomping back down the stairs and out into the night.

32

FINAL PREPARATIONS

{VIOLA}

I HIDE BEHIND THE TREE, my heart pounding.

I have a gun in my hand.

I listen hard for the snap of twigs, the sound of any footsteps, any sign that'll tell me where the soldier is. I know he's there because I can hear his Noise but it's so flat and wide I only get a general idea of the direction he's going to come after me.

Because he *is* coming for me. There's no doubt about that.

His Noise grows louder. My back is to the tree and I hear him off to my left.

I'm going to have to leap at just the right second.

I ready my gun.

I see the trees around me in his Noise, along with asking marks wondering which one I'm hiding behind, narrowing it down to two, the one that I'm actually using and one a few feet away to my left.

If he chooses that one, I've got him.

I hear his steps now, quiet against the damp forest floor. I close my eyes and try to concentrate solely on his Noise, on exactly where he's standing, where he's placing his feet.

Which tree he's approaching.

He steps. He hesitates. He steps again.

He makes his choice–

And I make mine–

I jump and I'm ducking and twisting and sweeping my leg at his feet and I'm catching him by surprise and he's falling to the ground, trying to aim his rifle at me, but I'm leaping on him and pinning his rifle arm down with my leg and throwing my weight on his chest and holding the barrel of my gun under his chin.

I've got him.

"Well done," Lee says, smiling up at me.

"Indeed, well done," Mistress Braithwaite says, stepping out of the darkness. "And now comes the moment, Viola. What do you do with the enemy under your mercy?"

I look down into Lee's face, breathing hard, feeling his warmth underneath me.

"What do you do?" Mistress Braithwaite asks again.

I look down at my gun.

"I do what I have to do," I say.

I do what I have to do to save him.

I do what I have to do to save Todd.

"You're *sure* you want to do this?" Mistress Coyle asks for the hundredth time as we leave the breakfast area the next

more tea.

"I'm sure," I say.

"You've got one chance before we make our move. *One.*"

"He came for me once," I say. "When I was captive, he came for me and made the biggest sacrifice he could make to do it."

She frowns. "People change, Viola."

"He deserves the same chance he gave me."

"Hmm," Mistress Coyle hmms. She's still not convinced.

But I haven't given her any choice.

"And when he joins us," I say, "think of the information he can provide."

"Yes." She looks away, looks out at the camp of the Answer preparing itself. Preparing itself for war. "Yes, so you keep saying."

Even with how well I know Todd, I can also see how anyone else would see him on horseback, would see him in that uniform, would see him riding with Davy, and they would think he's a traitor.

And in the dead of night, when I'm under my blankets, unable to sleep.

I think it, too.

(what's he doing?)

(what's he doing with *Davy*?)

And I try to put it out of my mind as best I can.

Because I'm going to save him.

She's agreed that I can. She's agreed I can risk myself and go to the cathedral the night before the Answer makes its final attack and try one last time to save him.

She agreed because I said if she didn't, I wouldn't help her with anything more, not with the bombs, not with the final attack, not with the ships when they land, now eight weeks away and counting. Nothing, if I couldn't try for Todd.

Even with all that, I think the only reason she agreed is for what he could tell us when he got here.

Mistress Coyle *likes* to know things.

"You're brave to try," Mistress Coyle says. "Foolish, but brave." She looks me up and down once more, her face unknowable.

"What?" I ask.

She shakes her head. "Just how much of myself I see in you, you exasperating girl."

"Think I'm ready to lead my own army?" I say, almost smiling.

She just gives me a last look and starts walking off into the camp, ready to give more orders, make more preparations, put the final touches to the plans for our attack.

Which happens tomorrow.

"Mistress Coyle," I call after her.

She turns.

"Thank you," I say.

She looks surprised, her forehead furrowed. But she nods, accepting it.

"Got it?" Lee calls over the top of the cart.

"Got it," I say, twisting the final knot and locking the clamp into place.

"'At's all of 'em," Wilf says, smacking some dust off his

hands. We look at the carts, eleven of them now, packed to bursting with supplies, with weapons, with explosives. Almost the entire stash of the Answer.

Eleven carts doesn't seem like much against an army of a thousand or more, but that's what we have.

"Bin done before," Wilf says, quoting Mistress Coyle, but he's always so dry you never know if he's making fun. "Only a matter a tactics."

And then he smiles the same mysterious smile Mistress Coyle always gives. It's so funny and unexpected, I laugh out loud.

Lee doesn't, though. "Yes, her top secret plan." He pulls a rope on the cart to test that it holds.

"I expect it has to do with him," I say. "*Getting* him, somehow, and then once he's gone–"

"His army will fall apart and the town will rise up against his tyranny and we'll save the day," Lee says, sounding unconvinced. He looks at Wilf. "What do you think?"

"She says it'll be the end," Wilf shrugs. "Ah want it to be done."

Mistress Coyle does keep saying that, that this could end the whole conflict, that the right blow in the right place right *now* could be all we need, that if even just the women of the town join us we could topple him before winter comes, topple him before the ships land, topple him before he finds us.

And then Lee says, "I know something I shouldn't."

Wilf and I both look at him.

"She passed by the kitchen window with Mistress Braithwaite," he says. "They were talking about where the attack will come from tomorrow."

"Lee–" I say.

"Don't say it," Wilf says.

"It's from the hill to the south of town," he presses on, opening his Noise so we can't *not* hear it, "the one with the notch in it, the one with the smaller road that leads right into the town square."

Wilf's eyes bulge. "Yoo shouldn'ta *said*. If Hildy gets caught–"

But Lee's only looking at me. "If you get into trouble," he says. "You come running toward that hill. You come running and that's where you'll find help."

And his Noise says, That's where you'll find me.

"And with burdened hearts, we commit you to the earth."

One by one, we throw a handful of dirt on the empty coffin that doesn't contain anything of the body of Mistress Forth, blown to pieces when a bomb went off too early as she was planting it on a grain house.

The sun is setting when we finish, dusk shining cold across the lake, a lake that had a layer of ice around the edges this morning that didn't melt all day. People start to spread out for the night's work, last minute packing and orders to be received, all the women and men who will soon be soldiers, marching with weapons, ready to strike the final blow.

All they look like now are ordinary people.

I'll leave tonight as soon as it's fully dark.

They'll leave tomorrow at sunset, no matter what happens to me.

"It's time," Mistress Coyle says, coming to my side.

371

There's something else that has to happen first.

"Are you ready?" she asks.

"As I'll ever be," I say, walking along with her.

"This is a huge risk we're taking, my girl. *Huge*. If you're caught–"

"I won't be."

"But if you are." She stops us. "If you are, you know where the camp is, you know when we're attacking and I'm going to tell you now that we're attacking from the east road, the one by the Office of the Ask. We're going to march into town and ram it down his throat." She takes both my hands and stares hard into my eyes. "Do you understand what I'm telling you?"

I do understand. I do. She's telling me wrong on purpose, she's telling me so I can truthfully give the wrong information if I'm caught, like she did before about the ocean.

It's what I'd do if I were her.

"I understand," I say.

She pulls her cloak further shut against a freezing breeze that's come up. We walk in silence for a few steps, heading towards the healing tent.

"Who did you save?" I ask.

"What?" She looks at me, genuinely confused.

We stop again. Which is fine with me. "All those years ago," I say. "Corinne said you were kicked off the Council for saving a life. Who did you save?"

She looks at me thoughtfully and rubs her fingers across her forehead.

372

"I may not return," I say. "You may never see me again. It'd be nice to know something good about you so I don't die thinking you're just a huge pain in my ass."

She almost grins but it disappears quickly, her eyes looking troubled again. "Who did I save?" she says to herself. She takes a deep breath. "I saved an enemy of the state."

"You *what*?"

"The Answer was never exactly authorized, you see." She walks us off in a different direction, towards the shore of the freezing lake. "The men fighting the Spackle War didn't really approve of our methods, effective as they might have been." She looks back at me. "And they were *very* effective. Effective enough to get the heads of the Answer onto the ruling Council when Haven was being put back together."

"That's why you think it'll work now. Why you think it'll work against a bigger force."

She nods and rubs her forehead again. I'm surprised she hasn't built a callus up there. "Haven restarted itself," she continues, "using the captured Spackle to rebuild and so on. But some people weren't happy with the new government. Some people didn't have as much power as they thought they should." She shivers under her cloak. "Some people in the Answer."

She lets me realize what this might mean. "Bombs," I say.

"Quite so. Some people get so caught up in warfare, they start doing it for its own sake."

She turns away, so that maybe I can't see her face or that maybe she can't see mine, see the judgement on it.

"Her name was Mistress Thrace." She's talking to the lake now, to the cold night sky. "Smart, strong, respected, but with one wanted her on the Council, including the Answer, and why she reacted so strongly to being left off."

She turns back to me. "She had her supporters. And she had her bombing campaign. Not unlike the one we're giving the Mayor now, except of course, that was meant to be peacetime." She glances up at the moons. "She specialized in what we took to calling a Thrace bomb. She'd leave it somewhere soldiers were gathered and it would look like an innocent package. Wouldn't arm itself until it felt the heartbeat in the skin of the hand picking it up. Your own pulse would make it dangerous, and at that point, you knew it was a bomb and that it would only go off when you let it go. So if you dropped it or couldn't disarm it." She shrugs. "Boom."

We watch a cloud pass between the two rising moons. "Meant to be bad luck, that is," Mistress Coyle murmurs.

She loops her arm in mine again and we start walking back towards the healing tent. "And so there wasn't another war exactly," she says. "More of a skirmish. And to the delight of everyone, Mistress Thrace was mortally wounded."

There's a silence where you can only hear our footsteps and the Noise of the men, crisp in the air.

"But not mortally wounded after all," I say.

She shakes her head. "I'm a very good healer." We reach the opening of the healing tent. "I'd known her since we were girls together on Old World. As far as I saw it, I had no choice." She rubs her hands together. "They kicked me off the Council for it. And then they executed her anyway."

I look at her now, trying to understand her, trying to understand all that's good in her and all that's difficult and conflicted and all the things that went into making her the person that she is.

We are the choices we make. And *have* to make. We aren't anything else.

"Are you ready?" she says again, finally this time.

"I'm ready."

We go into the tent.

My bag is there, packed by Mistress Coyle herself, the one I'll carry on the cart with Wilf, the one I'll carry into town. It's full of food, completely innocent food which, if all goes according to plan, will be my entry into town, my entry past the guards, my entry into the cathedral.

If all goes well.

If it doesn't, there's a pistol in a secret pouch at the bottom.

Mistresses Lawson and Braithwaite are also in the tent, healing materials at the ready.

And Lee is there, as I'd asked him to be.

I sit down on the chair facing him.

He takes my hand and squeezes it and I feel a note in the palm of his hand. He looks at me, his Noise filled with what's about to happen.

I open the note, keeping its contents out of view of all three mistresses around me, who no doubt think it's something romantic or stupid like that.

Don't react, it reads. *I've decided I'm coming with you. I'll meet your cart in the woods. You want to find your family, I want to find mine, and neither of us should do it alone.*

375

giving him the smallest of nods.

"Good luck, Viola," Mistress Coyle says, words echoed rapidly by everyone else there, ending with Lee.

I wanted him particularly to do this. I couldn't stand for it to have been Mistress Coyle, and I know Lee will take the best care.

Because there's only one way I'm going to be able to move around New Prentisstown without getting caught. Only one way based on the intelligence we've gathered.

Only one way I can find Todd.

"Are you ready?" Lee asks, and it feels different coming from him, so much so that I don't mind being asked yet again.

"I'm ready," I say.

I hold out my arm and roll up my sleeve.

"Just make it quick." I look into Lee's eyes. "Please."

"I will," he says.

He reaches into the bag at his feet and takes out a metal band marked 1391.

33

FATHERS AND SONS

[TODD]

"DID HE TELL YOU what he wanted?" Davy asks.

"When would I have talked to him when you weren't there?" I say.

"Duh, pigpiss, you live in the same *building*."

We're riding to the Office of the Ask, the sun setting on the end of our day. Two hundred more women labelled. It goes faster with Mr Hammar watching over it all with a gun. With the other teams around town led by Mr Morgan and Mr O'Hare, word is we've got nearly every one of 'em, tho the bands don't seem to be healing as fast on women as they do on sheep or Spackle.

I look up at the dusky sky as we move along the road and I realize something. "Where do *you* live?"

"Oh, *now* he asks." Davy slaps the reins on Deadfall/Acorn, causing him to canter for about two steps and then drop back into a trot. "Five months we're working together almost."

Davy's Noise is buzzing a little. He don't wanna answer, I can tell.

"You don't have to–"

"Above the stables," he says. "Little room. Mattress on a floor. Smells like horseshit."

We keep on riding. "Forward," Angharrad nickers. "Forward," Deadfall nickers back. Todd, Angharrad thinks. "Angharrad," I say.

Davy and I ain't talked about my ma's book since he brought it to me four nights back. Not a word. And any sign of it in either of our Noises gets ignored.

But we're talking more.

I begin to wonder what sort of man I'd be if I'd had the Mayor as a father. I begin to wonder what sort of man I'd be if I'd had the Mayor as a father and wasn't the son he wanted. I wonder if I'd be sleeping in a room over the stables.

"I try," Davy says, quiet. "But who knows what he effing *wants*?"

I don't know so I don't say nothing.

We tie up our horses at the front gates. Ivan tries to catch my eye again as I go inside but I don't let him.

"Todd," he says as we pass, trying harder.

"That's Mr Hewitt to you, *Private*," Davy spits at him.

I keep on walking. We take the short path from the gates to the front doors of the Office of the Ask building. Soldiers guard those doors, too, but we walk on past 'em into the entryway, across the cold concrete floor, still uncovered, still unheated, and go into the same viewing room as before.

"Ah, boys, welcome," the Mayor says, turning away from the mirror to greet us.

Behind him, in the Arena of the Ask, is Mr Hammar, wearing a rubber apron. Seated in front of him, a naked man is screaming.

The Mayor presses a button, cutting off the sound mid-cry.

"I understand the identification scheme is complete?" he asks, bright and clear.

"As far as we know," I say.

"Who's that?" Davy asks, pointing at the man.

"Son of the exploded terrorist," the Mayor says. "Didn't run when his mother did, foolish man. Now we're seeing what he knows."

Davy curls his lip. "But if he didn't run off when she did–"

"You both have done a tremendous job for me," the Mayor says, clasping his hands behind his back. "I'm very pleased."

Davy smiles and the pink rush fills his Noise.

"But the threat is finally upon us," the Mayor continues. "One of the original terrorists caught in the prison attack finally told us something useful." He looks back thru the mirror. Mr Hammar is blocking most of the view but the man's bare feet are curling tightly against whatever Mr Hammar's doing to him. "Before she unfortunately passed away, she was able to tell us that, based on the patterns

major move by the Answer within days, perhaps as soon as tomorrow."

Davy glances over to me. I keep looking at a middle point beyond the Mayor on the blank wall behind.

"They'll be defeated, of course," says the Mayor. "Easily. Their force is so much smaller than ours that I can't see it lasting more than a day at most."

"Let us fight, Pa," Davy says eagerly. "You know we're ready."

The Mayor smiles, smiles at his own son. Davy's Noise goes so pink you can't hardly look at it.

"You're being promoted, David," the Mayor says. "Into an army position. You will be Sergeant Prentiss."

Davy's smile almost explodes off his face in a little boom of pleased Noise. "Hot damn," he says, as if we weren't there.

"You will be at Captain Hammar's side as he rides into battle at the front of the first wave," the Mayor says. "You will get your fight exactly as you want."

Davy's practically glowing. "Aw, man, *thanks*, Pa!"

The Mayor turns to me. "I'm making you Lieutenant Hewitt."

Davy's Noise gives a sharp change. "*Lieutenant?*"

"You will be my personal bodyguard from the moment the fighting starts," the Mayor goes on. "You will remain by my side, protecting me from any threats that may approach while I superintend the battle."

I don't say nothing, just keep my eyes on the blank wall.

I am the Circle and the Circle is me.

"And this is how the Circle turns, Todd," says the Mayor.

"Why does he get to be a lieutenant?" Davy asks, Noise crackling.

"Lieutenant isn't a battle rank," the Mayor says smoothly. "Sergeant is. If you weren't a sergeant, you wouldn't be able to fight."

"Oh," Davy says, looking back and forth to each of us to see if he's being made a fool of. I don't think nothing about that.

"There's no need to thank me, Lieutenant," the Mayor teases.

"Thank you," I say, my eyes still on the wall.

"It keeps you from doing what you don't want," he says. "It keeps you from having to kill."

"Unless someone comes after you," I say.

"Unless someone comes after me, yes. Will that be a problem for you, Todd?"

"No," I say. "No, sir."

"Good," says the Mayor.

I look back thru the mirror. The naked man's head has lolled lifelessly onto his chest, drool dripping from his slack jaw. Mr Hammar is angrily taking off his gloves and slapping them on a table.

"I am very blessed," the Mayor says warmly. "I have achieved my ambition to put this planet back on track. Within days, maybe even hours, I will crush the terrorists. And when the new settlers come, it will be me who puts out a proud and peaceful hand to welcome them."

He raises his hands, like he can't wait to start putting 'em out. "And who will be right beside me?" He holds his

Davy, buzzing pink all over, reaches out and takes his pa's hand.

"I came into this town with one son," the Mayor says still holding out his hand to me, "but it has blessed me with another."

And his hand is out, waiting for me to take it.

Waiting for his second son to shake his hand.

"Congrats, *Lieutenant* Pigpiss," Davy says, hopping back into Deadfall's saddle.

"Todd?" Ivan says, stepping away from his post as I climb onto Angharrad. "Can I have a word?"

"He outranks you now," Davy says to him. "You'll address him as Lieutenant if you don't want to be digging bogs on the front lines."

Ivan takes in a deep breath, as if to calm himself. "Very well, *Lieutenant*, may I have a word with you?"

I look down on him from Angharrad's back. Ivan's Noise is busting with violence and the gunshot to his leg and conspiracies and resentments and ways to get back at the Mayor, openly thought, as if to impress me.

"You should keep that quiet," I say. "You never know who might hear."

I slap Angharrad's reins and off we go back down the road. Ivan's Noise follows me as I go. I ignore it.

Feeling nothing, taking nothing in.

* * *

"He called you *son*," Davy says, looking ahead as the sun disappears behind the falls. "Guess that makes us brothers."

I don't say nothing.

"We should do something to celebrate," Davy says.

"Where?" I say. "*How?*"

"Well, we're officers now, ain't we, brother? It's my understanding officers get *privileges*." He looks over at me sideways, his Noise bright as a flare, filled with things I used to see all the time in old Prentisstown.

Pictures of women with no clothes.

I frown and send him back a picture of a woman with no clothes and a band on her arm.

"So?" Davy says.

"Yer sick."

"No, brother, yer talking to *Sergeant* Prentiss. I may finally be *well*."

He laughs and laughs. He feels so good some of it actually touches my own Noise, brightening it whether I want it brightened or not.

"Oh, come *on*, Lieutenant Pigpiss, you ain't still pining for yer girl, are ya? She left you *months* ago. We need to get you someone new."

"Shut up, Davy."

"Shut up, *Sergeant* Davy." And he laughs again. "Fine, fine, you just stay at home, read yer book–"

He stops himself suddenly. "Oh, damn, sorry, no, I didn't mean that. I forgot."

And the weird thing is, he seems sincere.

There's a moment of quiet where his Noise pulses again with that strong feeling he's hiding–

383

And then he says, "You know…" and I can see the offer coming and I don't think I can bear it, I don't think I could live another minute if he says it out loud. "If you ever wanted me to read it for–"

"No, Davy," I say quickly. "No, thanks, no."

"You sure?"

"*Yes.*"

"Well, the offer's there." His Noise goes bright again, blooming as he thinks about his new title, about women, about me and him as brothers.

And he whistles happily all the way back to town.

I lay on my bed with my back turned to Mayor Ledger, who's chomping down his dinner as usual. I'm eating, too, but I've also got my ma's book out, just looking at it, lying on the blankets.

"People are wondering when the big attack's gonna happen," Mayor Ledger says.

I don't answer him. I run my hand over the cover of the book like I do every night, feeling the leather, touching the tear where the knife went in with the tips of my fingers.

"People are saying it'll be soon."

"Whatever you say." I open the cover. Ben's folded map is still inside, still where I stashed it. It don't even look like Davy bothered to open the book, not once in the whole time he had it. It smells a bit like stables, now that I know where it's been, but it's still the book, still *her* book.

My ma. My ma's words.

Look what's become of yer son.

Mayor Ledger sighs loudly. "They're going to attack here, you know," he says. "You'll have to let me out if that happens."

"Can't you keep quiet for five seconds?" I turn to the first page, the first entry my ma wrote on the day I was born. A page full of words I once heard read out.

(read out by–)

"No gun, no weapon." Mayor Ledger's standing now, looking out the windows again. "I'm defenceless."

"I'll take care of you," I say, "now *shut the hell up.*"

I'm still not turned to him. I'm looking at my ma's first words, the ones written in her hand. I know what they say but I try to sound them out across the page.

Muh-y. My. It's *My.* I take a deep breath. *Dee. Dee-arr. Dee-arr-ess. Dee-arr-ess-tuh.* Which is *Dearest*, which seems mostly right. *My Dearest.* And the last word is *Son*, which I know, having heard it so clearly today.

I think about his outstretched hand.

I think about when I took it.

My Dearest Son.

"I've offered to read that for you," Mayor Ledger says, not able to hide his groan at the sound of my reading Noise.

I turn round to him, looking fierce. "I said, *shut up!*"

He holds his hands up. "Fine, fine, whatever you say." He sits back down and adds a last sarcastic word under his breath. "*Lieutenant.*"

I sit up. Then I sit up higher. "What did you say?"

"Nothing." He won't meet my eye.

"I didn't tell you that," I say. "I didn't say a word."

"It was in your Noise."

I ain't been thinking bout nothing since I came in for dinner except my ma's book. "*How did you know?*"

He looks up at me but there ain't no words coming outta his mouth and his Noise is scrambling for something to say.

And it's failing.

I take a step towards him.

There's a *ker-thunk* at the door and Mr Collins lets himself in. "There's someone here for you," he says to me, then he notices my Noise. "What's going on?"

"I ain't expecting no one," I say, still staring at Mayor Ledger.

"It's a girl," Mr Collins says. "She says Davy sent her."

"Dammit," I say. "I *told* him."

"Whatever," he says. "Says she won't talk to no one but you." He chuckles. "Pretty little piece, too."

I turn at the tone of his voice. "Leave her alone, whoever she is. That ain't right."

"Best not take too long up here then." He's laughing as he shuts the door.

I stare back at Mayor Ledger, my Noise still high. "I ain't thru with you."

"It was in your *Noise*," he says, but I'm already out the door and locking it behind me. *Ker-thunk.*

I stomp my way down the stairs, thinking of ways to get the girl away without Mr Collins bothering her, without her having to go thru any of that for any reason, and my Noise is boiling with suspishuns and wonderings about Mayor Ledger and things beginning to come clear when I get to the bottom of the steps.

Mr Collins is waiting, leaning against the wall of the lobby with his legs crossed, all relaxed and smiling. He points with his thumb.

I look over.

And there she is.

34

LAST CHANCE

{VIOLA}

"LEAVE US," Todd says to the man who let me in, not looking away from me when he says it.

"*Told* you she was a piece," the man says, smirking as he disappears into a side office.

Todd stands there staring. "It's you," he says.

But he isn't moving towards me.

"Todd," I say and I take a step forward.

And he takes a step back.

I stop.

"Who's this?" he says, looking at Lee, who's doing his best to act like a real soldier behind me.

"That's Lee," I say. "A friend. He's come with me to–"

"What are you doing here?"

"I've come to get you," I say. "I've come to rescue you."

I see him swallow. I see his throat working. "Viola," he finally says. My name is all over his Noise, too. Viola Viola Viola.

He puts his hands up to the sides of his head, grabbing his hair, which is longer and shaggier than when I saw it last.

He looks taller, too.

"Viola," he says again.

"It's me," I say and I take another step forward. He doesn't step back so I keep coming, crossing the lobby, not running, just getting closer and closer to him.

But when I get to him, he steps back again.

"Todd?" I ask.

"What are you *doing* here?"

"I've come for you." I feel my stomach sink a little. "I said I would."

"You said you wouldn't leave without me," he says and in his Noise I can hear loud irritation at how he sounds. He clears his throat. "You *left* me here."

"They took me," I say. "I had no choice."

His Noise is getting louder now and though I can feel happiness in it–

Oh, Jesus, Todd, there's *rage*, too.

"What have I done?" I say. "We need to go. The Answer are going–"

"So yer part of the Answer now?" he snaps, bitterness suddenly rising. "Part of those *murderers*."

"Are you a soldier now then?" I say back, surprised, heat growing in my voice, too, pointing to the A on his sleeve. "Don't talk to me about *murder*."

"The Answer killed the Spackle," he says, his voice low and angry.

And the bodies of the Spackle in his Noise.

Piled high, one upon the other, tossed there like garbage.

And Todd in the middle of it.

"They might as well have killed me along with them," he says.

He closes his eyes.

I am the Circle and the Circle is me, I hear.

"Viola?" Lee says from behind me. I turn. He's crossed half the lobby.

"Wait outside," I say.

"Viola–"

"*Outside.*"

He looks so concerned, so ready to fight for me, my heart skips a little. He broadcast as loud as he could that I was his prisoner on the way here, so loud other soldiers thought he was covering up for a rape he was going to commit and whistled him good luck as we passed. Then we hid by the cathedral, seeing Davy Prentiss riding away from here, thinking things I wouldn't want to see again, thinking about how a *celebration* was due to him and Todd.

And so we pretended to be the celebration.

And it worked.

Kind of upsetting how easily it worked, frankly.

Lee shifts from foot to foot. "You call me if you need me."

"I will," I say, and he waits a second, then steps out the front door, keeping it open to watch us.

Todd's eyes are still closed and he repeats **I am the Circle and the Circle is me** which I have to say sounds an awful lot like something from the Mayor.

"We didn't kill the Spackle," I say.

"*We?*" he says, opening his eyes.

"I don't know who did it, but it wasn't us."

"You sent a bomb to kill them the day *you* blew up the tower." He's almost spitting the words. "Then you came back on the day of the prison break and finished the job."

"Bomb?" I say. "What bomb–?"

But then I remember–

The first explosion that made the soldiers run away from the communications tower.

No.

She wouldn't.

No, not even her. *What kind of people do you think we are?* she said–

But she never did answer the asking.

No, *no*, it's not true and besides–

"Who told you that?" I say. "Davy Prentiss?"

He blinks. "What?"

"What do you mean *what*?" My voice is harder now. "Your new best friend. The man who *shot* me, Todd, and who you ride to work with laughing every morning."

He clenches his hands into fists.

"You been *spying* on me?" he says. "Three months I don't see you, three months I don't hear *nothing* from you and you been *spying*? Is that what yer doing in yer spare time when yer not blowing people up?"

"Yeah!" I yell, my voice getting louder to match his. "Three months of defending you to people who'd be only too happy to call you enemy, Todd. Three months of wondering why the hell you're working so hard for the Mayor and how he knew to go right for the ocean the day after we spoke." He winces, but I keep going, thrusting out my arm and pulling

on women!"

His face changes in an instant. He actually calls out as if he felt the pain himself. He puts a hand over his mouth to stifle it but his Noise is suddenly washed with blackness. He moves the fingertips of his other hand within reach of the band, hovering over my skin, over the band that'll never be removed unless I lose my arm. The skin is still red, and band 1391 still throbs, despite the healing of three mistresses.

"Oh, no," he says. "Oh, no."

The side door opens and the man who let me in leans out. "Everything all right out here, Lieutenant?"

"Lieutenant?" I say.

"We're fine," Todd chokes a little. "We're fine."

The man waits for a second, then goes back inside.

"*Lieutenant?*" I say again, lowering my voice.

Todd's leant down, his hands on his knees, staring at the floor. "It wasn't me, was it?" he says, his voice quiet, too. "I didn't–" He gestures again at the band without looking up. "I didn't do it without knowing it was you, did I?"

"No," I say, reading things in his Noise, reading his numbness at them, reading all the horror that sits way down below that he's working so hard to ignore. "The Answer did it."

He looks up fast, filled with asking marks.

"It was the only way I could come and find you safely," I say. "The only way I could get past all the soldiers marching around town was if they thought I'd already been banded."

His face changes again as this sinks in. "Oh, Viola."

I breathe out heavily. "Todd," I say. "Please come with me."

His eyes are wet but I can see him now, I can see him finally, I can see him in his face and in his Noise and in his arms as they drop to his sides in defeat.

"It's too late," he says and his voice is so sad my own eyes start to wet. "I've been dead, Viola. I've been dead."

"You haven't," I say, moving a bit closer to him. "These are impossible times."

He's looking down now, his eyes not focused on anything.

Feeling nothing, his Noise says. Taking nothing in.

I am the Circle and the Circle is me.

"Todd?" I say and I'm close enough to reach his hand. "Todd, look at me."

He looks up and the loss in his Noise is so great it feels like I'm standing on the edge of an abyss, that I'm about to fall down *into* him, into blackness so empty and lonely there'd never be a way out.

"Todd," I say again, a catch in my voice. "On the ledge, under the waterfall, do you remember what you said to me? Do you remember what you said to save me?"

He's shaking his head slowly. "I've done terrible things, Viola. *Terrible* things–"

"*We all fall*, you said." I'm gripping him hard now. "We all fall but that's not what matters. What matters is picking yourself up again."

But he shakes me off.

"No," he says, turning away. "No, it was easier when you weren't here. It was easier when you couldn't see–"

"Todd, I've come to save you–"

"It's not too late."

"It *is* too late," he says, shaking his head. "It is!"

And he's moving away.

Away from me.

I'm losing him–

And I get an idea.

A dangerous, dangerous idea.

"The attack's coming tomorrow at sundown," I say.

He blinks again in surprise. "What?"

"That's when it happens." I swallow and step forward, trying to keep my voice steady. "I'm only supposed to know the fake plan, but I found out the real one. The Answer are coming over the hill with the notch in it just to the south of here, just to the south of this *cathedral*, Todd. They're coming right here and I'm sure they're coming right for the Mayor."

He looks nervously at the side door but I'm keeping my voice down. "There are only two hundred of them, Todd, but they're fully armed with guns and bombs and a plan and a hell of a leader who isn't going to stop until she topples him."

"Viola–"

"They're *coming*," I say, moving closer again. "And now you know when and from where and if that information gets to the Mayor–"

"You shouldn't have told me," he says, not meeting my eye. "I hide things but he figures them out. *You shouldn't have told me!*"

I keep moving forward. "Then you have to come with me, don't you? You *have* to or he wins for ever and ever and he'll be the one to rule this planet and he'll be the one who greets the new settlers–"

"With his hand outstretched," Todd says, his voice suddenly soft.

"What?"

But he just extends his hand out into the empty air, staring at it. "Greeting it with his son."

"Well, we don't want that either." I look nervously round to the front door. Lee is sticking his head in, trying not to look too out of place, but there are soldiers marching by out front. "We don't have much time."

Todd's hand is still outstretched.

"I've done bad things, too," I say. "I wish everything was different but it isn't. There's only now and here and you *have* to come with me if we have any chance of making this come out any good at all."

He doesn't say anything but his hand is still out and he's looking at it and so I move forward another step and I take it in my own.

"We can save the world," I say, trying to smile. "You and me."

He looks into my eyes, searching, trying to read me, trying to see if I'm actually here, if it's actually true, if the things I say are real, he searches and he searches–

But he doesn't find me.

Oh, Todd–

"Going somewhere?" says a voice from across the room.

A voice from a man holding a gun.

395

It's a different man from the one who let us in, a man I've never seen before.

Except once, in Todd's Noise.

"How did you get out?" Todd says, surprise rippling through him.

"You wouldn't leave without *this*, would you?" he says. In his non-gun hand, he's got the journal of Todd's mother.

"You *give* that to me!" Todd says.

The man ignores him and waves his gun at Lee. "Come inside now," he says. "Or I will ever so happily shoot our dear friend Todd."

I look back. Lee's got flight all over his Noise but he sees the gun pointed at Todd, sees my face, and comes forward, his Noise saying so loud that he won't leave me here that it almost distracts me from the gun.

"Drop it," the man says, referring to Lee's rifle. Lee sends it clattering to the floor.

"You liar," Todd says to the man. "You coward."

"For the good of the town, Todd," the man says.

"All that moaning," Todd says, his voice and Noise fiery. "All that bitching and moaning about how he's ruining everything and yer just another spy."

"Not at first," the man says, walking towards us. "At first I was just how you saw me, the former Mayor disgraced and left alive in all his inconvenience." The man passes Todd and comes up to me, putting Todd's book under one arm. "Give me your pack."

"What?" I say.

"Give it to me." He swings his arm back and points the gun right at Todd's head. I slide the pack off my shoulders and give it to him. He doesn't even open it the regular way, just feels along the bottom, feeling right for the secret pouch, the secret pouch where if you press right, you can feel my gun.

The man smiles. "There it is," he says. "The Answer don't change, do they?"

"You touch a hair on her head," Todd says, "and I'll kill you."

"So will I," Lee says.

The man keeps smiling. "I think you have a competitor, Todd."

"Who *are* you?" I say, annoyance at all this protection making me brave.

"Con Ledger, Mayor of Haven, at your service, Viola." He gives a little bow. "Since that's who you must be, isn't it?" He walks around Todd. "Oh, the President was very interested in the Noise of your dreams, my boy. *Very* interested in what you thought about while you were sleeping. About how much you miss your Viola, how you would do anything to find her."

I see Todd's face starting to glow red.

"And suddenly he became far more agreeable to me, asking me to pass along certain information to you, see if we could get you to do what he wanted." Mayor Ledger looks ridiculous, all the things he's carrying, a gun in one hand, pack in the other, book under his arm, and still trying to appear threatening. "I must say, it worked a treat." He winks at me. "Now that I know when and where the Answer are going to attack."

Lee's Noise rises and he takes a furious step forward.

"Like it?" asks the Mayor. "The President gave it to me when he gave me my own key."

He smiles again then sees how we're all looking at him. "Oh, stop it," he says. "If the President defeats the Answer then all this will be over. All the bombings, all the restrictions, all the curfews." His smile's a bit weaker now. "You have to learn how to work *within* the system for change. When *I'm* his deputy, I'll work very hard to make things better for everyone." He nods at me. "Women, too."

"You'd better shoot me," Todd says, Noise coming off him like flame. "Cuz there ain't no way yer life is safe if you ever put down that gun."

Mayor Ledger sighs. "I'm not going to shoot *anyone*, Todd, not unless–"

The side door suddenly opens and the man who let me in steps out, surprise lighting up his face and Noise. "What're you–"

Mayor Ledger points the gun at him and pulls the trigger three times. The man falls back into the doorway and all the way to the floor until only his feet are sticking out.

We all stand there, shocked, echoes of gunfire still ringing off the marble floors.

There's a clear picture in Mayor Ledger's Noise, of himself with a black eye and split lip, of the man on the floor giving him the beating.

He looks back at us, sees us staring at him. "*What*?"

"Mayor Prentiss ain't gonna like that," Todd says. "He knows Mr Collins from old Prentisstown."

"I'm sure the prize of Viola and the Answer's attack

will make up for any other misunderstandings." Mayor Ledger's looking around now, trying to find a place to free up his hands. He finally just tosses the book to Todd, as if he doesn't want it any more. Todd bobbles it in his hands but catches it.

"Your mother wasn't much of a writer, Todd," Mayor Ledger says, bending forward and zipping open the pack with his free hand. "Barely literate."

"You're going to pay for that." Todd looks back at me and I realize I'm the one who said it out loud.

Mayor Ledger digs around in my bag. "Food!" he says, his face lighting up. He takes out a crested pine from the top and immediately shoves it in his mouth. He digs some more, finding bread and more fruit, taking bites of almost everything. "How long were you planning on *staying*?" he asks, his mouth full.

I see Todd starting to edge forward.

"It's not like I can't hear you," Mayor Ledger says, waving the gun again, digging down to the bottom of the bag. He stops, his hand deep inside, and looks up. "What's this?" He feels around a little more and starts to drag something larger out of the pack. At first I assume it's the gun but then he shakes it free of the bag.

He stands up.

And looks curiously at the Thrace bomb in his hand.

There's a second where it can't be true. There's a second where my eyes can't be seeing what they're seeing, not believing that I know what a bomb looks like by now. There's

it doesn't mean anything at all.

But then Lee gasps beside me and it all makes sense, it all makes the worst goddam sense I can even think of.

"*No*," I say.

Todd spins around. "What? What is it?"

Time slows down to nothing. Mayor Ledger turns it over in his hand and a beeping starts, a fast beeping, a beeping obviously set to go whenever anyone searched through my bag and picked it up, the pulse in his hand setting it off, a bomb you know is going to kill you if you let go of it.

"This isn't–" says Mayor Ledger, looking up–
    But Lee is already reaching for my arm–
    Trying to grab it so we can bolt for the front door–
    "Run!" he's yelling–
    But I'm jumping forward, not back–
    And I'm pushing Todd sideways–
    Stumbling towards the room where the dead man fell–
    Mayor Ledger isn't trying to shoot us–
    Isn't doing anything–
    He's just standing there, realization dawning–
    And as we're falling through the doorway–

And rolling over the dead man–

And curling into each other for protection–

Mayor Ledger tries to throw the bomb away from himself–

Releasing it from his hand–

And–

BOOM

– it blasts him into a thousand pieces, tearing out the walls behind him and most of the room we're falling into and the heat from the explosion singes our clothes and our hair and rubble comes tumbling down and we force ourselves under a table but something hits Todd hard in the back of the head and a long beam falls across my ankles and I feel both of them break and all I can think as I yell out at the impossible pain is *she betrayed me she betrayed me she betrayed me* and it wasn't a mission to save Todd, it was a mission to *kill* him, and the Mayor, too, if she was lucky–

She betrayed me–

And then there's darkness.

Some time later, there are voices, voices in the dust and rubble, voices drifting into my pain-addled head.

One voice.

His voice.

Standing over me.

"Well, well," says the Mayor. "Look who we have here."

PART VI

THE ASK AND THE ANSWER

35

VIOLA IS ASKED

[TODD]

"LET HER GO!"

I pound my fists on the glass but no matter how hard I hit it, it ain't breaking.

"LET HER GO!"

My voice is cracking from the strain but I'll go and go till it gives out completely.

"YOU LAY A FINGER ON HER, I'LL KILL YOU!"

Viola is strapped to the frame in the Arena of the Ask, her arms back and up, the skin around the metal band burning red, her head twixt the little buzzing rods that keep her from hearing Noise.

The tub of water is below her, the table of sharp tools to her side.

Mr Hammar stands there waiting, arms crossed, and Davy, too, watching nervously from the far door, across the room.

And the Mayor is there, calmly walking round her in a circle.

All I remember is the *BOOM* and Mayor Ledger disappearing in a fury of fire and smoke.

I woke up here, my head aching, my body filthy from dirt and rubble and dried blood.

And I got to my feet.

And there she was.

Beyond the glass.

Being Asked.

I press the button again for the speaker in the room. "LET HER GO!"

But no one acts like they can hear me at all.

"I do this with the greatest reluctance, Viola," says the Mayor, still walking in his slow circle. I can hear *him* perfectly clear. "I thought we might be friends, you and I. I thought we had an understanding." He stops in front of her. "But then you blew up my home."

"I didn't know there was a bomb," she says and I can see the pain across her face. There's dried blood all over her, too, cuts and scratches from the explozhun.

But it's her feet that look the worst. Her shoes are off and her ankles are swollen and twisted and black and I just know the Mayor ain't given her nothing for the pain.

I can see it on her face.

See how much she's hurting.

I try to pull up the bench behind me so I can smash it thru the window but it's bolted into the concrete.

"I believe you, Viola," says the Mayor, re-starting his walk. Mr Hammar stands there smirking, watching it all, once in a while looking up to the mirror where he knows I'm standing and smirking some more. "I believe your dismay at your betrayal by Mistress Coyle. Though you can hardly be surprised."

Viola don't say nothing, just hangs her head.

"Don't hurt her," I whisper. "Please, please, please."

"If it helps," says the Mayor. "I'm not entirely sure I would take it personally. Mistress Coyle saw a way to get a bomb right into the heart of my cathedral, destroying it, perhaps destroying me in the process."

He glances up to me at the mirror. I pound my fists on it again. There's no way they can't hear *that* but he ignores me.

Davy looks over, tho, his face as serious as I've seen it.

And even from here I can hear the worry in his Noise.

"You presented her with an opportunity she couldn't pass up," the Mayor continues. "Your extreme loyalty to Todd might actually get you inside where any other bomber might not. She probably didn't wish to kill you, but there it was, a chance to take me down, and weighed up against that, you were finally expendable."

And I'm looking at her face.

It's pulled down sad, pulled down so sad and defeated.

And I feel her silence again, feel the yearning and the loss that I first felt out in the swamp a lifetime ago. I feel it so much my eyes get wet and my stomach tightens and my throat clenches.

"Viola," I say. "Please, Viola."

But she don't even look up.

407

leaning down in front of her now, looking into her face. "Then maybe you finally know who your real enemy is." He pauses. "And who your real friends are."

Viola says something real quiet.

"What was that?" the Mayor asks.

She clears her throat and says it again. "I only came for Todd."

"I know." The Mayor stands again and starts his walk. "I've grown fond of Todd, too. He's become like a second son to me." He looks over at Davy, whose face flushes. "Loyal and hardworking and truly making a contribution to the future of this town."

I start pounding my fists again. "YOU SHUT UP!" I scream. "YOU *SHUT UP!*"

"If *he's* with us, Viola," the Mayor says, "and your Mistress is against you, then surely your path is clear."

But she's already shaking her head. "I won't tell you," she says. "I won't tell you anything."

"But she betrayed you." The Mayor comes round to her front again. "She tried to kill you."

And at that, Viola lifts her head.

She looks him right in the eye.

And says, "No, she tried to kill *you.*"

Oh, good girl.

My Noise swells with pride.

That's my girl.

The Mayor gives a signal to Mr Hammar.

Who takes hold of the frame and plunges her into the water.

"NO!" I scream and start pounding again. "NO, GODDAMMIT!" I go to the door of the little room and start kicking it as hard as I can. "VIOLA! *VIOLA!*"

I hear a gasp and run back to the mirror–

She's up outta the water, coughing up liquid and spitting hard.

"We are running short on time," says the Mayor, picking a speck of lint off his coat, "so perhaps we should come right to it."

I'm still pounding on the mirror and shouting while he talks. He turns and looks over to me. He can't see me from his side but his eyes lock right on mine.

"VIOLA!" I scream and pound the glass again.

He's frowning a little–

"*VIOLA!*"

And he strikes me with his Noise.

It's *way* stronger than before.

Like a shout of a million people right in the middle of my brain, so far inside I can't reach it to protect myself and they're screaming YER NOTHING YER NOTHING YER NOTHING and it feels like my blood is boiling and my eyes are popping outta my skull and I can't even stand and I stagger back from the mirror and sit down hard on the bench, the slap ringing and ringing and ringing, like it ain't never gonna stop–

When I can open my eyes again, I see the Mayor stopping Davy from leaving the Arena and then Davy looking back towards the mirror.

And in his Noise he's worried.

409

"Tell me when the Answer is going to attack," the Mayor says to Viola, his voice colder now, harder. "And from where."

She shakes her head, sending water drops flying. "I won't."

"You will," says the Mayor. "I truly am afraid you will."

"No," she says. "Never."

And she's still shaking her head.

The Mayor glances up to the mirror, finding my eye again tho he can't see me. "Unfortunately," he says, "we don't have time for your refusals."

He nods at Mr Hammar.

Who plunges her into the water again.

"STOP!" I shout and pound. "STOP IT!"

He holds her there–

And holds her there–

I pound so hard my hands are bruising–

"LET HER UP! LET HER UP! LET HER UP!"

And she's thrashing in the water–

But he's still holding her there–

She's still under water–

"*VIOLA!*"

Her hands are pulling hard against the binds–

The water is splashing everywhere with her struggling against it–

Oh jesus oh jesus oh jesus oh jesus viola viola viola viola–

I can't–

I can't–

"NO!"

Forgive me–

Please forgive me–

"IT'S TONIGHT!" I shout. "AT SUNSET! OVER THE NOTCH IN THE HILL SOUTH OF THE CATHEDRAL! TONIGHT!"

And I'm pressing the button as I shout it again and again–

"TONIGHT!"

As she struggles under the water–

But no one looks like they hear me.

He's turned the sound off–

He's turned the *effing sound off*–

I go back to the window and pound–

But no one's moving–

And still she's underwater–

No matter how hard I slam my fists against the glass–

Why ain't it breaking–

Why ain't it ruddy *breaking*–

The Mayor gives a signal and Mr Hammar lifts up the frame. Viola swallows air in huge raking gulps, her hair (longer than I remember) stuck against her face, twisting in her ears, the water falling off her in great ropes.

"You're in control here, Viola," the Mayor says. "Just tell me when the Answer are attacking and this will all stop."

dried mud. "FROM THE SOUTH!"

But she's shaking her head.

And no one can hear me.

"But she betrayed you, Viola." The Mayor's making his voice do that fake surprised thing. "Why save her? Why–?"

He stops, as if realizing something. "You have people you care about in the Answer."

She stops shaking her head. She don't look up but she stops shaking her head.

The Mayor kneels down in front of her. "All the more reason to tell me. All the more reason to let me know where I can find your mistress." He reaches forward and pulls a few wet strands of hair away from Viola's face. "If you help me, I guarantee they won't be harmed. I only want Mistress Coyle. Any other mistresses can remain in prison and everyone else, innocent victims of inflamed rhetoric no doubt, can be released once we've had a chance to talk to them."

He gestures for Mr Hammar to hand him a towel which he uses to wipe Viola's face. She still don't look at him.

"If you tell me, you'd be saving lives," he says, gently sponging away the loose water. "You have my word on that."

She finally raises her head.

"Your word," she says, looking right past him at Mr Hammar.

And her face is so angry even *he* looks surprised.

"Ah, yes," the Mayor says, standing. He hands the towel back to Mr Hammar. "You should look upon Captain Hammar as an example of my mercy, Viola. I spared his life." He's walking again but when he passes behind her he looks over to me. "Just as I shall spare the lives of your friends and loved ones."

"It's tonight," I say, but my voice is a rasp.

How can he not hear me?

"Then again," he's saying, "if you don't know, perhaps your good friend Lee will tell us."

Her head goes right up, eyes wide, breath heavy.

I don't know how he coulda survived the explozhun–

"He doesn't know anything," she says quickly. "He doesn't know when or where."

"Even if I believed that," the Mayor says, "I'm sure we would have to Ask him long and hard before we could possibly be sure."

"Leave him alone!" Viola says, trying to turn her head to follow him.

The Mayor stops just in front of the mirror, his back to Viola, his face to me. "Or perhaps we should just ask Todd."

I pound the glass right at his face. He don't even flinch.

And then she says, "Todd would never tell you. Never."

And the Mayor just looks at me.

And he *smiles*.

My stomach sinks, my heart drops, my head feels so light I feel like I'm going to drop right to the ground.

Oh, Viola–

Viola, please–

Forgive me.

"Captain Hammar," the Mayor says and Viola's plunged

down she goes.

"NO!" I shout, pressing myself against the mirror.

But the Mayor ain't even looking at her.

He's looking right at me, as if he could see me even if I was behind a brick wall.

"STOP IT!" I shout as she's thrashing again–

And more–

And more–

"VIOLA!"

And I'm pounding even tho I think my hands are breaking–

And Mr Hammar is grinning and holding her there–

"*VIOLA!*"

And her wrists are starting to bleed from where she's pulling–

"I'LL KILL YOU!"

I'm shouting into the Mayor's face–

With all my Noise–

"I'LL *KILL* YOU!"–

And still holding her there–

"VIOLA! *VIOLA!*"–

But it's Davy–

Of all people–

It's Davy who stops it.

"Let her up!" he suddenly shouts, striding forward from his corner. "Jesus, yer gonna kill her!" And he's grabbing the frame and lifting it outta the water and the Mayor gives Mr

Hammar a sign to let him and Davy gets Viola back up and out, her throat roaring from taking in the air and coughing it right back out again with all the water.

No one says nothing for a minute, the Mayor just staring at his son like he was some new kinda fish.

"How can she help us if she's dead?" Davy says, his voice wobbly, his eyes not meeting no one's. "Is all I meant."

The Mayor stays quiet. Davy backs away from the frame and returns to his spot near the door.

Viola coughs and hangs from her bindings and I'm pressed so close against the window it's like I'm trying to crawl *thru* it to get to her.

"Well," the Mayor says, clasping his hands behind his back, looking at Davy. "I think perhaps we've learnt what we need to know anyway."

He walks over to a button on the wall and presses it. "Would you please repeat what you said earlier, Todd?"

Viola looks up at the sound of my name.

The Mayor walks back over to the frame, lifting up the little Noise-baffling rods from the sides of her face and she looks all around as she can suddenly hear my Noise.

"Todd?" she says. "Are you there?"

"I'm here!" I yell, my voice now booming thru the Arena so everyone can hear me.

"Please tell us again what you said a few moments ago, Todd." The Mayor's looking at me again. "Something about tonight at sunset?"

Viola looks up to where the Mayor's looking, surprise on her face, surprise and shock. "No," she whispers and it's as loud as any shouting.

Mayor says.

He knew. He could hear my Noise the whole time, *course* he could, he could hear my shouting, even if she couldn't.

"Viola?" I say and it sounds like I'm begging.

And she looks into the mirror, searching for where I might be. "Don't tell him!" she says. "Please, Todd, don't—"

"One more time, Todd," the Mayor says, putting his hand on the drowning frame, "or she goes back into the water."

"Todd, no!" Viola shouts.

"You bastard!" I yell. "I'll kill you. I swear it, I'll KILL YOU!"

"You won't," he says. "And we both know it."

"Todd, please, no—"

"Say it, Todd. Where and when?"

And he starts lowering the frame.

Viola's trying to look brave but her body is curling and twisting, trying to keep any part of it outta the water. "No!" she's yelling. "NO!"

Please please please—

"NO!"

Viola—

"Tonight at sunset," I say, my voice amplified over her shouts, over Davy's Noise, over my own Noise, just my voice filling everything. "Over the notch in the valley south of the cathedral."

"*NO!*" Viola screams—

And the look on her face—

The look on her face about *me*—

And my chest tears right in two.

416

* * *

The Mayor pulls back the frame, lifting her away from the water and setting her back down.

"No," she whispers.

And it's only then that she actually starts to cry.

"Thank you, Todd," the Mayor says. He turns to Mr Hammar. "You know where and when, Captain. Pass on the orders to Captains Morgan, Tate and O'Hare."

Mr Hammar stands to attenshun. "Yes, sir," he says, sounding like he just won a prize. "I'll take every single man, sir. They won't know what hit 'em."

"Take my son," the Mayor says, nodding at Davy. "Let him see all the battle he can stomach."

Davy's looking nervous but proud and excited, too, not noticing the odd twist Mr Hammar's smile has taken.

"Go," the Mayor says, "and leave none alive."

"Yes, *sir*," Mr Hammar says as Viola lets out a little sob.

Davy snaps a salute at his father, trying to make his Noise look brave. He sends the mirror a look meant for me, a look of sympathy, his Noise full of fear and excitement and more fear.

Then he's following Mr Hammar out the door.

And then there's just me, Viola and the Mayor.

I can only look at her, hanging from the frame, her head down, crying, still tied up and soaking wet and so much sorrow coming from her I can practically feel it on my skin.

"Tend to your friend," the Mayor says to me, just on the other side of the glass again, his face close to mine. "I return to my burnt-out home to prepare for the new dawn."

blink, don't even act like nothing's even happened.

He ain't human.

"All too human, Todd," he says. "The guards will escort both of you to the cathedral." He raises his eyebrows. "We have much to discuss about your futures."

36

DEFEAT

(VIOLA)

I HEAR TODD come into the room, hear his Noise come first, but I can't look up.

"Viola?" he says.

I still don't look up.

It's over.

We've lost.

I feel his hands on the binds at my wrists, pulling at them, finally getting one free, but my arm is so stiff from being held back it hurts more when it's released than it did when it was bound.

Mayor Prentiss has won. Mistress Coyle tried to sacrifice me. Lee's a prisoner if that wasn't a lie and he's not already dead. Maddy died for nothing. Corinne died for *nothing*.

And Todd–

He comes around in front of me to take off the second bind and when it's loose and I fall from the frame, he catches me, kneeling us gently down to the floor.

against his chest, the water on me soaking into his dusty uniform, my arms out, not able to grab anything, the metal band throbbing.

And I glance up to see the shiny silver *A* on his shoulder.

"Let me go," I say.

But he still holds me there.

"Let me *go*," I say, louder.

"No," he says.

I try to push him away but my arms are so weak and I'm so tired and everything is over. Everything is over.

And still he holds me.

And I start to cry again and I feel him hold me tighter and I cry harder and when my arms can move a little I put them around him and cry even harder because of how he feels and how he smells and how his Noise sounds and how he's holding me and his worry and his fretting and his care and his softness–

And I didn't know until just now how much I missed him.

But he told the Mayor–

He *told* him–

And I have to try and push him away again, even though I can hardly bear to do it.

"You told him," I say, choking it out.

"I'm sorry," he says, his eyes wide and terrified. "He was drowning you and I couldn't, I just couldn't–"

And I look at him and there I am in his Noise, dropping down into the water with him pounding on the other side of the mirror and worse, I can see what he felt, see the hopeless *rage* of it, see him unable to save me–

And his face is so worried.

"Viola, please," he says, begging me. "*Please.*"

"He'll kill them," I say. "Every one of them. Wilf is there, Todd. *Wilf.*"

He looks horrified. "Wilf?"

"And Jane," I say. "And so many others, Todd, *all* of them. He'll slaughter them and that'll be the end. That'll be the end of *everything.*"

His Noise goes black and barren and he sort of crumples down next to me, splashing in the little puddle that's formed around us. "No," he says. "Aw, no."

I don't want to say it but I hear my voice saying it anyway. "You did exactly what he wanted. He knew exactly how to get it out of you."

He looks at me. "What choice did I have?"

"You should have let him kill me!"

And he's looking at me and I can see his Noise trying to find me, trying to find the real Viola that's deep down in this mess and pain, I can see him looking–

And for a minute I don't want him to find me.

"You should have let him kill me," I say again quietly.

But he couldn't, could he?

He couldn't and still be himself.

He couldn't and still be Todd Hewitt.

The boy who can't kill.

The *man* who can't.

We are the choices we make.

"We have to warn them," I say, feeling ashamed and not looking into his eyes. "If we can." I grab the edge of the tub of water to pull myself up. Pain shoots up my legs from my ankles. I call out and fall forward again.

And once more, he catches me.

"My feet," I say. We look at them, bare and swollen badly, turning ugly shades of blue and black.

"We'll get you to a healer." He puts an arm around me to lift me.

"No," I say, stopping him. "We have to warn the Answer. That's the most important thing."

"Viola—"

"Their lives are more important than my—"

"She tried to *kill* you, Viola. She tried to blow you up."

I'm breathing hard, trying not to feel the pain from my legs.

"You don't owe her nothing," he says.

But I feel his arms on me and I'm realizing things don't seem so impossible any more. I feel Todd touching me and there's anger rising in my gut but it's not at him and I grunt and I pull myself up again, leaning on him to keep me there as I stand. "I *do* owe her," I say. "I owe her the look on her face when she sees me alive."

I try to take a small step but it's too much. I cry out again.

"I have a horse," he says. "I can put you on her."

"He's not just going to let us leave," I say. "He said guards would escort us back to him."

"Yeah," he says. "We'll see about *that*."

He puts his arm further around me and leans down to put his other arm under my knees.

And he lifts me in the air.

The pull on my ankles makes me cry out again but then he's holding me up, carrying me like he did down the hillside into Haven.

Holding me up.

He remembers it, too. I can see it in his Noise.

I put my arm around his neck. He tries to smile.

And it's crooked like it always is.

"We just keep on having to save each other," he says. "We ever gonna be even?"

"I hope not," I say.

He frowns again and I see the clouds roiling in his Noise. "I'm sorry," he says quietly.

I grab the cloth of his shirt front and squeeze it tight. "I'm sorry, too."

"So we forgive each other?" The crooked smile climbs up one more time. "Again?"

And I look right into his eyes, right into him as far as I can see, because I want him to hear me, I want him to hear me with everything I mean and feel and say.

"Always," I say to him. "Every time."

He carries me to a chair and then goes over to the door and starts pounding on it. "Let us out!" he shouts.

"This does mean something, Todd," I say, taking as little breath as possible because my feet are throbbing. "Something we have to remember."

"What's that?" He pounds on the door again and says "ow" quietly with how it's hurting his hands.

"The Mayor knows I'm your weakness," I say. "All he has to do is threaten me and you'll do what he wants."

"Yeah," Todd says, not looking back. "Yeah, I knew that already."

"He'll keep trying it."

He turns around to face me, fists clenched at his sides. "He won't be laying his eyes on you. Not never again."

"No." I shake my head and wince at the pain. "It can't be that way, Todd. He has to be stopped."

"Well, why's it have to be *us* that stops him?"

"It's got to be somebody." I arch my back a certain way to keep any weight off my feet. "He can't win."

Todd starts kicking at the door. "Then let yer Mistress do it. We'll get to her somehow, warn 'em if we can, and then we're outta here."

"Out of here where?"

"I don't know." He starts looking around for something that might knock down the door. "We'll go to one of the abandoned settlements. We'll hide out till yer ships get here."

"He'll beat Mistress Coyle and then he'll go right for the ships." I gasp a little as I turn my head to follow him. "There's only a small number of people awake when they land, Todd. He can overpower them and keep everyone else asleep as long as he wants. He doesn't ever have to wake them up if he doesn't want to."

He stops his search. "Is that true?"

I nod. "Once he destroys the Answer, who's left to stop him?"

He clenches and unclenches his fists again. "We have to do it."

"We find the Answer first," I say, trying to pull myself upright. "We warn them–"

"And tell 'em exactly what kinda leader they got."

I sigh. "We're going to have to stop both of them, aren't we?"

"Well, that's easy, ain't it?" Todd says. "We tell the Answer all about yer mistress and then someone new will lead 'em." He looks at me. "Maybe you."

"Maybe *you*." I take a minute to try and catch my breath. It's getting harder. "Either way, we have to get out of here."

And then the door suddenly opens.

A soldier stands there with a rifle.

"I have orders to take you both to the cathedral," he says.

And I think I recognize him.

"Ivan," Todd says.

"Lieutenant," Ivan nods. "I've got my orders."

"You're from Farbranch," I say, but he's staring at Todd, not blinking. I can hear something in his Noise, something–

"*Lieutenant*," he says again in a way that seems like some kind of signal.

I look at Todd. "What's he doing?"

"You have orders," Todd says, concentrating on Ivan. I can hear stuff flying between their Noises, fast and blurry. "*Private* Farrow."

"Yes, sir," Ivan says, standing at attention. "Orders from my superior officer."

425

"What's going on?" I say.

I see Lee rise in Todd's Noise. He turns back to Ivan. "Is there another prisoner? A boy? Blond shaggy hair?"

"There is, sir," Ivan says.

"And if I ordered you to take me to him, you'd do it?"

"You *are* my superior officer, *Lieutenant*." Ivan's looking harder at Todd now. "I'd have to follow any orders you gave me."

"Todd?" I say, but I'm beginning to understand.

"I've been a-trying to tell you this for some time, Lieutenant," Ivan says, impatience in his voice.

"Are there any higher ranking officers on the premises than me?" Todd asks.

"No, sir. Just myself and the guards. Everyone else has gone off to fight the war."

"How many guards?"

"Sixteen of us, sir."

Todd licks his lips, thinking. "Would they regard me as their superior officer, too, Private?"

Ivan looks away for the first time, glancing quickly behind him before saying again in a lower voice, "There is some concern with our current leadership, sir. They might be persuaded."

Todd stands up straighter, pulling at the hem of his uniform jacket. I notice again how tall he is, how much taller than the last time I saw him, how his face is lined in a way that's not at all boyish, how his voice is deeper and fuller.

I look at him, and I begin to see a man.

He clears his throat and stands at attention before Ivan.

426

"Then I order you to take me to the prisoner called Lee, Private."

"Even though I have been instructed to take you straight to the President," Ivan says in an official voice, "I feel I cannot disobey your direct order, *sir*."

He steps back out of the door to wait. Todd comes to my chair and kneels down in front of me.

"What are you planning?" I ask, trying to read his Noise, but it's spinning so fast I can hardly keep up with it.

"You said it's us who has to stop him cuz no one else will," he says, the crooked smile inching higher. "Well, maybe there's a way we can."

37

THE LIEUTENANT

[TODD]

I FEEL VIOLA WATCHING ME as I leave and follow Ivan down the hallway. She's wondering whether we can trust him.

I wonder it, too.

Cuz the answer's no, ain't it? Ivan joined the army as a volunteer, saving his own skin in Farbranch, and I remember him slinking up to me all those months ago even before it happened and telling me he was on the side of Prentisstown. He probably couldn't wait to join the army when it marched into town and then he led troops here and was even a Corporal.

Till Mayor Prentiss shot him in the leg.

You go where the power is, he said to me once. *That's how you stay alive.*

So maybe he thinks he's found the new power.

"Exactly what I'm a-thinking, *sir*," Ivan says, stopping outside a door. "He's in here."

"Can he walk?" I say as Ivan unlocks the door–

But Lee's already jumping out with an *AAAAAAAAHHHHHHHH!!!* and knocking Ivan over and punching him again and again in the face and I have to grab his shoulders and pull him back and he turns to me fists ready till he sees who it is.

"Todd!" he says, surprised.

"We need–" I start.

"Where is she?" he shouts, already looking round, and I have to step forward to keep Ivan from smashing the back of his head with a rifle.

"She's hurt," I say. "She needs bandages and splints." I turn to Ivan. "You got those here?"

"We got a first aid kit," Ivan says.

"That'll do. Give it to Lee and he'll take care of Viola. Then tell the men I wanna talk to 'em out front."

Ivan's glaring at Lee, Noise blaring.

"That's an order, *Private*," I say.

"Yes, *sir*," Ivan says, all sour, before he disappears down the hallway.

Lee goggles at me. "*Yes, sir?*"

"Viola'll explain." I push him after Ivan. "You get those bandages on her! She's hurting!"

That gets him moving. I turn about face and go towards the lobby. Two guards watch me walk past. "What's going on?" one of 'em asks.

"What's going on, *sir*," I snap without turning round. I walk out the front door of the Office of the Ask, down the little path and out the front gate.

Where it's almost peaceful.

Davy musta brought her.

"Hey, girl," I say, coming up on her slow, rubbing her nose. **Boy colt?** says her Noise. **Todd?**

"It's all right, girl," I whisper. "It's all right."

Hurt, she says, sniffing at the dried blood still on my face. She takes her big wet tongue and gives me the sloppiest lick right across my mouth and cheek.

I laugh a little and rub her nose again. "I'm okay, girl, I'm okay."

Her Noise keeps saying my name, **Todd Todd**, as I move to where my bag is still tied to the saddle. My rifle's still there.

So's my ma's book.

I'll bet Davy brought that, too.

I untie Angharrad's reins from the post and lead her out onto the road a little bit till she's pointing right at the gate with the big silver *A*. "Gotta give a little speech," I say, tightening the saddle. "Better from up top of you."

Boy colt, she says. **Todd**.

"Angharrad," I say.

I put my foot in a stirrup, hop up and swing my leg round till I'm sitting in the saddle, looking up at the sky. It's not darkening yet but the sun's getting down towards the falls. Afternoon is ticking away.

There ain't much time.

"Wish me luck," I say.

"Forward," Angharrad whinnies. "Forward."

* * *

The guards look up at me and back to Ivan who's trying to get 'em to stop talking, which would only help if they shut up the clatter of their Noise, too, cuz it's wailing like sheep on fire.

"He's a *lieutenant*," Ivan's saying to 'em.

"He's a *boy*," another guard says, one with ginger hair.

"He's the *President's* boy," Ivan responds.

"Yeah, and you were sposed to take him into town, Private," says another with a big pot belly and Corporal stripes on his sleeve. "Don't tell me yer disobeying a direct order."

"The Lieutenant gave me a different direct order," Ivan says.

"And he overrules the President, does he?" says Ginger Hair.

"Come on!" Ivan shouts. "How many of you got this assignment as punishment for something?"

That quiets 'em.

"Yer an idiot if you think I'm following a boy to face the President," says Corporal Pot Belly.

"Prentiss *knows* stuff," says Ginger Hair. "Stuff he shouldn't."

"He'd have us shot," says another soldier, a tall one this time, with sallow skin.

"By who?" says Ivan. "The army's all off fighting the war while the President sits in his blown-up cathedral a-waiting for me to show up with Todd here."

"What's he doing there?" asks Ginger Hair. "Why ain't he with the army?"

"Ain't his style," I say. They all look up at me again. "The

431

triggers and he don't get his hands dirty." Angharrad feels my nervousness and steps a little to one side. "He gets other people to do it for him."

Plus, I try to hide in my Noise, *he wants to talk to me*.

Which in a way feels worse than war.

"And yer gonna overthrow him, are ya?" asks the Corporal, crossing his arms.

"He's just a man," I say. "A man can be defeated."

"He's more'n a man," Ginger Hair says. "People say he uses his Noise as a weapon."

"And if you get too close to him, he can control your mind," says Sallow Skin.

Ivan scoffs. "That's all just grandmothers' tales. He can't do nothing of the sort–"

"Yes, he can," I say, and once again, all eyes turn on me. "He can hit you with his Noise and it hurts like hell. He can look into yer mind and try to force you to do and say the stuff he wants. Yeah, he can do all that."

They're staring at me now, wondering when I'm gonna get to the part that's helpful.

"But I think he's gotta make eye contact to do it–"

"You *think*?" says Ginger Hair.

"And the Noise hit ain't fatal and he can only do it to one person at a time. He can't beat all of us, not if we all come at once."

But I'm also hiding in my Noise how much stronger it was when he hit me in the Arena just now, how much more potent.

He's been working on it, sharpening his weapons.

"Don't matter," says Sallow Skin. "He'll have his own guards. We'd be walking right into our deaths."

"He'll be expecting you to escort me," I say. "We can walk right past the guards to where he's waiting."

"And why should we follow you, *Lieutenant*?" asks the Corporal, getting sarcastic on my rank. "What's in it for us?"

"Freedom from tyranny!" Ivan says.

The Corporal rolls his eyes. He ain't the only one.

Ivan tries again. "Because as soon as he's gone, *we* take over."

Less eye-rolling this time, but Sallow Skin says, "Anyone wanna be ruled by President Ivan Farrow?"

He says it to get a laugh but it don't get any.

"What about President Hewitt?" Ivan says, looking up at me with a weird glint in his eye.

Corporal Pot Belly scoffs and says again, "He's a *boy*."

"I'm not," I say. "Not no more."

"He's the only one a-willing to go after the President," Ivan says. "That speaks for *something*."

The guards look from one to another. I can hear all the askings in their Noise, all the doubts rattling around, all the fears confirming one another, and in their Noise I hear the idea being defeated.

But in their Noise I also hear how it can be saved.

"If you help me," I say, "I'll get you the cure."

They all shut right up.

"You can do that?" Ginger Hair asks.

"Naw," says the Corporal. "He's bluffing."

"It's stockpiled in the cellars of the cathedral," I say. "I saw the Mayor put it there himself."

asks.

"You come with me," I say. "You help me take him prisoner and every man here gets all the cure he can carry." They're listening to me now. "It's about ruddy time Haven became Haven again."

"He's taken it from the entire army," Ivan says. "We bring down the President, give 'em the cure, and who do you think they'll start a-listening to?"

"It won't be you, Ivan."

"No," says Ivan, giving me that look again. "But it could be *him*."

The men look up at me, up on top of Angharrad, with my rifle and my dusty uniform and my idea and my promises and there's a rustle thru their Noise as each man asks himself, is he desperate enough to take the chance?

I think of Viola, sitting in the Arena, sitting there as everything I want to save, everything I'd do anything for.

I think of her and I know exactly how to convince 'em.

"All the women are banded," I say. "Who do you think's gonna be next?"

Lee's pulling the last bandages round Viola's feet when I come back in and her face is looking way less pained.

"Can you stand?" I ask.

"Only a little."

"Don't matter," I say. "Angharrad's outside. She'll take you and Lee to find the Answer."

"What about you?" Viola says, sitting up.

434

"I'm gonna face him," I say. "I'm gonna take him down."

She *really* sits up at that.

"I'm coming with you," Lee says instantly.

"No, yer not," I say. "Yer telling the Answer to call off their attack *and* yer telling them just how Mistress Coyle works."

Lee's mouth sets firm but I can see his Noise roiling in anger over the bomb. He woulda died, too. "Viola says you can't kill."

I send her a dirty look. She's got the good grace to look away.

"I'm gonna kill him," Lee says. "I'm gonna kill him for what he did to my sister and mother."

"If you don't warn the Answer," I say, "there'll be a lot more dead people to make him pay for."

"He can *have* Mistress Coyle," Lee says but I can already see other people churning in his Noise, Wilf and Jane and other men and other women and Viola and Viola and Viola and Viola.

"What are you going to do, Todd?" she asks. "You can't just face him one on one."

"It won't be one on one," I say. "I got some of the guards to come with me."

Her eyes open wide. "You *what*?"

I smile. "Got me a little mutiny going."

"How many?" Lee asks, his face still serious.

I hesitate. "Seven," I say. "I couldn't get 'em all to agree."

Viola's face drops. "You're going to fight the Mayor with seven men?"

435

their final battle. The Mayor's *waiting* for me. It's the least guarded he's ever gonna be."

She watches me for a second, then she puts one hand on Lee's shoulder and one hand on mine and lifts herself to her feet. I can see her catch herself at the pain but Lee's wound the bandages tight and even if they ain't bone-fixers then at least they let her stand for a second or two.

"I'm coming with you," she says.

"No, yer not," I say at the same time as Lee yells, "Not a chance!"

She sets her jaw. "And what makes either of you think you have a say in the matter?"

"You can't walk," I say.

"You have a horse," she says.

"It's yer chance to get *safe*," I say.

"He's expecting *both* of us, Todd. You walk in there without me, your plan is over before you even speak."

I put my hands on my hips. "You said yerself the Mayor will use you against me if he gets the chance."

She kisses her teeth as she tests the weight on her ankle. "Then your plan had better work, hadn't it?"

"Viola—" Lee starts but she stops him with a look.

"Find the Answer, Lee. Warn them. You haven't got much time."

"But—"

"*Go*," she says again, more firmly.

And we both see her rise in his Noise, we both *feel* how much he don't wanna leave her. It's so strong, I have to look away from him.

436

But it sorta makes me wanna hit him, too.

"I'm not leaving Todd," she says. "Not now I've found him again. I'm sorry, Lee, but that's the way it is."

Lee takes a step back, unable to keep the hurt outta his Noise. Viola's voice softens. "I'm sorry," she says again.

"Viola–" Lee says.

But she's shaking her head. "The Mayor thinks he knows everything. He thinks he knows what's coming. He's just sitting there *waiting* for me and Todd to show up and try and stop him."

Lee tries to interrupt but she don't let him.

"But what he's forgetting," she says. "What he's forgetting is that me and Todd, we ran halfway across this planet together, by *ourselves*. We beat his craziest preacher. We outran an entire army and survived being shot and beaten and chased and we bloody well *stayed alive* this whole time without being blown up or tortured to death or dying in battle or anything."

She takes her hand off Lee so she's balancing just against me.

"Me and Todd? Together against the Mayor?" She smiles. "He doesn't stand a chance."

38

MARCH TO THE CATHEDRAL

{VIOLA}

"DID YOU MEAN what you said in there?" Todd says, pulling the strap on the saddle. His voice is low and he's keeping his eyes on the horse work. "Bout him not standing a chance against us?"

I shrug. "It helped, didn't it?"

He smiles to himself. "I gotta go talk to the men." He nods over to Lee, standing away from us, hands in his pockets, watching us chat. "You try and make this easy on him, okay?"

He gives Lee a wave and goes to where our escort of seven soldiers stands huddled by the big stone gate. Lee comes over.

"Are you sure about this?" he says.

"No," I say, "but I'm sure of Todd."

He breathes out through his nose, looking at the ground, trying to keep his Noise flat. "You love him," he says. Not an asking, just a fact.

"I do," I say. Also a fact.

"In *that* way?"

We both look over at Todd. He's gesturing with his arms and telling the men what we're planning and what they should do.

He's looking like a leader.

"Viola?" Lee asks.

I turn back to him. "You need to find the Answer before the army does, Lee, if you can at all."

He frowns. "They may not believe me about Mistress Coyle. A lot of people need her to be right."

"Well," I say, gently taking up the reins of the horse. **BQy Colt?** she thinks, watching Todd, too. "Think of it this way. If you can reach them and we can take care of the Mayor, this could all be over today."

Lee squints into the sun. "And if you don't take care of him?"

I try to smile. "Well, then, you're just going to have to come rescue us, aren't you?"

He tries to smile back.

"We're ready," Todd says, coming back over.

"This is it," I say.

Todd holds out his hand to Lee. "Good luck."

Lee takes his hand. "And to you," he says.

But he's looking at me.

After Lee's set off into the woods, running to scale the hills and intercept the Answer before the army does, the rest of us start our march down the road. Todd leads Angharrad, who keeps saying **BQy Colt** over and over again in her Noise, nervous at someone new on her back. Todd murmurs things keep her calm, rubbing her nose and petting her flank as we go.

"How do you feel?" he asks me as we approach the first set of dormitories.

"My feet hurt," I say. "My head, too." I rub my hand on my sleeve where the band is hiding. "And my arm."

"Other than that?" He smiles.

I look at the guards around us, marching in formation, as if they really are escorting me and Todd to the Mayor as ordered: Ivan and another in front, two behind, two to my right and the last to my left.

"Do you believe we can beat him?" I ask Todd.

"Well," he says and laughs, low, "we're going, ain't we?"

We're going.

Up the road and into New Prentisstown.

"Let's pick it up," Todd says, a bit louder.

The men pick up the pace.

"It's deserted," whispers the guard with flaming red hair as we pass through areas with more and more buildings.

Buildings but no people.

"Not deserted," another guard says, one with a big belly poking out in front of him. "In hiding."

"It's spooky without the army," the red-haired one says. "Without soldiers marching up and down the street."

"*We're* marching, Private," Ivan says. "We're soldiers, too."

We pass houses with shutters closed tight, store fronts with locked shutters, roads with no carts or fissionbikes or even people walking. You can hear the ROAR from behind closed doors but it's half the volume.

And it's *scared*.

"They know it's coming," Todd says. "They know this could be the war they've been waiting for."

I look around from atop Angharrad. No homes have any lights on, no faces peep out of windows, no one even curious as to what this band of guards is doing around a horse carrying a girl with bandaged feet.

And then the road bends and there's the cathedral.

"Holy moly," says the red-haired guard, as we come to a stop.

"You lived through *that*?" the pot belly says to Todd. He whistles in appreciation. "Maybe you *are* a bit blessed."

The bell tower still stands, though it's hard to see how, teetering on top of an unsteady ladder of bricks. Two walls of the main building stand, too, including the one with the coloured glass circle.

But the rest of it.

The rest of it's just a pile of stone and dust.

Even from behind, you can see that most of the roof has caved in and the largest parts of two walls have been blown out onto the road and the square in front of it. Arches lean dangerously out of balance, doors are twisted off their hinges, and most of the inside lies open to the world, receiving the last of the sun as it heads down to the horizon.

And there's not one soldier guarding it.

"He's unprotected?" says the red-haired one.

"That sounds like something he'd do," Todd says, staring at the cathedral as if he can see the Mayor somewhere through the walls.

"He is," Todd says. "Trust me."

The red-haired soldier starts backing away down the road. "No way," he says. "We're walking to our deaths here, boys. No way."

And with a final frightened look, he takes off running back the way we came.

Todd sighs. "Anyone else?" The men look to each other, their Noises wondering why they came in the first place.

"He'll put the band on you," Ivan says. He nods up at me. I pull up my sleeve and show them. The skin is still red and hot to the touch. Infection, I think. The first aid creams aren't doing what they're supposed to.

"And then he'll enslave you," Ivan continues. "I don't know about you, but that's not why I joined the army."

"Why *did* you join?" asks another guard but it's clear he doesn't want an answer.

"We take him down," Ivan says. "And we're heroes."

"Heroes with the cure," says the pot belly, nodding. "And he who controls the cure–"

"Enough talking," Todd says and I hear the discomfort in his Noise about how this is going. "Are we gonna do this or not?"

The men look to one another.

And Todd raises his voice.

Raises it so it commands.

Raises it so even *I* look at him.

"I said, are we *ready*?"

"Yes, sir," the men say, seeming almost surprised to hear it coming out of their mouths.

"Then let's go," Todd says.

And the men start marching again, *step step step*, crunching through the loose gravel scattered across the road, down a small slope, through the town and towards the cathedral, getting bigger and bigger the closer we get.

We file past some trees and I look to our left, to the hills on the southern horizon.

"Sweet Jesus," Pot Belly says.

Even from here you can see the army marching in the distance, a single black arm twisting up a path too narrow for them, up to the summit of the hill with the notch on top, up to where they'll meet The Answer.

I look at the setting sun.

"Maybe an hour," Todd says, seeing me check. "Probably less."

"Lee won't get to them in time," I say.

"He might. There must be short cuts."

The snake of the army slithers up the hillside. So many there's no way the Answer will be able to fight them if it comes to open battle.

"We can't fail," I say.

"We won't," Todd says.

And we reach the cathedral.

We march up the side. This is where most of the damage is, the whole north wall having collapsed straight onto the road.

"Remember," Todd murmurs to the men, as we climb over rubble. "Yer taking two prisoners to see the President like you

443

that."

We pick our way down the road. The pile of stones is so high you can't see into the cathedral. The Mayor could be in there anywhere.

We come around the corner to where the front used to be, now just a gaping hole into the vast lobby and sanctuary, still watched over by the bell tower and by that circle of coloured glass. The sun, behind us, shines right into it. Open rooms hang from upper walls, their floors crumbling. Half a dozen redbirds pick through the remains of food and worse in amongst the stones. The rest of the structure leans in on itself, like it's grown suddenly tired and might fall down to rest at any time.

And inside its shell–

"No one," Ivan says.

"That's why there aren't any guards," says Pot Belly. "He's with the army."

"He's not," Todd says, looking around, frowning.

"Todd?" I ask, sensing something–

"He told us *himself* to bring Todd here," Ivan says.

"Then where is he?" asks Pot Belly.

"Oh, I'm here," says the Mayor, stepping out of a shadow that shouldn't have been able to hide him, almost seeming to step straight out of the brick, out of a shimmer where he couldn't be seen.

"What the devil–?" says Pot Belly, stepping back.

"Not the Devil," the Mayor says, taking his first steps down the rubble towards us, his hands open at his sides. The guards all raise their rifles at him. He doesn't even look like he's armed.

But here he comes.

"No, not the Devil," he says, smiling. "Much worse than that."

"Stop where you are," Todd says. "There are men here who would happily shoot you."

"I know it," the Mayor says, stopping on the bottom step of the cathedral entrance, resting one foot on a large stone toppled there. "Private Farrow, for example." He nods at Ivan. "Still seething for being punished for his own incompetence."

"You shut your mouth," Ivan says, looking down the barrel of his rifle.

"Don't look into his eyes," Todd says quickly. "Nobody look into his eyes."

The Mayor slowly puts his hands in the air. "Am I to be your prisoner then?" He takes a look around at the soldiers, at all the guns pointed at him. "Ah, yes, I see," he says. "You have a plan. Returning the cure to the people, capitalizing on their resentment to install yourselves in power. Yes, *very* clever."

"That ain't how it's gonna be," Todd says. "Yer gonna call off the army. Yer gonna let everyone be free again."

The Mayor puts a hand to his chin like he's thinking about it. "The thing is, Todd," he says, "people don't really *want* freedom, no matter how much they might bleat on about it. No, I should think what will happen is that the army will crush the Answer, that the soldiers accompanying you will be put to death for treason, and that you and I and Viola will have that little chat about your future I promised."

do you?"

"Yer our prisoner and that's the end of it," Todd says, taking out a length of rope from Angharrad's saddle bag. "We'll just have to see how the army reacts to that."

"Very well," the Mayor says, sounding almost cheerful. "But I should send one of your men to the cellar so you can start taking the cure immediately. I can read all your plans perfectly clearly, and you wouldn't want that."

Pot Belly looks back. Todd nods at him and Pot Belly jogs on up the steps past the Mayor. "Just back and down," the Mayor points. "The way's quite clear."

Todd takes the rope and walks towards the Mayor, moving past the guns pointed at him. My hands are sweating into the reins.

It can't be this easy.

It can't–

The Mayor holds out his wrists and Todd hesitates, not wanting to actually get near him. "He tries anything funny," Todd says, without looking back. "Shoot him."

"Gladly," Ivan says.

Todd reaches forward and starts winding the rope around the Mayor's wrists.

We hear footsteps in the cathedral. Pot Belly comes jogging back, out of breath, his Noise a storm.

"You said it was in the cellar, *Lieutenant*."

"It is," Todd says. "I saw it there."

Pot Belly shakes his head. "Empty. Completely empty."

Todd looks back at the Mayor. "Then you moved it. Where is it?"

"Or what?" the Mayor says. "You'll shoot me?"

"I'd actually *prefer* that option," Ivan says.

"*Where did you move it?*" Todd says again, his voice strong, angry.

The Mayor looks at him, then looks around at all the men, and finally looks up to me on horseback.

"It was you I was worried about," he says. "But you can hardly walk, can you?"

"Don't you look at her," Todd spits, stepping closer to him. "You keep yer filthy eyes *off* her."

The Mayor smiles again, his hands still out, loosely bound by rope. "Very well," he says. "I'll tell you."

He looks around at everyone again, still smiling.

"I burnt it," says the Mayor. "After the Spackle sadly left us, there was no more need and so I burnt every last pill, every last plant that the pills were made from, and then I blew up the processing lab and blamed it on the Answer."

There's a shocked silence. We can hear the ROAR of the army in the distance, marching up that hill, keeping on towards their goal.

"You're a *liar*," Ivan finally says, stepping forward, gun still raised. "And a stupid one, at that."

"We can't hear yer Noise," Todd says. "You can't have burnt it all."

"Ah, but Todd, my son," the Mayor says, shaking his head. "I have never taken the cure."

Another silence. I hear suspicions rising in the Noise of the men. I even see a few of them step back, thoughts of the

447

control his Noise. And if he can do *that—*

"He's lying," I say, remembering Mistress Coyle's words. "He's the President of Lies."

"Well, at least you finally called me *President*," the Mayor says.

Todd gives the Mayor a shove. "Tell us where it is."

The Mayor stumbles back a step, then regains his balance. He looks around at us all again. I can hear everyone's Noise rising, Todd's most of all, red and loud.

"I tell no lies, gentlemen," says the Mayor. "If you only have the right discipline, Noise can be controlled. It can be silenced." He looks around at each of us again, his smile reappearing. "It can be used."

I AM THE CIRCLE AND THE CIRCLE IS ME, I hear.

But I can't tell if it's from his Noise—

Or Todd's.

"I've had just about enough of this!" Ivan shouts.

"You know, Private Farrow," says the Mayor, "so have I."

And that's when he attacks.

19

YER OWN WORST ENEMY

[TODD]

I FEEL THE FIRST STRIKE of Noise fly by me, a *whooshing* of concentrated words and sound and pictures rushing over my shoulder, straight for the men with rifles. I flinch away and dive for the ground–

Cuz the men start firing their guns–

And I'm right in the way–

"Todd!" I hear Viola shout but the rifles are firing and the men are screaming and I roll on the rubble, jarring my elbow, and whip round to see Corporal Pot Belly on his knees in front of Angharrad, his back turned, both hands on the sides of his head, screaming wordlessly down into the ground, Viola watching him, wondering what the hell is going on. Another guard has fallen on his back, fingers in his eyes, as if he's trying to dig them out, and a third lies unconshus on his stomach. Two others are already running back into the city.

The Noise flies from the Mayor, louder and stronger than anything I've seen before.

Loud enough to take out five men at once.

Only Ivan still stands, one hand up to his ear and the other trying to aim his rifle at the Mayor but weaving it dangerously around–

BANG

A bullet smacks the ground in front of my eyes, sending dust and dirt up into them–

BANG

Another bounces off stones deep in the cathedral–

"IVAN!" I shout.

BANG

"Stop firing! Yer gonna get us killed!"

BANG

His rifle goes off right by Angharrad's head. She rears up and I see Viola grab the reins, surprised, holding on for dear life–

And then I see the Mayor is walking forward and forward and forward–

His eyes on the men he's attacking–

Coming past me–

And I don't even think–

I leap from the ground to stop him–

And he turns and sends his Noise straight at me–

The world goes all bright, terribly, painfully bright, like everyone can see how much you hurt, everyone watching and laughing and nowhere to hide and YER NOTHING YER NOTHING YER NOTHING all bound up tight like a bullet right thru you, telling you everything that's wrong with you, everything you ever done bad in yer life, telling you yer worthless, yer dirt, YER NOTHING, yer life ain't got no point nor reason nor purpose and you should just tear down the walls of yerself, ripping apart who you are and either die or give it up as a gift, as a gift to the one who can save you, as a gift to the man who can control you, who can take it all away, who can make everything fine fine fine–

But not even Noise can stop a body when it's moving.

I feel all these things and I'm still flying at him and I still hit him and I still knock him over on the steps of the cathedral.

He grunts as the air is crushed out of him and the Noise attack stops for a second. Corporal Pot Belly calls out and falls over and Ivan's gasping for breath and Viola's calling out "Todd!" and then a hand is around my neck and it's pushing my head up and the Mayor is looking right into my eyes–

And this time it hits me full blast.

"Give me the rifle!" the Mayor is shouting, standing over Ivan, who's crouched on the ground below him, hand over his ear again but the rifle still pointed up at the Mayor. "Give it to me!"

I blink, grit and dust in my eyes, wondering for a second where I am–

YER NOTHING YER NOTHING YER NOTHING YER NOTHING

"Give me the rifle, *Private*!"

But his rifle's still aimed–

"Todd!"

I see horse legs beside my head. Viola's still up on Angharrad. "Todd, wake up!" she's yelling. I look up at her. "Thank God!" she yells and her face is a picture of frustrayshun. "My stupid feet! I can't get off the goddam horse!"

"I'm okay," I say, tho I don't know if I am, and I lean myself up, my head spinning.

YER NOTHING YER NOTHING YER NOTHING YER NOTHING

"Todd, what's going on?" Viola says as I grab a rein to help me stand. "I hear Noise but–"

"The rifle!" shouts the Mayor, stepping closer to Ivan. "Now!"

"We have to help him," I say–

But I flinch back at the strongest attack yet–

A flare of Noise so white you can almost see the air bending twixt the Mayor and Ivan–

And Ivan grunts sharply and bites his tongue–

Blood spilling from his mouth–

Before he screams like a child and falls back–

Dropping the rifle–

Dropping it right into the Mayor's hands.

He lifts it, cocks it and aims it at us in one fluid move. Ivan lies twitching on the ground.

"What just happened?" Viola says, too angry it seems to care much about the rifle.

I put my hands in the air, still holding the reins.

"He can use Noise," I say, keeping my eyes on him. "He can use it like a weapon."

"Just so," says the Mayor, smiling again.

"All I heard was shouting," she says, looking at the men lying on the ground, still breathing but out cold. "What do you mean, a weapon?"

"The truth, Viola," the Mayor answers. "The best weapon of all. You tell a man the truth about himself and, well," he nudges Ivan with his boot, "they find they have trouble accepting it." He frowns. "You can't kill him with it, though." He looks back up at us. "Not yet, anyway."

"But…" She's not believing this. "How? How can you–?"

"I have two maxims that I believe, dear girl," the Mayor says, coming slowly towards us. "One, if you can control yourself, you can control others. Two, if you can control *information*, you can control others." He grins, his eyes flashing. "It's been a philosophy that's worked out rather well for me."

I think about Mr Hammar. About Mr Collins. About the chanting I used to hear coming from the Mayor's house back in my old town.

"You taught the others," I say. "The men from Prentisstown, you taught them how to control their Noise."

"With varying degrees of success," he says, "but yes, none of my officers has ever taken the cure. Why should they? It's a weakness to have to rely on a drug."

He's nearly on us now. "I am the Circle and the Circle is me," I say.

"Yes, you were certainly making an impressive beginning,

453

_____ Todd? Controlling yourself while you did the most unspeakable things to those _____"

My Noise turns red. "You *shut up* about that," I say. "I was only doing what you told me—"

"*I was only following orders*," the Mayor mocks. "The refuge of scoundrels since the dawn of time." He stops two metres away from us, rifle pointed firmly at my chest. "Help her off the horse, please, Todd."

"What?" I say.

"Her ankles, I believe the problem was. She'll need your help walking."

I still have the reins in my hand. I have a thought I try to bury.

Boy colt? Angharrad asks.

"I assure you, Viola," the Mayor says to her. "If you think about running on that beautiful animal, I will put more than one bullet through Todd." He looks back at me. "However much pain it might cause me."

"You let her go," I say. "I'll do anything you want."

"Now where have I heard that before?" he says. "Help her down."

I hesitate, wondering if I should slap Angharrad's flanks anyway, wondering if I should send Viola riding off into the distance, wondering if I could get her safe—

"No," Viola says and she's already working her leg round the saddle. "Not a chance. I'm not leaving you."

I take her arms and help her down. She has to lean on me to stand but I keep her up.

"Splendid," says the Mayor. "Now let's go inside and have that chat."

* * *

"Let us start with what I know."

He's brought us into what used to be the room with the round coloured glass window in it but it's now open to the air on two sides and above, the window still there, looking down, but looking down on rubble.

Looking down on a little cleared area with a broken table and two chairs.

Where me and Viola sit.

"I know, for example," the Mayor says, "that you did not kill Aaron, Todd, that you never took your final step towards becoming a man, that it was Viola here who put the blade in all along."

Viola takes my arm and squeezes it tight, letting me know it's okay that he knows.

"I know that Viola told you the Answer were hiding at the ocean when I let you escape to go speak with her."

My Noise rises in anger and embarrassment. Viola squeezes my arm harder.

"I know that you've sent the boy called Lee to warn the Answer." He leans against the broken table. "And of course I also know the exact time and place of their attack."

"Yer a monster," I say.

"No," the Mayor says. "Just a leader. Just a leader who can read every thought you have, about yourself, about Viola, about me, about this town, about the secrets you think you're keeping, I can read *everything*, Todd. You're not listening to what I'm saying." He's still holding the rifle, watching us sit before him. "I knew everything about the

455

Answer's attack this morning before you even opened your
mouth."

I sit up in my chair. "You what?"

"I had the army gathering before we even started Asking Viola."

I start to rise. "You tortured her for *nothing*?"

"Sit down," the Mayor says and a little flash from him weakens my knees enough that I sit right back down. "Not for nothing, Todd. You should know me well enough by now to know that I do not do *anything* for nothing."

He sits up from the broken table, showing again that he likes to walk and talk.

"You are completely transparent to me, Todd. From our first proper meeting here in this very room until how you sit before me today. I've known everything. *Always.*"

He looks at Viola. "Unlike your good friend here, who's a little tougher than I imagined."

Viola frowns. If she had Noise I'm sure she'd be slapping him around a bit.

I get a thought–

"Don't try it," the Mayor says. "You're not nearly that advanced yet. Even Captain Hammar has yet to master it. You'd merely end up hurting yourself very badly." He looks at me again. "But you *could* learn, Todd. You could advance far, farther than any of those poor imbeciles who followed me from Prentisstown. Poor Mr Collins barely worth more than a butler and Captain Hammar just another garden-variety sadist, but you, Todd, *you.*" His eyes flash. "You could lead armies."

"I don't wanna lead armies," I say.

He smiles. "You may have no choice."

"There's always a choice," Viola says by my side.

"Oh, people like to say that," the Mayor says. "It makes them feel better." He approaches me, looking into my eyes. "But I've been watching you, Todd. The boy who can't kill another man. The boy who'd risk his own life to save his beloved Viola. The boy who felt so guilty at the horrible things he was doing that he tried to shut off all feeling. The boy who still felt every pain, every twitch of hurt he saw on the face of the women he banded."

He leans down closer to my face. "The boy who refused to lose his soul."

I feel him. He's in my Noise now, rummaging around, turning things over, upending the room inside my head. "I've done bad things," I say and I don't even mean to say it.

"But you *suffer* for them, Todd." His voice is softer now, almost tender. "You're your own worst enemy, punishing yourself far more than I could ever hope to. Men have Noise and the way they handle it is to make themselves just a little bit dead, but *you*, even when you *want* to, you can't. More than any man I've ever met, Todd, you *feel*."

"Shut up," I say, trying to look away, not being able to.

"But that makes you *powerful*, Todd Hewitt. In this world of numbness and information overload, the ability to feel, my boy, is a rare gift indeed."

I put my hands to my ears but I can still hear him in my head.

"You're the one I couldn't break, Todd. The one who wouldn't fall. The one who stays innocent no matter the blood on his hands. The one who *still* calls me Mayor in his Noise."

457

"You could rule by my side. You could be my second in command. And when you learn to control your Noise, you may have power to overtake even *mine*."

And then the words thunder thru my whole body.

I AM THE CIRCLE AND THE CIRCLE IS ME.

"Stop it!" I hear Viola shout but it's from miles away.

The Mayor puts a hand on my shoulder. "You could be my son, Todd Hewitt," he says. "My real and true heir. I've always wanted one that wasn't–"

"Pa?" we all hear, cutting thru everything like a bullet thru fog.

The Noise in my head stops, the Mayor steps abruptly back, I feel like I'm able to breathe again.

Davy stands behind us, rifle in one hand. He's led Deadfall up to the steps and is looking over the rubble to the three of us here. "What's going on? Who are the men out there on the ground?"

"What are you doing here?" the Mayor snaps, frowning. "Is the battle already won?"

"No, Pa," Davy says, climbing over the rubble towards us. "It was a trick." He plants his feet next to my chair. "Hey, Todd," he says, nodding in greeting. He glances at Viola but he can't hold her eye.

"*What* was a trick?" the Mayor demands but he's already looking angry.

"The Answer ain't coming over the hill," Davy says. "We marched way back deep into the forest but there ain't no sign, not nowhere."

I hear Viola take a little gasp, a bit of pleased surprise

escaping from her even as she tries to hold it back.

The Mayor looks her way, his eyes fierce, his face thinking and thinking.

And he raises his rifle at her.

"Something you'd like to tell us, Viola?"

40

NOTHING CHANGES, EVERYTHING CHANGES

{VIOLA}

TODD'S ALREADY UP and out of his chair, standing between me and the Mayor, his Noise raging so loud and furious the Mayor takes a step back.

"You see the power in you, my boy?" he says. "This is why you watched her being Asked. Your suffering makes you *strong*. I'll teach you how to harness it and together we'll–"

"You hurt her," Todd says, clearly and slowly, "and I'll tear every limb from yer body."

The Mayor smiles. "I believe you." He hoists the rifle. "Nevertheless."

"Todd," I say.

He turns to me. "This is how he wins. Playing us off each other. Just like you said. Well, it stops here–"

"Todd–" I'm trying to stand up but my stupid ankles won't hold me and I stumble. Todd reaches for me–

But it's Davy–

Davy catches me by the arm, stopping the fall and then lowering me back into the chair. He won't meet my eye. Or Todd's. Or his father's. His Noise flushes yellow with embarrassment as he lets me go and steps back.

"Why, thank you, David," the Mayor says, unable to mask his surprise. "Now," he says, turning back to me, "if you would please be so kind as to inform me of the Answer's *real* plan of attack."

"Don't tell him nothing," Todd says.

"I don't *know* anything," I say. "Lee must have reached–"

"There wasn't sufficient time and you know it," the Mayor says. "It's obvious what's happened, isn't it, Viola? Your Mistress misled you once more. If the bomb went off as it should have, it wouldn't have mattered if you had the wrong information because you and, she hoped, *I* would be dead. But if you were caught, well, then. The best liar is the one who believes her lie is true."

I don't say anything because how could she have misled me if it was only something Lee overheard–

But then I think–

She *wanted* him to overhear it.

She *knew* he wouldn't be able to not tell me.

"Her plan worked perfectly, didn't it, Viola?" The shadow from the setting sun reaches the Mayor's face, covering him in black. "One twist after another, lies building on lies. She played you exactly how she wanted, didn't she?"

I glare at him. "She'll beat you," I say. "She's as ruthless as you are."

He grins. "Oh, *more*, I should say."

"Pa?" Davy asks.

461

David?"

"Um, the *army*?" Davy's Noise is full of bewilderment and exasperation, trying to make sense of what his father's doing but not finding much relief. "What're we sposed to do *now*? Where're we sposed to go? Captain Hammar's waiting for yer orders."

All around us the low, frightened **ROAR** of New Prentisstown seeps out of the houses, but still no faces at the windows, and from over the hill with the notch, the blacker, twistier buzz of the army. You can still see them up the hillside, shiny like a trail of black beetles sliding off one another's shells.

And here we sit, alone with the Mayor and his son, in the open ruins of the cathedral, like we're the only people on the planet.

The Mayor looks back at me. "Yes, Viola, tell us. What are we supposed to do now?"

"You're supposed to fall," I say, staring back at him, not blinking. "You're supposed to lose."

He smiles at me. "Where are they coming from, Viola? You're a clever girl. You must have heard *something*, seen some clue as to her real plans."

"She ain't telling you," Todd says.

"I *can't*," I say, "because I don't *know*."

And I'm thinking, I really *don't* know–

Unless the thing she told me about the east road–

"I'm waiting, Viola." The Mayor raises the rifle at Todd's head. "On pain of his life."

"Pa?" Davy says, shock coming out of his Noise. "What're you *doing*?"

"Never you mind, David. Get back on your horse. I'll have a message for you to take to Captain Hammar presently."

"Yer pointing the gun at *Todd*, Pa."

Todd turns around to look at him. So do I. So does the Mayor.

"You ain't gonna shoot him," Davy says. "You can't." Davy's cheeks are red now, so dark you can even see them in the sunset. "You said he's yer second son."

There's an uncomfortable silence as Davy tries to hide his Noise.

"You see what I mean by power, Todd?" the Mayor says. "Look at how you've influenced my son. You've already got yourself a follower."

Davy looks at me, right in the eyes. "Tell him where they are." There's worry all over his Noise, anxiety at how things are playing out. "C'mon, just tell him."

I look back at Todd.

He's looking at Davy's rifle.

"Yes, Viola, tell me, why don't you?" the Mayor says. "Your best speculation. Are they coming from the west?" He looks up towards the falls, the highest point on the horizon, where the sun's disappearing behind the zigzag road carved down the hill, the hill I've only been down once and never gone back up. The Mayor turns. "The north, perhaps, though they'd have to cross the river somehow? Or a hill to the east? Yes, maybe even over the hill where your Mistress blew up the tower and any chance you had of communicating with your people."

I clench my teeth again.

"Still loyal, after all that?"

I don't say anything.

463

"We could send out troops, Pa," Davy says. "To different parts. They gotta come from *somewhere.*"

The Mayor waits for a minute, staring us down. He finally turns to Davy and says, "Go tell Captain Hammar–"

He's interrupted by a distant *BOOM*.

"That's due east," Davy says, as we all look up even though there's a wall of the cathedral in the way.

It *is* east.

It's exactly the road she told me it was going to be.

She made me think the truth was a lie and a lie was the truth.

If I get out of this, we're going to have words, her and me.

"The Office of the Ask," the Mayor says. "Of course. Where else would they–"

He stops again, cocking his head, listening out. We hear it several seconds after he does. The Noise of someone running full out towards the cathedral from the back, up the road we took to get here, around the side of the cathedral and up to the front, coming upon us, gasping.

It's the red-haired guard, the one who fled. He's obviously barely registering who he's seeing as he stumbles into the wreckage of the building. "They're coming!" he shouts. "The Answer is coming!"

There's a burst of Noise from the Mayor and the red-haired soldier falls back, catching himself. "Calm down, Private," the Mayor says, his voice slinky, snake-like. "Tell us clearly."

The guard pants, seemingly unable to catch his breath. "They've taken the Office of the Ask." He looks up at the

464

Mayor, caught by his eyes. "They killed all the guards."

"Of course they did," the Mayor says, still holding the red-haired soldier's gaze. "How many are there?"

"Two hundred." The red-haired soldier isn't blinking now. "But they're releasing the prisoners."

"Weapons?" asks the Mayor.

"Rifles. Tracers. Launchers. Siege guns on the backs of carts." Still the stare.

"How goes the battle?"

"They're fighting fierce."

The Mayor cocks an eyebrow, still staring at him.

"They're fighting fierce, *sir*," the guard says, still not blinking, like he couldn't look away from the Mayor if he tried. There's another *BOOM* in the distance and everyone except the Mayor and the soldier flinches. "They're coming for war, sir," says the soldier.

The Mayor keeps the stare. "Then you should be trying to stop them, shouldn't you?"

"Sir?"

"You should be taking your rifle and preventing the Answer from destroying your town."

The soldier looks confused but he's still not blinking. "I should..."

"You should be on the front line, soldier. This is our hour of need."

"This is our hour of need," the soldier mumbles, like he's not hearing himself.

"Pa?" Davy says but the Mayor ignores him.

"What are you waiting for, soldier?" the Mayor says. "It's time to fight."

"Go!" the Mayor suddenly barks and the red-haired guard springs away, back down the road towards the Answer, his rifle up, yelling incoherently, running back to the Answer as fast as he ran away from them.

We watch him go in stunned silence.

The Mayor sees Todd staring at him, mouth agape. "Yes, dear boy, better at *that*, too."

"You as good as killed him," I say. "Whatever you did–"

"What I did was make him see his duty," the Mayor says. "No more, no less. Now, as *fascinating* as this discussion is, we're going to have to settle it later. I'm afraid I'm going to have to have Davy tie you both up."

"*Pa?*" Davy says again, startled.

The Mayor looks at him. "Then you'll ride to Captain Hammar, tell him to bring the army down the road with all speed and fury." The Mayor casts his eyes to the far hillside where the army waits. "It's time we brought this to an end."

"I can't tie him up, Pa, it's *Todd*."

The Mayor doesn't look at him. "I've had just about enough of this, David. When I give you a direct order–"

Boom!

He stops and we all look up.

Because it's different this time, a different kind of sound. We hear a low *whoosh* and a rumble starts to fill the air, getting louder as the seconds pass.

Todd looks at me, confused.

I just shrug. "Nothing I ever heard before."

The roar starts to get louder, filling the darkening sky.

"That don't sound like no bomb," Davy says.

The Mayor looks at me. "Viola, is there–"

He stops and then turns his head.

And we all realize–

It's not coming from the east.

"Over there," Davy points, raising his hand towards the falls, towards where the sky is bright pink with sunset.

The Mayor looks at me again. "That's too loud for a simple tracer." His face tightens. "Have they got missiles?" He takes a step so big he's almost on top of me. "*Have they built missiles?*"

"You *back off*!" Todd yells, trying to get between us again.

"I will *know* what this is, Viola!" the Mayor says. "You will tell me!"

"I don't *know* what it is!" I say.

Todd's shouting and threatening, "You lay a *finger* on her–"

"It's getting louder!" Davy shouts, putting his hands to his ears. We all turn and watch the western horizon, watch as a dot rises, getting lost in the last of the sun before reappearing, growing larger as it comes.

As it comes straight for the city.

"*Viola!*" the Mayor shouts, through clenched teeth, sending some Noise at me but I don't feel whatever it is that men feel.

"I DON'T KNOW!" I yell.

And then Davy, who hasn't stopped watching it, says, "It's a ship."

41

THE MOMENT OF DAVY PRENTISS

[TODD]

IT'S A SHIP.

It's a ruddy *ship*.

"Yer people," I say to Viola.

But she's shaking her head, tho not to say no, just staring at it as it rises over the falls.

"Too small for a settler ship," Davy says.

"And too early," the Mayor says, aiming his rifle at it as if he could shoot it from this distance. "They're not due for another two months at least."

But Viola still ain't looking like she can hear any of this, hope rising on her face so painful it hurts my heart just to see it. "A scout," she whispers, so quiet I'm the only one who hears it. "Another scout. Sent to look for me."

I turn back to the ship.

It clears the crest of the falls, soaring out over the river.

A scout ship, just like the one she crashed in back in the

swamp, killing her parents and stranding her here all those months and lifetimes ago. It still looks as big as a house, stubby wings looking too short to keep it in the air, flames coming outta the tail end as it flies flies flies down the river, using it as a road hundreds of metres below.

We watch it come.

"David," the Mayor says, his eyes still on it. "Get my horse."

But Davy's got his face up to the sky, his Noise opening up in wonder and amazement.

And I know exactly how he feels.

Nothing flies on New World except the birds. We got machines that go down the roads, fissionbikes, a few fissioncars, but mainly we just got horses and oxes and carts and our feet.

We don't got *wings*.

The ship comes down the river, nearing the cathedral and flying almost right over us, not stopping, so close you can see lights on the underside and the sky above the exhaust shimmering with the heat. It flies right on past, down the river.

Down east towards the Answer.

"*David!*" the Mayor says sharply.

"Help me up," Viola whispers. "I have to get to them. I have to *go*."

And her eyes are wild and her breath is heavy and she's staring at me so hard it's like a solid thing I can feel.

"Oh, he'll help you up," the Mayor says, pointing the gun. "Because you're coming with me."

"*What?*" Viola says.

"They're going to be wondering where you are. I can either bring you to them right away." He looks at me. "Or I can sadly inform them that you died in the crash. Which would you prefer?"

"I'm not going with *you*," she says. "You're a liar and a murderer—"

He cuts her off. "David, you'll remain guard over Todd while I take Viola to her ship." He looks back at her. "I think you know first-hand my son's eagerness with a gun if you don't cooperate."

Viola looks furiously at Davy. I look at Davy, too, standing there, rifle in hand, looking back and forth twixt me and his pa.

His Noise roiling.

His Noise saying clearly there ain't no way he's *ever* gonna shoot me.

"Pa?" he says.

"Enough of this, David," the Mayor frowns, trying to catch Davy's eye—

And catching it.

"You will do what I say," he says to his son. "You will tie Todd up with the rope he so helpfully brought and you will stand guard over him and when I return with our newly arrived guests, everything will be peaceful and happy. The new world will begin."

"New world," Davy mumbles, his eyes glazing over, just like the ginger-haired soldier, askings and doubt being pushed outta his Noise.

As he bends to the will of another.

470

I get an idea.

Forgive me, Davy.

"You gonna let him talk to you like that, Davy?"

He blinks. "What?"

He looks away from his pa.

"You gonna let him point a gun at me and Viola?"

"Todd," the Mayor warns.

"All that Noise you say you hear," I say to the Mayor but I still look at Davy, still hold his eye. "All the way you say you know *everything*, but you don't know yer own son very well, now, do ya?"

"David," the Mayor says.

But *I* got Davy's eye now.

"You gonna let him get his way again?" I say to him. "You gonna let him boss you round with no reward?"

Davy watches me nervously, trying to blink away the mess his pa's put in his head.

"That ship changes everything, Davy," I say. "A whole new batch of people. A whole city's worth to try and make this place something better than the stinking boghole it is."

"*David*," the Mayor says. There's a flash of Noise and Davy flinches.

"Stop it, Pa," he says.

"Who do you want to get to that ship first, Davy?" I say. "Me and Viola to get some help? Or yer pa so he can rule them, too?"

"Be *quiet*!" says the Mayor. "Are you forgetting who has the gun?"

"Davy has one, too," I say.

There's a bit of a pause as we all see Davy remember he's holding a rifle.

There's another flash of Noise from the Mayor and another flinch from Davy. "Jesus, *Pa*, effing quit it already!"

But he looks at his pa to say it.

And his pa catches his eyes again.

"Tie Todd up and get my horse, David," the Mayor says, holding his stare.

"Pa?" Davy says, his voice gone quiet.

"My horse," says the Mayor. "He's out back."

"Get between them," Viola hisses at me. "Break the eye contact!"

I move but the Mayor turns the gun on her without taking his eyes off Davy. "One move, Todd."

I stop.

"Bring me my horse, son," says the Mayor, "and we'll greet the new settlers side by side." He smiles at his son. "You'll be my prince."

"He said that before," I say to Davy. "But not to you."

"He's controlling you," Viola shouts. "He's using his Noise to—"

"Please tell Viola to be quiet," the Mayor says.

"Be quiet, Viola," Davy says, his voice soft, his eyes not blinking.

"*Davy!*" I shout.

"He's just trying to control you, David," the Mayor says, his voice rising. "Like he's done from the start."

"*What?*" I say.

472

"From the start," Davy mumbles.

"Who do you think's held you back from promotion, son?" the Mayor's saying it and he's saying it right into the middle of Davy's brain. "Who do you think tells me all the things you do wrong?"

"Todd?" Davy says weakly.

"He's *lying*," I say. "Look at me!"

But Davy's overloading. He's just staring frozen at his pa, not moving at all.

The Mayor gives a heavy sigh. "I see I have to do this myself."

He comes forward, gesturing us back with his rifle. He grabs Viola and lifts her to her feet. She cries out from the pain in her ankles. I move automatically to help but he pushes her forward so she's right in front of him, his rifle at her back.

I open my mouth to shout, to threaten, to damn him–

But it's Davy who speaks first.

"It's landing," he says quietly.

We all turn eastward. The ship is taking a slow circle, flying around a hilltop east of town–

Maybe even the one where the tower once stood–

It comes round again and hovers above the treetops–

Before slowly starting to lower itself out of sight–

I turn to Davy, too, see his eyes fogged and confused–

But he ain't looking at his pa no more–

He's looking at the ship–

And then he's turning his head and looking at me–

And his rifle is just there, just hanging from his hand–

And one more time–

Forgive me.

I lunge forward and snatch it from him. He don't even put up any resistance, just lets it go, lets it go right into my fingers and I'm already raising it and cocking it and pointing it at the Mayor.

Who's already smiling, his gun still in Viola's back.

"So it's a stand-off, is it?" he says, grinning from ear to ear.

"Let her go," I say.

"Please take your gun back from Todd, David," the Mayor says, but he has to keep looking at me, watching me with the gun.

"Don't you do no such thing, Davy."

"Stop it!" Davy says, his voice thick, his Noise rising. I sense him putting his hands to the sides of his head. "Can't you both just effing *stop it*?"

But the Mayor's still looking at me and I'm still looking at the Mayor.

The sound of the ship landing screams over the city, over the Noise of the army marching its way back down the hill, over the distant *booms* of the Answer making its way up the road, and over the terrified, hidden **ROAR** of New Prentisstown all around us, not knowing that their whole future depends on this, right now, right this second, me and the Mayor with our rifles.

"Let her go," I say.

"I don't think so, Todd." I hear a rumble of Noise coming from him.

"My finger's on this trigger," I say. "You try to hit me with yer Noise and yer a dead man."

The Mayor smiles. "Fair enough," he says. "But what you need to ask yourself, my dear friend Todd, is if, when you decide to finally pull that trigger, can you pull it fast enough so that I don't also pull my own? Will killing me kill your beloved Viola, too?" He lowers his chin. "Could you live with that?"

"You'd be dead," I say.

"So would she."

"Do it, Todd," Viola says. "Don't let him win."

"That ain't happening neither," I say.

"Are you going to let him point a gun at your own father, David?" the Mayor asks.

But he's still looking at me.

"Times are changing, Davy," I say, eyes still on the Mayor. "This is where we all decide how it's gonna be. Including you."

"Why's it have to be like this?" Davy asks. "We could all go together. We could all ride up on horseback and–"

"No, David," says the Mayor. "No, that won't do at all."

"Put the gun down," I say. "Put it down and end this."

The Mayor's eyes flash and I know what's coming–

"You stop that," I say, blinking furiously and looking over his shoulder.

"You cannot win this," the Mayor says and I hear his voice twice over, three times, a legion of him inside my head. "You cannot shoot me and guarantee her life, Todd. We all know you'd never risk that."

out at the pain in her ankles.

But I find myself taking a step back.

"Don't look in his eyes," she says.

"I'm trying," I say, but even the *sound* of his voice is getting inside me.

"This isn't a loss, Todd," the Mayor is saying, so loud in my head it feels like my brain's vibrating. "I wish for your death no more than I wish for my own. Everything I said earlier was true. I want you by my side. I want you as part of the future we're going to create here with whoever steps out of that ship."

"Shut *up*," I say.

But he's still stepping forward.

I'm still stepping back.

Till I'm behind even Davy.

"I want no harm to come to Viola, either," the Mayor says. "All along I promised both of you a future. That promise still stands."

Even without looking right at him, his voice is buzzing in my head, weighing it down, making it seem like it's easier just to—

"Don't listen to him!" Viola shouts. "He's a liar."

"Todd," says the Mayor. "I think of you as my son. I really do."

And Davy turns to me, his Noise rising all hopeful, and he says, "C'mon, Todd, you hear that?"

And his Noise is reaching for me, too, eagerness and worry coming forward like fingers and hands, asking me, *begging* me to put the gun down, put it down and make everything all right, make it so all this stops–

And he says, "We could be brothers–"

And I cast my eyes to Davy's–

And I see myself in them, see myself in his Noise, see the Mayor as my father and Davy as my brother and Viola as our sister–

See the hopeful smile rising to Davy's lips–

And for the third time, I have to ask–

Forgive me.

I point the rifle at Davy.

"Let her go," I say to the Mayor, not quite able to look Davy in the face.

"Todd?" Davy asks, his forehead furrowing.

"Just do it!" I snap.

"Or you'll what, Todd?" the Mayor teases. "You'll shoot him?"

Davy's Noise is spilling over with more asking marks, with surprise and shock–

With a betrayal that's rising–

"Answer me, Todd," the Mayor says. "Or you'll *what*?"

"Todd?" Davy says again, his voice lower this time.

I look him briefly in the eyes and look away again.

"Or I'll shoot Davy," I say. "I'll shoot yer son."

Davy's Noise is pouring with disappointment, disappointment so thick it falls off him like mud. I don't even read no anger in his Noise, which makes it worse. He ain't even thinking of jumping me or punching me or wrestling the gun away.

The only thing in his Noise is me holding a gun on him.

His only friend holding a gun on him.

"I'm sorry," I whisper.

But he don't look like he hears.

"I gave you yer book," he says. "I gave you back yer book."

"You let Viola go!" I shout, looking away from Davy, anger at myself snapping my voice loud. "Or I swear to God–"

"Go ahead then," the Mayor says. "Shoot him."

Davy looks at the Mayor. "Pa?"

"Never much use as a son anyway," the Mayor says, still pushing Viola forward with the rifle. "Why do you think I sent him to the front line? I was at least hoping he'd die a *hero*'s death."

There's pain on Viola's face still but it ain't all her ankles.

"Never mastered his Noise," the Mayor continues, looking at Davy, whose Noise–

I can't say what his Noise is like.

"Never followed an order he couldn't get out of. Couldn't capture you. Couldn't take care of Viola. Only ever showed improvement because of *your* influence, Todd."

"Pa–" Davy starts.

But his pa ignores him.

"*You* are the son I want, Todd. Always you. *Never* this waste of space."

And Davy's Noise–

Oh, Jesus, Davy's Noise–

"LET HER GO!" I shout so I don't have to hear it. "I'll shoot him, I'll do it!"

"You won't," says the Mayor, smiling again. "Everyone knows you aren't a killer, Todd."

He pushes Viola forward again–

She calls out from the pain of it–

Viola, I think–

Viola–

I grit my teeth and raise the rifle–

I cock it–

And I say what's true–

"I would kill to save her," I say.

The Mayor stops edging forward. He looks twixt me and Davy and back again.

"Pa?" says Davy. His face is twisted and crumpled.

The Mayor looks back at me, reading my Noise.

"You would, wouldn't you?" he says, almost under his breath. "You'd kill him. For her."

Davy looks back at me, his eyes wet but anger rising there, too. "Don't, Todd. Don't do it."

"Let her go," I say again. "*Now*."

The Mayor's still looking twixt me and Davy, seeing that I'm serious, seeing that I'd really do it.

"Just put the gun down," I growl, not looking at Davy's eyes, not looking at his Noise. "*This is over*."

The Mayor takes in a long breath and lets it out.

He steps away from Viola.

My shoulders relax.

And he fires his gun.

42

ENDGAME

{VIOLA}

"TODD!" I shout, the sound of the rifle shot blasting past my ear, erasing everything but him, the whole world reduced to not knowing if he's all right or not, if he's been hit, if–

But it's not him–

He's still holding up his gun–

Unfired–

Standing next to Davy–

Who falls to his knees–

Sending up two small clouds of dust as he hits the rubble–

"Pa?" he asks, his voice pleading, like a little kitten–

And then he coughs, spilling blood down his lips–

"Davy?" Todd says, his Noise rising like he's the one that's been shot–

And I see it–

A hole high in Davy's chest, in the fabric of his uniform, just below the base of his throat–

"*Davy!*" he shouts–

But Davy's Noise is staring at his father–

Asking marks sent everywhere–

His expression shocked–

His hand reaching up to the wound–

He coughs again–

And gags–

Todd's looking at the Mayor, too–

His Noise railing–

"*What did you do?*" he shouts–

[TODD]

"*WHAT DID YOU DO?!*" I shout.

"I removed him from the equation," the Mayor says calmly.

"Pa?" Davy asks again, holding out a bloodied hand towards him–

But his pa is only looking at me.

"You were always the truer son, Todd," the Mayor says. "The one with the potential, the one with the power, the one I'd be proud to have serve by my side."

Pa? Davy's Noise says–

And he's hearing *all* of this–

"You effing *monster*," I say. "I'll *kill* you–"

"You'll *join* me," the Mayor says. "You know you will. It's only a matter of time. David was weak, an embarrassment–"

"*SHUT UP!*" I shout.

482

Todd? I hear–

I look down–

Davy's looking up at me–

His Noise swirling–

Swirling with askings and confuzhun and fear–

And **Todd?**–

Todd?–

I'm sorry–

I'm sorry–

"Davy, don't–" I start to say–

But his Noise is still swirling–

And I see–

I see–

I see the truth–

Here at the last–

He's showing me the truth–

The thing he's been hiding from me–

About Ben–

All in a messy rush–

Pictures of Ben racing up the road towards Davy–

Pictures of Davy's horse rearing–

Pictures of Davy firing his gun as he falls–

Pictures of the bullet hitting Ben in the chest–

Pictures of Ben staggering out into the bushes–

Davy too scared to go after him–

Davy too scared to tell me the truth after–

After I became his only friend–

I didn't mean it, his Noise is saying–

"Davy–" I say–

I'm sorry, he thinks–

And that's the truth all over–

He *is* sorry–

For everything–

For Prentisstown–

For Viola–

For Ben–

For every failure and every wrong–

For letting his pa down–

And he's looking up at me–

And he's begging me–

He's begging me–

Like I'm the only one who can forgive him–

Like it's only me who's got the power–

Todd?–

Please–

And all I can say is "Davy–"

And the fright and the terror in his Noise is too much–

It's too much–

And then it stops.

Davy slumps, eyes still open, eyes still staring back at me, eyes still asking (I swear) for me to forgive him.

And he lies there, still.

Davy Prentiss is dead.

{VIOLA}

"You're insane," I say to the Mayor behind me.

"No," he says. "You've been right all along, both of you. Never love something so much it can be used to control you."

484

The sun is down now but the sky is still pink, the Noise of the town still *ROAR*s, there's another *Boom!* in the distance as the Answer approaches, and the ship must have landed by now. Its doors must be opening. Someone, probably Simone Watkin or Bradley Tench, people I know, people who know *me*, must be looking out, wondering what sort of place they've landed in.

And Todd kneels over the body of Davy Prentiss.

And then Todd looks up–

His Noise is boiling and burning and I can hear the grief in it and the shame and the *rage*–

And he gets to his feet–

And he raises his rifle–

I see myself in his Noise, I see the Mayor there, too, behind me, rifle pointed, eyes glinting with triumph.

And I know exactly what Todd is going to do.

"Do it," I say, my stomach dropping but it's right right right–

And Todd raises the rifle to his eye–

"*Do it!*"

And the Mayor shoves me hard, sending lightnings of pain up my legs, and I can't help it and I scream out and fall forward, forward towards Todd, forward towards the ground–

And the Mayor does it again–

Uses me to control Todd–

Because Todd can't help it either–

He jumps to catch me–

To catch me when I'm falling–

And the Mayor attacks.

485

My brain explodes, burning and raging with everything he fires at it and it ain't nothing like a slap at all, it's like fiery metal poked right into the centre of who I am, and as I jump forward to catch Viola, it hits me so hard my head snaps back and here it comes again, the Mayor's voice but somehow *my* voice, too, somehow *hers* as well and all of 'em saying YER NOTHING YER NOTHING YER NOTHING YER NOTHING—

Our bodies are still moving together and I feel us tumble into one another, feel the top of her skull crack into my mouth, and YER NOTHING YER NOTHING YER NOTHING she falls into my chest and my fumbling arms and we twist down onto the rubble together, a siren ripping off the roof of my head YER NOTHING YER NOTHING YER NOTHING and I feel the rifle fall and bounce away and I feel the weight of her against me and I hear her as if from the other side of the moons and she's calling my name and YER NOTHING she's saying "Todd" YER NOTHING YER NOTHING she's saying "Todd!" and it's as if I'm watching her from under water and I see her try to rise up on her hands to protect me but the Mayor's above her and swinging his rifle by the barrel and smacking her across the back of her head and she's falling to one side—

And my brain is boiling—

My brain is boiling—

My brain is boiling—

YER NOTHING YER NOTHING YER NOTHING YER NOTHING YER NOTHING—

And I see her eyes as they're closing—

And I feel her against me–

And I think *Viola*–

I think *VIOLA!*

I think **VIOLA!!!!**

And the Mayor steps away from me like he's been stung.

"Whoo," he says, shaking his head as I blink away the buzz still rocketing from my brain, as my eyes refocus and my thoughts are mine again. "Told you you had some power in you, boy."

And his eyes are wide and bright and eager.

And he hits me again with his Noise.

I fling my hands up to my ears (not holding the gun, not holding the gun) as if that'll stop it but it ain't thru yer ears that you hear Noise and he's in there, inside my head, inside my self, invading it like I don't have any self at all YER NOTHING YER NOTHING YER NOTHING my own Noise swept up and hit against me, like I'm punching myself with my own fists YER NOTHING YER NOTHING YER NOTHING–

Viola, I think but I'm disappearing, I'm falling deeper into it, I'm weaker and my brain is rattling–

Viola–

{VIOLA}

Viola, I hear, as if from the bottom of a canyon. My head is aching and bleeding from the Mayor's blow and my face is in the dust and my eyes are half-open but they aren't seeing anything–

Viola, I hear again.

I open my eyes wide.

Todd's scooting back into the rocks, his hands over his
ears, eyes squeezed shut–

And the Mayor is standing over him and I can hear the same shouting as before, the same kind of clanging, laser-bright Noise firing right at him and–

Viola, I hear in amongst all the clatter–

And I open my mouth–

And I shout–

[TODD]

"TODD!" I hear screamed from somewhere out there–

And it's her–

It's her–

It's her–

And she's alive–

And her voice is coming for me–

Viola–

Viola–

VIOLA–

I hear a grunt and the Noise in my head stops again and I open my eyes and the Mayor is staggering back, one hand up to his ear, the same reflex that everyone does–

That everyone does when they hear an attack of Noise.

VIOLA, I think again, right at him, but he ducks his head and raises the rifle at me. I think it again–

VIOLA

And again–

VIOLA

And he steps back and stumbles over Davy's body, falling

488

backwards along it and down into the rubble–

I push myself up–

And I run to her–

{Viola}

He runs to me, his hands open and reaching for me, taking my shoulders and rolling me up to a sitting position and saying, "Are you hurt, are you hurt, are you hurt–"

And I'm saying, "He's still got the gun–"

And Todd turns–

[Todd]

And I turn and the Mayor's getting to his feet and he's looking at me and here comes his Noise again and I roll outta the way and I hear it following me as I scramble over rocks, scramble back to where I dropped my rifle and–

And there's a gunshot–

And dust flies up in the air in front of my hands–

Hands that were reaching for the rifle–

And I stop–

And I look up–

And he's staring right back at me–

And I hear her call my name again–

And I know she's understanding–

Understanding that I need to hear her say my name–

And that way I can use hers as a weapon–

"Don't try it, Todd," the Mayor says, looking down the barrel at me–

Not an attack–

The slinky, snaky, twisty verzhun of his voice–

The one that's him taking hold of my choices–

The one that's him turning them into his–

"You won't fight any more," he says–

He takes a step closer–

"You won't fight any more and that'll be the end of it–"

I turn away from him–

But I have to turn back–

Have to look into his eyes–

"Listen to me, Todd–"

And his voice is hissing twixt my ears–

And it would be so easy just to–

Just to–

Just to fall back–

Fall back and do what he says–

"No!" I shout–

But my teeth are locked together–

And he's still in there–

Still trying to get me to–

And I will–

I will–

YER NOTHING–

I'm nothing–

"That's right, Todd," the Mayor says, stepping forward, rifle bearing down on me. "You are nothing."

I'm nothing–

"But," he says–

And his voice is a whisper scratching across the deepest

490

part of me–

"But," he says–

"I will make you *something*."

And I look right up into his eyes–

Eyes that are an abyss I feel myself falling into–

Up and into the blackness–

And outta the corner of my eye–

{VIOLA}

I throw the stone as hard as I can, praying as it leaves my
hand that my aim's as good as Lee said–

Praying, Please, God–

If you're there–

Please–

And *wham!*

It hits the Mayor right in the temple–

[TODD]

There's a terrible *ripping* feeling, like a strip is being torn
right outta my Noise–

And the abyss is gone–

It's turned away–

And the Mayor lurches to the side, holding his temple,
blood already dripping from it–

"*TODD!*" Viola shouts–

And I look at her–

Look at her arm outstretched where she threw the rock–

And I see her–

491

And I get to my feet.

{Viola}

He gets to his feet.

He stands up tall–

And I shout his name again–

"TODD!"

Because it does something–

It does something to him–

It does something *for* him–

The Mayor's wrong–

He's wrong for ever and ever–

It's not that you should never love something so much it can control you.

It's that you *need* to love something that much so you can *never be controlled*.

It's not a weakness–

It's your best strength–

"TODD!" I shout again–

And he looks at me–

And I hear my name in his Noise–

And I know it–

I know it in my heart–

Right now–

Todd Hewitt–

There's nothing we can't do together–

And we're gonna *win*–

The Mayor is looking up now, half crouched, blood seeping from twixt his fingers held against the side of his head–

He turns to look at me, a scowl on his face–

And here comes his Noise–

And–

VIOLA

I beat it back–

He flinches away–

But he tries again–

VIOLA

"You can't beat us," I say–

"I can," he says, clenching his teeth. "I will."

VIOLA

He flinches again–

He tries to raise the rifle–

I hit him extra hard–

VIOLA

He drops the rifle and staggers back–

I can hear his Noise buzzing at me, trying to twist its way in–

But his head is hurting–

From my own attacks–

From one well-thrown rock–

"What exactly do you think this proves?" he spits. "You've got power, but you don't know what to do with it."

VIOLA

"Looks like I'm doing fine," I say.

And he smiles, teeth still clenched. "Are you?"

And I notice my hands are shaking–

I can't feel my feet below me–

"It takes practice," the Mayor says. "Or you'll blow your mind apart." He stands up a little straighter, trying to lock my eyes again. "I could show you."

And right on cue, Viola yells *"TODD!"*

And I hit him with everything I got–

Every bit of her behind me–

Every piece of anger and frustrayshun and nothingness–

Every moment I didn't see her–

Every moment I worried–

Everything–

Every little tiny thing I know about her–

I send it right into the centre of him–

VIOLA

And he falls–

Back and back and back–

His eyes rolling up–

His head twisting round–

His legs buckling–

Falling falling falling–

Right to the ground–

And lying there still.

{VIOLA}

"Todd?" I say.

He's shaking all over, almost to the point of not being able to stand, and I can hear an unhealthy-sounding whine cutting through his Noise. He wobbles a little as he takes a step.

"Todd?" I try to get to my feet but my ankles–

"Jeez," he says, crumpling down beside me. "That takes it outta you."

He's breathing heavy, his eyes unfocused.

"Are you all right?" I ask, putting a hand on his arm.

He nods. "I think so."

We look back at the Mayor.

"You did it," I say.

"*We* did it," he says and his Noise is getting a little clearer and he sits up a little straighter.

His hands are still shaking, though.

"Poor bloody Davy," he says.

I grip his arm. "The ship," I say quietly. "She's going to get there first."

"Not if I can help it," he says. He stands up and he swoons for a second but I hear him call Acorn with his Noise.

Boy colt, I hear clearly and Davy's horse tugs free of where he's tied and walks up over the rubble, boy colt, boy colt, boy colt.

Todd, I hear from farther out and there's more clopping of hooves as Angharrad follows Acorn in and stands beside him. "Forward," she nickers. "Forward," Acorn nickers.

"Absolutely forward," Todd says to them.

He puts an arm under my shoulders to lift me up. Acorn sees in his Noise and kneels down so it's easier for me to get up top. When I'm sat in the saddle, Todd slaps his flank gently and up he stands.

but, "No, girl," he says, petting her nose.

"*What*?" I say, alarmed. "What about you?"

He nods at the Mayor. "I have to take care of him," he says and doesn't meet my eye.

"What do you mean, take care of him?"

He looks past me. I turn. The beetle march of the army has reversed its course and stretches to the bottom of the hill now.

It'll be marching here next.

"Go," he says. "Get to the ship."

"Todd," I say. "You can't kill him."

He looks at me and his Noise is a muddle and he's still struggling to stay upright. "He deserves it."

"He does but–"

But Todd's already nodding. "We are the choices we make."

I nod back. We understand each other. "You'd stop being Todd Hewitt," I say. "And I ain't losing you again."

[TODD]

I give a little snort when she says *ain't*.

"I'm gonna have to stay with him, you know," I say. "Yer gonna have to go to the ship as fast as you can and I'm gonna have to wait for the army to come."

She nods, even tho there's sadness there. "And what'll you do then?"

I look over at the Mayor, still sprawled on the rocks, unconshus and moaning slightly.

I feel so *heavy*.

But I say, "I reckon they might not be too unhappy to see him beaten. I reckon they just might be on the lookout for a new leader."

She smiles. "And that'll be you?"

"And if you meet the Answer?" I say, smiling back. "What'll you do then?"

She brushes her hair outta her eyes. "I reckon they may need a new leader, too."

I step forward and I put my hand near hers on Acorn's side. She don't look at my face, just slides her hand till the tips of our fingers are touching.

"Just cuz yer going there and I'm staying here," I say. "It don't mean we're parting."

"No," she says and I know she understands. "No, it certainly doesn't."

"I ain't parting from you again," I say, still looking at our fingers. "Not even in my head."

She pushes her hand forward and laces her fingers in mine and we both look at 'em wrapped together.

"I have to go, Todd," she says.

"I know."

I look deep into Acorn's Noise and I show him where the road is, where the ship landed, and how fast fast fast he's gotta run.

"Forward," he whinnies, loud and clear.

"Forward," I say.

I look back up at Viola.

"I'm ready," she says.

"Me, too," I say.

"I reckon we just might."

One last look.

One last look where we know each other.

Right down to our souls.

And I slap Acorn hard on the flanks.

And off they go, over the rubble, right down the road, tearing hard towards the people who (I hope I hope I hope) can help us.

I look down at the Mayor, still lying on the ground.

I hear the army marching down the hill, three kilometres away, if that.

I look for the rope.

I see it but before I pick it up, I take a second to close Davy's eyes.

{VIOLA}

We fly down the road, and it's all I can do not to fall off and break my neck.

"Watch for soldiers!" I shout in the space between Acorn's flattened-back ears.

I have no idea how far into town the Answer's managed to march, no idea if they'll wait to see who I am before they blow me off the road.

No idea what her reaction will be if she sees me–

When she sees me–

When I tell her and everyone else the things I've got to tell them–

"Faster if you can!" I shout and there's a jolt like an engine firing and Acorn goes even faster.

She'll head for the ship. No doubt about that. She'll have seen it land and gone straight for it. And if she gets there first, she'll tell them how sorry she is that I died so tragically, how I fell so cruelly at the hands of the tyrant the Answer are trying to overthrow, how if the scout ship has any weapons that can be used from the air–

Which it does.

I lean down farther in the saddle, biting hard against the pain in my ankles, trying to make us go even faster.

We get well past the cathedral, down through the rows of shuttered-up shops and bolted-in houses. The sun is completely down, everything turning to silhouette against the darkening of the sky.

And I think about how the Answer will respond when they find out the Mayor's fallen–

And what they'll think when they find out *Todd* did it–

And I think of him–

I think of him–

I think of him–

Todd, Acorn thinks.

And we race down the road–

And I nearly tumble off as a *BOOM* rises in the distance.

Acorn judders to a halt, twisting round to keep me on his back. We turn and I look–

And I see the fires burning down the road.

I see houses on fire.

And stores.

And grain sheds.

And I see people running this way through the smoke, not

Passing us so fast they don't even stop to look at us.

They're fleeing from the Answer.

"What is she *doing*?" I say out loud.

𝖥𝗂𝗋𝖾, Acorn thinks, nervously clattering his hooves.

"She's burning everything," I say. "She's burning it all."

Why?

Why?

"Acorn—" I start to say.

And a horn blows a deep, long call across the entire valley.

Acorn whinnies sharply, no words in his Noise, just a flash of fear, of terror so sharp I feel my heart leap, echoed by the disbelieving gasps of some of the people running past me, many of them shouting out and stopping, looking behind me, back towards the city and beyond.

I turn, even though the sky's too dark to see much.

There are lights in the distance, lights coming down the zigzag road by the falls—

Not the road the army is on.

"What is it?" I say to no one, to anyone. "What are those lights? What was that *sound*?"

And then a man, stopped next to me, his Noise bright and circling with amazement, with disbelief, with fright as clear as a knife, whispers, "No."

He whispers, "No, it can't be."

"*What*?" I shout. "What's happening?"

And the long, deep horn sounds again across the valley.

And it's a sound like the end of the world.

THE BEGINNING

THE MAYOR WAKES before I even finish tying his hands.

He moans, pure, real Noise ratcheting from him, the first I've ever heard outta his head, now that he's off guard.

Now that he's been beaten.

"Not beaten," he murmurs. "Temporarily waylaid."

"Shut up," I say, pulling the ropes tight.

I come round the front of him. His eyes are still misty from my attack but he manages a smile.

I smack him cross the face with the butt of the rifle.

"I hear one stitch of Noise coming from you," I warn, pointing the barrels at him.

"I know," says the Mayor, a grin still coming from his bloody mouth. "And you would, wouldn't you?"

I don't say nothing.

And that's my answer.

The Mayor sighs, leaning his head back as if to stretch

503

standing, impossibly, in a wall all its own. The moons are rising behind it, lighting up their glass verzhuns just a little.

"Here we are again, Todd," he says. "The room where we first properly met." He looks around himself, at how he's the one tied to the chair now and I'm the one out here. "Things change," he says, "but they stay the same."

"I don't need to hear you talking while we wait."

"Wait for what?" He's growing more alert.

His Noise is disappearing.

"And you'd like to be able to do that, too, wouldn't you?" he says. "You'd like just for once to have no one know what you're thinking."

"I said, shut up."

"Right now, you're thinking about the army."

"Shut *up*."

"You're wondering if they really *will* listen to you. You're wondering if Viola's people can really help you—"

"I'll hit you again with the damn rifle."

"You're wondering if you've really won."

"I have really won," I say. "And you know it."

We hear a *BOOM* in the distance, another one.

"She's destroying everything," the Mayor says, looking towards the sound. "Interesting."

"Who is?" I ask.

"You never met Mistress Coyle, did you?" He stretches one shoulder and then the other against his binds. "Remarkable woman, remarkable opponent. She might have beaten me, you know. She might really have done it." He smiles wide again. "But you've done it first, haven't you?"

"What do you mean *She's destroying everything*?"

"As always," he says, "I mean what I say."

"Why would she do that? Why would she just blow things up?"

"Twofold," he says. "One, she creates chaos so it's harder to fight her as an orderly enemy. And two, she obliterates the safety of those who won't fight, creating the impression that she cannot be beaten, so that everyone's that much easier to rule when she's done." He shrugs. "Everything's a war to people like her."

"People like you," I say.

"You'll be swapping one tyrant for another, Todd. I'm sorry to be the one to tell you."

"I won't be swapping nothing. And I told you to be quiet."

I keep the rifle pointed at him and go to Angharrad, watching us both from a cramped space in the rubble. **Todd**, she thinks. **Thirsty**.

"Is there a trough still out front?" I ask the Mayor. "Or did it get blown up?"

"It did," the Mayor says. "But there's one round the back where my own horse is tied. She can go there."

Morpeth, I think to Angharrad, the name of the Mayor's horse, and a feeling rises in her.

Morpeth, she thinks. **Submit**.

"Attagirl," I say, rubbing her nose. "Damn right he'll submit."

She pushes me playfully once or twice then clops off outta the rubble, making her way round the back.

There's another *BOOM*. I have a little flash of worry for

505

must be getting near where the Answer is, she must be—

I hear a little stirring of Noise from the Mayor.

I cock the gun.

"I *said*, don't try it."

"Do you know, Todd?" he says, like we were having a nice lunch. "The attacking Noise was easy. You just wind yourself up and slam someone with it as hard as you can. I mean, yes, you have to be focused, tremendously focused, but once you've got it, you can pretty much do it at your will." He spits away a little blood pooling on his lip. "As we saw with you and your *Viola*."

"Don't you say her name."

"But the other thing," he continues. "The *control* over another's Noise, well, I must say, that's a *lot* trickier, a *lot* harder. It's like trying to raise and lower a thousand different levers at once and sure on some people, some *simple* people, it's easier than others and it's surprisingly easy on crowds, but I've tried for years to get it to work as a useful tool and it's only recently I've had any level of success at all."

I think for a minute. "Mayor Ledger."

"No, no," he says brightly. "Mayor Ledger was *eager* to help. Never trust a politician, Todd. They have no fixed centre, so you can never believe them. *He* came to *me*, you see, with your dreams and things you said. No, no control there, just ordinary weakness."

I sigh. "Would you just be *quiet* already?"

"My point is, Todd," he presses on, "that it's only today that I've been able to even come close to forcing *you* to do what I want you to do." He looks at me, to see if I'm getting it. "Only today."

Another *BOOM* in the distance, another thing destroyed by the Answer for no good reason at all. It's too dark to see the army but they must be marching into town by now, down the road straight to here.

And night is falling.

"I know what yer saying," I say. "I know what I've done."

"It was all you, Todd." He keeps his eyes on me. "The Spackle. The women. All your own action. No control needed."

"I know what I've done," I say again, my voice low, my Noise getting a warning sizzle to it.

"The offer's still open," the Mayor says, his voice low, too. "I'm quite serious. You have power. I could teach you how to use it. You could rule this land by my side."

I AM THE CIRCLE AND THE CIRCLE IS ME, I hear.

"That's the source," he says. "Control your Noise and you control yourself. Control yourself," he lowers his chin, "and you can control the world."

"You killed *Davy*," I say, stepping up to him, gun still pointed. "Yer the one with no fixed centre. And now yer *really* gonna shut the hell up."

And then a low and powerful sound rumbles thru the sky, like some giant, deep horn.

A sound God would make when he wanted yer attenshun.

I hear whinnies from the horses out back. I hear a filament of shock race thru the still-hiding Noise from the people of feet collapse into a racket of sudden confuzhun.

I hear the Mayor's Noise spike and pull back.

"What the hell was that?" I say, looking up and around.

"No," the Mayor breathes.

And there's *delight* in it.

"What?" I say, poking the rifle at him. "What's going on?"

But he's just smiling and turning his head.

Turning it towards the hill by the falls, by the zigzag road coming down into town.

I look there, too.

Lights are at the top.

Lights are starting to come down the zigzag.

"Oh, Todd," the Mayor says, amazement and, yeah, it's *joy* coming thru his voice. "Oh, Todd, my boy, what *have* you done?"

"What is it?" I say, squinting into the dark, as if that'll help me see it clearer. "What's making that—"

A second horn blast comes, so loud it's like the sound of the sky folding in half.

I can hear the ROAR of the town rising, so many asking marks you could drown in 'em.

"Tell me, Todd," the Mayor says, his voice still bright. "What exactly were you planning on doing when the army arrived?"

"What?" I say, my forehead furrowing, my eyes still trying to see what's coming down the zigzag road, but it's too far and too dark to tell. Just lights, individual points of 'em, moving down the hill.

"Were you going to offer me up for ransom?" he goes on,

508

still sounding cheerful. "Were you going to give me to them for execution?"

"What were those blasts?" I say, grabbing him by the shirt front. "Is that the settlers landing? Are they invading or something?"

He just looks in my eyes, his own sparkling. "Did you think they'd elect you leader and you'd single-handedly usher in a new era of peace?"

"I'll lead them," I hiss into his face. "You watch me."

I let him go and climb up one of the higher piles of rubble. I see people poking their heads outta their houses now, hear voices calling to one another, see people start running to and fro.

Whatever it is, it's enough to get the people of New Prentisstown out of hiding.

I feel a buzz of Noise at the back of my head.

I whip round, pointing the gun at him again, climbing back down the rubble and saying, "I *told* you, none of that!"

"I was just trying to keep our conversation going, Todd," he says, false innocence everywhere. "I'm very curious to know your plan for leadership now that you'll be head of the army and President of the planet."

I want to punch the smile off his face.

"What's going on?" I shout at him. "*What's coming down that hill?*"

There's a third blast of the horn sound, even louder this time, so loud you can feel it humming thru yer body.

And now people in town are really starting to scream.

"Reach in my front shirt pocket, Todd," the Mayor says. "I think you'll find something that once belonged to you."

there is that stupid grin.

Like he's winning again.

I push the rifle at him and use my free hand to dig in his pocket, my fingers hitting something metal and compact. I pull it out.

Viola's binos.

"Really remarkable little things," the Mayor says. "I do so look forward to the rest of the settlers landing, seeing what new treats they bring us."

I don't say nothing to him, just climb back up the rubble and hold the binos to my eyes with my free hand, clumsily trying to get the night vision to work. It's been a long time since I–

I get the right button.

Up pops the valley, in shades of green and white, cutting thru the dark to show me the town.

I raise them up the road, up the river, to the zigzag on the hill, to the points of lights coming down it–

And–

And–

And oh my God.

I hear the Mayor laugh behind me, still tied to his chair. "Oh, yes, Todd. You're not imagining it."

I can't say nothing for a second.

There ain't no words.

How?

How can this be *possible*?

An army of Spackle is marching for the town.

Some of 'em, the ones near the front, are riding on the backs of these huge, wide creachers covered in what looks like armour and a single curving horn coming out the end of their noses. Behind 'em are troops, cuz this ain't a friendly march, nosiree, it ain't nothing like that at all, there are troops marching down the zigzag road, troops marching over the lip of the hill at the top of the falls.

Troops that are coming for battle.

And there are thousands of 'em.

"But," I say, gasping, hardly able to get the words out. "But they were all *killed*. They were all killed during the Spackle War!"

"All of them, Todd?" the Mayor asks. "Every single one of them on this whole planet when all we live on is one little strip? Does that make sense to you?"

The lights I've been seeing are torches carried by the Spackle riding on the creachers' backs, burning torches to lead the army, burning torches that light up the spears that the troops carry, the bows and arrows, the clubs.

All of 'em carrying weapons.

"Oh, we beat them," says the Mayor. "Killed them in their thousands, certainly, every one within miles of here. Though they out-numbered us by a considerable margin, we had better weapons, stronger motivation. We drove them out of this land on the understanding that they would never return, never get in our way ever again. We kept some of them as slaves, of course, to rebuild our city after that war.

The town is really **ROAR**ing now. The marching of the army has stopped and I can hear people running about and screaming to each other, stuff that don't make no sense, stuff of disbelief, stuff of fear.

I run back down the rubble to him, pushing the gun hard into his ribs. "Why did they come back? Why *now*?"

And still he grins. "I expect they've had time to work on how they might get rid of us once and for all, don't you? All these years? I expect they were only looking for a reason."

"What reason?!" I shout at him. "Why–"

And I stop.

The genocide.

The death of every slave.

Their bodies piled up like so much rubbish.

"Quite right, Todd," he says, nodding like we're talking about the weather. "I suspect that must certainly be it, don't you?"

I look down at him, understanding coming too late like always. "You did it," I say. "Of *course* you did it. You killed every Spackle, every single one, made it look like it was the Answer." I push the rifle into his chest. "You were *hoping* they'd come back."

He shrugs. "I was hoping I'd have the chance to beat them once and for all, yes." He purses his lips. "But it's you I have to thank for speeding the plan along."

"Me?" I say.

"Oh, yes, definitely you, Todd. I set the stage. But you sent them the messenger."

"The messen–?"

512

No.

No.

I turn and run up the rubble again, binos back on, looking and looking and looking.

There's too many, they're too far away.

But he's there, ain't he?

Somewhere in that crowd.

1017.

Oh, no.

"I should say, *Oh, no* is right, Todd," the Mayor calls up to me. "I left him alive for you to find, but even with your *special relationship*, he wasn't very fond of you, was he? No matter how much you tried to help him. You're the face of his torturers, the face he took back to his brothers and sisters." I hear a low laugh. "I really wouldn't want to be you right now, Todd Hewitt."

I spin round, looking at the horizon on all sides. I spin round again. There's an army to the south, one to the east, and now one marching down from the west.

"And here we sit," says the Mayor, still sounding calm. "Right in the middle of it all." He scratches his nose on his shoulder. "I wonder what those poor people on the scout ship must be thinking."

No.

No.

I spin round once more, as if I could see them all coming. Coming for me.

My mind is racing.

What do I do?

What do I *do*?

the world.

And Viola's out there–

Oh, Jesus, she's out there in it–

"The army," I say. "The army's gonna have to fight them."

"In their spare time?" the Mayor says, raising his eyebrows. "When they've got a few free minutes from fighting the Answer?"

"The Answer will have to join us."

"Us?" says the Mayor.

"They'll have to fight alongside the army. They'll *have* to."

"You really think that's how Mistress Coyle is going to play it?" He's smiling but I can see his legs starting to bounce up and down now, energy coursing thru him. "She'll see herself and them as having a common enemy, now won't she? You mark my words. She'll try to negotiate." He catches my eye again. "And where will that leave you, Todd?"

I'm breathing heavy. I don't got no answer.

"And Viola's out there," he reminds me, "all on her own."

She is.

She is out there.

And she can't even *walk*.

Oh, Viola, what have I done?

"And under these circumstances, my dear boy, do you really think the army is going to want you as leader?" He laughs as if it was always the dumbest idea anywhere. "Do you think they'll trust *you* to lead them into battle?"

I spin round again with the binos. New Prentisstown is

514

in chaos. Buildings burn to the east. People run thru the streets, running away from the Answer, running away from the Mayor's army, and now running away from the Spackle, running all direkshuns with nowhere to go.

The horn blasts again, shaking glass outta some of the windows.

I spy it in the binos.

A great long trumpet, longer than four Spackle put together, carried on the backs of two of the horned creachers, being blown by the biggest Spackle I've ever seen.

And they've reached the bottom of the hill.

"I think it's time you untied me, Todd," the Mayor says, his voice a low buzz in the air.

I spin around to him, aiming the gun one more time. "You won't control me," I say. "Not no more."

"I'm not trying to," he says. "But I think we both know it's a good idea, don't you?"

I hesitate, breathing heavy.

"I've beaten the Spackle before, you see," he says. "The town knows it. The army knows it. I don't think they'll be quite so eager to discard me and unite behind you now that they know what we're up against."

I still don't say nothing.

"And after all this betrayal from you, Todd," he says, looking right up at me. "I *still* want you by my side. I *still* want you fighting next to me." He pauses. "We can win this together."

"I don't want to win this with you," I say, looking down the barrel. "I *beat* you."

He nods as if in agreement, but then he says one more

515

I hear marching feet getting closer to the church. A troop from the army's finally pulled itself together enough to come into town. I can hear them heading down a side road, towards the square.

There ain't much time.

"I don't even mind that you tied me up, Todd," the Mayor says, "but you have to let me go. I'm the only one who can beat them."

Viola–

Viola, what do I do?

"Yes, Viola, again," he says, his voice slinky and warm. "Viola out there among them, all by herself." He waits till I'm looking him in the eye. "They'll kill her, Todd. They will. And you know I'm the only one who can save her."

The horn blasts again.

There's another *BOOM* to the east.

The feet of the Mayor's soldiers getting closer.

I look at him.

"I beat you," I say. "You remember that. I beat you and I'll do it again."

"I have no doubt you will," he says.

But he's smiling.

VIOLA I think right at him, and he flinches.

"You save her," I say, "and you live. She dies, you die."

He nods. "Agreed."

"You try to control me, I shoot you. You try to attack me, I shoot you. Got it?"

"I've got it," he says.

I wait a second more but there ain't no more seconds.

There ain't no more time to decide nothing.

Only that the world's marching to meet up right here, right now.

And she's out there.

And I ain't never parting from her again, not even when we're not together.

Forgive me, I think.

And I go behind the Mayor and untie the rope.

He stands up slowly, rubbing his wrists.

He looks up at another blast of the horn.

"At last," he says. "No more of this slinking, secret fight, no more running after shadows and all this undercover cloak and dagger nonsense." He turns to me, catches my eye, and I see behind his smile the real glint of madness. "Finally, we come to the real thing, the thing that makes men men, the thing we were *born* for, Todd." He rubs his hands together and his eyes flash as he says the word.

"*War*."

END OF BOOK TWO

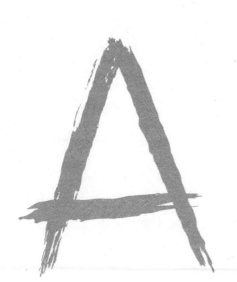

MORE CHAOS WALKING

A BONUS SHORT STORY BY PATRICK NESS

THE WIDE, WIDE SEA

13 YEARS AGO

"It has to end, Declan. You know this. We're leaving."

"Mistress–"

"Are you going to live here alone? I know you think sixteen is old enough but–"

"I wouldn't *be* alone–"

"Declan–"

"You never told me to stop. You just said to keep out of everyone's way–"

"It was never going to work. I was waiting for you to see that–"

"Why? Just because Eli Pinchin says–"

"Eli Pinchin is a racist and hateful man–"

"So why should I–?"

"Because there are other reasons than what Eli Pinchin spouts about!"

She got to her feet and started making the angriest cup of tea Declan might have ever seen.

"Mistress–"

as clear as day that you're not listening to a word I'm saying."

Declan frowned. "All right, then listen to this."

And he opened his Noise and he showed her.

The last remaining residents of Horizon were loading their carts in the small, sandy town square. Declan walked past them, avoiding eye contact as he headed to the house he shared with his mum.

Though that isn't true any more, is it? he thought as he went. His mum had already gone to Haven with the pen-ultimate group this morning, and before she left, she'd yelled at him even worse than Mistress Coyle had just now. They'd exchanged ugly words and hadn't made them right. It sat on him like an open wound, one that he couldn't help poking. He didn't want to be having these disagreements, not with his mother, not with the Mistress, not with the *town*. He wasn't the disagreeing sort.

But he just couldn't make them see. And if they couldn't see, then–

"Declan Lowe." The voice of Eli Pinchin always sounded like a whisper, even when it boomed across the dunes. Despite himself, Declan turned. Eli was in charge of the final clear-out, loading up the last and most vital of the town's possessions – its generators, its remaining medicines and supplies – onto the four ox-carts and the fissioncar that shuttled back and forth from here to Haven.

Eli Pinchin *was* the disagreeing sort, his face the wrath of God under a hat. The men and women helping him with the

524

work had all stopped, too. A wall of Noise churned from the men, Eli's own striding along the top, like a general marching his parapet.

It wasn't pleasant. Full of Declan and the things they imagined him doing, things they professed to be disgusted by, but which they sure seemed to have fully-fledged pictures of floating around their heads.

It's nothing like that, his own Noise said, though he knew from experience they wouldn't listen. *It's not like that at all.*

He spoke out loud. "I have nothing to say to you, Eli."

"Your time's a-coming, boy," Eli replied.

"Everybody's time is coming," Declan said, his stomach clenched with the nerve of talking back. Eli had twenty kilos and five inches on Declan. A fight, if it came to it, wouldn't last long. "Even yours."

"We leave in the morning, boy," Eli said. "All of us. You are not the exception you think you are."

Eli's Noise showed a picture of Declan being dragged behind the cart, his hands bound, his mouth gagged.

Declan shoved his hands into his pockets and turned away. But as he walked along the beach, he swore he could feel the gaze of Eli stabbing into him, like the barrel of a shotgun pressed between his shoulder blades. He forced himself to keep walking, veering towards the slope down to the water.

Though staying well away from the actual waves.

Eat, he could hear the fish saying, see their long black shadows moving through the water like torpedoes. They were the primary reason Horizon was closing itself down. For over ten years, the people of the town had tried to carve out a living as fishermen and -women, providing food not only for themselves but also – they hoped – a vital trading resource to the rest of New World. They'd come here, like all the arriving settlers had, dreaming of a home free of the stains of the Old World they'd left.

But of course, no one had ever expected the *new* world to be filled with Noise. Or its oceans to be filled with monsters.

The fish – if you could really call them that, when they'd look you in the eye and tell you they were going to eat you just before they did – weren't invincible. They could be caught, they could even be eaten, if you didn't mind flesh that tasted of iron no matter how much you seasoned it. But there were just too many out there, despite a ten-year war against them, too many to make fishing barely *safe*, much less viable. Worse, the fish turned out to be farmers themselves, fiercely tending and defending the shoals of the smaller fish they ate, shoals the humans on the beach would like to have eaten, too. Each day out on a boat was like jumping into a lion's den to catch a frightened lamb.

The town had started with optimism, moved into defiance, before slowly, slowly, slowly collapsing into defeat. A month ago, Mistress Coyle had *finally* won her argument that it was time to pack up what they could and move back to Haven, where they could at least count on eating regularly. Fishermen would have to become farmers, that was the way of it. Eli Pinchin, the sole remaining hold-out, had at long last agreed with her, having lost a second son this summer to a fish that had rammed their boat and knocked him into the water, where he didn't stand a chance.

The town felt they finally had nothing left to keep them here. In this, they were mostly right.

But only mostly.

Declan zipped up his jacket as he passed around the back of the church. Winter wasn't quite here yet, but it promised itself in the icy gusts coming off the sea. A coldness in the air, deeper than usual. All the more reason for the town to leave tomorrow morning, get away before the first hard freeze.

Tomorrow morning, Declan thought, walking up the small pathway to his house.

He still had no idea what he was going to do. Why him? Why him of all the boys in the town? He was the least likely, the most reserved, the one who was never going to cause a fuss.

Until the fuss found him, he guessed.

He opened his front door. "Hello?" he called.

There was no answer. The house, more of a shack really, the three little rooms marked off by hanging curtains, was mostly bare. His mother had taken her belongings with her this morning, and Declan didn't have many of his own. Clothes, obviously, a few pictures, his fishing gear, kept clean and polished. He hadn't packed any of it, but it was all so meagre he could reverse that intention in less than five minutes.

But he wasn't going to. No, he wasn't.

"Hello?" he asked again, a slight anxiety taking him now. They wouldn't have *done* anything...

Would they?

He crossed to the back door, pushing it open harder than

he'd intended so that it slammed open against the back wall of the house–

Startling her from where she sat in a corner of the thread-bare garden, wearing the same light lichen clothing as ever, heedless of the frigid breeze. She was reading a book on his pad, he saw, her strange attraction to the written words of his people still unabated, still amazed at how anyone could pack so much of themselves into lines on a page. It was a reduction, as she saw it, when expansion seemed so much more natural. And yet here she was again, spending time decoding a language not her own.

Maybe she was trying to decode *him*, he thought.

If she did, he'd be happy to hear what she discovered.

Her Noise trilled with warmth at seeing him, but it was followed immediately by sadness. She'd read him in an instant, though it was news they'd known was coming for weeks.

Tomorrow morning, she showed.

"We'll find a way," he said.

And he opened his Noise for her in an embrace.

"It's un*natural*!" his mother had shouted at him, again, just last night. "She's an animal."

"She's *not* an animal!" he'd shouted back. "She thinks. She speaks. She *feels*–"

"They only feel things in mimicry of us, you know that."

"*I* don't know that. That's what Eli Pinchin says, but since when did you start listening to him–"

"You have brought shame on yourself. On *me*–"

"It has nothing to do with you–"

"And what small town have you been living in your whole life that you think what you do doesn't matter? Doesn't get noticed?"

"It's nobody's business–"

"There's no such thing as nobody's business. Not any more. You've got to leave her behind. That's it, that's all. There's no other choice."

"I won't–"

"What exactly do you think's going to happen, Declan? Eli Pinchin's just going to welcome her on board as your equal? Give you his blessing to marry her–"

"I don't *need* his blessing. Or *yours*–"

"I would hope you'd want my blessing. Son, the Spackle are *dangerous*. There's rumours of attacks coming in from the west, even talk of war–"

"Rumours from Eli Pinchin. *Talk* from Eli Pinchin. He's not even Mayor–"

"Mistress Coyle isn't too thrilled about it either."

"And who are they to tell me how to live my life? Wasn't the whole point of flying all the way to this stupid planet was because it was free?"

"She is not coming to Haven with us."

"But they've got more of them there. They work side by side–"

"I will not have her in my house."

"Then I'll get my own house."

And this, for some reason, had been the last straw for her. She had used very bad words, very bad names for Spackle, and he had said very strong, very angry things back until she had thrown him out of the house. He'd slept outdoors, neither

529

or them willing to speak to the other, neither of them willing to be the first to try and resolve their argument. This morning, he had watched her drive off from a distance, not waving at her, her not waving back, and he had returned to their empty house.

Which, for him, wasn't empty at all.

Her name – a noun that wasn't even remotely accurate, but they had to find *some* common ground – was something like Stone Centre or Resolute Intention or Rock Against The Tide, which weren't the insults in Spackle they might have been in human. "Stone" and "Rock" in their wordless language signified, among a whole bunch of other things, something steadfast. A Rock Against The Tide wasn't a hard thing, or at least not always; it was something that was strong, something that could withstand.

But it is still not quite what you think, she had shown. This name, the layers of it, is more encouragement than fact.

"They think your centre should be stonier?"

While at the same time already being somewhat stony.

"Ah," he'd said, "so kind of like everybody else then."

She had laughed at that, one of the rare physical sounds the Spackle made, a kind of joyous clicking. They'd agreed that, as Rock Against The Tide was a bit of a mouthful, he could just call her Ti.

Spackle-human contact had started with as much optimism as everything else in New World. The natives had been another surprise, not registering in the usual scans from orbit before they landed, or if they did, registering as nothing more than wildlife. Or at least that's what the settlers had chosen to believe while they dealt with the other surprises of this place.

Declan was too young to remember the trauma of the Noise when the settler ships had first landed, but by the time his mother had joined the group that moved out to found Horizon, a kind of grudging understanding had taken hold, with many of the settlers spreading out as far as they could to give themselves relative peace and quiet. A few families had always planned on trying their hand at fishing; a few more joined them, Declan's mother included, and down the river they went to the ocean, growing more and more used to the Noise as the years passed.

Only growing slightly more used to the Spackle, though. Initial relations had been hit and miss, with some early disasters that the settlers never liked to talk about but whose gory details Declan had read in their Noise. Eventually, a sort of distant peace held. The two groups avoided each other for the most part, and by the time the founders of Horizon reached the ocean, the Spackle there knew to keep their distance from a people whose weapons were better, sharper, more effective at killing.

Except that the Spackle knew how to fish. Knew how to navigate both the ocean waves and the creatures beneath them in flat, small, one-man boats that looked barely substantial enough to withstand a light breeze. While the humans fumbled and drowned and were eaten from their heavy wooden vessels, the Spackle – hunting with intimidatingly sophisticated spear and net combinations – could be seen on the ocean to the north, standing up in their precarious crafts, loading them with enormous catches of fish.

Horizon had been forced to trade with the Spackle just to survive. Nicola Coyle, the town's Mayor and only healing Mistress, had set up the first negotiations, offering mostly iron-work and blacksmithing – which the Spackle used with their livestock – in exchange for fish and some fishing expertise that the humans failed badly to master. Still, the two groups had eked out a kind of co-existence, one that had lasted nearly a decade, though one that had always seemed dependent on the clear division between Horizon south of the river-mouth and the Spackle settlements north of it.

Until Declan was reading a book up on the riverbank six months ago. He had begged off sick from fishing duties that day, as he'd overslept and Eli Pinchin's was the only boat left to leave that morning. Fishing with Eli was a misery for any-one, but especially Declan, who was perfectly fine at ship duties unless the scornful eye of Eli was on him. When that happened, Declan found he couldn't tie a knot, couldn't load a reel, couldn't hoist a net, his Noise raging pink with embar-rassment all the while, so much so it threatened to crowd out everyone else on the boat. His professions of a bad cough had been welcomed possibly too eagerly by Eli and his crew.

So that morning, he'd snuck back to a place he liked by the river, secluded, quiet, the rush of the water drowning out most of the Noise of the town. His Noise painted his read-ing in the air, and he was happily lost within it all. Until he reached the end of a chapter and stopped.

But what happens to the boy? asked a voice through the trees in an accent not human. A Spackle was above him, stretched across the length of the branch, watching him intently. *Surely he does not ... starve? Is this the right showing?*

"The right what?" he asked.

She slid off the branch with an ease and nimbleness he'd never be able to match if he practised for a hundred years. She pointed at his reading pad. *This boy,* she showed. *He is not real. He is a memory-twist. A conduit for meaning.*

"A story," Declan answered.

Her Noise had glowed at this word. *A story. Yes.*

They stared at one another then, his Noise telling her who knew what, hers in better order, more curious, reaching out but also consulting with itself, assessing the situation. The fact that she was a young female with Noise was enough to stun him for a moment. Human women didn't have it, of course, something that had caused no end of difficulty, given how eager humans were to be outraged about difference.

But here she was, trying to communicate, wanting to connect.

So what happens next? she showed, and it took him a moment to realize she meant the book.

What actually happened next was that they met the following day to finish the story. And the day after that to start a new one. And somehow, it was as simple and impossible as that.

They'd quickly moved through his small library, uploading more and more texts from the town's reserves. She picked up written language with breathtaking speed, and he eventually let her borrow his reading pad so often he no longer really considered it his own. When their respective days' work had been

533

accomplished – they were both fishers, which was gruelling enough to make them want to talk about *anything* else – they would meet at the riverbank and read together, her watching the story unfold in his Noise, or the even more amazing reverse, where her Noise would recast the story through a Spackle's perspective. It was better than any vid he'd ever seen.

Faster than he could have ever expected, she grew to mean something to him, something more than just friendship, despite all their differences, despite the simple physical incompatibilities, the vastly different life experiences, the undeniably enormous fact that they weren't the same species.

His heart moved when he saw her, that was as far as he could explain it. He could see her heart move when she saw him, too, and if they couldn't be physical in the way that the whole stupid town seemed to spend far too much time trying to imagine, then there were other ways they could invent. Even better, in their shared Noise, they could be intimate in a way completely different than anything he'd ever known. Enough to stop the world.

What will happen? she asked him now, setting the pad down on a small garden table.

"I don't know," he said. "Are you still willing to try? To strike out on our own?"

Yes, she said, but the thing about talking to a Spackle was that there was more than just words in the words they said. She said **Yes** but it contained all the sadness at leaving her own family behind, the worry that things wouldn't be any easier if they went to Haven or – his preferred option – they found a remote spot, maybe on their own, where they could just be, the two of them. As unlikely as that sounded. It wasn't much of a plan, but it was what they had.

Because neither side were very happy about Declan and Rock Against The Tide.

You couldn't keep a thing like that out of your Noise, of course, but Declan had never been a boy the town took much notice of. A few weeks had managed to pass before Eli Pinchin caught him in an idle thought in church. Nothing particularly bad, just that he'd taken her hand for the first time the day before, feeling the somehow surprising warmth of her skin against his own.

He'd looked up from the pew to find Eli staring at him, the faces around him following suit.

The pressure had started then. The name-calling. Even the sermons at the church started warning against the dangers of "impurity". The Mistress, while clearly disapproving herself, had still shielded them some when things threatened to get out of hand, but his mother had just cried, then shouted, then cried some more, despite his protestations that they were "just friends, that's it, that's all, nothing's happened".

Which hadn't been quite true, even then.

For Ti's part, she'd convinced her people that she regarded Declan as little more than a pet. She'd laughed when he was insulted at this. But I have seen the way your people love their pets.

And there had been the word for the first time. Love.

Do you not wonder sometimes, she showed now, sadly, if in some ways they are correct? That we are asking too much of the world?

535

"No," he said. "They're the ones who are asking for too little."

Her Noise warmed, she liked this answer, but there was no disguising her anxiety beneath it.

And there was something new to it, too.

"What?" he asked, trying to read her. "What is it?"

He could sense her fighting with her Noise, wondering how much was safe to reveal.

"You can tell me," he said. "You can tell me anything."

His first indication of how dangerously bad things had got came out on the water one day on Eli Pinchin's skip. Two of Eli's sons – the younger of which would be taken by a monster later that summer – were on lances, guarding against the one large fish who had taken an interest in their boat. Another boy, Andrew, was helping Declan with the nets, and there was a girl called Deborah on the engines and rudder. Declan was clumsily pulling up a heavy line, not coiling it as fast as Eli would have liked.

"How can you have reached this age and still be so talentless, boy?" Eli said.

Declan heard the others laugh. He kept pulling in the line.

"Mind elsewhere?" Eli said. "Mind on your little wench out by the river?"

Declan paused momentarily, but went back to his work.

Eli's hot breath beat against his ear, suddenly close. "You are an abomination."

Declan spun around, his back against the low wall of the skip. Eli towered over him, the rest of the crew watching.

"I'm not sure how I feel about having a pervert on my boat," Eli said, loud enough for everyone to hear.

"I'm not a pervert," Declan said. "She's just a friend–"

"Well, now, that's obviously a lie, isn't it, boy? We can see it in your Noise. All of us."

"What's it to you, anyway?" Declan said, his face burning.

Eli leaned down, his breath stinking, his eyes wide. "The Mistress may be fine with it–"

"She isn't really–"

"But out here on the water, it's the captain who's in charge. And *this* captain isn't sure he wants someone like you stinking up the place for the rest of us."

For a moment, there was only the sound of the waves sloshing against the low skip and the Noise of the monster that swam around them. But deep within Eli, Declan could see an intention forming.

"Don't–" he started to say, but it was too late. Eli grabbed the front of his tunic, hoisted him up with alarming ease and flung him out of the boat–

But didn't let go.

Declan hung well out over the side of the skip, all his weight above the water, only his feet and ankles still inside. Eli's brute strength suspended him there, above the monster now saying **𝐄𝐚𝐭** as it sensed it might be about to be fed.

"No one would miss you, boy," Eli said. "Your ma would weep and wail, but in her heart she'd be glad to be free of your stain–"

"Captain–" one of Eli's sons said, nervously holding his lance.

Eli ignored him. "They're vermin," he spat at Declan. "They're slaughtering people out west. *War* is coming. And you think you have the right to shack up with one of them?"

Declan struggled in his grasp, the water perilously close now. "She's not *like* that—"

"Dad!" Eli's son said, louder this time.

"What is it?" Eli roared.

"There are two," the son said.

"Three," Deborah said, staring into the water.

"More will come if you keep hanging him there," Eli's son said. "Put him in the water or pull him back in the boat."

Eli sneered, but looked down past Declan. Declan twisted to look, too. Indeed, three dark shapes were circling in the deep.

And now a fourth.

Eli and Declan looked back at each other. In Eli's Noise, Declan could see Eli letting him go, could see his plunge into the water, into the mouths of the monsters that awaited—

But with a grunt, he pulled Declan back into the boat, dropping him roughly to the wooden bench. "Back to shore!" Eli called, in a tone that brooked no disagreement. Deborah revved the small fission engine, steering them towards Horizon's docks.

No one in the boat would meet Declan's eye as they went.

The moons rose on one horizon, while the sun started its descent on the other.

Declan couldn't quite get his Noise around what Ti had just told him.

"If that's the way it has to be," he finally said, not looking at her, feeling the words strain against his throat, "then maybe we *should* give each other up, maybe—"

My earlier words remain true, she showed. *We will find a way.*

"But, Ti—"

You think you are the only one who will make a sacrifice. But this is not true.

Declan kept his face in his hands, not knowing what to do. She would be cast out. That's what she'd told him. She would become an enemy to Spackle. Her people had been waiting when she docked her fishing craft this afternoon. They no longer believed Declan was anything like a "pet". They had seen the depth of her feeling in her Noise all along, of course, but had thought it a passing fancy. They tolerated it because the village – and therefore Declan – was meant to be leaving. When they had read in her Noise that the two of them intended to stay together, they had informed her of the consequences in no uncertain terms.

A war is coming, she showed him, *between my people and yours.*

"But if *that's* true, where could we go? Where could we ever get away from it?"

Across the sea. There are different lands, with different voices—

"How would we ever cross the sea?"

We would do what we must. The world is big. Surely there is space in it for one like you and one like me.

"You'd think so," he said. "But it never seems to turn out that way." He looked around the small back garden, with its tumble-down fence, the weeds that no one had time to remove properly, all at the back of a wood-framed house that leaned more than it should, now emptied after a life in a village they'd all moved to, filled with hope. Of which there was none to be found.

She read all of this in an instant, and he could already sense her Noise moving to rebuke him.

"I'll give you up," he said again, not meeting her eyes, "if I have to. If it keeps you safe."

But what makes you think I will give you up? she showed. Her Noise changed again, and he saw that she had made a space for him inside it. He tried to do the same for her, but he couldn't get his hope to work strongly enough. He could only lean into her arms and look for an escape for them both in a future that seemed to offer none.

A knock on his front door jolted them both upright. The sun was setting behind the hills, dusk falling with an even stronger chill. Winter was definitely coming, and a bitter one it would be.

The knock came again.

"I know you're in there, Declan," shouted a voice. "A blind person could see the Noise of you."

"Mistress Coyle," Declan whispered.

She has been sympathetic, Ti showed back.

"Up to a point." Declan got to his feet. Ti followed him inside. They went through and opened the front door. Mistress Coyle took them both in with a glance.

"I need to talk to you, Declan," she said. "Alone."

"I've told you, Mistress. I'm not going anywhere."

"That's not why I'm here." Her face was hard. She said nothing more.

Declan tried to outwait her, but no one could do that to

Mistress Coyle. He looked to Ti, then back to the Mistress. "Will she be safe here?"

"As safe as anywhere else," Mistress Coyle said.

Which is not especially safe, is it? Ti showed.

"If what you two were trying to do wasn't monumentally stupid," said the Mistress, "I'd say that you otherwise seem pretty smart." She turned to Declan. "Come with me."

Go, Ti showed. I will be all right.

He waited a moment, then stepped out of his front door to follow the Mistress–

Who turned back before the door shut, reaching a hand round to stop it. She leaned in to address Ti. "Keep out of sight. Just stay inside and do your reading, since I know you like it so much."

She ignored the questions rising in Declan's Noise as she stomped away, before looking back at him. "You coming?"

"Where are we going?" Declan said, as they climbed further up the trail.

"Where does it look like?" Mistress Coyle grunted, pulling herself up with a tree branch. They had followed a path into the hills that walled the town on the side opposite the ocean. The main road followed the river all the way back into Haven, but there were a number of informal trails into the woods, used for hunting, both by human and Spackle, and the Mistress had taken him nearly all the way up the steepest one until they could look out over the ramshackle buildings of the town – its one store, its church, the sad little town square meant to echo the larger one in Haven – as well as the vast ocean beyond, stretching north, south and east literally as far as the eye could see, as if this one plot of beach was the very last step before eternity.

"It looks like you're trying to get me as far from the town as possible," he said.

She sat in the nook of a low tree. "I repeat what I said about you being smart if you weren't also obviously so very, very dumb."

"I'm not leaving her, Mistress. I don't even know if I could."

She sighed, angrily. "Do you really think this is the first time this has ever happened, Declan? Do you honestly think in the admittedly short history of this blasted world, a human and a Spackle haven't found each other more interesting than decent people think is right?"

"You mean–?"

"You put people together, no matter how different, and nature sometimes takes surprising courses. But guess how many happy endings I've heard about from similar situations, Declan?"

He didn't answer, which seemed good enough for her.

"I brought you up here because I have something to tell you," she said, her voice as hard as any tidal rock the Spackle might choose as an example. "And when I do, I don't want anyone else hearing your Noise." She hugged herself in the increasing cold. "Things are bad enough as it is."

"What things?" he said.

She sat in shadow and he could see only the smallest of reflections in the wet of her eyes. There was something there to read, he knew it, if only she had Noise–

"I've got news, Declan," she said. "Hard news."

He swallowed. "Tell me."

He could see her nod in the shadows. "The group that left this morning never arrived in Haven."

He waited for more, but that was all she said. And then he knew. "My mother. What happened to my mother?"

"Things have got very bad, Declan. Even worse than the rantings of Eli Pinchin would have you believe–"

"What happened to my mother?"

Mistress Coyle raised her chin, as if to accept an unjust blow. "She's gone, Declan. I'm sorry. They were attacked. By Spackle."

He could say nothing for a moment. There were so many implications here he couldn't even begin to look at them just yet.

"War has begun," she continued. "War is *here*. And the rights and wrongs of it, who started it and why, well, that's all just words now. We're at war. And blows are being struck. This was just one." She looked down at her hands. "One, I'm afraid, of many more to come."

Declan stood there, fists clenched, trying to read her. "I don't believe it," he said. "I don't believe they would do that."

"They did, Declan," she said. "I'm sorry, but that's what war is. I've been in constant contact with the Mistresses in Haven and we're in deep discussions about how we might proceed, but things are going to get worse before they get better."

"My mother," Declan said, thinking of how they'd left things, all the last things they never said–

"We're sticking to the plan," Mistress Coyle said. "The rest of us are leaving for Haven at first light. It'll be dangerous, but less so than staying here." She leaned forward. "You need to

543

be with us, Declan. Now more than ever. You cannot stay. You can't stay with her."

He shook his head, but more out of confusion than refusal. "It was nothing to do with her. I'd have seen something if she was even *remotely*–"

"Maybe it wasn't her particular people," said the Mistress. "Or maybe they can hide things better than we can. You showed me you loved her. You showed me how much she meant to you. But how well do you really know her, Declan?"

He looked up at that and thought about the question. How well *did* he know her? He'd spent more time with her in the past six months than with any other person he'd ever known, save his mother – and the pain of *that* waited there, almost separate from himself, waiting to be felt, waiting to overwhelm him when he let it – but Ti was so different than him. So different. Maybe there were bridges they could never cross, maybe there was always going to be some distance, some doubt–

He stopped as a light flashed in Mistress Coyle's eyes.

A small dot of bright white in the middle of the growing darkness–

But the sun was behind her, so where–

He spun round and looked down at the town.

Across the trees and dunes, near the bank of the river, not a hundred metres from the ocean itself–

His house was on fire.

He ran, without looking back once at the Mistress.

It was dark and the trail was steep. He had to grab tree trunks several times to keep from falling. He knocked his head on an overhanging branch, but that didn't stop him. Blood dripped into his eyes. Still he ran.

↑í, said his Noise, and that was all it needed to say.

He could see the fire all the way down the trail. The flames lifting into the air from the roof of his house were a lighthouse on the shore, casting long bright stripes across the sea.

"Declan!" he heard the Mistress yelling behind him, but there was no way he was going to stop. He reached the bottom of the hill and ran down the little lane towards his house.

He could see it was already gone. The wooden frame, dried and cracked from the sea wind, burnt like so much kindling. The flames reached higher than the tops of the nearby trees. The circle of people around his house were having to stand back from the surprising heat of it.

The circle of people carrying torches.

They watched as Declan broke through them, racing up to the house, but it was completely engulfed.

"Is she inside?!" he screamed, racing frantically back and forth, looking for a way in.

But there was no way in, the fire too strong, every door burning.

He ran up to Eli Pinchin. "IS SHE INSIDE?!" he yelled, inches away from Eli's face.

Eli didn't flinch. "You brought this on yourself, boy," he said in that carrying whisper of his, and though Declan could read shock in the Noise of the rest of the people – gathered all the way around his house, he saw, so she'd have no chance to escape – shock at how high the fire burned, shock at what they had found themselves caught up in, there was also still defiance and anger–

Anger that wasn't just the usual at Declan being familiar with a Spackle.

"You knew," Declan said. "You knew about the attack on the road to Haven–"

"Your mother is dead, boy," Eli said, "and yet your Noise still rages for the vermin that killed her."

"She's not *vermin*!" Declan said. "And *she* didn't attack the travellers. That was–"

But he was stopped by Eli's fist clubbing him across the face. He fell backwards into the sandy dirt that made up most of Horizon's ground. He spat out a bloody tooth and wondered for a moment if his jaw had been broken.

"You need to pick a side!" Eli said, standing over him, and Eli's Noise, his hard, unrelenting Noise, roiled, showing the start of the fire–

Echoing the shouts of Ti as she was trapped inside–

Shouts that died as the fire raged.

Declan's anger forced him to his feet and he flew at Eli, fists up–

And was punched aside again, easily, toppling to the ground, his head spinning. The fire burned so heavily behind him he could smell his clothes start to scorch.

Ti, he thought. *Ti*.

But he couldn't rise this time. He could sense more than actually see the crowd of people withdrawing, melting into the night.

As behind him, his house burned, his mother dead, Ti gone.

That quickly, in less than the course of a day, he had nothing.

* * *

He woke to a bandage across his face. It was fully dark, and the fire still burned, though it had lessened in height, if not in the intensity of the heat. He had been pulled away from it, so it didn't burn him.

Pulled away by Mistress Coyle.

"You couldn't have saved her, Declan," the Mistress said, kneeling above him, wiping the blood from his face. "There was never a chance to do that."

He looked up at her, his jaw almost too sore to speak. But he was figuring things out now, and he would not be silent. "You..." he said. "You brought me up there—"

"It was the best I could do," she said, applying another bandage to his forehead. "I could either save one of you or neither of you. That choice had to be made, and I made it."

"They knew about the attack on the road. You said they didn't. You got me away so they could..."

He turned back to the fire. *Ti*, he thought, and it felt as if his body would curl in on itself with the grief that punched him.

"Everything I told you was true," Mistress Coyle said. "Your mother is dead. We're at war with the Spackle. Eli Pinchin found out before I could help it, and they were ready to hang you both from the highest tree." Her face held firm. "I talked him out of that part and let him settle on burning the house down instead."

"With her in it," Declan stared at the Mistress, unbelieving, his eyes watering. "And somehow you think that makes you a hero."

547

Mistress Coyle shook her head. "Sometimes leaders have to do hideous things, Declan, horrible things, inhuman things."

He sat up, slower than he'd like, but still, he sat up. Then he dragged himself to his feet. Mistress Coyle stayed kneeling. "She's gone, Mistress," he said.

"I'm very, very sorry about that, Declan."

"She's gone," he said again, his fists clenching. "And your life is forfeit."

Mistress Coyle didn't move, didn't even blink. "So be it."

And more than anything, it was her *certainty* that made him move, the rightness even now written across her face. He looked around, finding a short, thick plank that had fallen from the house. It was blackened but not burning. He picked it up.

He thought he knew what he was going to do with it, and the idea shocked him, but only in a distant way.

Declan hefted the plank. It was heavy enough to do a lot of damage. He approached the Mistress with it, as if watching himself from a distance. They were alone, the people who had caused the fire hiding in their own houses, awaiting the morning when they would abandon this place for good.

"What're you planning, Declan?" the Mistress said, annoyingly calmly. "The choice is yours now."

"You took me away so they could kill her," he said, turning the plank in his hands. "We could have run away. We could have been together–"

"Her people don't want you either, Declan. *War* has started–"

"You killed her. You as good as set the fire yourself."

She was still on the ground before him, and for the first time there was a nervous look in her eye. "Declan," she said.

"Stop using my name," he said. "We no longer know each other."

"*Declan*," she said again, then looked back to the other houses, seeing the Noise there, reading it, seeing nothing there that would come to her aid. She turned back to him, squaring her shoulders. "Do what you will."

He stopped. "Do what I will?"

She looked up into his eyes, defiant. "Everything you say is true. I have made monstrous choices. They had to be made. I deserve to suffer the consequences of them."

He hefted the plank again, looking down on her. His Noise raged around them, tangling itself up in the fire behind him and the still-shocking news of his mother and the terrible, awful, yawning gap that was the loss of Ti.

And here was the Mistress, offering herself as a release for all that rage.

She stared back up at him, probably not even afraid.

He raised the plank–

Her eyes squinted shut a little, but that was the only reaction she gave–

Until he threw the plank down next to her so hard she flinched.

"There'll come a day, Mistress," he said, "when you'll stop being so sure of everything. And that'll be the day when you crumble. That'll be the day you collapse. I only hope I'm there to see it."

He turned back to the fire, sank to his knees, and began to weep.

* * *

When the rest of the town left the next morning, no one came to get him. He didn't see anyone, not Eli Pinchin, not even the Mistress, from where he still lay, curled into the ashy grass in front of the remains of his house. He was ready to refuse them, ready to tell them exactly what they could do with themselves and their trip to Haven, but no one even came to ask.

He wondered if that was the Mistress's doing.

Shortly after daybreak, he heard the fissioncar start up in the square, heard the ox-drawn carts begin to creak their way to the river road, heard the Noise of the last townfolk gather itself together in fear of what they might face before they reached Haven.

He hoped they'd be slaughtered.

And then he didn't, as much as he wanted to. There were people he knew in that group, people who might not have been as much a part of it, people who were maybe just weak in the face of Eli Pinchin, someone who – he had to admit – he *did* wish slaughter on.

The sounds of the engine and the carts and the Noise all dimmed until only the usual, too familiar crashing of the waves remained.

He didn't know what to do. Didn't know where he could go. Wondered if he could make a life here, by himself.

Or if he should just walk down into the surf, arms open, and greet with relief the creatures who wanted to **Eat** him–

Then all of our trouble would be for nothing, Ti showed, placing an arm around his hunched shoulders and wrapping him in her Noise.

* * *

He lay, still stunned, in the bow of her terrifyingly shallow fishing craft. She'd uncovered it near the river mouth, encouraging him in, encouraging him to hurry, encouraging him to please lie flatter and stiller as she pushed the boat out into the waves.

He turned the old communicator over and over in his hands. "I didn't think these even worked any more."

Stay inside and do your reading, Mistress Coyle had said as she led Declan away. And that was because she'd managed to send both a warning and a possibility of escape straight to Declan's pad for Ti to read.

She wrote that there was no time, Ti showed, feet planted on either side of the vessel in the way of Spackle fishers. She guided them with a single long paddle, pushing them towards the coral reef that acted as a breakwater to the deeper waters beyond. **And that I would have to be convincing.**

Mistress Coyle had left Ti *two* communicators underneath a brick out by the front door to Declan's house, one to leave inside the house as it burned, one to speak into from a safe distance. When the fire started, Ti was to scream into the one she held, and the one in the house was set to broadcast her cries, as if she was burning to death.

She did not think it would work, but that it was worth a try. She looked down to Declan. **In this, she was correct.**

"And she couldn't tell me, because it would be in my Noise for everyone to hear. I had to believe it." He looked up at Ti in wonder. "I was threatening her. I was ready to *kill* her." He turned the communicator over again. "She was willing to die rather than risk the town finding out and lynching us both."

They had to believe I was dead. *You* had to believe it. This was very difficult.

Yes, Declan said, quietly. "Yes, it was." He set the communicator down. "Tough old bird, isn't she?"

Yes. Even though she is mute, the poor thing.

They crossed over the coral reef. Larger fish began to circle, but warily, recognizing a Spackle boat with tricks up its sleeve.

I am sorry for your mother, Ti showed.

Declan said nothing, but his Noise curled in grief again.

Not all of us want this war, she said. Not all of us want the pain that it will bring.

Her settlement, for example, were peaceable and as the calls to war had remained voluntary, they had held back, hoping it would pass. Nevertheless, they had cursed her for wanting to leave with him, telling her of the atrocities committed by his people out in the west. They had turned their backs on her in disgust when she told them he was a person, not a whole people.

He read the pain of separation in her as she paddled them into the deeper waters.

So we're both grieving, he thought.

We are, she answered, reading his thought. But at least we grieve together.

They pushed out further and further from shore. The monstrous fish kept their distance for now, but the boat still felt amazingly flimsy beneath Declan.

"Tell me again where we're going," he said.

To a place where we can be, she showed, paddling still. Across the water.

"But that's impossibly far."

Far, she showed, but not impossible.

Declan turned back, watching Horizon shrink in the distance. It looked so small. Ahead of them, towards the other horizon, there was just water, an eternity of it, water they were somehow going to cross in their tiny, tiny boat, with monsters raging beneath it.

But for now, they remained together, alive and afloat, plunging ever further across the wide, wide sea.

PRAISE FOR
THE CHAOS WALKING TRILOGY

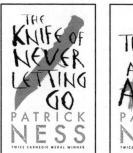 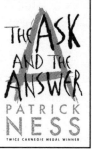 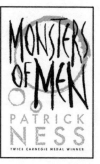

"We are convinced that this is a major achievement
in the making."
Costa Book Awards Judges

"I would press the Chaos Walking trilogy urgently
on anyone, anyone at all. It is extraordinary."
Guardian

"Chaos Walking is remarkable."
The Times

"Gripping, thrilling, hurtling stories."
Independent on Sunday

"One of the outstanding literary achievements
of the present century."
Irish Times

"Powerful and provocative."
Daily Mail

"A novel that triumphantly concludes what will almost certainly come to be seen as one of the outstanding literary achievements of the present century."
Irish Times

"Lives up to all expectations... An electrifying ending to a brilliant series."
Daily Express

"As addictive as its predecessors... It maintains a breakneck pace and ratchets up the suspense to almost unbearable levels."
Books Quarterly

"As in his preceding books, Ness offers incisive appraisals of violence, power, and human nature..."
Publishers Weekly

"This is science fiction at its best, and is a singular fusion of brutality and idealism that is, at last, perfectly human."
Booklist

"An explosive quality pervades *Monsters of Men*, the concluding instalment of the Chaos Walking trilogy. The breathtaking novel sees Todd and Viola ensnared in the ravages of war. It contains an enduring message regarding individual connections and communications and the danger of their failure. With the feel of prophetic epic, this is innovative, intense writing at its incendiary best."
Bookseller

A MONSTER CALLS

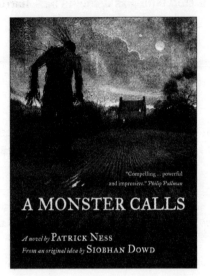

"Outstanding… Gripping, moving, brilliantly crafted."
The Times

"Compelling … powerful and impressive."
Philip Pullman

"Electrifying."
Telegraph

"This haunting and demanding book shines with
compassion, insight and flashes of humour."
Daily Mail

MORE THAN THIS

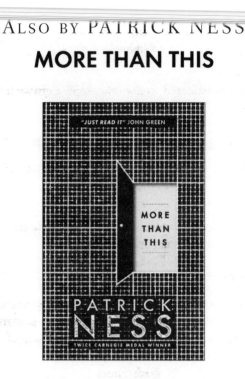

"Crackling dialogue, suspenseful action, twisty plots and big ideas."
Sunday Times

"A tense thriller and an impressively challenging and philosophical book... Captivating throughout."
Telegraph

"A powerfully unsettling but uplifting tale."
Observer

"Demanding and gripping."
Daily Mail

Enjoyed this book? Tweet us your thoughts.
#ChaosWalking @Patrick_Ness @WalkerBooksUK